Neuro Integrated for NIMHANS Entrance Examination

Neuro Integrated for NIMHANS Entrance Examination

5th Edition

Includes all Recent Questions

- Neuroanatomy
- Neuropathophysiology
- Neurology
- Neuropharmacology
- Neuro-ophthalmology
- Neuroanesthesia
- Neurosurgery
- Neuroradiology
- Psychiatry

Pramod KS MBBS MS (Orthopedics)
Fellow in Spine Surgery (ASSI)
Spine Surgeon
Bengaluru, Karnataka, India

K Gayathri MBBS MD
Psychiatrist
Senior Resident
Chennai, Tamil Nadu, India

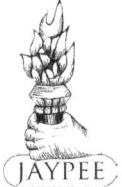

JAYPEE BROTHERS MEDICAL PUBLISHERS
The Health Sciences Publisher
New Delhi | London

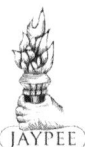 **Jaypee Brothers Medical Publishers (P) Ltd**

Headquarters
Jaypee Brothers Medical Publishers (P) Ltd
4838/24, Ansari Road, Daryaganj
New Delhi 110 002, India
Phone: +91-11-43574357
Fax: +91-11-43574314
Email: jaypee@jaypeebrothers.com

Overseas Office
J.P. Medical Ltd
83 Victoria Street, London
SW1H 0HW (UK)
Phone: +44 20 3170 8910
Fax: +44 (0)20 3008 6180
Email: info@jpmedpub.com

Website: www.jaypeebrothers.com
Website: www.jaypeedigital.com

© 2020, Jaypee Brothers Medical Publishers

The views and opinions expressed in this book are solely those of the original contributor(s)/author(s) and do not necessarily represent those of editor(s) of the book.

All rights reserved. No part of this publication may be reproduced, stored or transmitted in any form or by any means, electronic, mechanical, photocopying, recording or otherwise, without the prior permission in writing of the publishers.

All brand names and product names used in this book are trade names, service marks, trademarks or registered trademarks of their respective owners. The publisher is not associated with any product or vendor mentioned in this book.

Medical knowledge and practice change constantly. This book is designed to provide accurate, authoritative information about the subject matter in question. However, readers are advised to check the most current information available on procedures included and check information from the manufacturer of each product to be administered, to verify the recommended dose, formula, method and duration of administration, adverse effects and contraindications. It is the responsibility of the practitioner to take all appropriate safety precautions. Neither the publisher nor the author(s)/editor(s) assume any liability for any injury and/or damage to persons or property arising from or related to use of material in this book.

This book is sold on the understanding that the publisher is not engaged in providing professional medical services. If such advice or services are required, the services of a competent medical professional should be sought.

Every effort has been made where necessary to contact holders of copyright to obtain permission to reproduce copyright material. If any have been inadvertently overlooked, the publisher will be pleased to make the necessary arrangements at the first opportunity. The **CD/DVD-ROM** (if any) provided in the sealed envelope with this book is complimentary and free of cost. **Not meant for sale.**

Neuro Integrated for NIMHANS Entrance Examination

First Edition: 2011
Second Edition: 2012
Third Edition: 2015
Fourth Edition: 2017

Fifth Edition: 2020

ISBN: 978-93-90020-03-4

Dedicated to
My Parents
Vijaya Sudarshan and KS Sudarshan

PREFACE TO THE FIFTH EDITION

The overwhelming response to the previous edition of NIMHANS Neuro Integrated provided great encouragement in updating our current edition. In line with readers' responses, suggested changes have been made wherever required, new topics have been added to relevant chapters covering recent advances, high yield chapters with question banks for practice. The ever changing pattern of the competitive exam acts as a challenge for us to improve and adapt new editions with relevant updates in accordance with the changing times. Additionally, as supplement to the text, pictures and tabular columns, have been provided as an assist to condense extensive topics. Along with questions provided at the end of select chapters, to serve as self assessment, question banks have been provided at the end of the book acting as mock tests for the final exam. This book will help as supplement to mainstream subject books in the preparation for the competitive exams by providing a template and focusing on high yield chapters. This book is the result of the efforts of many minds over several months; any errors in text or MCQ are unintentional and deeply regretted. Suggestions and comments are most welcome.

K Gayathri

PREFACE TO THE FIRST EDITION

Neurosciences—probably the toughest topics to crack questions from, in any PG entrance exam. And when more than half of the paper comprises of questions from these topics, it can make the answering minds miserable. NIMHANS PG entrance exam is one such exam where more than half of the paper comprises of questions from Neurosciences, be it the February paper for MD/Dip in Psychiatry or the June paper for DM Neuro/MCh Neurosurgery. The lack of depth of knowledge in these topics accompanied by the lack of time devoted for the exam (since it comes with a bunch of exams following AIPGMEE) makes the aspirants tough to crack the paper.

This book comes as a breather for such aspirants. It integrates high yield topics from embryology to surgery pertaining to the neurosciences and psychiatry. The topics are concise, yet comprehensive. They carry reliable information from widely followed and accepted reference books. Each subject is organized into topics for clear reading and understanding. Each topic is covered in view of questions asked in PG entrance exams and arranged pointwise for quick memorization.

High yield topics are followed by multiple choice questions. These MCQs are primarily intended to test the student after reading the high yield topics of a subject, and hence is arranged subject-wise. They also help to answer repeat questions covering questions of the PG entrance examinations held at All India level in the recent years (Including AIIMS May 2010 and NIMHANS Feb/June 2010), as well as few potential questions for the future. This book cannot replace answering year-wise papers of the exams conducted, but practice of attempting these questions is highly recommended as it makes it much easier to answer in the actual exam.

A plus point of this book is the chapters in the Appendix A to Z in neurology covers an extensive list of symptoms, signs and syndromes in neurology. A list of differential diagnosis covers etiological differentials for important diseases in Neurology. These are indispensable in preparation for any PG entrance exam.

This book will also be useful for other PGMEEs like AIPG, AIIMS, PGI, etc. since 20–25% of questions in these exams are asked from the neurosciences. Aspirants of other Neurosciences institutes and specialty exams like CMC Vellore will be benefitted.

I hope this book will make life much easier for PG aspirants and helps to achieve their goals by clearing the exams in flying colors. Wish you all the best.

Remember the quote:

"Most of the things worth doing in the world had been declared impossible before they were done."

Nothing is impossible.
Suggestions and comments are most welcome.

Pramod KS

ACKNOWLEDGMENTS

I would like to express my heartfelt gratitude

To God, for being my anchor and constant source of strength,

To my parents, for always providing guidance on the right way ahead,

To my sister and brother-in-law, for being my perennial source of inspiration,

To my husband, for his unwavering support and constant encouragement,

To all my teachers, who have imparted the very knowledge I wish to share,

To Dr. Pramod for giving me this wonderful opportunity, to realize an unknown potential.

Thanks to Shri Jitendar P Vij (Group Chairman), M/s Jaypee Brothers Medical Publishers (P) Ltd, New Delhi, India, Mr Venugopal and Mr Palani for their professional approach and for helping this book to take its shape.

Finally, thanks to all the readers of this book. I regret for any unintentional mistakes in the book. However, I request your valuable feedback if any gross errors are found, either in the subject as a whole, or in the answers given for MCQs. I request you to send your suggestions and comments, as it is invaluable for the success of the book.

K Gayathri

CONTENTS

Chapter	1. Neuroanatomy	1
Chapter	2. Neuropathophysiology	25
Chapter	3. Neurology	53
Chapter	4. Neuropharmacology	145
Chapter	5. Neuro-ophthalmology	169
Chapter	6. Neuroanesthesia	192
Chapter	7. Neurosurgery	200
Chapter	8. Neuroradiology	227
Chapter	9. Psychiatry	239
Question Bank		*313*

CHAPTER 1

Neuroanatomy

FORMATION OF THE BRAIN

- The central nervous system (CNS) appears at the beginning of the third week as an infolding of thickened ectoderm, the neural plate, in the mid-dorsal region in front of the primitive node. Its lateral edges soon elevate to form the neural folds. With further development, the neural folds continue to elevate, approach each other in the midline, and finally fuse, forming the neural tube.
- Fusion begins in the cervical region and proceeds in cephalic and caudal directions. Once fusion is initiated, the open ends of the neural tube form the cranial and caudal neuropores that communicate with the overlying amniotic cavity. Closure of the cranial neuropore proceeds cranially from the initial closure site in the cervical region. Final closure of the cranial neuropore occurs at the 18- to 20-somite stage (25th day); closure of the caudal neuropore occurs approximately at 26–28 days.
- **The cephalic end of the neural tube shows three dilations, the primary brain vesicles:**
  - The prosencephalon, or forebrain;
  - The mesencephalon, or midbrain; and
  - The rhombencephalon, or hindbrain.
- **When the embryo is 5 weeks old, the prosencephalon consists of two parts:**
  - The telencephalon, formed by a midportion and two lateral outpocketings, the primitive cerebral hemispheres, and
  - The diencephalon, characterized by outgrowth of the optic vesicles.
- **A deep furrow, the rhombencephalic isthmus, separates the mesencephalon from the rhombencephalon. The rhombencephalon also consists of two parts:**
  - The metencephalon, which later forms the pons and cerebellum, and
  - The myelencephalon, forming the medulla.
- The lumen of the spinal cord, the central canal, is continuous with that of the brain vesicles. The cavity of the rhombencephalon is the fourth ventricle, that of the diencephalon is the third ventricle, and those of the cerebral hemispheres are the lateral ventricles. The lumen of the mesencephalon connects the third and fourth ventricles and is known as the *aqueduct of Sylvius*. The lateral ventricles communicate with the third ventricle through *the interventricular foramina of Monro*.

HINDBRAIN

The rhombencephalon consists of the myelencephalon, the most caudal of the brain vesicles, and the metencephalon, which extends from the pontine flexure to the rhombencephalic isthmus.

Myelencephalon

The myelencephalon is a brain vesicle that gives rise to the medulla oblongata. The roof plate of the myelencephalon consists of a single layer of ependymal cells covered by vascular mesenchyme, the pia mater. The two combined are known as the tela choroidea. Because of active proliferation of the vascular mesenchyme, a number of saclike invaginations project into the underlying ventricular cavity. These tuftlike invaginations form the choroid plexus, which produces cerebrospinal fluid.

Metencephalon

The metencephalon, similar to the myelencephalon, is characterized by basal and alar plates. Two new components form: the cerebellum and the pons. The marginal layer of the basal plates of the metencephalon expands as it makes a bridge for nerve fibers connecting the cerebral cortex and cerebellar cortex with the spinal cord. Hence, this portion of the metencephalon is known as the pons (bridge).

Cerebellum

- The dorsolateral parts of the alar plates bend medially and form the rhombic lips. Immediately below the mesencephalon they approach each other in the midline. The rhombic lips compress cephalocaudally and form the cerebellar plate. In a 12-week embryo, this plate shows a small midline portion, the vermis, and two lateral portions, the hemispheres. A transverse fissure soon separates the nodule from the vermis and the lateral flocculus from the hemispheres. This flocculonodular lobe is phylogenetically the most primitive part of the cerebellum.
- Cells of the external granular layer retain their ability to divide and form a proliferative zone on the surface of the cerebellum which migrate toward the differentiating Purkinje cells and give rise to granule cells. Basket and stellate cells are produced by proliferating cells in the cerebellar white matter.

MIDBRAIN

- The marginal layer of each basal plate enlarges and forms the crus cerebri. These crura serve as pathways for nerve fibers descending from the cerebral cortex to lower centers in the pons and spinal cord. Initially the alar plates of the mesencephalon appear as two longitudinal elevations separated by a shallow midline depression. A transverse groove divides each elevation into an anterior (superior) and a posterior (inferior) colliculus.

FOREBRAIN

The prosencephalon consists of the telencephalon, which forms the cerebral hemispheres, and the diencephalon, which forms the optic cup and stalk, pituitary, thalamus, hypothalamus, and epiphysis.

Diencephalon

- The diencephalon, which develops from the median portion of the prosencephalon consists of a roof plate and two alar plates but to lack floor and basal plates. The roof plate of the diencephalon consists of a single layer of ependymal cells covered by vascular mesenchyme, together which they form the choroid plexus of the third ventricle. The most caudal part of the roof plate develops into the pineal body, or epiphysis. This body begins to evaginate and becomes a solid organ on the roof of the mesencephalon. The alar plates form the lateral walls of the diencephalon. A groove, the hypothalamic sulcus, divides the plate into a dorsal and a ventral region, the thalamus and hypothalamus, respectively. The thalamus gradually projects into the lumen of the diencephalon. The hypothalamus, forming the lower portion of the alar plate, differentiates into a number of nuclear areas that regulate the visceral functions, including sleep, digestion, body temperature, and emotional behavior.
- The hypophysis, or pituitary gland, develops from two completely different parts: (a) an ectodermal outpocketing of the stomodeum immediately in front of the buccopharyngeal membrane, known as Rathke's pouch, and (b) the infundibulum.
- Rathke's pouch appears as an evagination of the oral cavity and subsequently grows dorsally toward the Infundibulum. Cells in the anterior wall of Rathke's pouch increase rapidly in number and form the anterior lobe of the hypophysis, or adenohypophysis. The pars tuberalis, grows along the stalk of the infundibulum and surrounds it. The infundibulum gives rise to the stalk and the pars nervosa, or posterior lobe of the hypophysis (neurohypophysis).

Telencephalon

- The telencephalon, consists of two lateral outpockets, the cerebral hemispheres, and a median portion, the lamina terminales. The cerebral hemispheres arise at the beginning of the fifth week of development as bilateral evaginations of the lateral wall of the prosencephalon. The basal part of the hemispheres begins to grow and bulges into the lumen of the lateral ventricle and into the floor of the foramen of Monro. Immediately above the choroidal fissure, the wall of the hemisphere thickens, forming the hippocampus which bulges into the lateral ventricle.
- The corpus striatum being a part of the wall of the hemisphere expands posteriorly and is divided into two parts, the caudate nucleus, and the lentiform nucleus.
- The medial wall of the hemisphere and the lateral wall of the diencephalon fuse so that the caudate nucleus and thalamus come into close contact. Continuous growth of the cerebral hemispheres in anterior, dorsal, and inferior directions results in the formation of frontal, temporal, and occipital lobes, respectively. The surface of the cerebral hemispheres grows so rapidly that a great many convolutions (gyri) separated by fissures and sulci appear on its surface.
- The commissures, which cross the midline, connect the right and left halves of the hemispheres. The most important fiber bundles make use of the lamina terminalis. The first of the crossing bundles to appear is the anterior commissure. It consists of fibers connecting the olfactory bulb and related brain areas of one hemisphere to those of the opposite side. The hippocampal commissure fibers arise in the hippocampus and converge on the lamina terminalis close to the roof plate of the diencephalon. The fibers continue, forming an arching system immediately outside the choroid fissure, to the mammillary body and the hypothalamus. The corpus callosum appears by the 10th week of development and connects the nonolfactory areas of the right and the left cerebral cortex.

Formation of the Spinal Cord
- Once the neural tube closes, neuroepithelial cells begin to give rise to another cell type characterized by a large round nucleus with pale nucleoplasm and a dark-staining nucleolus, the primitive nerve cells, or neuroblasts. They form the mantle layer, a zone around the neuroepithelial layer. The mantle layer later forms the gray matter of the spinal cord.
- The outermost layer of the spinal cord, the marginal layer, contains nerve fibers emerging from neuroblasts in the mantle layer. As a result of myelination of nerve fibers, this layer is called the white matter of the spinal cord.
- Due to continuous addition of neuroblasts to the mantle layer, each side of the neural tube shows a ventral and a dorsal thickening. The ventral thickenings, the basal plates, which contain ventral motor horn cells, form the motor areas of the spinal cord; the dorsal thickenings, the alar plates, form the sensory areas.

DIFFERENTIATION OF CELLS

Nerve Cells
- Neuroblasts, or primitive nerve cells, arise by division of the neuroepithelial cells. A transient dendrite, migrates into the mantle layer and become temporarily round and apolar. With further differentiation, they form a bipolar neuroblast. The process at one end of the cell elongates rapidly to form the primitive axon and the process at the other end, the primitive dendrites. The cell is then known as a multipolar neuroblast and with further development becomes the adult nerve cell or neuron.
- Axons of neurons in the basal plate break through the marginal zone and become visible on the ventral aspect of the cord as the ventral motor root of the spinal nerve. Axons of neurons in the dorsal sensory horn (alar plate) penetrate into the marginal layer of the cord, where they ascend to either higher or lower levels to form association neurons.

Glial Cells
- The majority of primitive supporting cells are formed by neuroepithelial cells after production of neuroblasts cease. In the mantle layer, they differentiate into protoplasmic astrocytes and fibrillar astrocytes. Another type of supporting cell, the oligodendroglial cell is found primarily in the marginal layer, forms myelin sheaths around the ascending and descending axons in the marginal layer.
- The microglial cell is a highly phagocytic cell type derived from mesenchyme.
- When neuroepithelial cells cease to produce neuroblasts and supporting cells, they differentiate into ependymal cells lining the central canal of the spinal cord.

Neural Crest Cells
- During elevation of the neural plate, a group of cells appears along each edge of the neural folds. These neural crest cells are ectodermal in origin and extend throughout the length of the neural tube. Crest cells migrate laterally and give rise to sensory ganglia (dorsal root ganglia) of the spinal nerves and other cell types.
- Neuroblasts of the sensory ganglia derived from neural crest cells give rise to the dorsal root neurons. In addition to forming sensory ganglia, cells of the neural crest differentiate into sympathetic neuroblasts, Schwann cells, pigment cells, odontoblasts, meninges, and mesenchyme of the pharyngeal arches.

Spinal Nerves
- Motor nerve fibers begin to appear in the fourth week, arising from nerve cells in the basal plates of the spinal cord and collect into bundles known as ventral nerve roots.
- Dorsal nerve roots form as collections of fibers originating from cells in dorsal root ganglia (spinal ganglia). Central processes from these ganglia form bundles that grow into the spinal cord opposite the dorsal horns. Distal processes join the ventral nerve roots to form a spinal nerve.

Myelination
- Schwann cells myelinate the peripheral nerves. These cells originate from neural crest, migrate peripherally, and wrap themselves around axons, forming them neurilemma sheath.
- The myelin sheath surrounding nerve fibers in the spinal cord has a different origin, the oligodendroglial cells. Myelination completes at the first year of postnatal life. Tracts in the nervous system become myelinated at about the time they start to function.

Cranial Nerves
- By the fourth week of development, nuclei for all 12 cranial nerves are present. All except the olfactory (I) and optic (II) nerves arise from the brainstem, and of these only the oculomotor (III) arises outside the region of the hindbrain.

- In the hindbrain, proliferation centers in the neuroepithelium give rise to motor nuclei of cranial nerves IV, V, VI, VII, IX, X, XI, and XII. Establishment of this segmental pattern is directed by mesoderm collected into somitomeres beneath the overlying neuroepithelium. Motor neurons for cranial nuclei are within the brainstem, while sensory ganglia are outside of the brain.
- Cranial nerve sensory ganglia originate from ectodermal placodes and neural crest cells. Parasympathetic (visceral efferent) ganglia are derived from neural crest cells, and their fibers are carried by cranial nerves III, VII, IX, and X

Autonomic Nervous System (ANS)

Functionally the ANS can be divided into a sympathetic portion in the thoracolumbar region and a parasympathetic portion in the cephalic and sacral regions.

Sympathetic Nervous System

- In the fifth week, cells originating in the neural crest of the thoracic region migrate on each side of the spinal cord toward the region immediately behind the dorsal aorta where they form a bilateral chain of segmentally arranged sympathetic ganglia interconnected by longitudinal nerve fibers. Together they form the sympathetic chains on each side of the vertebral column.
- From the thorax, neuroblasts migrate toward the cervical and lumbosacral regions, extending the sympathetic chains to their full length. Some sympathetic neuroblasts migrate in front of the aorta to form preaortic ganglia, the celiac and mesenteric ganglia. Other sympathetic cells migrate to the heart, lungs, and gastrointestinal tract, where they give rise to sympathetic organ plexuses.
- Nerve fibers originating in the intermediate horn of the thoracolumbar segments (T1-L1,2) of the spinal cord penetrate the ganglia of the chain and synapse at the same levels in the sympathetic chains known as preganglionic fibers, have a myelin sheath, and stimulate the sympathetic ganglion cells. They form the white communicating rami, found only at level of the first thoracic to the second or third lumbar segment of the spinal cord.
- Axons of the sympathetic ganglion cells, the postganglionic fibers, have no myelin sheath. They either pass to other levels of the sympathetic chain or extend to the heart, lungs, and intestinal tract. The gray communicating rami, pass from the sympathetic chain to spinal nerves. Gray communicating rami are found at all levels of the spinal cord.

Parasympathetic Nervous System

Neurons in the brainstem and the sacral region of the spinal cord give rise to preganglionic parasympathetic fibers. Fibers from nuclei in the brainstem travel via the oculomotor (III), facial (VII), glossopharyngeal (IX), and vagus (X) nerves. Postganglionic fibers arise from neurons (ganglia) derived from neural crest cells and pass to the structures they innervate.

SUMMARY

Embryonic Layers

- Embryonic disk consists of ectoderm, mesoderm and endoderm
    - Virtually entire central nervous system (CNS) is derived by an infolding of the ectoderm
    - Microglia, one of the supporting cells of the CNS, thought to be derived from mesoderm.

Neural Tube Formation

- Occurs roughly between days 18 and 21 of embryonic development
- Tube forms from the neural plate, a thickened region of ectoderm on midline of embryonic disk
    - Cells at lateral margins of plate grow and accumulate to form neural folds, between which is found the neural groove
    - Folds grow to meet each other across the midline, forming a tube which begins at the fourth somite and continues rostrally and caudally
    - Neural groove enclosed as a cavity which will become the ventricles and connecting passages of the CNS
    - Tube sinks beneath the surface ectoderm, after which the specialized neural crest cells split off and come to lie on either side of the tube
    - Neural crest cells will form the sensory neurons of the dorsal root ganglia, the neurons of the sensory portions of CN V, VII, IX and X, the bipolar neurons of in the peripheral ganglia of CN VIII, and the postganglionic motor neurons of the autonomic nervous system.

Neural Tube Differentiation

- Closed neural tube consists of single layer of pseudostratified columnar epithelium, considered to be neuroepithelium
    - This neuroepithelium is the source of all the cells in the CNS, both neurons and glia, except for the microglia
    - Neuroepithelium adjacent to central canal begins to divide and migrate laterally, until a three layered structure is formed.

- Three layers of neural tube
  - Ependymal layer—Layer nearest the central canal
  - Mantle layer—Primitive neuroblasts derived from neuroepithelium
  - Marginal layer—Processes derived from cells in mantle layer
- Fate of neural tube layers
  - Ependymal layer will become the lining cells of the cavities of the CNS
  - Mantle layer will become the gray matter (cell bodies and their dendrites) of the CNS
  - Marginal layer will become the white matter (axons of neurons) of the CNS

Formation of Spinal Cord from Neural Tube

- Mantle layer proliferates producing dorsal, or alar plate, and ventral, or basal plate. Alar and basal plates are separated by lateral evagination of central cavity, the sulcus limitans.
- Dorsal and ventral regions of tube thin to form roof plate and floor plate
- Neural crest cells come to lie laterally adjacent to tube. This stage reached at about end of fourth week of development
- Correlates in the adult condition of regions seen in differentiating neural tube
  - Alar plate—Dorsal horn of cord: Sensory region
  - Basal plate—Ventral horn of cord: Motor region
  - Marginal layer—White matter of cord: Ascending and descending tract systems
  - Neural crest—Sensory neurons in dorsal root ganglion: Pseudounipolar

Formation of Brain from Neural Tube

- Begins by expansion of cranial end of the neural tube
  - By end of fourth week of development, expansion results in production of the three vesicle stage: Prosencephalon, mesencephalon and rhombencephalon
  - Subsequent subdivision of vesicles produces the five vesicle stage Telencephalon and diencephalon from the prosencephalon, mesencephalon, and metencephalon and myelencephalon from the rhombencephalon
- Five vesicle stage includes all the major regions of the adult brain
  - Telencephalon—Cerebral hemispheres: Lateral ventricles
  - Diencephalon—Thalamus, hypothalamus: Third ventricle
  - Mesencephalon—Midbrain: Cerebral aqueduct
  - Metencephalon—Pons and cerebellum: Fourth ventricle
  - Myelencephalon—Medulla oblongata
- Expansion of cephalic end of tube into vesicles accompanied by formation of bends, or flexures, in the tube
  - Three vesicle stage includes two flexures: cephalic and cervical
  - Five vesicle stage includes three flexures: cephalic, pontine and cervical
  - The cervical and pontine flexures eventually straighten out, but cephalic flexure remains with result that axis of forebrain is at an angle to the rest of the CNS
- Telencephalic portion of the brain continues to grow and expand
  - Eventually comes to surround the diencephalon; growth accounts for very large size of human cerebral hemispheres
  - Cells in mantle layer of neural tube migrate to surface of hemisphere, forming the gray matter which constitutes the cerebral cortex.

CEREBRAL HEMISPHERES

The cerebral hemispheres comprise the cerebral cortex, the basal ganglia, and their afferent and efferent connections. The lateral ventricles, containing CSF, are at their centre.

CEREBRAL CORTEX

The cortex of the cerebral hemispheres is divided on topographical and functional grounds into four lobes—frontal, parietal, temporal and occipital.

Frontal Lobe

Cortex anterior to the central sulcus of Rolando. The lateral aspect of the frontal lobe is related to 'intellectual activity' (i.e. cognitive functions—analysis, judgement and planning), the medial and orbital surfaces to affective (or emotional) behavior and the control of autonomic activity
- *Motor cortex*—Occupies a large part of the precentral gyrus. It receives afferents from the premotor cortex, thalamus and cerebellum and is concerned with voluntary movements.
- *Premotor cortex*—Lies anterior to the precentral gyrus and the adjoining lower part of the frontal gyri.
- *Eye motor field*—Lies in the middle frontal area anterior to the premotor cortex.
- *Broca's speech area*—area around the posterior part of the inferior frontal gyrus of the dominant (usually the left) hemisphere
- *Frontal association cortex (*the prefrontal cortex)— Its afferents are derived from the thalamus, limbic area and also from other cortical areas; it sends efferents to the thalamus and hypothalamus.

Parietal Lobe

Bounded anteriorly by the central sulcus and behind by a line drawn from the parieto-occipital sulcus to the posterior end of the lateral (Sylvian) sulcus. The lower part of the parietal lobe in the subject's dominant hemisphere interacts with the somato-sensory visual and auditory associations and has a key role in language.
- *Primary somato-sensory cortex*—the postcentral gyrus receives afferent fibers from the thalamus and is concerned with all forms of somatic sensation.
- *Parietal association cortex*—concerned largely with the recognition of somatic sensory stimulation and their integration with other forms of sensory information. It also receives afferents from the thalamus

Temporal Lobe

Arbitrarily separated from the occipital lobe by a line drawn vertically downwards from the upper end of the lateral sulcus. The visual area of the occipital lobe connects with the temporal lobe and is concerned with visual recognition. The antero-inferior aspect of the frontal lobe connects with the medial aspect of the temporal lobe and is concerned with behavior.
- *Auditory cortex*—lies in the superior temporal gyrus on the lateral and superior surfaces of the hemisphere. Its afferent fibers are from the medial geniculate body and it is concerned with the perception of auditory stimuli.
- *Temporal association cortex*—area surrounding the auditory cortex is responsible for the recognition of auditory stimuli and for their integration with other sensory modalities. The cortical region just above and behind this area on the dominant hemisphere (Wernicke's area) is of considerable importance in the sensory aspects of language comprehension.
- The cortex of the most medial part of the undersurface of the temporal lobe is known as the parahippocampal gyrus, much of which is referred to as the *entorhinal cortex*. It receives widespread association cortical afferents and is a significant source of inputs to the hippocampus. Its relations are:
  - **Anterior:** Olfactory cortex of the uncus
  - **Medially:** In direct continuity with the *hippocampus*
- *Limbic system*—this is an important substrate for emotions, behaviour and memory. The circuit is completed by projections of the hypothalamus to the thalamus, from the thalamus to the cingulate gyrus and from thence back to the hippocampus. The hippocampus occupies the whole length of the floor of the inferior horn of the lateral ventricle and extends to the amygdala. It sends its efferents into the overlying layer of white matter known as the *alveus*. The fibers of the alveus collect on the medial margin of the hippocampus to form a compact bundle, the *fimbria*, which, as it arches under the corpus callosum, becomes known as the *fornix*. The fornix passes forwards and then downwards in front of the interventricular foramen and finally backwards into the hypothalamus to terminate in the *mammillary body*. It also gives fibers to the thalamus and the hypothalamus.
- Amygdaloid nuclear complex—a prominent temporal lobe structure, situated immediately rostral to the hippocampus. It is divided into three groups of nuclei: corticomedial, central and basolateral, which receive largely olfactory, gustatory, and association cortical afferents respectively.

Occipital Lobe

It lies behind the parietal and temporal lobes.
- *Visual cortex*—surrounds the calcarine and postcalcarine sulci and receives its afferent fibers from the lateral geniculate body of the thalamus of the same side.
- *Occipital association cortex*—it lies anteriorly to the visual cortex and is particularly concerned with the recognition and integration of visual stimuli.

BASAL GANGLIA

Compact masses of gray matter situated deep in the substance of the cerebral hemisphere and comprise the *corpus striatum* (composed of the caudate nucleus, the putamen and the globus pallidus) and the *claustrum*.

Corpus Striatum

It receives afferent connections from the cerebral cortex and sends efferents to the globus pallidus, projecting to the thalamus and back to the premotor cortex. Dopaminergic fibers project from the substantia nigra to the corpus striatum and efferent fibers also pass to the thalamus, hypothalamus, red nucleus, substantia nigra and the inferior olivary nucleus

- *Caudate nucleus*—large homogeneous mass of gray matter consisting of a head, anterior to the interventricular foramen and forming the lateral wall of the anterior horn of the lateral ventricle; a body, forming the lateral wall of the body of the ventricle; and an elongated tail, which forms the roof of the inferior (temporal) horn of the ventricle.
- *Putamen and the Globus pallidus (together called the Lentiform nucleus)*
- *Basal ganglia components are supplied by the striate (medial and lateral) arteries which are branches from the roots of anterior and middle cerebral arteries. The posteroinferior part of the lentiform complex is supplied by the thalamostriate branches of the posterior cerebral artery, with additional contributions from anterior choroidal artery.*

HYPOTHALAMUS

The hypothalamus forms the floor of the 3rd ventricle:

- It includes, from before backwards, the *optic chiasma*, the *tuber cinereum*, the *infundibular stalk* (leading down to the posterior lobe of the pituitary), the *mammillary bodies* and the posterior *perforated substance.*
- The medial forebrain bundle which runs throughout the length of the hypothalamus and serves to link it with the midbrain posteriorly and the basal forebrain areas anteriorly.
- It is largely concerned with autonomic activity and can be divided into a posteromedial sympathetic area and an anterolateral area concerned with parasympathetic activity.
- It plays an important part in endocrine control by the formation of releasing factors or release-inhibiting factors.
- The *Papez circuit* links the limbic system to the hypothalamus and the thalamus and is concerned with the expressive side of emotions. It consists of fornix (Hippocampus) – mammillary body (Hypothalamus) – Anterior nucleus (Thalamus) – Cingulate gyrus – Hippocampus.
- **The hypothalamus comprises three main nuclear groups:**
    - The anterior group, which includes the preoptic, supraoptic, and paraventricular nuclei;
    - The middle group, which includes the tuberal, arcuate, ventromedial, and dorsomedial nuclei; and
    - The posterior group, comprising the mammillary and posterior hypothalamic nuclei.

PITUITARY GLAND (HYPOPHYSIS CEREBRI)

It lies in the cavity of the pituitary fossa covered over by the diaphragma sellae, which is a fold of dura mater.

- The pituitary comprises a larger anterior and smaller posterior lobe, the latter connected by the hollow infundibulum (pituitary stalk) to the tuber cinereum in the floor of the 3rd ventricle. The two lobes are connected by a narrow zone termed the pars intermedia.
- **Relations:**
    - Below is the body of the sphenoid,
    - Laterally lies the cavernous sinus and its contents separated by dura mater and intercavernous sinuses communicating in front, behind and below.
    - The optic chiasma lies above, immediately in front of the infundibulum.
- The anterior lobe is extremely cellular and consists of chromophobe, eosinophilic and basophilic cells. The pars intermedia contain large colloid vesicles reminiscent of the thyroid. The posterior lobe is made up of nerve fibers whose cell stations lie in the hypothalamus.

THALAMUS

It is an oval mass of gray matter which forms the lateral wall of the 3rd ventricle; it extends from the interventricular foramen rostrally to the midbrain caudally.

- **Relations:**
    - Laterally, it is related to the internal capsule (and through it to the basal ganglia), and dorsally to the floor of lateral ventricle.
    - Medially, it is connected with its fellow of the opposite side through the *massa intermedia* (interthalamic connexus).
    - Posteriorly, it presents three distinct eminences, the *pulvinar*, and the *medial* and *lateral geniculate bodies*, which are the thalamic relay nuclei of hearing and vision respectively.

- LGN receives a major sensory input from the retina and is the main central connection for the optic nerve to the occipital lobe. Each LGN has 6 layers of neurons (gray matter) alternating with optic fibers (white matter).
- LGN is a small ovoid ventral projection at the termination of the optic tract on either side of the brain.
- MGN is a part of the auditory thalamus and represents the thalamic relay between inferior colliculus and the auditory cortex.

- The blood supply of the thalamus is derived principally from the posterior cerebral artery through its thalamostriate branches, which pierce the posterior perforated substance to supply also the posterior part of the internal capsule.
- It is the principal sensory relay nucleus which projects impulses from the main sensory pathways onto the cerebral cortex via thalamic radiations in the internal capsule.

CEREBELLUM

Largest part of the hind-brain and occupies most of the posterior cranial fossa.

- It is made up of two lateral *cerebellar hemispheres* and a median *vermis*. Inferiorly, the vermis is clearly separated from the two hemispheres and lies at the bottom of a deep cleft, the *vallecula*; superiorly, it is only marked off from the hemispheres as a low median elevation.
- A small ventral portion of the hemisphere lying on the middle cerebellar peduncle is almost completely separated from the rest of the cerebellum as the flocculus.
- Surface of the cerebellum is divided into numerous narrow *folia* and, by a few deep fissures, into a number of lobules to give the cerebellum in section the appearance of a branched tree (the *arbor vitae*).

Internal Structure

- Consists of a *cortex* of gray matter (in which all the afferent fibers terminate) covering a mass of white matter, in which deep nuclei of gray matter are buried.
- Of these, the *dentate nucleus* is the largest and occupies the central area of each hemisphere. The other nuclei are *emboliformis*, *globosus* and *fastigii*.
- It is connected to the brainstem by way of three pairs of *cerebellar peduncles*. The *inferior peduncles* connect it to the dorsolateral aspect of the medulla; the *middle cerebellar peduncles* to the pons, and the *superior peduncles* to the caudal midbrain.

Connections

Peduncle	Afferent	Efferent
Superior	Anterior spinocerebellar (uncrossed)	From dentate nucleus (crossed) to: 1. Thalamus 2. Cerebral cortex 3. Red nucleus
Middle	Pontocerebellar (crossed)—relays from cerebral cortex via pontine nuclei	—
Inferior	1. Vestibulocerebellar (uncrossed) 2. Posterior spinocerebellar (uncrossed) 3. Olivocerebellar (crossed)	From cerebellar cortex and nucleus to vestibular nuclei

- **Relations:**
    - Ventrally, the cerebellum is related to the 4th ventricle and to the medulla and pons;
    - Laterally, to the sigmoid sinus and the mastoid antrum and air cells;
    - Dorsally, it is separated from the cerebral hemispheres by the *tentorium cerebelli*.
- The *blood supply* of the cerebellum is derived from three pairs of arteries, the *posterior inferior cerebellar* branches of the vertebral arteries supply the posterior aspect of the vermis and hemispheres, and the *anterior inferior* and *superior cerebellar branches of the basilar artery* supply the anterolateral part of the under surface and the superior aspect of the cerebellum respectively.

THE MEDULLA

It is 25 mm in length and about 18 mm in diameter. It is continuous below, through the foramen magnum, with the spinal cord and above with the pons; posteriorly, it is connected with the cerebellum by way of the inferior cerebellar peduncles.

External Features

- The anterior surface of the medulla is grooved by an anteromedian fissure, on either side of which are the swellings due to the pyramidal tracts. These *pyramids*, in turn, are separated from the *olivary eminences* by the anterolateral sulcus along which the rootlets of the XIIth cranial nerve emerge.

- Between the olive and the inferior cerebellar peduncle there is another groove corresponding to the posterolateral sulcus of the spinal cord; emerging from this groove are the rootlets of cranial nerves IX, X and XI.
- The posteromedian sulcus of the cord is continued half-way up the medulla, where it widens out to form the posterior part of the IVth ventricle.
- Internal arcuate fibers of the medulla comes from nucleus gracilis and cuneatus
- The *blood supply* of the medulla is derived from the vertebral arteries directly and from their posterior inferior cerebellar branches.

THE PONS

- It is 25 mm in length and 38 mm in width. The *blood supply* of the pons is derived from the basilar artery formed by the junction of the two vertebral arteries, by way of a number of small pontine branches.

External Features

- The pons lies between the medulla and the midbrain and is connected to the cerebellum by the middle cerebellar peduncles.
- Its ventral surface presents a shallow median groove and numerous transverse ridges, which are continuous laterally with the middle cerebellar peduncle.
- The dorsal surface of the pons forms the upper part of the floor of the IVth ventricle
- Its junction with the medulla is marked close to the ventral midline by the emergence of the VIth cranial nerves and, in the angle between the pons and the cerebellum, by the VIIth and VIIIth nerves.
- The motor and sensory roots of V leave the lateral part of the pons near its upper border.

Internal Structure

- It consists for the most part of a number of cell masses (the *pontine nuclei*), scattered amongst the long ascending and descending pathways and the decussating pontocerebellar fibers, the pontine *tegmentum* (the pontine component of the reticular formation) and the central connections of the Vth, VIth and VIIth cranial nerves.

The Midbrain

It is the shortest part of the brainstem; it is just 25 mm long and connects the pons and cerebellum to the diencephalon. It lies in the gap in the tentorium cerebelli and is largely hidden by the surrounding structures.

External Features

- There are two *cerebral peduncles*, which emerge from the substance of the cerebral hemisphere and pass downwards and medially, connecting the internal capsule to the pons.
- The fibers of the 3rd nerves emerge between the two cerebral peduncles in the *interpeduncular fossa*.
- Consists of three distinct portions: the basis pedunculi ventrally, the midbrain *tegmentum* centrally and the *tectum* dorsally.
- The trochlear nerve (IV), the optic tract and the posterior cerebral artery wind around this aspect of the midbrain.
- The dorsal surface of the midbrain presents the four *colliculi* (or *corpora quadrigemini*) and the superior *medullary velum* between the two superior cerebellar peduncles.
- The *pineal gland* rests between the two superior colliculi and is attached by a stalk to the posterior dorsal thalamus.

Internal Structure

- The sections pass through the midbrain at the level of the decussation of the superior cerebellar peduncle and the nucleus of the 4th nerve, on the one hand, and through the red nucleus and the nucleus of III on the other.
- Above the level of the cerebral aqueduct lies the *tectum* and between the aqueduct and the basis pedunculi is the gray matter of the *tegmentum* separated from basis pedunculi by the deeply pigmented lamina of the *substantia nigra*.

VASCULAR SUPPLY OF THE CEREBRAL HEMISPHERES

- The aortic arch gives rise to three major vessels: the brachiocephalic, the left common carotid, and the left subclavian arteries. The brachiocephalic in turn gives rise to the right subclavian and the right common carotid arteries. The two common carotid arteries run upward lateral to the trachea to approximately the level of the fourth cervical vertebra, where each bifurcates into the external and internal carotid arteries.
- The two vertebral arteries arise from their respective subclavian arteries medial to the anterior scalene muscle and join to form the basilar artery.
- The basilar artery has a relatively constant course, beginning at or slightly below the pontomedullary junction and stretching the length of the pons, tapering to its termination at the pons and midbrain junction where it bifurcates into its two terminal branches, the right and left posterior cerebral arteries (PCA), at the level of the interpeduncular cistern.

- The blood supply of the upper spinal cord, brainstem (medulla, pons, and midbrain), labyrinth, cochlea, cerebellum, subthalamus, portion of the thalamus, and temporo-occipital areas originates from the vertebral and basilar system.
- The carotid and vertebral artery systems join at the base of the brain to form the circle of Willis.

Internal Carotid Artery

- The internal carotid artery (ICA) may be divided into three main segments: cervical, petrosal, and intracranial.
  - The cervical segment of the ICA has no branches. It ascends vertically in the neck, extending from the common carotid bifurcation to the base of the skull. It then enters the base of the skull through the carotid canal in the petrous portion of the temporal bone. The artery crosses the foramen lacerum and enters the cavernous sinus.
  - The petrosal segment gives off a caroticotympanic branch (to the tympanic cavity) and a vidian branch (artery to the pterygoid canal).
  - The intracranial segment begins distal to the petrous segment and proximal to the anterior clinoid process.
- The ICA then pierces the dura mater medial to the anterior clinoid process, where it becomes the supraclinoid. The ophthalmic artery, the first major branch of the ICA, arises at the level of the anterior clinoid process.
- After giving off the ophthalmic branch, the ICA gives rise to the posterior communicating artery and then to the anterior choroidal artery (AChA). The posterior communicating artery joins the posterior cerebral artery to form the posterolateral portion of the circle of Willis.
- After giving off the AChA, the ICA then bifurcates to form the anterior cerebral and middle cerebral arteries.

Collateral Circulation

- There are three main sources of collateral circulation to the brain that compensate in cases of carotid or basilar occlusion:
  - The circle of Willis, located on the ventral surface of the brain, which connects the internal carotid and vertebrobasilar arterial systems with each other,
  - Anastomoses between branches of the extracranial and intracranial arteries, and
  - Leptomeningeal anastomoses between the terminal branches of the major arteries of the cerebrum and cerebellum.
- The **circle of Willis** (named after Sir Thomas Willis) is a confluence of vessels that gives rise to all of the major cerebral arteries. It is fed by the paired internal carotid arteries and the basilar artery. When the circle is complete, it contains a posterior communicating artery on each side and an anterior communicating artery. The circle of Willis shows many variations among individuals and is completely formed in only 40% of the individuals.
- Each major artery supplies a certain territory, separated by border zones (watershed areas) from other territories; sudden occlusion in a vessel affects its territory immediately, sometimes irreversibly.

VENOUS DRAINAGE

- The venous drainage of the brain and coverings includes the veins of the brain itself, the dural venous sinuses, the dura's meningeal veins, and the diploic veins between the tables of the skull.
- Emissary veins drain from the scalp, through the skull, into the larger meningeal veins and dural sinuses. Unlike systemic veins, cerebral veins have no valves and seldom accompany the corresponding cerebral arteries.

Internal Drainage

- The interior of the cerebrum drains into the single midline great cerebral vein (of Galen), which lies beneath the splenium of the corpus callosum. The internal cerebral veins (with their tributaries, the septal, thalamostriate, and choroidal veins) empty into this vein, as do the basal veins (of Rosenthal), which wind (one right and one left) around the side of the midbrain, draining the base of the forebrain.
- The precentral vein from the cerebellum and veins from the upper brainstem also empty into the great vein, which turns upward behind the splenium and joins the inferior sagittal sinus to form the straight sinus. The venous drainage of the base of the cerebrum is also into the deep middle cerebral vein (coursing in the lateral fissure) and then to the cavernous sinus.

Cortical Veins

- Venous drainage of the brain surface is generally into the nearest large vein or sinus, from there to the confluence of the sinuses, and ultimately to the internal jugular vein.

Venous Sinuses

- Venous channels are lined by mesothelium and they lie between the inner and outer layers of the dura, called intradural (or dural) sinuses. Their tributaries come mostly from the neighboring brain substance. All sinuses ultimately drain into the internal jugular veins or pterygoid plexus. The sinuses may also communicate with extracranial veins via the emissary veins.

- The blood can flow through them in either direction, and infections of the scalp may extend by this route into the intracranial structures.

Of the venous sinuses, the following are considered most important:
- **Superior sagittal sinus:** between the falx and the inside of the skull cap.
- **Inferior sagittal sinus:** in the free edge of the falx.
- **Straight sinus:** in the seam between the falx and the tentorium.
- **Transverse sinuses:** between the tentorium and its attachment on the skull cap.
- **Sigmoid sinuses:** curved continuations of the transverse sinuses into the jugular veins; a transverse and a sigmoid sinus together form a lateral sinus.
- **Sphenoparietal sinuses:** drain the deep middle cerebral veins into the cavernous sinuses.
- **Cavernous sinuses:** on either side of the sella turcica. The cavernous sinuses receive drainage from multiple sources, including the ophthalmic and facial veins. Blood leaves the cavernous sinuses via the petrosal sinuses. The cavernous sinuses are convoluted, with different chambers separated by fibrous trabeculae giving the appearance of a cavern. The internal carotid artery runs through the cavernous sinus. In addition, the oculomotor, trochlear, and abducens nerves run through the cavernous sinus, as does the ophthalmic division of the trigeminal nerve, together with the trigeminal ganglion.
- **Inferior petrosal sinuses:** from the cavernous sinus to the jugular foramen.
- **Superior petrosal sinus:** from the cavernous sinus to the beginning of the sigmoid sinus.

The spinal cord is about 45 cm long. It is continuous above with the medulla oblongata at the level of the foramen magnum and ends below at the lower level of the 1st, or the upper level of the 2nd lumbar vertebra. Up to the 3rd month of fetal life the spinal cord occupies the full extent of the vertebral canal. The vertebrae then outpace the cord in the rapidity of their growth so that, at birth, the cord reaches only the level of the 3rd lumbar vertebra. Further differential growth up to the time of adolescence brings the cord to its definitive position at the approximate level of the disk between the 1st and 2nd lumbar vertebrae.

- The cord bears a deep longitudinal *anterior fissure*, a narrower *posterior septum* and on either side, a *posterolateral sulcus* along which the *posterior (sensory) nerve roots* (which bear a ganglion constituting the first cell-station of the sensory nerves) are serially arranged.
- The *anterior (motor) nerve roots* emerge serially along the anterolateral aspect of the cord on either side.
- At each intervertebral foramen the anterior and posterior nerve roots unite to form a *spinal nerve* which immediately divides into its *anterior* and *posterior primary rami*, each transmitting both motor and sensory fibers.
- The length of the roots increases progressively from above downwards due to the disparity between the length of the cord and the vertebral column; the lumbar and sacral roots below the termination of the cord at vertebral level L2 continue as a leash of nerve roots termed the *cauda equina.*
- Inferiorly, the cord tapers into the *conus medullaris* from which a prolongation of pia mater, the *filum terminale*, descends to be attached to the back of the coccyx.
- The *anterior* and *posterior spinal arteries* descend in the pia from the intracranial part of the vertebral artery. They are reinforced serially by branches from the ascending cervical, the cervical part of the vertebral, the intercostals and the lumbar arteries.

Internal Structure

- In transverse section of the cord is seen the *central canal* around which is the H-shaped *gray matter*, surrounded in turn by the *white matter* which contains the long ascending and descending tracts.
- Within the *posterior horns* of the gray matter, capped by the *substantia gelatinosa*, terminate many of the sensory fibers entering from the posterior nerve roots. The motor cells which give rise to the fibers of the anterior roots lie in the large *anterior horns*.

In the thoracic and upper lumbar cord are found the *lateral horns* on each side, containing the cells of origin of the sympathetic system
- **Descending tracts**
  - The pyramidal (lateral cerebrospinal or crossed motor) tract—the motor pathway commences at the pyramidal cells of the motor cortex, decussates in the medulla, then descends in the pyramidal tract on the contralateral side of the cord.
  - The direct pyramidal (anterior cerebrospinal or uncrossed motor) tract—small tract descending without medullary decussation.
- **Ascending tracts**
  - The posterior and anterior spinocerebellar tracts—ascend on the same side of the cord and enter the cerebellum through the inferior and superior cerebellar peduncles respectively.
  - The Lateral and Anterior Spinothalamic tracts—Pain and temperature fibers enter the posterior roots, ascend a few segments, relay in the substantia gelatinosa, then cross to the opposite side to ascend in these tracts to the thalamus, where they are relayed to the sensory cortex.

- The posterior columns [*fasciculus gracilis* (*of Goll*) and *fasciculus cuneatus* (*of Burdach*)]
- They convey 1st order sensory fibers subserving fine touch and proprioception (position sense), mostly uncrossed, to the gracile and cuneate nuclei in the medulla where, after synapse, the 2nd order fibers decussate, pass to the thalamus and the 3rd order fibers are relayed to the sensory cortex.

Membranes of the Cord

- Cord is closely ensheathed by the *pia mater* which is thickened on either side between the nerve roots to form the *denticulate ligament*, which passes laterally to adhere to the dura. Inferiorly, the pia continues as the *filum terminale*, which pierces the distal extremity of the dural sac and becomes attached to the coccyx.
- The *arachnoid mater* lines the *dura matter*, leaving an extensive *subarachnoid space*, containing cerebrospinal fluid (C.S.F.), between it and the pia.
- The dura itself forms a tough sheath to the cord. It ends distally at the level of the 2nd sacral vertebra.
- The *extradural* (or *epidural*) *space* is the compartment between the dural sheath and the spinal canal. It extends downwards from the foramen magnum (above which the dura becomes two-layered) to the sacral hiatus.
- The extradural veins form a plexus which communicate freely and also receive the *basivertebral veins*, which emerge from each vertebral body on its posterior aspect. In addition, the veins link up with both the pelvic veins below and the cerebral veins above—a pathway for the spread of both bacteria and tumor cells termed Batson's valveless vertebral venous plexus, which accounts for the ready spread of prostatic cancer to the sacrum and vertebrae.

Spinal Cord Level Relative to the Vertebral Bodies

Spinal cord level	Corresponding vertebral body
Upper cervical	Same as cord level
Lower cervical	1 level higher
Upper thoracic	2 levels higher
Lower thoracic	2 to 3 levels higher
Lumbar	T10-T12
Sacral	T12-L1

Long Ascending and Descending Pathways

Somatic Afferent Pathways

- Proprioceptive and tactile impulses pass uninterruptedly through the posterior root ganglia, through the ipsilateral *posterior columns* of the spinal cord to the *gracile* and *cuneate nuclei* in the lower part of the medulla. In the posterior columns those from sacral and lumbar segments are situated medially in the tracts while fibers from thoracic and cervical levels are successively added to their lateral aspect. This arrangement according to body segments is maintained in the gracile and cuneate nuclei and in the efferents from these nuclei to the contralateral thalamus. The fibers arising from the gracile and cuneaten nuclei immediately cross over to the opposite side in the *sensory decussation* of the medulla and continue up to the thalamus as a compact contralateral bundle—the *medial lemniscus*.
- Dorsal root fibers subserving pain and temperature, together with some tactile afferents, end ipsilaterally in the *substantia gelatinosa* of the posterior horn. They then synapse and cross to the contralateral anterior lateral columns of the cord and are relayed to the contralateral thalamus. The fiber crossing occurs in the anterior white commissure of the spinal cord.
  - In the brainstem these fibers come to lie immediately lateral to the medial lemniscus and are sometimes known as the *spinal lemniscus* which terminates in the thalamus.
  - These somatic afferents are relayed from the thalamus, through the posterior limb of the internal capsule to the somatic sensory cortex of the *postcentral gyrus*.
  - In the internal capsule the fibers are arranged in the sequence 'face, arm, trunk and leg' from before backwards, and this segregation persists in the sensory cortex, where the leg is represented on the dorsal and medial part of the cortex, the trunk and arm in its middle portion and the face most inferiorly. Since the size of the area of cortical representation reflects the density of the peripheral innervation and hence complexity of the function being performed rather than the area of the receptive field, there is a distortion of the body image in the cortex, the cortical representation of the face and hand being much greater than that of the limbs and trunk.

MOTOR PATHWAYS

Pyramidal Tract

- The pyramidal system is the main 'voluntary' motor pathway and derives its name from the fact that projections to the motor neurons in the spinal cord are grouped together in the medullary pyramids.
- The fibers in this pathway arise from a wide area of the cerebral cortex. About two-thirds derive from the motor and premotor cortex of the frontal lobes; however, about one-third arises from the primary somatosensory cortex. In both the motor and premotor cortex there is an organization comparable to that seen in the sensory area. Again, the body is inverted so that the 'leg area' is situated in the dorsomedial part of the precentral gyrus encroaching on the medial surface of the hemisphere, supplied by the anterior cerebral artery. The 'face area' is near the lateral sulcus, while the 'arm area' occupies a central position, both supplied by the middle cerebral artery. The body image is greatly distorted; the area representing the hand, lips, eyes and foot are exaggerated out of proportion to the rest of the body and in accordance with the complexity of the tasks they perform.
- From the cortex, the motor fibers pass through the posterior limb of the internal capsule where they are again organized in the sequence of 'face, arm, leg', anteroposteriorly. From the internal capsule the fibers form a compact bundle which occupies the central third of the cerebral peduncle. Hence, they pass through the ventral pons, where they are broken up into a number of small bundles between the cells of the pontine nuclei and the transversely disposed pontocerebellar fibers. Near the lower end of the pons they again collect to form a single bundle which comes to lie on the ventral surface of the medulla and forms the elevation known as the 'pyramid'. As it passes through the brainstem, the pyramidal system gives off, at regular intervals, contributions to the somatic and branchial arch efferent nuclei of the cranial nerves. Near the lower end of the medulla the great majorities of the pyramidal tract fibers cross over to the opposite side and come to occupy a central position in the lateral white column of the spinal cord. This is hence called 'crossed pyramidal tract'. A small proportion of the fibers of the medullary pyramid, however, remain uncrossed until they reach the segmental level at which they finally terminate. This is the *direct* or *uncrossed pyramidal tract*, which runs downwards close to the anteromedian fissure of the cord, with fibers passing from it at each segment to the opposite side.

Extrapyramidal System

The extrapyramidal motor system includes all those motor projections which do not pass physically through the medullary pyramids.

- Components of the extrapyramidal system include the red nuclei, vestibular nuclei, superior colliculus and reticular formation in the brainstem, all of which project via discrete pathways to influence spinal cord motor neurons. Cerebellar projections act via the dentatothalamic projection.
- The neostriatum (caudate and putamen) receives widespread cortical afferents, including those from high order sensory association and motor areas, and projects mainly to the globus pallidus. The latter nucleus is the major outflow for the basal ganglia and, via the ventral anterior thalamus, exerts its major influence on premotor and hence the motor cortices. This pattern of connections suggests that the basal ganglia are involved in complex aspects of motor control, including motor planning and the initiation of movement.
- The membranes of the brain (the meninges)
- The three membranes surrounding the spinal cord, the dura mater, arachnoid mater and pia mater, are continued upwards as coverings to the brain.

The *dura* is a dense membrane which, within the cranium, is made up of two layers. The outer layer is intimately adherent to the skull; the inner layer is united to the outer layer except where separated by the great dural venous sinuses and where it projects to form four sheets:

- The falx cerebri;
- The falx cerebelli;
- The tentorium cerebelli;
- The diaphragma sellae.

The *arachnoid* is a delicate membrane separated from the dura by the potential *subdural space*. It projects only into the longitudinal fissure and the stem of the lateral fissure.

The *pia* is closely moulded to the outline of the brain; it dips down into the cerebral sulci leaving the *subarachnoid space* between it and the arachnoid. This space is broken up by trabeculae of fine fibrous strands and contains the cerebrospinal fluid.

Nerve Supply

- *Anterior cranial fossa:* Meningeal branches of anterior and posterior ethmoidal nerves, maxillary nerve and mandibular nerve
- *Middle cranial fossa:* Meningeal branches of recurrent tentorial nerve, maxillary and mandibular nerves.
- *Posterior cranial fossa:* Tentorial nerve, vagus nerve and the upper 3 cervical nerves.

The Ventricular System and the Cerebrospinal Fluid Circulation

The cerebrospinal fluid (CSF) is formed by the secretory activity of the epithelium covering the choroid plexuses in the lateral, 3rd and 4th ventricles; it circulates through the ventricular system of the brain and drains into the subarachnoid space from the roof of the 4th ventricle before being reabsorbed into the dural venous system.

- The two *lateral ventricles*, which are the largest components of the system, occupy a considerable part of the cerebral hemispheres. Each has an *anterior horn* (in front of the interventricular foramen), a *body*, above and medial to the body of the caudate nucleus, a *posterior horn* in the occipital lobe and an *inferior horn* reaching down into the temporal lobe. The choroid plexuses of the lateral ventricles, which are responsible for the production of most of the CSF, extend from the inferior horn, through the body, to the interventricular foramen where they become continuous with the plexus of the 3rd ventricle.
- The *3rd ventricle* is a narrow midline slit-like cavity between the two thalami in its upper portion and the hypothalamus in its lower part. Its floor is formed by the hypothalamus. From the 3rd ventricle the CSF passes through the narrow *cerebral aqueduct* (*of Sylvius*) in the midbrain to reach the 4th ventricle.
- The *4th ventricle* is diamond-shaped when viewed from above and tentshaped as seen from the side.
  Relations:
    - Its floor is diamond shaped, lined by ependyma and is formed below by the medulla and above by the pons. It has the median sulcus, vestibular area, stria medularis, facial colliculus and the vagus triangle.
    - It is bounded laterally by the superior and inferior cerebellar peduncles, cuneate and gracile tubercles and fasciculus cuneatus.
    - Its roof is formed by the cerebellum and the superior and inferior medullary vela.
    - The CSF escapes from the 4th ventricle into the subarachnoid space by way of the *median* and *lateral apertures* (of *Magendie* and *Luschka* respectively) and then flows over the surface of the brain and spinal cord.
- About one-fifth of the CSF is absorbed along similar spinal villi or escapes along the nerve sheaths into the lymphatics. This absorption of CSF is passive, depending on its hydrostatic pressure being higher than that of the venous blood.

BROADMANN AREAS

A Broadmann area is a region of the cortex defined based on its cytoarchitecture, or organization of cells.

Major Areas

Motor

- Area 4—Primary *Motor Cortex*
- Area 6—*Premotor cortex* and supplementary motor cortex (secondary motor cortex)(supplementary motor area)

Sensory

- Areas 3, 1 and 2—Primary *somatosensory cortex*
- Area 5 and 7—Somatosensory *association cortex*

Visual

- Area 8—Includes *Frontal eye fields*
- Areas 11 and 12—Orbitofrontal area (orbital and rectus gyri, plus part of the rostral part of the superior frontal gyrus)
- Area 17—*Primary visual cortex* (V1)
- Area 18—Secondary visual cortex (V2)
- Area 19—Associative visual cortex (V3)

Auditory

- Area 22—Superior temporal gyrus, of which the caudal part is usually considered to contain the *Wernicke's area*
- Area 39—Angular gyrus, considered by some to be part of Wernicke's area
- Area 40—Supramarginal gyrus considered by some to be part of Wernicke's area
- Areas 41 and 42—Primary and *Auditory association cortex*.

Speech

- Area 44—pars opercularis, part of *Broca's area*
- Area 45—pars triangularis Broca's area

Others
- Area 9 and 10—prefrontal cortex
- Area 13 and 14—Insular cortex
- Area 23 and 24—cingulate cortex
- Area 27—Piriform cortex
- Areas 28, 34, 35 and 36—Part of Limbic system
- Area 48—Retrosubicular area (a small part of the medial surface of the temporal lobe)
- Area 52—Parainsular area (at the junction of the temporal lobe and the insula)

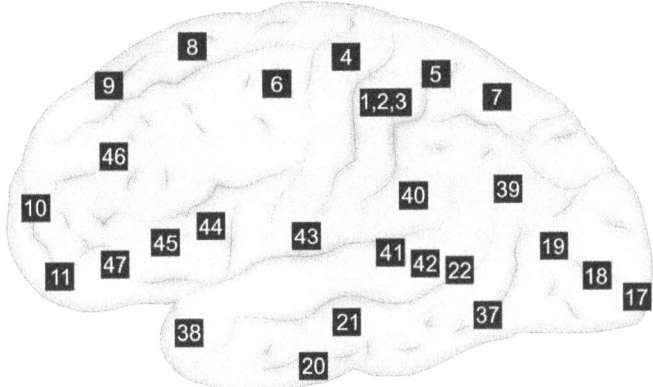

Fig. 1.1: Broadmann areas[1]

Cranial nerve fibers with motor (efferent) functions arise from collections of cells (motor nuclei) that lie deep within the brain stem; they are homologous to the anterior horn cells of the spinal cord. Cranial nerve fibers with sensory (afferent) functions have their cells of origin (first-order nuclei) outside the brainstem, usually in ganglia that are homologous to the dorsal root ganglia of the spinal nerves. Second-order sensory nuclei lie within the brainstem.

Cranial nerves can be functionally divided into:
- Nerves I, II, and VIII are devoted to special sensory input.
- Nerves III, IV, and VI control eye movements and pupillary constriction.
- Nerves XI and XII are pure motor (XI: sternocleidomastoid and trapezius; XII: muscles of tongue).
- Nerves V, VII, IX, and X are mixed.
- Note that nerves III, VII, IX, and X carry parasympathetic fibers.

OLFACTORY NERVE (I)

The fibers of the olfactory nerve, unlike other afferent fibers, are unique in being the central processes of the olfactory cells and not the peripheral processes of a central group of ganglion cells.

The central processes of the olfactory receptors pass upwards from the olfactory mucosa in the upper part of the superior nasal concha and septum, through the cribriform plate of the ethmoid bone to end by synapsing with the dendrites of mitral cells in the olfactory bulb. The mitral cells in turn send their axons back in the olfactory tract to terminate in the cortex of the uncus, the adjacent inferomedial temporal cortex and the region of the anterior perforated space. The further course of the olfactory pathway is uncertain in humans.

OPTIC NERVE (II)

The optic nerve is the nerve of vision. It is not a true cranial nerve but should be thought of as a brain tract which has become drawn out from the cerebrum. Embryologically, it is developed, together with the retina, as a lateral diverticulum of the forebrain. Devoid of neurilemmal sheaths, its fibers, like other brain tissues, are incapable of regeneration after division. From a functional point of view the retina can be regarded as consisting of three cellular layers: a layer of receptor cells — the *rods* and *cones* — an intermediate layer of *bipolar cells*, and a layer of *ganglion cells*, whose axons form the optic nerve. From all parts of the retina these axons converge on the *optic disk* whence they pierce the sclera to form the optic nerve.

The Visual Pathway and Defects are explained in Neuro-ophthalmology.

OCULOMOTOR NERVE (III)

In addition to supplying most of the extrinsic eye muscles, the oculomotor nerve conveys the preganglionic parasympathetic fibers for the sphincter of the pupil via the ciliary ganglion. Its nucleus of origin lies in the floor of the cerebral aqueduct at the level of the superior colliculus and consists essentially of two components: the *somatic efferent nucleus*, which supplies the ocular muscles, and the *Edinger–Westphal nucleus* from which the preganglionic parasympathetic fibers are derived.

From these nuclei, fibers pass vertically through the midbrain tegmentum to emerge just medial to the cerebral peduncle. Passing forwards between the superior cerebellar and posterior cerebral arteries, the nerve pierces the dura mater to run in the lateral wall of the cavernous sinus as far as the superior orbital fissure. Before entering the fissure it divides into a superior and inferior branch; both branches enter the orbit through the tendinous ring from which the recti arise. The superior branch passes lateral to the optic nerve to supply the superior rectus muscle and levator palpebrae superioris; the inferior branch supplies three muscles, the medial rectus, the inferior rectus and the inferior oblique, the nerve to the last conveying the parasympathetic fibers to the ciliary ganglion.

The ciliary ganglion lies near the apex of the orbit just lateral to the optic nerve. It receives, in addition to the preganglionic parasympathetic fibers from the Edinger–Westphal nucleus, a sympathetic (postganglionic) root ultimately from the plexus on the internal carotid artery, and a sensory root from the nasociliary nerve. The postganglionic efferent fibers from the ganglion pass to the ciliary muscle and the muscles of the iris by way of about ten *short ciliary nerves*.

TROCHLEAR NERVE (IV)

The trochlear nerve is the most slender of the cranial nerves and supplies only one eye muscle, the *superior oblique*. Its nucleus of origin lies in a similar position to that of the 3rd nerve at the level of the inferior colliculus, but from here its fibers pass dorsally around the cerebral aqueduct and decussate in the superior medullary velum.

Emerging on the dorsum of the pons (being the only cranial nerve to arise from the dorsal aspect of the brainstem), the nerve winds round the cerebral peduncle and then passes forwards between the superior cerebellar and posterior cerebral arteries to pierce the dura. It then runs forwards in the lateral wall of the cavernous sinus between the oculomotor and ophthalmic nerves to enter the orbit through the superior orbital fissure, lateral to the tendinous ring from which the recti take origin. It then passes medially over the optic nerve to enter the superior oblique muscle.

TRIGEMINAL NERVE (V)

As the name suggests, this nerve consists of three divisions. Together they supply sensory fibers to the greater part of the skin of the head and face, the mucous membranes of the mouth, nose and paranasal air sinuses and, by way of a small motor root, the muscles of mastication. In addition it is associated with four autonomic ganglia, the ciliary, pterygopalatine, otic and submandibular.

The trigeminal ganglion also termed the *semilunar ganglion*, is equivalent to the dorsal sensory ganglion of a spinal nerve. It is crescent-shaped and is situated within an invaginated pocket of dura in the middle cranial fossa. It lies near the apex of the petrous temporal bone. The motor root of the trigeminal nerve and the greater superficial petrosal nerve both pass deep to the ganglion. Above lies the hippocampal gyrus of the temporal lobe of the cerebrum; medially lies the internal carotid artery and the posterior part of the cavernous sinus. The trigeminal ganglion represents the 1st cell station for all sensory fibers of the trigeminal nerve except those subserving proprioception.

Divisions

- **V1: The ophthalmic division:** This is the smallest division of the trigeminal nerve; it is wholly sensory and is responsible for the innervation of the skin of the forehead, the upper eyelid, cornea and most of the nose. Passing forwards from the trigeminal ganglion, it immediately enters the lateral wall of the cavernous sinus where it lies beneath the trochlear nerve. Just before entering the orbit it divides into three branches, frontal, lacrimal and nasociliary.
    - The *frontal nerve* runs forward just beneath the roof of the orbit for a short distance before dividing into its two terminal branches, the *supratrochlear* and *supra-orbital nerves*, which supply the upper eyelid and the scalp as far back as the lambdoid suture.
    - The *lacrimal nerve* supplies the lacrimal gland (with postganglionic parasympathetic fibers from the pterygopalatine ganglion which reach it by way of the maxillary nerve) and the lateral part of the conjunctiva and upper lid.
    - The *nasociliary nerve* gives branches to the ciliary ganglion, the eyeball, cornea and conjunctiva the medial half of the upper eyelid, the dura of the anterior cranial fossa, and to the mucosa and skin of the nose.

- **V2: The maxillary nerve:** The maxillary nerve is again purely sensory. Passing forwards from the central part of the trigeminal ganglion, close to the cavernous sinus, it leaves the skull by way of the *foramen rotundum* and emerges into the upper part of the pterygopalatine fossa. It continues through the inferior orbital fissure and the infraorbital canal as the *infraorbital* nerve which supplies the skin of the cheek and lower eyelid. The maxillary nerve has the following named branches:
    1. The *zygomatic nerve*, whose zygomaticotemporal and zygomaticofacial branches supply the skin of the temple and cheek respectively;
    2. *Superior alveolar (dental) branches* to the teeth of the upper jaw; and
    3. The *branches from the pterygopalatine ganglion*, which run a descending course and are distributed as follows: the *greater and lesser palatine nerves*, which pass through the corresponding palatine foramina to supply the mucous membrane of the hard and soft palates, the uvula and the tonsils, and the mucous membrane of the nose and a *pharyngeal branch* supplying the mucosa of the nasopharynx. The *nasopalatine nerve* (long sphenopalatine) supplies the nasal septum then emerges through the incisive canal of the hard palate to supply the gum behind the incisor teeth. The *posterior superior lateral nasal nerves* (short sphenopalatine) supply the posterosuperior lateral wall of the nose.
- **V3: The mandibular nerve:** This is the largest of the three divisions of the trigeminal nerve and the only one to convey motor fibers. In addition to supplying the skin of the temporal region, part of the auricle and the lower face, the mucous membrane of the anterior two-thirds of the tongue and the floor of the mouth, it also conveys the motor root to the muscles of mastication and secretomotor fibers to the salivary glands. Passing forwards from the trigeminal ganglion, it almost immediately enters the foramen ovale through which it reaches the infratemporal fossa.
    - It gives off the *nervus spinosus* to supply the dura mater and the *nerve to the medial pterygoid muscle* from which the *otic ganglion* is suspended and through which motor fibers are transmitted to tensor palati and tensor tympani and then it divides into a small anterior and a larger posterior trunk.
- **The anterior trunk gives off:**
    - A sensory branch, the *buccal nerve*, which supplies part of the skin of the cheek and the mucous membrane on its inner aspect; and
    - Motor branches to the masseter, temporalis and lateral pterygoid muscles.
- **The posterior trunk, which is principally sensory, divides into three branches:**
    1. The *auriculotemporal nerve*, which conveys sensory fibers to the skin of the temple and auricle and secretomotor fibers from the otic ganglion to the parotid gland;
    2. The *lingual nerve*, which passes downwards under cover of the ramus of the mandible to the side of the tongue, where it supplies the mucous membrane of the floor of the mouth, the anterior two-thirds of the tongue (including the taste buds by way of fibers which join it from the chorda tympani), and the sublingual and submandibular salivary glands;
    3. The *inferior alveolar (dental) nerve*, which passes down into the mandibular canal and supplies branches to the teeth of the lower jaw. It then emerges from the mental foramen to supply the skin of the chin and lower lip. This branch also conveys the only motor component of the posterior trunk: the *nerve to the mylohyoid*, supplying the muscle of that name and the anterior belly of the digastric.

The central processes of the trigeminal ganglion cells enter the lateral aspect of the pons and divide into ascending and descending branches which terminate in one or other component of the sensory nucleus of V nerve. This nucleus consists of three parts, each of which appears to subserve different sensory modalities: a chief sensory nucleus in the pontine tegmentum concerned with touch; a descending, or spinal, nucleus subserving pain and temperature; and a mesencephalic nucleus receiving proprioceptive afferents. The *motor root of the trigeminal nerve* lies just medial to the sensory nucleus in the upper part of the pons; its efferents pass out with the sensory fibers and are distributed by way of the mandibular division of the nerve.

ABDUCENT NERVE (VI)

Like the trochlear nerve, the abducent nerve supplies only one eye muscle, the *lateral rectus*. Its nucleus lies in the caudal part of the pons and from there its fibers pass through the pontine tegmentum to emerge on the base of the brain at the junction of the pons and medulla. The nerve then passes forwards to enter the cavernous sinus. Here it lies lateral to the internal carotid artery and medial to the 3rd, 4th and 5th nerves. Passing through the tendinous ring just below the 3rd nerve, it enters the orbit to pierce the deep surface of the lateral rectus.

FACIAL NERVE (VII)

In addition to supplying the muscles of facial expression, the facial nerve conveys secretomotor fibers to the sublingual and submandibular salivary glands and the lacrimal gland as well as the nasal mucosa; it also carries taste fibers from the anterior two-thirds of the tongue.

- The fibers innervating the facial muscles have their nucleus of origin in the ventral part of the caudal pons; the secretomotor fibers for the salivary glands are derived from the superior salivary nucleus. The sensory fibers associated with the nerve have their cells of origin in the facial (geniculate) ganglion.
- From the motor nucleus, fibers of the facial nerve run a devious course over the nucleus of the abducent nerve, where they form an elevation on the floor of the 4th ventricle known as the *facial colliculus*. Then pass downwards and forwards to emerge from the lateral aspect of the pons together with VIII in the cerebellopontine angle.
- The sensory and motor fibers pass together into the internal auditory meatus, at the bottom of which they leave the 8th nerve and enter the facial canal. Here they run laterally over the vestibule before bending sharply backwards over the promontory of the middle ear. This bend, or *genu of the facial nerve*, as it is called, marks the site of the facial ganglion and the point at which the secretomotor fibers for the lacrimal gland leave to form the greater superficial petrosal nerve. The facial nerve then passes downwards, medial to the middle ear, to reach the stylomastoid foramen.
- Just before entering this foramen it gives off the branch, known as the *chorda tympani*, which runs back through the middle ear between the incus and malleus, exits via the fissure between the tympanic and petrous parts of the temporal bone to enter the infratemporal fossa where it joins the lingual nerve. Hence, its taste fibers reach the anterior two-thirds of the tongue and its secretomotor fibers are conveyed to the submandibular ganglion, and then to the submandibular and sublingual salivary glands.
- On emerging from the stylomastoid foramen, the nerve supplies the stylohyoid and the posterior belly of digastric muscle. It then enters the parotid gland where it divides into five divisions for the supply of the facial muscles: the temporal, zygomatic, buccal, mandibular, and cervical branches.

AUDITORY (VESTIBULOCOCHLEAR) NERVE (VIII)

- The 8th nerve consists of two sets of fibers: cochlear and vestibular.
- The *cochlear fibers* (concerned with hearing) represent the central processes of the bipolar spiral ganglion cells of the cochlea which traverse the internal auditory meatus to reach the lateral aspect of the medulla, at the cerebellopontine angle (together with VII), where they terminate in the *dorsal* and *ventral cochlear nuclei*. The majority of the projection fibers from these nuclei cross to the opposite side, those from the dorsal nucleus forming them auditory striae in the floor of the 4th ventricle, those from the ventral nucleus forming the trapezoid body in the ventral part of the pons. Most of these efferent fibers terminate in nuclei associated with the trapezoid body, either on the same or the opposite side, and then ascend in the lateral lemniscus to the *inferior colliculus* and the *medial geniculate body*; from the former, fibers reach the motor nuclei of the cranial nerves and form the pathway of auditory reflexes; from the latter, fibers sweep laterally in the *auditory radiation to the auditory cortex* in the superior temporal gyrus.
- The *vestibular fibers* (concerned with equilibrium) enter the medulla just medial to the cochlear division and terminate in the *vestibular nuclei*. Many of the efferent fibers from these nuclei pass to the cerebellum in the inferior cerebellar peduncle together with fibers bypassing the vestibular nuclei and passing directly to the cerebellum. Other vestibular connections are to the nuclei of III, IV, VI and XI and to the upper cervical cord (via the vestibulospinal tract). These connections bring the eye and neck muscles under reflex vestibular control.

GLOSSOPHARYNGEAL NERVE (IX)

- The glossopharyngeal nerve contains sensory fibers for the pharynx and the posterior one-third of the tongue (including the taste buds), motor fibers for the stylopharyngeus muscle and secretomotor fibers for the parotid gland. It is attached to the upper part of the medulla by four or five rootlets along the groove between the olive and the inferior cerebellar peduncle and leaves the skull by way of the jugular foramen in which it gives off its tympanic branch. Below the jugular foramen the nerve courses downwards and forwards between the internal carotid artery and the internal jugular vein to reach the styloid process. From here it passes along the stylopharyngeus muscle to enter the pharynx between the superior and middle constrictors where it breaks up into its terminal branches which supply the posterior one-third of the tongue and the mucous membrane of the pharynx (including the tonsil).

- The *tympanic branch*, which is continued as the *lesser superficial petrosal nerve*, conveys the preganglionic parasympathetic fibers to the otic ganglion (parotid secretomotor fibers).
- The only other branch of significance is the *carotid nerve* which arises just below the skull and runs down on the internal carotid artery to supply both the carotid body and carotid sinus. This branch serves as the afferent limb of the baroreceptor and chemoreceptor reflexes from the carotid sinus and body respectively.

VAGUS NERVE (X)

The vagus has the most extensive distribution of all the cranial nerves, innervating the heart and the major part of the respiratory and alimentary tracts.

The *dorsal nucleus* of the vagus in the medulla is a mixed visceral afferent and efferent nucleus. It receives sensory fibers from the heart, the lower respiratory tract and the alimentary tract down to the transverse colon; in addition it gives rise to preganglionic parasympathetic motor fibers to the heart and the smooth muscles of the bronchi and gut. From the *nucleus ambiguus* efferent fibers pass to the striped muscles of the pharynx and larynx.

- The nerve is connected to the side of the medulla by about ten filaments which lie in series with the glossopharyngeal nerve along the groove between the olive and the inferior cerebellar peduncle. These filaments unite to form a single bundle which passes beneath the cerebellum to the jugular foramen. Two sensory ganglia are associated with this part of the nerve: a superior, within the jugular foramen, and an inferior, immediately beneath the skull.
- The vagus then passes vertically downwards to the root of the neck, lying in the posterior part of the carotid sheath between the internal jugular vein and the internal and then common carotid arteries. There are a number of important branches in the neck: *pharyngeal* to the pharyngeal and palatal musculature by way of the pharyngeal plexus; *superior laryngeal*, supplying the interior of the larynx above the vocal folds and the cricothyroid and inferior constrictor muscles; and the superior and inferior *cardiac branches* which are inhibitory to the heart.
- Below the level of the subclavian arteries the course and relations of the nerve on the two sides differ.
- On the *right side* the *recurrent laryngeal branch* is given off as it crosses the subclavian artery; beyond this the nerve descends through the superior mediastinum in close association with the great veins. Behind the root of the lung it takes part in the formation of the *pulmonary plexus* and then passes on to the esophagus to form, with its fellow, the *esophageal plexus*. The *left vagus* enters the thorax in close association with the great arteries, lying at first lateral to the common carotid and then crossing the arch of the aorta.
- The *left recurrent laryngeal branch*, which is given off as the vagus crosses the aortic arch, passes below the ligamentum arteriosum, behind the arch and then ascends in the groove between the trachea and the esophagus. The vagus then passes behind the root of the lung, enters into the formation of the pulmonary plexus and passes on to the esophagus to form a plexus from which emerge two trunks, each comprising fibers from both the left and right vagus.
- The two vagi then enter the abdomen through the esophageal opening in the diaphragm, the anterior vagus passing on to the anterior surface and the posterior passing to the posterior aspect of the stomach. Then, branches are given to the *coeliac*, *hepatic* and *renal plexuses* and, by way of these plexuses, are distributed to the foregut, midgut and to the kidneys.

Functional Division of Cranial Nerve Nuclei

- **Sensory/Afferent**
  1. *General Somatic:* Sensory nucleus of trigeminal nerve
  2. *General Visceral:* Nucleus of tractus solitaries
  3. *Special Somatic:* 4 vestibular nuclei, 2 cochlear nuclei
- **Motor/Efferent**
  1. *General Somatic:* Nuclei of 3rd, 4th, 6th and 12th nerves
  2. *General visceral:* Edinger-Westphal nucleus of 3rd nerve, Superior salivatory nucleus of 7th nerve, Inferior salivatory nucleus of 9th nerve and Dorsal nucleus of Vagus nerve.
  3. *Special Visceral:* Nuclei of 5th, 7th, 9th and 11th nerves.

ACCESSORY NERVE (XI)

The accessory nerve is conventionally described as having a cranial and a spinal root. The cranial root is formed by a series of rootlets that emerge from the medulla between the olive and the inferior cerebellar peduncle. These rootlets are considered to join the spinal root, travel with it briefly, then separate within the jugular foramen and are distributed with the vagus nerve to supply the musculature of the palate, pharynx and larynx.

- The accessory nerve has *no* cranial component and consists only of the spinal root of the accessory nerve. This spinal root is formed by the union of fibers from an elongated nucleus in the anterior horn of the upper five cervical segments, which leave the cord mid-way between the anterior and posterior roots, join, and then pass upwards through the foramen magnum. The accessory nerve and the converging rootlets of the vagus nerve then enter the jugular foramen in a shared sheath of dura. The glossopharyngeal nerve enters the jugular foramen anterior to the vagus through a separate dural sheath.
- The nerve passes backwards over the internal jugular vein to the sternocleidomastoid muscle which it pierces (and supplies) and then crosses the posterior triangle of the neck to enter and supply the deep surface of the trapezius.

HYPOGLOSSAL NERVE (XII)

The hypoglossal nerve is entirely motor and supplies all the intrinsic and extrinsic muscles of the tongue (with the exception of the palatoglossus). From its nucleus, which lies in the floor of the 4th ventricle, many rootlets leave the side of the medulla in the groove between the pyramid and the olive. These rootlets unite to leave the skull by way of the anterior condylar, or hypoglossal, canal.

Lying at first deep to the internal carotid artery and the jugular vein, the nerve passes downwards between these two vessels to just above the level of the angle of the mandible. Here it passes forwards over the internal and external carotid arteries, and gives off its descending and thyrohyoid branches. It then crosses the hyoglossus and genioglossus muscles to enter the tongue.

Its descending branch (*descendens hypoglossi*) actually derives from a twig of the 1st cervical nerve and therefore transmits C1 fibers. It passes more or less vertically downwards upon the internal carotid artery to join the descending cervical nerve (C2 and C3) to form a loop known as the *ansacervicalis* (or *ansa hypoglossi*) just above the omohyoid muscle. From this loop branches are given to three infrahyoid muscles—sternothyroid, sternohyoid and omohyoid.

COMMON FEATURES OF CRANIAL NERVES (REPEATEDLY ASKED QUESTIONS)

- *Oculomotor nerve:* Commonly involved in intracranial aneurysm.
- *Trochlear nerve:* Emerges dorsally from the brainstem, has the longest intracranial course.
- *Trigeminal nerve:* Largest cranial nerve.
- *Vagus nerve:* Has the most extensive distribution.
- *Facial nerve:* Most commonly paralyzed nerve, has the longest intraosseous course.
- *Abducent nerve:* Most commonly involved in raised ICT, nerve with the longest course.

COMMON SITES OF CRANIAL NERVE ENTRAPMENT

- *Cranial nerves 3,4,5,6:* Sphenoid fissure, lateral wall of cavernous sinus and the retrosphenoid space
- *Cranial nerves 5,6:* Apex of the petrous bone
- *Cranial nerves 7, 8:* Internal auditory meatus and the pontocerebellar angle.
- *Cranial nerves 9, 10, 11:* Jugular foramen, posterior laterocondylar space and the posterior retroparotid space.

CINGULATE CORTEX

- Part of limbic cortex (medial part of cerebral hemisphere)—considered part of limbic lobe
- Receives input from the thalamus and neocortex and projects to the entorhinal cortex via the cingulum
- It is involved in emotion formation and processing, learning and memory; plays an important role in executive function and respiratory control.

Superior Temporal Gyrus

One of 3 gyri in the temporal lobe

Boundaries
- Lateral sulcus above
- Superior temporal sulcus below
- Imaginary line drawn from the preoccipital notch to the lateral sulcus poteriorly

Structures
- Broadmann areas 41 and 42 – auditory cortex
- Wernicke's area, Broadmann 22p – processing speech.

Inferior Frontal Gyrus
Boundaries
- Superior border – inferior frontal sulcus
- Inferior border – lateral fissure
- Posterior border – inferior precentral sulcus

Structures:
- Broca's area, which comprises of Broadmann area 44 and 45, is located in the opercular and triangular sections of the inferior frontal gyrus
- Broca's area is connected to the Wernicke's area by arcuate fasciculus and both are found unilaterally in the left hemisphere.

CRANIAL STRUCTURES AND PAIN SENSITIVITY

Pain Sensitive Structures
- Scalp
- Aponeurotica
- Dura mater/dural sinuses
- Middle meningeal artery, superficial temporal artery
- Falx cerebri
- Proximal segment of large pial arteries

Pain Insensitive Structures
- Most of brain parenchyma
- Pial arteries over convexities and veins
- Cerebral ventricular ependyma
- Choroid plexus

Pain Producing Viscera
- Heart, parietal pleura of lung, intestine, liver capsule, gallbladder, ureter, urinary bladder

Pain Insensitive Viscera
- Liver parenchyma and alveoli of lung
  - Cerebellum
- Cerebellum has 3 parts:
  - Archicerebellum (vestibulocerebellum)–it includes the flocculonodular lobe located in t medial zone. It is closely interconnected with the vestibular nuclei; helps to maintain equilibrium and coordinate eye, head and neck movements
  - Paleocerebellum: midline vermis; helps to coordinate trunk and leg movements; lesions result in abnormalities in stance and gait
  - Neocerebellum (lateral hemispheres) – control quick and finely coordinated limb movements, predominantly of the arms

Anatomy Involved in Cerebellar Dysfunction
Cerebellar lesion in the
- **Posterior (flocculonodular lobe archicerebellum)** – eye movement disorders, nystagmus, vestibule ocular reflex
- **Midline (vermis, paleocerebellum)** – truncal and gait ataxia
- **Hemisphere (neocerebellum)** – limb ataxia: dysmetria, dysdiadochokinesis, intention tremor, dysarthria, hypotonia

BASAL GANGLIA COTD
- Striatum—caudate nucleus and putamen
- Lenticular nucleus—globus pallidus and putamen

- Neurotransmitters and related dysfunctional disorders
    - Substantia nigra (dopamine) – Parkinson's disease
    - Caudate nuclueus (GABA) – Huntington chorea
    - Putamen (GABA)
    - Globus pallidus (GABA) – athetosis
    - Subthalamic nucleus (glutamate) – hemiballismus

Ventricular System COTD CSF

- CSF Pressure: 150 mm H_2O/ 5–15 mm Hg
- It is regulated by rate of CSF absorption by arachnoid
- Below a pressure of 68 mm H_2O, CSF absorption stops
- 500–550 mL/day is the rate of production.

Composition

- The osmolarity and Na^+ concentration is same that of plasma chloride, H^+, concentration is higher and K^+, Glucose concentration is lower
- *Specific Gravity:* 1.007
- *Cellular:* No neutrophils, < 5 cells/mm mostly lymphocytes

Neurotransmitters

Excitatory: Glutamate (chief in CNS and spinal cord), aspartate cortical pyramidal cells).
Inhibitory: Glycine (spinal cord), GABA (CNS)

Small Molecules

- A.ch
- *AMINES: NE,* E, Dopamine, Serotonin
- *Amino acid:* glutamate, glycine, aspartate, GABA

Large Molecules

- Neuropeptides: Substance P, Enkephalins, Endorphins

Substance P

- Pain transmission (dorsal horn of spinal cord)
- Skinaxon reflex
- Intestine—peristalsis

BRAIN LOBES AND DYSFUNCTION

Parietal Lobe Dysfunction

- Paroxysmal localized paresthesia affecting contralateral side of the body also known as sensory seizures.
- Sensory deficits to the contralateral side of the body can occur leading to astereognosis, agraphesthesia, loss of proprioception, vibration and fine touch
- Mild hemiparesis may also occur; primary sensory modalities may return but the discriminative sense may not return
- Dominant lobe dysfunction: aphasia, alexia, Gerstmann syndrome, apraxia
- Nondominant lobe dysfunction: hemispatial neglect, sensory and visual inattention, constructional and dressing apraxia
- Bilateral lobe dysfunction: visuospatial disorientation, Balint syndrome

Fusiform Gyrus

- Part of temporal lobe and occipital lobe in Broadmann area 37; also known as occipitotemporal gyrus
- Located between the inferior temporal gyrus and parahippocampal gyrus
- Mid fusiform sulcus separates the lateral and medial portions.

- **Functions:**
  - Processing of color information
  - Face and body recognition
  - Word recognition
  - Within category identification
- Lesions result in: prosopagnosia, William's syndrome
- Increased neurophysiological activity in the fusiform face area may produce hallucinations of faces as seen in Charles Bonnet syndrome, hypnagogic hallucinations, peduncular hallucinations or drug induced hallucinations.

INTERNAL CAPSULE

- It has the following divisions: anterior limb, genu and posterior limb
- *Anterior limb* contains axons that send information between the thalamus and the cingulate gyrus and prefrontal cortex
- It also contains axons in the frontopontine pathway; it is supplied by lenticulostriate branches of the middle cerebral artery and recurrent artery of heubner
- *Genu* contains the corticobulbar tract, which originate in the motor areas of the frontal lobes and extend to the cranial nerve nuclei in the brainstem. It also contains axons that connect the motor section of the thalamus with the motor areas of the frontal cortex; it is supplied by lenticulostriate branches of the middle cerebral artery and recurrent artery of Heubner
- *Posterior limb* contains the corticospinal tract which are axons that come from the motor area of the frontal cortex and extend to the anterior horns of the spinal cord where alpha motor neurons are located. It also contains sensory information coming from the body via the medial lemniscus and the anterolateral systems; it is supplied by lenticulostriate branches of the middle cerebral artery and anterior choroidal artery (branch of the internal carotid).

FRONTAL LOBE PATHOLOGY

Foster-Kennedy Syndrome

It is caused by tumor of frontal lobe and gives rise to ipsilateral optic atrophy and contralateral papilledema; frontal disinhibition syndrome, Rett syndrome and ADHD. It is produced from frontal lobe damage often due to tumors. They are socially disinhibited and show severe impairment of judgment, insight; antisocial behavior is a characteristic feature of frontal disinhibition syndrome.

Abulia—frontal Lobe Pathology

- Loss of initiative, creativity and curiosity
- Pervasive emotional apathy and blandness
- Akinetic mutism.

REFERENCE

1. NOCH: a framework for biologically plausible models of neural motor control.

Multiple Choice Questions

1. **Which is NOT true about Internal capsule ?**
   a. Continues above as corona radiata
   b. Continues below as tectum
   c. Corticobulbar and corticonuclear fibres occupy genu and anterior part of posterior limb
   d. Corticospinal tract is carried by posterior limb of internal capsule

2. **Lateral geniculate body is a part of:**
   a. Pons
   b. Midbrain
   c. Thalamus
   d. Hypothalamus

3. **The Broca's area is situated in the:**
   a. Temporal lobe
   b. Posterior part of inferior frontal gyrus
   c. Occipital calcarine fissure
   d. Mammillary body region

Answers

1. c   2. c   3. b

Neuropathophysiology

NEURONS

- The major function of neurons is to receive, integrate, and transmit information to other cells. Neurons consist of three parts: dendrites, which are elongated processes that receive information from the environment or from other neurons; the cell body, which contains the nucleus; and the axon, which may be up to 1 m long and conducts impulses to muscles, glands, or other neurons.
- Most neurons are multipolar, containing one axon and several dendrites. Bipolar neurons have one dendrite and one axon and are found in the cochlear and vestibular ganglia, retina, and olfactory mucosa.
- Spinal sensory ganglia contain pseudounipolar neurons that have a single process that emanates from the cell body and divides into two branches, one extending to the spinal cord and the other extending to the periphery.
- Axons and dendrites usually branch extensively at their ends. Dendritic branching can be very complex, with the result that a single neuron may receive thousands of inputs. Axon branching allows several target cells to simultaneously receive a message from one neuron. Each branch of the axon terminates on the next cell at a synapse, which is a structure specialized for information transfer from the axon to muscle, to glands, or to another neuron.

Synapses between neurons most often occur between axons and dendrites but may occur between an axon and a cell body, between two axons, or between two dendrites.

TRANSMISSION IN NEURONS

- Signals are propagated electrically along axons. Like other cells, neurons maintain cell size and osmolarity primarily through the action of Na^+–K^+ ATPase, which actively pumps Na^+ out of cells in exchange for K^+. This results in the formation of concentration gradients for Na^+ and K^+ across the cell membrane. The membrane is practically impermeable to Na^+, but the presence of K^+ leak channels permits the flow of K^+ out of cells. This produces a difference in electrical charge across the membrane that counters transport of K^+ from the cell. The flow of ions continues until the opposing electrical force reaches a value that balances the diffusional force and the membrane reaches the equilibrium potential for K^+ which is calculated by the Nernst equation.
- The membrane potential may be altered by increasing the permeability of the membrane to another ion, which drives the resting membrane potential toward the equilibrium potential for that ion. Neurons are highly specialized to use rapid changes in membrane potential to generate electrical signals. This is accomplished by ligand-gated and voltage-gated ion channels that allow the passage of Na^+, K^+, Ca^{2+}, or Cl^- ions in response to electrical or chemical stimuli. These channels are composed of protein complexes embedded in the lipid membrane to form aqueous pores to the inside of the cell. In general, channels are selective for a particular species of ion. An array of charged amino acids within voltage-dependent channels detects changes in voltage and induces a conformational change in the channel to alter ion permeability. Binding sites for neurotransmitters such as glutamate, Gamma-aminobutyric acid (GABA), glycine, and acetylcholine exist on ligand-gated channels and, when occupied, induce a conformational change to open the channel.
- Electrical signals are propagated in neurons because a voltage change across the membrane in one part of a neuron is propagated to other parts. Passive spread of a voltage disturbance weakens with increasing distance from the source unless energy-dependent processes amplify the signal. Passive spread of electrical signals works well over short distances and is a major mechanism of signal propagation in dendrites. However, long-distance communication down axons to nerve terminals requires amplification which is accomplished through the generation of self-propagating waves of excitation known as action potentials.

- An action potential arises primarily from voltage-dependent changes in membrane permeability to Na⁺ and K⁺. If a depolarizing stimulus raises the membrane potential, allowing influx of Na⁺, areas of membrane are depolarized to the threshold for Na⁺ channel activation, propagating a wave of depolarization from the initial site.
- The resting potential is restored quickly by a combination of events. First, Na⁺ channels close rapidly and remain in an inactive state until the membrane potential returns to negative levels for several milliseconds. Voltage-dependent K⁺ channels open as the membrane potential peaks, speeding the efflux of K⁺ from cells and driving the membrane potential back to E_K. K⁺ channels are also inactivated, but more slowly than Na⁺ channels, and this may transiently hyperpolarize cells. Plasma membrane ion exchangers and ion pumps then counteract the ion fluxes and eventually restore the resting state.
- Neurons transmit signals chemically to other cells at synapses. Presynaptic and postsynaptic cells are electrically isolated from each other and separated by a narrow synaptic cleft. Signaling across the cleft occurs through the release of neurotransmitters from the terminal of the presynaptic neuron. Most neurotransmitters are stored in membrane-bound synaptic vesicles and are released into the synaptic cleft by Ca^{2+}-dependent exocytosis. Depolarization of the nerve terminal opens voltage-gated Ca^{2+} channels, stimulating Ca^{2+} influx and neurotransmitter release.
- In general, excitatory neurotransmitters such as glutamate open cation channels that allow influx of Na⁺ or Ca^{2+} and generate a depolarizing excitatory postsynaptic potential. Inhibitory neurotransmitters such as GABA and glycine open Cl⁻ channels and generate an inhibitory postsynaptic potential. Termination of the signal is achieved by removal of the neurotransmitter from the synaptic cleft. Acetylcholine is hydrolyzed by acetylcholinesterase at the postsynaptic membrane. Other neurotransmitters such as glutamate are removed by specific membrane transporters on nerve terminals or glial cells.
- Temporal summation occurs if repeated afferent stimuli cause new EPSPs before previous EPSPs have decayed. A longer time constant for the EPSP allows for a greater opportunity for summation. When activity is present in more than one synaptic knob at the same time, spatial summation occurs and activity in one synaptic knob summates with activity in another to approach the firing level.

EXCITATORY NEUROTRANSMITTERS

- Glutamate is a major excitatory neurotransmitter in the central nervous system (CNS). Its activation depolarizes neurons, increasing the number of action potentials generated.
  - There are three major ionotropic glutamate receptors – AMPA, Kainate and NMDA. The AMPA and kainate receptors are attached to ion channels that allow Na and K to pass through them; a small number of AMPA receptors are also permeable to Ca. The NMDA channels activated when neurons are already depolarized are permeable to Na, K, and Ca. Activation of NMDA channels has been associated with long-term changes in neuronal activity that may be cellular correlates of learning and memory.
  - Metabotropic receptors are also activated by glutamate. These receptors act via GTP – second messenger pathway [cAMP /IP3] which in turn can alter ionic conductance, cell Ca levels, and a host of other biochemical changes.

INHIBITORY NEUROTRANSMITTERS

- Gamma-aminobutyric acid (GABA) and glycine are major inhibitory neurotransmitters in the CNS. Their activation hyperpolarizes neurons, decreasing the number of action potentials generated. Inhibition is important for the brain and spinal cord to function.
  - GABA is a major inhibitory transmitter in the brain and spinal cord. The $GABA_A$ receptor contains a chloride channel that is opened when GABA binds. This activity is augmented by benzodiazepines, volatile anesthetics, and barbiturates. The $GABA_B$ receptor acts via a second messenger to open K channels.
  - Glycine is a major inhibitory transmitter in the spinal cord. Strychnine blocks the action of glycine.

ASTROCYTES

- Astrocytes serve a variety of metabolic, immunologic, structural, and nutritional support functions required for normal function of neurons. They possess numerous processes that radiate from the cell body, surrounding blood vessels and covering the surfaces of the brain and spinal cord. Foot processes form part of the blood-brain barrier. Astrocytes express voltage- and ligand-gated ion channels and regulates K⁺ and Ca^{2+} concentrations within the interstitial space. Many synapses are invested with astrocytic processes, and this allows astrocytes to modulate neurotransmission by regulating extracellular concentrations of these cations.
- Astrocytes provide structural and trophic support for neurons through the production of extracellular matrix molecules such as laminin and through release of growth factors such as nerve growth factor, fibroblast growth factors, and brain-derived neurotrophic factor. End-feet of astrocytic processes at blood vessels provide sites for release of cytokines and chemoattractants during CNS injury.

- Astrocytes respond to brain injury by increasing in size and in some cases in number through a process called reactive astrocytosis. This phenotypic change is characterized by an increase in cells expressing glial-fibrillary acidic protein and by synthesis and release of cytokines that regulate inflammatory responses and entry of hematogenous cells into the CNS.
- Astrocytes play an important role also in terminating neuronal responses to glutamate, the most abundant excitatory neurotransmitter in the brain. In cell cultures, neurons die in the presence of high levels of glutamate unless astrocytes are present. Glutamate transporters present on astrocyte cell membranes remove glutamate from the synapse. Astrocytes also contain glutamine synthase, which converts glutamate to glutamine, detoxifying the CNS of both glutamate and ammonia.

OLIGODENDROCYTES AND SCHWANN CELLS

- Plasma membranes of oligodendrocytes in the CNS and Schwann cells in the peripheral nervous system envelop axons. For many axons, the membranes of these glial cells are wrapped layer on layer around the axon, forming a myelin sheath.
- Gaps form between myelin sheaths from neighboring glia and produce nodes of Ranvier where a small portion of the axon is exposed to the interstitial space and where voltage-dependent Na^+ channels are clustered in the axonal membrane. Between the nodes, myelin insulates the axon from the extracellular space, allowing efficient spread of depolarization from one node to another. This allows action potentials to propagate rapidly by jumping from node to node in a process called saltatory conduction.

MICROGLIA

- Microglia which reside in the CNS, function as the main immune effector cells.
- They appear to be derived from bone marrow precursors of macrophage-monocyte lineage and invade the CNS during the perinatal period. Microglia cells are activated by brain injury, infection, or neuronal degeneration. Activation is characterized by proliferation, migration into damaged tissue, increased or de novo expression of surface receptors, including CD45 (leukocyte common antigen), MHC class I and class II and immunoglobulin Fc receptors, and secretion of several cytokines, reactive oxygen intermediates, and proteinases. This response functions to remove dead tissue and destroy invading organisms but may contribute to CNS damage, particularly in certain CNS inflammatory and degenerative diseases.

LOWER MOTOR NEURONS AND SKELETAL MUSCLES

- Each alpha motor neuron axon contacts up to about 200 muscle fibers, and together they constitute the motor unit. Axons of the motor neurons intermingle to form spinal ventral roots, plexuses, and peripheral nerves. Muscles are innervated from specific segments of the spinal cord, and each muscle is supplied by at least two roots. Motor fibers are rearranged in the plexuses so that most muscles are supplied by one peripheral nerve. Thus, the distribution of muscle weakness differs in spinal root and peripheral nerve lesions.
- The lower motor neurons are the final common pathway for all voluntary movement. Therefore, damage to lower motor neurons or their axons causes flaccid weakness of innervated muscles. In addition, muscle tone or resistance to passive movement is reduced, and deep tendon reflexes are impaired or lost.
- Each point of contact between nerve terminal and skeletal muscle forms a specialized synapse known as a neuromuscular junction composed of the presynaptic motor nerve terminal and a postsynaptic motor end plate. Presynaptic terminals store synaptic vesicles that contain the neurotransmitter acetylcholine. The amount of neurotransmitter within a vesicle constitutes a quantum of neurotransmitter. Action potentials depolarize the motor nerve terminal, opening voltage-gated calcium channels and stimulating calcium-dependent release of neurotransmitter from the terminal. Released acetylcholine traverses the synaptic cleft to the postsynaptic (end plate) membrane, where it binds to nicotinic cholinergic receptors. These receptors are ligand-gated cation channels, and, on binding to acetylcholine, they allow entry of extracellular sodium into the motor end plate. This depolarizes the motor end plate, which in turn depolarizes the muscle fiber. After activation, cholinergic receptors are rapidly inactivated, reducing sodium entry. They remain inactive until acetylcholine dissociates from the receptor. This is facilitated by the enzyme acetylcholinesterase, which hydrolyzes acetylcholine and is present in the postsynaptic zone.

UPPER MOTOR NEURONS

- The motor cortex is the region from which movements can be elicited by electrical stimuli. This includes the primary motor area (Brodmann area 4), premotor cortex (area 6), supplementary motor cortex (medial portions of 6), and primary sensory cortex (areas 3, 1, and 2). In the motor cortex, groups of neurons are organized in vertical columns, and discrete groups control contraction of individual muscles.
- Planned movements and those guided by sensory, visual, or auditory stimuli are preceded by discharges from prefrontal, somatosensory, visual, or auditory cortices, which are then followed by motor cortex pyramidal cell discharges that occur several milliseconds before the onset of movement.

- Cortical motor neurons contribute axons that converge in the corona radiata and descend in the posterior limb of the internal capsule, cerebral peduncles, ventral pons, and medulla. These fibers constitute the corticospinal and corticobulbar tracts and together are known as upper motor neuron fibers. As they descend through the diencephalon and brainstem, fibers separate to innervate extrapyramidal and cranial nerve motor nuclei. The lower brainstem motor neurons receive input from crossed and uncrossed corticobulbar fibers, although neurons that innervate lower facial muscles receive primarily crossed fibers.
- In the ventral medulla, the remaining corticospinal fibers course in a tract that on cross section is pyramidal in shape thus the name pyramidal tract. At the lower end of the medulla, most fibers decussate, although the proportion of crossed and uncrossed fibers varies somewhat between individuals. The bulk of these fibers descend as the lateral corticospinal tract of the spinal cord.
- Upper motor neurons are the final common pathway between cortical and subcortical structures, such as the basal ganglia, in the planning, initiation, sequencing, and modulation of all voluntary movement. Upper motor neuron lesions cause a characteristic pattern of limb weakness and change in tone. Antigravity muscles of the limbs become more active relative to other muscles. The arms tend to assume a flexed, pronated posture, and the legs become extended. In contrast, muscles that move the limbs out of this posture (extensors of the arms and flexors of the legs) are preferentially weakened. Tone is increased in antigravity muscles (flexors of the arms and extensors of the legs), and if these muscles are stretched rapidly, they respond with an abrupt catch, followed by a rapid increase and then a decline in resistance as passive movement continues. This sequence constitutes the clasp knife phenomenon. Clonus, a series of involuntary muscle contractions in response to passive stretch may be present.

The distribution of paralysis resulting from upper motor neuron lesions varies with the location of the lesion. Lesions above the pons impair movements of the contralateral lower face, arm, and leg. Lesions below the pons spare the face. Lesions of the internal capsule often impair movements of the contralateral face, arm, and leg equally, because motor fibers are packed closely together in this region. In contrast, lesions of the cortex or subcortical white matter tend to differentially affect the limbs and face, because the motor fibers are spread over a larger area of brain. Bilateral cerebral lesions cause weakness and spasticity of cranial and trunk muscles in addition to limb muscles and lead to dysarthria, dysphonia, dysphagia, bifacial paresis, and sometimes reflexive crying and laughing (pseudobulbar paralysis).

Tracts and Homunculus

Ascending tracts

Dorsal column:

a   Fasciculus Gracilis (Tract of Goll): Lower half of the body

b   Fasciculus Cuneatus (Tract of Burdach): Upper half of the body

- *Sensations:* Proprioception, fine touch, tactile localization, 2 point discrimination, stereognosis, position of joints and kinesthetic
- Anterior spinothalamic tract—crude touch
- Lateral spinothalamic tract—pain and temperature.
- Dorsal column CROSS to the opposite side in the thalamus whereas the anterolateral column CROSS to the opposite side in the spinal cord
- Therefore in lesion of spinal cord ipsilateral dorsal column and contralateral spinothalamic tract is involved.
- Second order neuron of dorsal column—thalamus.
- Second order neuron of spinothalamic tract—spinal cord
- First relay station of pain and temperature is—spinal cord
- First relay station of touch, proprioception and vibration—thalamus

Descending system is classified as medial and lateral descending system.

Medial: Lateral corticospinal tract, rubrospinal tract; they are involved in skilled voluntary movements of distal muscles

Medial pathways: Anterior white column of spinal cord; postural control (muscles of the trunk and proximal muscles of limb)

Ventral (anterior) corticospinal tract, vestibulospinal, reticulospinal, tectospinal tracts;

Lateral pathways: Lateral white column of spinal cord; fine skilled movements (distal muscles of limbs).

Lateral corticospinal tract and rubrospinal tract.

Body representation is vertical—upside down with face at the foot and legs and feet at the top.

Sensory homunculus: Lips, face tongue large representation.
- In the sensory cortex the part of the body represented is proportionate to the number of sensory receptors (innervations density)
- Fibres carrying tactile and proprioceptive information ascend through the thalamic radiation to the area 3 of primary somatic sensory cortex. If the somatosensory area is removed, tactile and proprioceptive sensations are lost, but pain and temperature persists, since they are appreciated primarily by the thalamus.

- The sensations that are most affected by cortical lesions are: proprioception and tactile sensation (fine touch, two point discrimination, and astereognosis).

Motor Cortex

a. Primary motor area (4)
b. Premotor area (6, 44, 45, 8)
c. Supplementary motor area
   - Body representation is vertical, each PMA controls contralateral side of the body
   - Face is presented B/L, rest all U/L
   - Cortical presentation is proportional to skilled movements

MOTOR HOMUNCULUS

Maximum representation: Muscles for vocalization and mastication.

Motor System

- Area of leg presentation is on the medial surface of cerebral hemisphere in the central sulcus (paracentral lobule)
- Regulation of voluntary movement:

Cortical association area: Ideas (commands) for voluntary movement originate.
Basal ganglia, lateral portion of cerebellum and cerebral cortex:

Planning and Programming

- **Supplementary motor area:** Programming the motor sequences (not visually/sensory guided)
- **Premotor cortex:** Setting a posture (sensory inputs)
- **Somatosensory area:** Aiming hands toward an object (5), hand-eye coordination (7)
- **Spinocerebellum:** Smoothens and coordinates the movement
- **Corticospinal and corticobulbar tracts:** Final pathway for skillful movements
- **Extrapyramidal tract:** Back ground posture

Cerebral Dominance and Handedness

91% of population is right handed, 95% dominant hemisphere is left
In left handed also, 60–70% of population hemisphere is left, only 15% right hemisphere is dominant.
15% no lateralization

Right/nondominant/Representational

- Left-handed control
- Spatial relationship between person and surrounding (visuospatial relation).
- Insight/imagination
- Music/art
- Recognition of faces
- Identification of object by forms and shapes.

Lesions of Right Lobe

- Agnosia
- Agraphia
- Asterognosis
- Anosognosia
- Visuo-spatial defects

Left/Dominant/Categorial

- Right-handed control
- Language function
- Mathematical and scientific skill
- Reasoning

Lesions

- Dyslexia
- Dyscalculia
- Fluent aphasia
- Loss of ability to think logically

Cerebellum

The cerebellum is responsible for the coordination of muscle groups, control of stance and gait, and regulation of muscle tone. Rather than causing paralysis, damage to the cerebellum interferes with the performance of motor tasks.

Basal Ganglia

Basal ganglia circuits regulate the initiation, amplitude, and speed of movements. Diseases of the basal ganglia cause abnormalities of movement and are collectively known as movement disorders.

Several neurotransmitters are found within the basal ganglia. Acetylcholine is present in high concentrations within the corpus striatum, where it is synthesized and released by large Golgi type 2 neurons. Acetylcholine acts as an excitatory transmitter at medium-sized spiny striatal neurons that synthesize and release the inhibitory neurotransmitter GABA and project to the globus pallidus. Dopamine is synthesized by neurons of the substantia nigra, whose axons form the nigrostriatal pathway that terminates in the corpus striatum. Dopamine released by these fibers inhibits striatal GABAergic neurons.

Somatosensory pathways confer information about touch, pressure, temperature, pain, vibration, and the position and movement of body parts. This information is relayed to thalamic nuclei and integrated in the sensory cortex of the parietal lobes to provide conscious awareness of sensation. Information is also relayed to cortical motor neurons to adjust fine movements and maintain posture. Some ascending sensory fibers, particularly pain fibers, enter the midbrain and project to the amygdala and limbic cortex, where they contribute to emotional responses to pain. In the spinal cord, painful stimuli activate local pathways that induce the firing of lower motor neurons and cause a reflex withdrawal. Thus, somatosensory pathways provide tactile information, guide movement, and serve protective functions.

Sensory receptors can be specialized dendritic endings of afferent nerve fibers, and they are often associated with non-neural cells that surround it, forming a sense organ. Touch and pressure are sensed by four types of mechanoreceptors.

- *Meissner corpuscles* are dendrites encapsulated in connective tissue and respond to changes in texture and slow vibrations.
- *Merkel cells* are expanded dendritic endings, and they respond to sustained pressure and touch.
- *Ruffini corpuscles* are enlarged dendritic endings with elongated capsules, and they respond to sustained pressure.
- *Pacinian corpuscles* consist of unmyelinated dendritic endings of a sensory nerve fiber, encapsulated by concentric lamellae of connective tissue. These receptors respond to deep pressure and fast vibration.

LAWS OF SENSORY SYSTEM

- *Weber–Fechner law:* The intensity of sensation is determined by the amplitude of the stimulus applied to the receptor. The magnitude of the sensation felt is proportional to the log of the intensity of the stimulus.
- *Law of specific nerve energies:* When the nerve pathways from a particular sense organ are stimulated, the sensation evoked is that for which the receptor is specialized no matter how or where along the pathway the activity is initiated.
- *Law of projection:* No matter where a particular sensory pathway is stimulated along its course to the cortex, the conscious sensation produced is referred to the location of the receptor.
- *Bell–Magendie law:* In the spinal cord the dorsal roots are sensory and the ventral roots are motor.

SENSORY MODALITIES

Pain

- Free nerve endings of unmyelinated C fibers and small-diameter myelinated fibers in the skin convey sensory information in response to chemical, thermal, and mechanical stimuli. Intense stimulation of these nerve endings evokes the sensation of pain. In contrast to skin, most deep tissues are relatively insensitive to chemical or noxious stimuli. Information from primary afferent fibers is relayed via sensory ganglia to the dorsal horn of the spinal cord and then to the contralateral spinothalamic tract, which connects to thalamic neurons that project to the somatosensory cortex.

- Neuropeptides released by injured nerves may recruit an inflammatory reaction that stimulates pain. In the dorsal horn, denervated spinal neurons may become spontaneously active. In the brain and spinal cord, synaptic reorganization occurs in response to injury and may lower the threshold for pain. In addition, inhibition of pathways that modulate transmission of sensory information in the spinal cord and brainstem may promote neuropathic pain.
- Pain-modulating circuits exert a major influence on the perceived intensity of pain. One such pathway is composed of cells in the periaqueductal gray matter of the midbrain that receive afferents from frontal cortex and hypothalamus and project to rostroventral medullary neurons. These in turn project in the dorsolateral white matter of the spinal cord and terminate on dorsal horn neurons. Additional descending pathways arise from other brainstem nuclei (locus ceruleus, dorsal raphe nucleus, and nucleus reticularis gigantocellularis).

Mechanisms of Pain and Nociception

- *Nociception* is the mechanism whereby noxious peripheral stimuli are transmitted to the central nervous system. *Pain* is a subjective experience not always associated with nociception. Allodynia is a sensation of pain in response to innocuous stimuli. It is due to sensitivity of nociceptive afferent fibres due to chemicals released during injury.
- Polymodal nociceptors (PMNs) are the main type of peripheral sensory neuron that responds to noxious stimuli. The majority are non-myelinated C fibres whose endings respond to thermal, mechanical and chemical stimuli.
- Chemical stimuli acting on PMNs to cause pain include bradykinin, protons, ATP and vanilloids (e.g. capsaicin). PMNs are sensitised by prostaglandins, which explains the analgesic effect of aspirin-like drugs, particularly in the presence of inflammation.
- The vanilloid receptor TRPV1 (transient receptor potential vanilloid receptor 1) responds to noxious heat as well as capsaicin-like agonists. The lipid mediator anandamide is an agonist at vanilloid receptors, as well as being an endogenous cannabinoid receptor agonist; other TRP channels: TRPM8 (M – menthol) cooling effect given by mint; activated by moderate cold; TRPV4 (V – vanilloid) activated by warm temperature 34°C; TRPV 3 – activated by slightly higher temperature (35–39°C); V – activated also by intense heat, acids, chemicals such as capsaicin (hot pepper)
- Nociceptive fibres terminate in the superficial layers of the dorsal horn, forming synaptic connections with transmission neurons running to the thalamus.
- PMN neurons release glutamate (fast transmitter) and various peptides (especially substance P) that act as slow transmitters. Peptides are also released peripherally and contribute to neurogenic inflammation.
- Neuropathic pain, associated with damage to neurons of the nociceptive pathway rather than an excessive peripheral stimulus, is frequently a component of chronic pain states and may respond poorly to opioid analgesics.
- *Causalgia:* Spontaneous burning pain sensation in injured area, due to release of NA from sympathetic nerve fibres, (alpha blockers relieve pain).
- *Hyperalgesia:* Exaggerated response to painful stimuli, is of two types:
  1. *Primary:* Directly due to noxious stimuli (hypersensitization of nociceptors)
  2. *Secondary:* Noxious stimuli also activating the silent receptors, (increase sensitization of spinothalamic tract due to continuous discharge of type C fibre (sensory facilitation).
- *Analgesic system:*
  - Endogenous analgesic system
  - Dorsal horn gating
  - Dorsal horn gating/segmental suppression: Rubbing/massage/application of cold, counter irritants/acupuncture/TENS activation of AB presynaptic inhibition of pain carrying fibres, (blocking Ca^{++} channels) of AB
- *Endogenous analgesic system:*
  - Raphe magnus nucleus (RMN)
  - Periaquaductal gray matter (PAG)
- *RMN:* They contain neurons serotonin and substance P serotoninergic neurons exert post synaptic inhibition on nociceptive afferents in the dorsal horn.
- *PAG:* It inhibits pain by stimulating the RMN, they have OPIOID receptors.
- *Opioid receptors:*
  1. Present in the spinal cord (substantia gelatinosa)
  2. PAG MORPHINE can act on both the (spinal and supraspinal receptors.

PROPRIOCEPTION AND VIBRATORY SENSE

Receptors in the muscles, tendons, and joints provide information about deep pressure and the position and movement of body parts. This allows one to determine an object's size, weight, shape, and texture. Information is relayed to the spinal cord via large myelinated fibers and to the thalamus by the dorsal column-lemniscal system. Detecting vibration requires sensing touch and rapid changes in deep pressure. This depends on multiple cutaneous and deep sensory fibers and is impaired by lesions of multiple peripheral nerves, the dorsal columns, medial lemniscus, or thalamus but rarely by lesions of single nerves. Vibratory sense is often impaired together with proprioception.

DISCRIMINATIVE SENSATION

- Primary sensory cortex provides awareness of somatosensory information and the ability to make sensory discriminations. Touch, pain, temperature, and vibration sense are considered the primary modalities of sensation and are relatively preserved in patients with damage to sensory cortex or its projections from the thalamus.
- In contrast, complex tasks that require integration of multiple somatosensory stimuli and of somatosensory stimuli with auditory or visual information are impaired. These include the ability to distinguish two points from one when touched on the skin (two-point discrimination), localize tactile stimuli, perceive the position of body parts in space, recognize letters or numbers drawn on the skin (graphesthesia), and identify objects by their shape, size, and texture (stereognosis).

HEARING AND BALANCE

- **There are three types of hearing loss:**
  1. Conductive deafness, which is due to diseases of the external or middle ear that impair conduction and amplification of sound from the air to the cochlea;
  2. Sensorineural deafness, resulting from diseases of the cochlea or eighth cranial nerve; and
  3. Central deafness, resulting from diseases affecting the cochlear nuclei or auditory pathways in the CNS. Because of the redundancy of central pathways, almost all cases of hearing loss are due to conductive or sensorineural deafness.
- Conductive and sensorineural deafness may be distinguished by examining hearing with a vibrating 512Hz tuning fork. In the Rinne test, the tuning fork is held on the mastoid process behind the ear and then is placed at the auditory meatus. If the sound is louder at the meatus, the test is positive. Normally the test is positive, because sound transmitted through air is amplified by middle-ear structures. In sensorineural deafness, although sound perception is reduced, the Rinne test is still positive because middle-ear structures are intact. In conductive deafness, sounds are heard less well through air and the test is negative. In the Weber test, the tuning fork is applied to the forehead at the midline. In conductive deafness, the sound is heard best in the abnormal ear, whereas with sensorineural deafness the sound is heard best in the normal ear. Audiometry can distinguish types of hearing loss. In general, sensorineural deafness causes greater loss of high-pitched sounds, whereas conductive deafness causes more loss of low-pitched sounds.

In contrast to hearing, vestibular function is commonly disturbed by small brainstem lesions. The vestibular nuclei occupy a large portion of the lateral brainstem, extending from medulla to midbrain. Although there are extensive bilateral connections between vestibular nuclei and other motor pathways, these connections are not redundant but are highly lateralized and act in concert to control posture, balance, and conjugate eye movement.

CONSCIOUSNESS AND AROUSAL

- Consciousness is awareness of self and the environment. It has two aspects: arousal, which is the state of wakefulness, and cognition, which is the sum of mental activities. This distinction is useful because neurologic disorders can affect arousal and cognition differently.
- Arousal is generated by activity of the ascending reticular activating system, which is composed of neurons within the central mesencephalic brainstem, the lateral hypothalamus, and the medial, intralaminar, and reticular nuclei of the thalamus. Widespread projections from these nuclei synapse on distal dendritic fields of large pyramidal neurons in the cerebral cortex and generate an arousal response. Cognition is the chief function of the cerebral cortex, particularly of prefrontal cortex and cortical association areas of the occipital, temporal, and parietal lobes. Some specialized mental functions are localized to specific cortical regions. Several subcortical nuclei in the basal ganglia and thalamus are intimately linked with cortical association areas, and damage to these nuclei or their interconnections with cortex may give rise to cognitive deficits similar to those observed with cortical lesions.
- The reticular activating system is excited by a wide variety of stimuli, especially somatosensory stimuli. It is most compact in the midbrain and can be damaged by central midbrain lesions, resulting in failure of arousal, or coma. Higher nuclei and projections are less localized, and lesions rostral to the midbrain, therefore, must be bilateral to cause coma.

COGNITION

- The prefrontal cortex generally refers to areas 9, 10, 11, 12, 45, 46, and 47 of Brodmann on the superior and lateral surfaces of the frontal lobes and the anterior cingulate, parolfactory, and orbitofrontal cortex inferiorly and mesially. These regions are

essential for orderly planning and sequencing of complex behaviors, attending to several stimuli or ideas simultaneously, concentrating and flexibly altering the focus of concentration, grasping the context and meaning of information, and controlling impulses, emotions, and thought sequences.
- The parietal association cortex is the region principally involved in visuomotor integration of constructional tasks. The visual cortex is required for observation, whereas the auditory cortex and the temporal language cortex are necessary for drawing objects on command. The inferior parietal cortex (areas 39 and 40) integrates visual and auditory information, and the output from this region is translated into motor patterns by motor cortex.

Calculation ability, abstract reasoning, problem solving, and several other aspects of intelligence are difficult to localize because they require integration of several cortical regions. They are frequently disturbed by diseases that cause widespread cortical dysfunction, such as those that cause dementia.

Hypothalamus and its Functions

The hypothalamus forms an integral part in maintaining the internal environment of the body.

Function	Corresponding areas
Temperature regulation	Anterior hypothalamus, response to heat; posterior hypothalamus, response to cold
Catecholamines	Dorsal and posterior hypothalamus
Vasopressin	Supraoptic and paraventricular nuclei
Oxytocin	Supraoptic and paraventricular nuclei
Thyroid-stimulating hormone (thyrotropin, TSH)	Paraventricular nuclei and neighboring areas
Adrenocorticotropic hormone (ACTH) and lipotropin (LPH)	Paraventricular nuclei
Follicle-stimulating hormone (FSH) and luteinizing hormone (LH)	Preoptic area; other areas
Prolactin	Arcuate nucleus
Growth hormone	Periventricular nucleus, arcuate nucleus
Thirst	Lateral superior hypothalamus
Hunger	Ventromedial, arcuate, and paraventricular nuclei; lateral hypothalamus
Sexual behavior	Anterior ventral hypothalamus plus, in the male, piriform cortex
Defensive reactions (fear, rage)	Diffuse, in limbic system and hypothalamus
Control of body rhythms	Suprachiasmatic nuclei
Hypothalamic functions	

TEMPERATURE REGULATION

Physiological changes to cold: (decrease heat loss)
- Cutaneous vasoconstriction: skin acts as a cold shell around a warm core and keeps the core warm, by reducing heat loss. (earliest response)
- Curling up posture
- Piloerection (animals)

Increase heat production:
- Shivering (major heat production)
- Hyperphagia and exercise
- Nonshivering thermogenesis
- *Hormones:* CA, Thyroxine

Nonshivering thermogenesis:
- *Organs:* Liver, abdominal viscera, skeletal muscle and brown fat.
- Activation of sympathetic nervous system (NE).
- *Human beings:* Very important in infants and neonates.
- Uncoupling of oxidative phosphorylation, UCP-1
- Mitochondria, B3 receptors.
- *Chemical thermogenesis:* Thyroxine.

Heat loss from the body, when the environmental temperature falls below the body temperature;
- Radiation and conduction: 70%
- Vaporization of sweat: 27%
- Respiration: 2%
- Urination and defecation: 1%

When the environmental temperature is > body temperature (heat stress), then the major route of heat loss is sweating.
Physiological changes to heat:
- Cutaneous vasodilatation (earliest response)
- Sweating (sympathetic cholinergic (most important)
- Panting (animals).

Learning and Memory

- Learning is acquisition of the information that gives humans the ability to alter behavior on the basis of experience. Memory is the retention and storage of that information.
- Explicit or declarative memory is associated with consciousness and is dependent on the hippocampus and other parts of the medial temporal lobes of the brain for its retention. Explicit memory is divided into episodic memory for events and semantic memory for facts.
- Implicit or nondeclarative memory does not involve awareness, and its retention does not usually involve processing in the hippocampus.
- Explicit memory and many forms of implicit memory involve (1) short-term memory, which lasts seconds to hours, during which processing in the hippocampus and elsewhere lays down long-term changes in synaptic strength; and (2) long-term memory, which stores memories for years and sometimes for life. Working memory is a form of short-term memory that keeps information available, usually for very short periods, while the individual plans action based on it.

Mechanisms

- Memory requires that information be registered by the primary somatosensory, auditory, or visual cortex. Posterior cortical areas involved in comprehension of language are needed for immediate processing of spoken or written events and recalling them immediately. The hippocampi and their connections to the dorsal medial nuclei of the thalamus and the mamillary nuclei of the hypothalamus constitute a limbic system network crucial for learning and processing of events for long-term storage. Memories that remain with a person for years are considered remote memories and are stored in corresponding association cortex areas.
- Short- and long-term changes in synaptic function can occur due to discharge at a synapse. They can be presynaptic or postsynaptic in location. One form of plastic change is post-tetanic potentiation, the production of enhanced postsynaptic potentials in response to stimulation. Habituation is a simple form of learning in which a neutral stimulus is repeated many times. The subject becomes habituated to the stimulus and ignores it after a period of time. This is associated with decreased release of neurotransmitter from the presynaptic terminal because of decreased intracellular Ca^{2+}. Sensitization is the prolonged occurrence of augmented postsynaptic responses after a stimulus to which one has become habituated is paired once or several times with a noxious stimulus. Sensitization is due to presynaptic facilitation.
- Long-term potentiation (LTP) is a rapidly developing persistent enhancement of the postsynaptic potential response to presynaptic stimulation after a brief period of rapidly repeated stimulation of the presynaptic neuron. It is initiated by an increase in intracellular Ca^{2+} in the postsynaptic neuron.
- A classic example of associative learning is a conditioned reflex. A conditioned reflex is a reflex response to a stimulus that previously elicited little or no response, acquired by repeatedly pairing the stimulus with another stimulus that normally does produce the response. The salivation normally induced by placing meat in the mouth of a dog was studied in the Pavlov's classic experiments. A bell was rung just before the meat was placed in the dog's mouth (the unconditioned stimulus (US) and this was repeated a number of times until the animal would salivate when the bell was rung (conditioned stimulus (CS). After the CS and US had been paired a sufficient number of times, the CS produced the response originally evoked only by the US.
- The encoding process for short-term explicit memory involves the hippocampus. Information from the senses is temporarily stored in various areas of the prefrontal cortex as working memory. From there, it enters the hippocampus. The hippocampus is closely associated with the overlying parahippocampal cortex in the medial frontal lobe. The connections of the hippocampus to the diencephalon are involved in memory. Some cases of memory loss correlate well with the presence of pathologic changes in the mamillary bodies, which have extensive efferent connections to the hippocampus via the fornix. The amygdala is closely associated with the hippocampus and is concerned with encoding and recalling emotionally charged memories.

- Output from the hippocampus leaves via the subiculum and the entorhinal cortex and somehow binds together and strengthens circuits in many different neocortical areas, forming over time the stable remote memories. Long-term memories are stored in various parts of the neocortex. Once long-term memories have been established, they can be recalled or accessed by a large number of different associations.
- The Wechsler Memory Scale-Revised (WMS-R) is the most widely used memory test battery for adults. The Benton Visual Retention Test is sensitive to short-term memory loss.

Language and Speech
- One group of functions localized to the neocortex in humans consists of those related to language, that is, understanding the spoken and printed word and expressing ideas in speech and writing.
- The hemisphere concerned with categorization and symbolization has been called the dominant hemisphere. The other hemisphere is not "nondominant;" but, is specialized in the area of spatiotemporal relations. It plays a primary role in the recognition of faces. The concept of "cerebral dominance" and a dominant and nondominant hemisphere has been replaced by a concept of complementary specialization of the hemispheres, one for sequential-analytic processes (the categorical hemisphere) and one for visuospatial relations (the representational hemisphere). The categorical hemisphere is concerned with language functions.
- In most of right-handed individuals, the left hemisphere is the dominant or categorical hemisphere, and in the remaining, the right hemisphere is dominant. However, in the majority of left-handers, the left hemisphere is the categorical hemisphere.
- The dominant cerebral hemisphere in right-handed individuals is highly developed in language function, understanding of spoken and written words and expressing speech; lesions of the left lobe is associated with aphasia; the nondominant or right hemisphere is representational hemisphere associated with music, art and spaciotemporal relationship; lesion of the nondominant hemisphere – agnosia, astereognosis.
- Language is one of the fundamental bases of human intelligence. The cortical regions most critical for language include Broca's area (area 44), Wernicke's area (area 22), the primary auditory cortex (areas 41 and 42), and neighboring frontal and temporoparietal association areas. Wernicke's area is concerned with comprehension of auditory and visual information. It projects via the arcuate fasciculus to Broca's area (area 44) in the frontal lobe.
- Broca's area processes the information received from Wernicke's area into a detailed and coordinated pattern for vocalization and then projects the pattern via a speech articulation area in the insula to the motor cortex, which initiates the appropriate movements of the lips, tongue, and larynx to produce speech. The angular gyrus behind Wernicke's area processes information from words that are read in such a way that they can be converted into the auditory forms of the words in Wernicke's area.

Wernicke's area(22): Posterior end of superior temporal gyrus (inferior branch of MCA)
- Area of comprehension (words are planned)
- Lesion: Sensory/fluent/receptive/Wernicke's aphasia.
- Comprehension" naming,* insight-Impaired
- Fluency, neologism* Present

Brocas area(44): Inferior frontal gyrus (superior branch of MCA)
- Motor centre for speech
- Lesion: Affluent/motor/expressive aphasia
- Insight, comprehension (except grammar)—Preserved fluency, naming-impaired
- Neologism-absent; motor writing centre—Middle frontal gyrus, Exner's area.
- Motor cortex for speech (area 4).
- **Conduction aphasia:** Understanding present, mistakes in framing a sentence; Lesion—arcuate fasciculus.
- **Anomic aphasia:** Difficulty in understanding written language and pictures; Lesion: Angular gyrus (Dejerine area, 38)
- **Causes:** Metabolic encephalopathy, head trauma and Alzheimer's

Nerve fibers have been divided into three types according to their diameters, conduction velocities, and physiologic characteristics.
1. A fibers are large and myelinated, conduct rapidly, and carry various motor or sensory impulses. They are most susceptible to injury by mechanical pressure or lack of oxygen.
2. B fibers are smaller myelinated axons that conduct less rapidly than A fibers. These fibers serve autonomic functions.
3. C fibers are the smallest and are nonmyelinated; they conduct impulses the slowest and serve pain conduction and autonomic functions.

Classification of nerve fibres			
Fiber type	Function	Fiber diameter (microm)	Conduction velocity (m/s)
A–alpha	Proprioception; somatic motor	12–20	70–120
Beta	Touch, pressure	5–12	30–70
Gamma	Motor to muscle spindles	3–6	15–30
Delta	Pain, temperature, touch	2–5	12–30
B	Preganglionic autonomic	<3	3–15
C–dorsal root sympathetic	Pain, reflex responses	0.4–1.2	0.5–2
	Postganglionic sympathetics	0.3–1.3	0.7–2.3

Number	Origin	Fiber type
Ia	Muscle spindle, annulospiral ending	A alpha
Ib	Golgi tendon organ	A alpha
II	Muscle spindle, flower-spray ending; touch, pressure	A beta
III	Pain and temperature receptors; some touch receptors	A delta
IV	Pain and other receptors	C

Muscle Spindles

- Each muscle spindle has three essential elements:
  1. A group of specialized intrafusal muscle fibers with contractile polar ends and a noncontractile center,
  2. Large diameter myelinated afferent nerves (types Ia and II) originating in the central portion of the intrafusal fibers, and
  3. Small diameter myelinated efferent nerves supplying the polar contractile regions of the intrafusal fibers
- Changes in muscle length are associated with changes in joint angle; thus muscle spindles provide information on position. The intrafusal fibers are positioned in parallel to the extrafusal fibers (the regular contractile units of the muscle) with the ends of the spindle capsule attached to the tendons at either end of the muscle. Intrafusal fibers do not contribute to the overall contractile force of the muscle, but rather serve a pure sensory function. There are two types of intrafusal fibers in mammalian muscle spindles. The first type contains many nuclei in a dilated central area and is called a nuclear bag fiber. The second intrafusal fiber type, the nuclear chain fiber, is thinner and shorter and lacks a definite bag.
- When the muscle spindle is stretched, its sensory endings are distorted and receptor potentials are generated. These in turn set up action potentials in the sensory fibers at a frequency proportional to the degree of stretching. Because the spindle is in parallel with the extrafusal fibers, when the muscle is passively stretched, the spindles are also stretched. This initiates reflex contraction of the extrafusal fibers in the muscle.
- When a stretch reflex occurs, the muscles that antagonize the action of the muscle involved (antagonists) relax. This phenomenon is said to be due to *reciprocal innervation*. Up to a point, the harder a muscle is stretched, the stronger is the reflex contraction. However, when the tension becomes great enough, contraction suddenly ceases and the muscle relaxes. This relaxation in response to strong stretch is called the *inverse stretch reflex*. The receptor for the inverse stretch reflex is in the Golgi tendon organ and it senses muscle tension.

ELECTROENCEPHALOGRAPHY (EEG)

- Summation of the excitatory postsynaptic potential generated by the pyramidal cells of the cerebral cortex gives rise to the electrical activity of the brain, which can be recorded as an electroencephalogram (EEG). The EEG comprises many underlying components with different frequencies and harmonics. The component waves are typically classified according to the respective frequencies. This electrical activity is volume conducted and can be recorded from the scalp and forehead, using surface or needle electrodes.
- Because the scalp has no electrically neutral area, EEG is typically recorded using a montage (electrode arrangement) with bipolar recording. Thus, both electrodes are active, and the polarity of the signal recorded depends on the arbitrary designation of recording versus referential electrode.
- The gold standard for raw EEG recording is 16-channel recording (eight channels for each hemisphere) with electrodes placed according to the International System. The EEG is a random activity reflecting the state of arousal and metabolic activity. The generation of electrical activity is an energy-requiring process that depends on an adequate supply of substrates including oxygen and glucose.

Types of EEG waves		
	Frequency	Description
Beta	13–30	High frequency, low amplitude, dominant during awake state
Alpha	9–12	Medium frequency, higher amplitude seen in occipital cortex with eyes closed while awake
Theta	4–8	Low frequency, not predominant in any condition
Delta	0–4	Very low frequency, low to high amplitude signifies depressed functions, consistent with deep coma (cause can be anesthesia, metabolic, or hypoxia)

- Awake EEG is dominated by beta activity with high-frequency and low-amplitude waves. With the onset of ischemia/hypoxia, initially a transient increase in beta activity occurs, followed by development of slow waves (theta and delta) with large amplitude, disappearance of beta activity, and eventually the occurrence of delta waves with low amplitude.
- The ischemic changes can progress to suppression of electrical activity with an occasional burst of activity (burst suppression) and finally to complete electrical silence with flat EEG, signaling the onset of irreversible damage.

Uses of EEG

- EEG is useful in evaluating patients with suspected epilepsy. The presence of electrographic seizure activity (abnormal, rhythmic electrocerebral activity of abrupt onset and termination) during a behavioral disturbance could represent a seizure. The interictal presence of epileptiform activity (abnormal paroxysmal activity containing some spike discharges) is of particular help in diagnosis.
- EEG findings may help in classifying the seizure disorder and thus in selecting appropriate anticonvulsant medication. For example, in patients with the typical absences of petit mal epilepsy, the EEG is characterized both ictally and interictally by episodic generalized spike-and-wave activity. In contrast, in patients with episodes of complex partial seizures, the EEG may be normal or show focal epileptiform discharges interictally.
- The EEG findings may provide a guide to prognosis and have been used to follow the course of seizure disorders.
- Certain neurologic disorders also produce characteristic but nonspecific abnormalities in the EEG. The presence of repetitive slow-wave complexes over one or both temporal lobes suggests a diagnosis of herpes simplex encephalitis. Similarly, the presence of periodic complexes in a patient with an acute dementing disorder suggests a diagnosis of Creutzfeldt-Jakob disease or subacute sclerosing panencephalitis.
- Electrocerebral silence in coma implies neocortical death, in the absence of hypothermia or drug overdose.

Evoked Potential Monitoring

Sensory Evoked Potentials (SEPs)

- SEP is a time-locked, event-related, pathway-specific electroencephalographic activity generated in response to a specific stimulus such as electrical stimuli applied to the median nerve. The typical peaks and troughs are described by their polarity and latency. For example, the cortical negative peak that typically occurs 20 msec after stimulation of the median nerve is called N20. Alternatively, it is numbered according to the sequence in which it is generated; thus, the first positive wave that occurs following posterior tibial nerve stimulation is called P1. The amplitude of evoked potential waves is small relative to conventional EEG and is not easily visualized without computer averaging of repetitive stimuli. SEPs are anatomically pathway specific and theoretically assess only the integrity of the pathway monitored. SEP can be recorded in response to stimulation of any sensory nerve, cranial or peripheral.
- The common modalities of evoked potentials used in clinical practice are:
  - Somatosensory evoked potentials (SSEPs),
  - Visual evoked potentials (VEPs), and
  - Brain stem auditory evoked potentials (BAEPs).
- As with EEG, ischemia/hypoxia leads to depression of conduction with resultant decrease in amplitude and increase in latency of the specific peaks.

Motor Evoked Potentials

Because SSEP monitors only the integrity of the sensory pathway, it is theoretically possible to miss an injury specifically affecting the motor pathway but sparing the sensory tracts. Thus, motor evoked potential (MEP) recording was introduced into clinical practice to complement SSEP recording. The MEP is basically an electromyographic potential recorded over muscles in the hand or foot in response to depolarization of the motor cortex. Depolarization can be achieved using transcranial magnetic or electrical stimulation.

Spontaneous Electromyography

Although not technically an evoked potential, spontaneous electromyography (EMG) is frequently recorded during surgical procedures of both the cervical spine and lumbar spine. Irritation of peripheral nerves, such as spinal nerve roots, invokes immediate motor activity in muscles that should otherwise be silent under general anesthesia.

Nerve Conduction Studies

Motor Nerve Conduction Studies

These studies are performed by recording the electrical response of a muscle to stimulation of its motor nerve at two or more points along its course. This permits conduction velocity to be determined in the fastest-conducting motor fibers between the points of stimulation.

Sensory Nerve Conduction Studies

These are performed by analogous means, by determining the conduction velocity and amplitude of action potentials in sensory fibers when these fibers are stimulated at one point and their responses are recorded at another point along the course of the nerve.

Uses of Nerve Conduction Studies

Nerve conduction studies provide a means of confirming the presence and extent of peripheral nerve damage. Nerve conduction studies are particularly helpful in:

- Determining whether sensory symptoms are caused by a lesion proximal or distal to the dorsal root ganglia and whether neuromuscular dysfunction relates to peripheral nerve disease.
- Detecting subclinical involvement of other peripheral nerves in patients who present with a mononeuropathy.
- Determining the site of a focal lesion and providing a guide to prognosis in patients with a mononeuropathy.
- Distinguishing between a polyneuropathy and a mononeuropathy multiplex.
- Prognosis of peripheral nerve disorders and their response to treatment.
- Indicating the predominant pathologic change in peripheral nerve disorders. In demyelinating neuropathies, conduction velocity is often markedly slowed and conduction block may occur; in axonal neuropathies, conduction velocity is usually normal or slowed only mildly, sensory nerve action potentials are small or absent, and electromyography shows evidence of denervation in affected muscles.
- Detecting hereditary disorders of the peripheral nerves at a subclinical stage in genetic and epidemiologic studies.

Repetitive Nerve Stimulation

- The size of the electrical response of a muscle to supramaximal electrical stimulation of its motor nerve depends on a number of factors but correlates with the number of activated muscle fibers.
- Neuromuscular transmission can be tested by recording (with surface electrodes) the response of a muscle to supramaximal stimulation of its motor nerve either repetitively or by single shocks or trains of shocks at selected intervals after a maximal voluntary contraction.

CNS INFECTIONS

- The most common bacteria that cause meningitis, *S. pneumoniae* and *N. meningitidis*, initially colonize the nasopharynx by attaching to nasopharyngeal epithelial cells. Bacteria are transported across epithelial cells in membrane-bound vacuoles to the intravascular space or invade the intravascular space by creating separations in the apical tight junctions of columnar epithelial cells.
- Once in the bloodstream, bacteria are able to avoid phagocytosis by neutrophils and classic complement–mediated bactericidal activity because of the presence of a polysaccharide capsule. Blood-borne bacteria can reach the intraventricular choroid plexus, directly infect choroid plexus epithelial cells, and gain access to the CSF.
- Some bacteria, such as *S. pneumoniae*, can adhere to cerebral capillary endothelial cells and subsequently migrate through or between these cells to reach the CSF. Bacteria are able to multiply rapidly within CSF because of the absence of effective host immune defenses.
- The inflammatory reaction is induced by the invading bacteria. The lysis of bacteria with the subsequent release of cell-wall components into the subarachnoid space is the initial step in the induction of the inflammatory response and the formation of a purulent exudate in the subarachnoid space. Bacterial cell-wall components, such as the lipopolysaccharide (LPS) molecules of gram-negative bacteria and teichoic acid and peptidoglycans of *S. pneumoniae*, induce meningeal inflammation by stimulating the production of inflammatory cytokines and chemokines by microglia, astrocytes, monocytes, microvascular endothelial cells, and CSF leukocytes.
- Bacterial meningitis is a direct consequence of elevated levels of CSF cytokines and chemokines. TNF and IL-1 act synergistically to increase the permeability of the blood-brain barrier, resulting in induction of vasogenic edema and the leakage of serum proteins into the subarachnoid space. The subarachnoid exudate of proteinaceous material and leukocytes obstructs the flow of CSF through the ventricular system and diminishes the resorptive capacity of the arachnoid granulations in the dural sinuses, leading to obstructive and communicating hydrocephalus and concomitant interstitial edema.

- Inflammatory cytokines upregulate the expression of selectins on cerebral capillary endothelial cells and leukocytes, promoting leukocyte adherence to vascular endothelial cells and subsequent migration into the CSF. The adherence of leukocytes to capillary endothelial cells increases the permeability of blood vessels, allowing for the leakage of plasma proteins into the CSF, which adds to the inflammatory exudate. Neutrophil degranulation results in the release of toxic metabolites that contribute to cytotoxic edema, cell injury, and death.
- The combination of interstitial, vasogenic, and cytotoxic edema leads to raised ICP and coma. Cerebral herniation usually results from the effects of cerebral edema, either focal or generalized; hydrocephalus and dural sinus or cortical vein thrombosis may also play a role.

BRAIN ABSCESS

- The intact brain parenchyma is relatively resistant to infection. Once bacteria have established infection, brain abscess frequently evolves through a series of stages, influenced by the nature of the infecting organism and by the immunocompetence of the host.
- The early cerebritis stage (days 1–3) is characterized by a perivascular infiltration of inflammatory cells, which surround a central core of coagulative necrosis. Marked edema surrounds the lesion at this stage.
- In the late cerebritis stage (days 4–9), pus formation leads to enlargement of the necrotic center, which is surrounded at its border by an inflammatory infiltrate of macrophages and fibroblasts. A thin capsule of fibroblasts and reticular fibers gradually develops, and the surrounding area of cerebral edema becomes more distinct than in the previous stage.
- The third stage, early capsule formation (days 10–13), is characterized by the formation of a capsule that is better developed on the cortical than on the ventricular side of the lesion.
- The final stage, late capsule formation (day 14 and beyond), is defined by a well-formed necrotic center surrounded by a dense collagenous capsule. The surrounding area of cerebral edema has regressed, but marked gliosis with large numbers of reactive astrocytes has developed outside the capsule. This gliotic process may contribute to the development of seizures as sequelae of brain abscess.

MOTOR NEURON DISEASE

- In ALS there is selective degeneration of motor neurons in the primary motor cortex and the anterolateral horns of the spinal cord. Many affected neurons show cytoskeletal disease with accumulations of intermediate filaments in the cell body and in axons. There is only a subtle glial cell response and little evidence of inflammation.
- In sporadic ALS, there is a large decrease in glutamate transport activity in the motor cortex and spinal cord but not in other regions of the CNS. This has been associated with a loss of the astrocytic glutamate transporter protein excitatory amino acid transporter 2 (EAAT2), perhaps resulting from a defect in splicing of its messenger RNA.
- About 10% of ALS cases are familial and few cases are due to missense mutations in the cytosolic copper-zinc superoxide dismutase (SOD1) gene on the long arm of chromosome 21. SOD1 catalyzes the formation of hydrogen peroxide from superoxide anion.
- A role for neurofilament dysfunction in ALS is supported by the finding that neurofilamentous inclusions in cell bodies and proximal axons are an early feature of ALS pathology. In addition, mutations in the heavy chain neurofilament subunit (NF-H) have been detected in some patients with sporadic ALS.

Multiple Sclerosis

- Multiple sclerosis (MS) is characterized by a triad of inflammation, demyelination, and gliosis (scarring); the course can be relapsing-remitting or progressive. Lesions of MS typically occur at different times and in different CNS locations (i.e., disseminated in time and space).
- The lesions of MS (plaques) vary in size from 1 or 2 mm to several centimeters. Acute MS lesions are characterized by perivenular cuffing with inflammatory mononuclear cells, predominantly T cells and macrophages, which also infiltrate the surrounding white matter. In many lesions, myelin-specific autoantibodies are present, presumably promoting demyelination directly as well as stimulating macrophages and microglial cells (bone marrow-derived CNS phagocytes) that scavenge the myelin debris. As lesions evolve, there is prominent astrocytic proliferation (gliosis).
- Ultrastructural studies of MS lesions suggest that fundamentally different underlying pathologies may exist in different patients. Although relative sparing of axons is typical of MS, partial or total axonal destruction can also occur, especially within highly inflammatory lesions.

- Nerve conduction in myelinated axons occurs in a saltatory manner, with the nerve impulse jumping from one node of Ranvier to the next without depolarization of the axonal membrane underlying the myelin sheath between nodes. This produces considerably faster conduction velocities (~70 m/s) than the slow velocities (~1 m/s) produced by continuous propagation in unmyelinated nerves. Conduction block occurs when the nerve impulse is unable to traverse the demyelinated segment. A temporary conduction block often follows a demyelinating event before sodium channels (originally concentrated at the nodes) redistribute along the naked axon. This redistribution ultimately allows continuous propagation of nerve action potentials through the demyelinated segment.
- MS is approximately threefold more common in women than men. The age of onset is typically between 20 and 40 years (slightly later in men than in women), but the disease can present across the lifespan. One proposed explanation for the latitude effect on MS is that there is a protective effect of sun exposure. Ultraviolet radiation from sun is the most important source of vitamin D in most individuals, and low levels of vitamin D are common at high latitudes where sun exposure may be low, particularly during winter months. Prospective studies have confirmed that vitamin D deficiency is associated with an increase in MS risk. Immunoregulatory effects of vitamin D could explain this possible relationship.
- Susceptibility to MS is polygenic, with each gene contributing a relatively small amount to the overall risk. The major histocompatibility complex (MHC) on chromosome 6 is the strongest MS susceptibility region in the genome. Studies implicate primarily the class II region of the MHC (encoding HLA molecules involved in presenting peptide antigens to T cells) and specifically the DR2 allele. Other recently identified MS susceptibility genes encode receptors for two proinflammatory cytokines, the IL-7 receptor alpha chain (CD127) and the IL-2 receptor alpha chain (CD25); the MS associated variant of the IL-7 receptor increases the amount of soluble compared to membrane bound receptor. It is also likely that genetic heterogeneity is present in MS, meaning that there are different causative genes in different individuals.
- Myelin basic protein (MBP) is an important T cell antigen in EAE and probably also in human MS. Activated MBP-reactive T cells have been identified in the blood, in cerebrospinal fluid (CSF), and within MS lesions. Moreover, DR2 may influence the autoimmune response because it binds with high affinity to a fragment of MBP, stimulating T cell responses to this self-protein.
- Myelin-specific autoantibodies, some directed against myelin oligodendrocyte glycoprotein (MOG), have been detected bound to vesiculated myelin debris in MS plaques. In the CSF, elevated levels of locally synthesized immunoglobulins and oligoclonal antibodies derived from expansion of clonally restricted plasma cells are also characteristic of MS. The pattern of oligoclonal banding is unique to each individual, and attempts to identify the targets of these antibodies have been largely unsuccessful, although one recent report indicated that some bands recognized EBV antigens.
- Axonal damage occurs in every newly formed MS lesion, and cumulative axonal loss is considered to be the major cause of progressive and irreversible neurological disability in MS. Demyelination can result in reduced trophic support for axons, redistribution of ion channels, and destabilization of action potential membrane potentials. Axons can initially adapt, but eventually distal and retrograde degeneration occurs.

PARKINSON'S DISEASE

- In Parkinson's disease, there is selective degeneration of monoamine-containing cell populations in the brainstem and basal ganglia, particularly of pigmented dopaminergic neurons of the substantia nigra. In addition, scattered neurons in basal ganglia, brainstem, spinal cord, and sympathetic ganglia contain eosinophilic, cytoplasmic inclusion bodies (Lewy bodies). These contain filamentous aggregates of alpha-synuclein, along with parkin, synphilin, neurofilaments, and synaptic vesicle proteins.
- MPTP is a by-product of synthesis of a synthetic opioid derivative of meperidine. Illicit use of opioid preparations heavily contaminated with MPTP led to several cases of parkinsonism. MPTP selectively injures dopaminergic neurons in the brain and produces a clinical syndrome very similar to Parkinson's disease.
- Genetic studies have identified causative mutations in five genes that provide important information about molecular pathways involved in the disease. These genes include the genes for alpha synuclein (PARK1), parkin (PARK2), DJ-1 (PARK7), ubiquitin-C-hydrolase-L1 (PARK5), and PTEN (phosphatase and tensin homolog deleted on chromosome 10)-induced kinase 1 (PARK6).
- Mutations in the gene for alpha-synuclein on chromosome 4q21-23 cause autosomal dominant Parkinson's disease. Alpha-synuclein is found in nerve terminals in close proximity to synaptic vesicles. Misfolded, damaged, or unassembled proteins are generally degraded by a process involving covalent attachment of ubiquitin. A missense mutation in one component of the ubiquitin-proteasome system, ubiquitin carboxyl terminal hydrolase L1, has been found in one family with autosomal dominant Parkinson's disease. Mutations in parkin on chromosome 6q25 have been identified in cases of autosomal recessive juvenile parkinsonism. Parkin is a ubiquitin E3 ligase that catalyzes the addition of ubiquitin to specific proteins to target them for degradation.

MYASTHENIA GRAVIS

- The major structural abnormality in myasthenia gravis is a simplification of the postsynaptic region of the neuromuscular synapse. The muscle end plate shows sparse, shallow, and abnormally wide or absent synaptic clefts. In contrast, the number and size of the presynaptic vesicles are normal. Scattered collections of lymphocytes, some within the vicinity of motor end plates, may be present.
- Electrophysiologic studies indicate that the postsynaptic membrane has a decreased response to applied acetylcholine. Circulating antibodies to the receptor are present in 90% of patients, and the disorder may be passively transferred to animals by administration of IgG from affected patients. The antibodies block acetylcholine binding and receptor activation. In addition, the antibodies cross-link receptor molecules, increasing receptor internalization and degradation. Bound antibody also activates complement-mediated destruction of the postsynaptic region, resulting in simplification of the end plate. Many patients who lack antibodies to the acetylcholine receptor have autoantibodies instead against the muscle-specific receptor tyrosine kinase, which is an important mediator of acetylcholine receptor clustering at the end plate. These antibodies inhibit clustering of receptors in muscle cell culture.
- During repetitive stimulation of a motor nerve, the number of quanta released from the nerve terminal declines with successive stimuli. Normally, this causes no clinical impairment because a sufficient number of acetylcholine receptor channels are opened by the reduced level of neurotransmitter. However, in myasthenia gravis, where there is a deficiency in the number of functional receptors, neuromuscular transmission fails at lower levels of quantal release.

EPILEPSY

- Seizures are paroxysmal disturbances in cerebral function caused by an abnormal synchronous discharge of cortical neurons. The epilepsies are a group of disorders characterized by recurrent seizures.
- Normal neuronal activity occurs in a nonsynchronized manner, with groups of neurons inhibited and excited sequentially during the transfer of information between different brain areas. Seizures occur when neurons are activated synchronously. The kind of seizure depends on the location of the abnormal activity and the pattern of spread to different parts of the brain.
- Interictal spike discharges are often observed on EEG recordings from epileptic patients. These are due to synchronous depolarization of a group of neurons in an abnormally excitable area of brain.
- Spread of a local discharge occurs by a combination of mechanisms. During the paroxysmal depolarizing shift, extracellular potassium accumulates, depolarizing nearby neurons. Increased frequency of discharges enhances calcium influx into nerve terminals, increasing neurotransmitter release at excitatory synapses by a process known as post-tetanic potentiation.
- This involves increased calcium influx through voltage-gated channels and through the N-methyl-d-aspartate (NMDA) subtype of glutamate receptor-gated ion channels. NMDA receptor-gated channels preferentially pass calcium ions but are relatively quiescent during normal synaptic transmission because they are blocked by magnesium ions.
- In secondary epilepsy, loss of inhibitory circuits and sprouting of fibers from excitatory neurons appear to be important for the generation of a seizure focus. In several of the idiopathic epilepsies, genetic studies have identified mutations in ion channels. For example, benign familial neonatal convulsions have been linked to mutations in two homologous voltage-gated K+ channels: KCNQ2 encoded by a gene on chromosome 20q13 and KCNQ3 encoded by a gene on chromosome 8q24.

ALZHEIMER'S DISEASE

- The pathology of Alzheimer's disease is characterized by extracellular neuritic plaques in the cerebral cortex and in walls of meningeal and cerebral blood vessels. These plaques contain a dense core of amyloid material surrounded by dystrophic neurites (axons, dendrites), reactive astrocytes, and microglia. Other structural changes include the formation of intraneuronal neurofibrillary tangles, neuronal and synaptic loss, reactive astrocytosis, and microglial proliferation.
- Neurofibrillary tangles are paired helical filaments composed of a hyperphosphorylated form of the microtubule protein tau. They are not specific for Alzheimer's disease and occur in several other neurodegenerative disorders. In general, all pathologic changes are most prominent in the hippocampus, entorhinal cortex, association cortex, and basal forebrain.
- The major protein in neuritic plaques is amyloid peptide which is proteolytically derived from a membrane protein, the alpha amyloid precursor protein (APP) encoded by a gene on chromosome 21q21. Almost all patients with trisomy 21 (Down syndrome) develop pathologic changes indistinguishable from those seen in Alzheimer's disease, suggesting that having an increased copy of the APP gene increases the metabolism of APP to Aβ.
- Almost 70% of familial cases of Alzheimer's disease have been linked to missense mutations in the gene PS-1/S182, which encodes a seven-transmembrane protein (presenilin 1) on chromosome 14q24.3. Another 20% of cases have been linked to mutations in another gene, STM2 (presenilin 2), on chromosome 1q31-42.

- The majority of patients with Alzheimer's disease are older than 60 years, and in about 50% of these patients the e4 isoform of apolipoprotein E (apoE4) has been identified as a risk factor. It is synthesized and secreted by astrocytes and macrophages and is thought to be important for mobilizing lipids during normal development of the nervous system and during regeneration of peripheral nerves after injury. The e4 allele is associated with increased risk and earlier onset of both familial and sporadic late-onset Alzheimer's disease. In contrast, inheritance of e2 is associated with decreased risk and later onset. It is important to note that Alzheimer's disease develops in the absence of e4 and also that many persons with e4 escape disease. Therefore, genotyping is not currently recommended as a useful genetic test.

Stroke

- The focal symptoms and signs that result from stroke correlate with the area of brain supplied by the affected blood vessel. Strokes may be classified into two major categories based on pathogenesis: ischemic stroke and hemorrhage. In ischemic stroke, vascular occlusion interrupts blood flow to a specific brain region, producing a fairly characteristic pattern of neurologic deficits resulting from loss of functions controlled by that region. The pattern of deficits resulting from hemorrhage is less predictable because it depends on the location of the bleed and also on factors that affect the function of brain regions distant from the hemorrhage (e.g., increased intracranial pressure, brain edema, compression of neighboring brain tissue, and rupture of blood into ventricles or subarachnoid space).
- Ischemic strokes result from thrombotic or embolic occlusion of cerebral vessels. Neurologic deficits caused by occlusion of large arteries result from focal ischemia to the area of brain supplied by the affected vessel and produce recognizable clinical syndromes. Thrombosis usually involves the internal carotid, middle cerebral, or basilar arteries. Symptoms typically evolve over several minutes and may be preceded by brief episodes of reversible focal deficits known as transient ischemic attacks. Emboli from the heart, aortic arch, or carotid arteries usually occlude the middle cerebral artery, because it carries more than 80% of blood flow to the cerebral hemisphere. Emboli that travel in the vertebral and basilar arteries commonly lodge at the apex of the basilar artery or in one or both posterior cerebral arteries.
- Most result from a degenerative change in the vessel, described pathologically as lipohyalinosis, that is caused by chronic hypertension and predisposes to occlusion. The most common vessels involved are the lenticulostriate arteries, which arise from the proximal middle cerebral artery and perfuse the basal ganglia and internal capsule. Also commonly affected are small branches of the basilar and posterior cerebral arteries that penetrate the brainstem and thalamus.

Vascular stroke features		
Artery	Territory	Symptoms and Signs
Anterior cerebral	Medial frontal and parietal cortex, anterior corpus callosum	Paresis and sensory loss of contralateral leg and foot
Middle cerebral	Lateral frontal, parietal, occipital, and temporal cortex and adjacent white matter, caudate, putamen, internal capsule	Aphasia (dominant hemisphere), neglect (nondominant hemisphere), contralateral hemisensory loss, homonymous hemianopia, hemiparesis
Vertebral (posterior inferior cerebellar)	Medulla, lower cerebellum	Ipsilateral cerebellar ataxia, Horner's syndrome, crossed sensory loss, nystagmus, vertigo, hiccup, dysarthria, dysphagia
Basilar (including anterior inferior cerebellar, superior cerebellar)	Lower midbrain, pons, upper and mid cerebellum	Nystagmus, vertigo, diplopia, skew deviation, gaze palsies, hemi- or crossed sensory loss, dysarthria, hemi- or quadriparesis, ipsilateral cerebellar ataxia, Horner's syndrome, coma
Posterior cerebral	Distal territory: medial occipital and temporal cortex and underlying white matter, posterior corpus callosum	Contralateral homonymous hemianopia, dyslexia without agraphia, visual hallucinations and distortions, memory defect, cortical blindness (bilateral occlusion)
	Proximal territory: upper midbrain, thalamus	Sensory loss, ataxia, third nerve palsy, contralateral hemiparesis, vertical gaze palsy, skew deviation, hemiballismus, choreoathetosis, impaired consciousness

- Epidural and subdural hematomas typically occur as sequelae of head injury. Epidural hematomas arise from damage to an artery, typically the middle meningeal artery, which can be ruptured by a blow to the temporal bone.
- Subarachnoid hemorrhage may occur from head trauma, extension of blood from another compartment into the subarachnoid space, or rupture of an arterial aneurysm. Cerebral dysfunction occurs because of increased intracranial pressure and from poorly understood toxic effects of subarachnoid blood on brain tissue and cerebral vessels. The most common cause of spontaneous (nontraumatic) subarachnoid hemorrhage is rupture of a berry aneurysm, which is thought to arise from a congenital weakness in the walls of large vessels at the base of the brain.

- Intraparenchymal hemorrhage may result from acute elevations in blood pressure or from a variety of disorders that weaken vessels. The resultant hematoma causes a focal neurologic deficit by compressing adjacent structures. In hypertensive patients, small Charcot-Bouchard aneurysms appear in the walls of small penetrating arteries and are thought to be the major sites of rupture.
- Neurons deep within an ischemic focus die from energy deprivation. However, at the edge of the ischemic region, neurons appear to die because of excessive stimulation of glutamate receptors. Glutamate is released at excitatory synapses, and glutamate levels in the extracellular space are normally tightly regulated by sodium-dependent reuptake systems in neurons and glia. Ischemia deprives the brain of oxygen and glucose, and the resultant disruption in cellular metabolism depletes neurons and glia of energy reserves required to maintain normal transmembrane ion gradients.
- Two energy-dependent transporters are particularly important for removal of extracellular K^+ by glia: a Na^+-K^+ ATPase and an anion transporter that cotransports K^+ and Na^+ with Cl^-. In ischemia, these energy-dependent mechanisms fail, and K^+ released into the extracellular space is no longer be taken up by glia. This depolarizes neurons because the gradient of K^+ across neuronal membranes determines the level of the resting membrane potential. Depolarization activates release of neurotransmitters, increasing accumulation of glutamate at excitatory synapses and in the extracellular space.
- The net effect of these events is a tremendous influx of Na^+ and Ca^{2+} into neurons through glutamate- and voltage-gated ion channels. The resultant overload in intracellular Ca^{2+} appears to be especially toxic and may exceed the ability of the neuron to extrude or sequester the cation. This results in sustained activation of a variety of calcium-sensitive enzymes, including proteases, phospholipases, and endonucleases, leading to cell death.

Speech Disorders

Type	Naming	Fluency	Auditory comprehension	Repetition	Location of lesion
Broca's	+/−	−	+	−	Broca's area (area 44 and 45)
Wernicke's	−	+	−	−	Wernicke's area (area 22)
Global	−	−	−	−	Large left hemispheric lesions
Conduction	+/−	+	+	−	Arcuate fasciculus
Motor transcortical	−	−	+	+	Surrounding Broca's area
Sensory transcortical	−	+	−	+	Surrounding Wernicke's area
Mixed transcortical	−	−	−	+	Surrounding Broca's and Wernicke's areas
Anomic	−	+	+	+	Anywhere within left (or right) hemisphere

(−: impaired; +: intact)

Channelopathies

Class	Disorder	Channel type
Ataxias	Episodic ataxia-1	K
	Episodic ataxia-2	
	Spinocerebellar ataxia-6	Ca
Migraine	Familial hemiplegic migraine 1	Ca
	Familial hemiplegic migraine 2	Na
Epilepsy	Benign neonatal familial convulsions	K
	Generalized epilepsy with febrile convulsions plus	Na
Periodic paralysis	Hyperkalemic periodic paralysis	Na
	Hypokalemic periodic paralysis	Ca
Myotonia	Myotonia congenita	Cl
	Paramyotonia congenita	Na
Deafness	Jorvell and Lange-Nielsen syndrome (deafness, prolonged QT interval, and arrhythmia)	K
	Autosomal dominant progressive deafness	K
Paraneoplastic	Limbic encephalitis	Kv1
	Acquired neuromyotonia	Kv1
	Cerebellar ataxia	Ca (P/Q type)
	Lambert-Eaton syndrome	Ca (P/Q type)

Amygdala

Window of the limbic system

Functions

- Autonomic functions
- Sexual behavior
- Fear (stimulation of hypothalamus and amygdaloid nuclei), placidity (lesions of amygdala)
- Memory (associated with emotions) and learning
- Punishment and reward centres
- Vital role in coordinating central and peripheral components

Lesion

- Visual agnosia
- Oral tendencies
- Emotionally dull
- Hypersexuality
- Hypermetamorphosis

Neuropeptides

Neuropeptides which increase food intake:
- Neuropeptide Y
- MCH
- Ghrelin
- Orexin
- Galanin
- AGRP

Neuropeptides which decrease food intake:
- CCK
- Glucagon
- Somatostatin
- CA
- RTII cocaine-amphetamine regulated transcript
- GRP
- alpha-MSH

Neuropeptide-Y
- Polypeptide—36 amino acids
- Increase in fasting/starvation
- Orexigenic and decreases thermogenesis
- Suppresses the activity of MSH
- Secreted by paraventricular and arcuate nucleus

Ghrelin

- Released from stomach (oxyntic) in fasting state.
- Increases hunger (inhibits satiety centre)
- Stimulates ghrelin secretion
- Induces lipolysis.

Multiple Choice Questions

NEUROPHYSIOLOGY

1. Which of the following sensory receptors is found in epidermis for determination of texture?
   a. Merkel disc
   b. Meissner's corpuscles
   c. Paccinian corpuscles
   d. Ruffini ending

2. Which of the following phrase adequately describes paccinian corpuscles?
   a. Type of pain receptor
   b. Slowly adapting touch receptor
   c. Rapidly adapting touch receptor
   d. Located in the joints.

3. Vanilloid receptors are activated by:
   a. Pain
   b. Vibration
   c. Touch
   d. Pressure

4. Intensity of sensory stimulation is directly related to:
   a. Duration of action potential
   b. Frequency of action potential
   c. Amplitude of action potential
   d. All of the above

5. Weber Fechner law is related to:
   a. Amplitude
   b. Surface area
   c. Number of sensory fibre involvement
   d. Stimulus discrimination

6. If a single spinal nerve is cut, the area of tactile loss is always greater than the area of painful sensations, because:
   a. Tactile information is carried by myelinated and conducting fibres
   b. Tactile receptors adapt quickly
   c. Degree of overlap of fibres carrying tactile sensations is much less
   d. In the primary sensory cortex, tactile sensation is represented by larger area

7. Kinesthetic sensation is:
   a. Transmitted by the beta type of fibre
   b. Located in Merkel's disc
   c. Transmitted by Meissner's corpuscles
   d. Means abnormal perception of sensation

8. Ventrolateral cordotomy for relief of pain in right lower limb is due to cutting:
   a. Left ventral spinothalamic tract
   b. Left lateral spinothalamic tract
   c. Right ventral spinothalamic tract
   d. Right lateral spinothalamic tract

9. All are features of Brown-sequard syndrome *except*:
   a. Ipsilateral pyramidal tract features
   b. Contralateral dorsal column
   c. Contralateral spinothalamic tract
   d. Ipsilateral planter extensor

10. Loss of proprioception and fine touch:
    a. Anterior spinothalamic tract
    b. Lateral spinothalamic tract
    c. Dorsal column
    d. Corticospinal tract

11. Cortical representation of the body in the cerebrum:
    a. Horizontal
    b. Vertical
    c. Tandem
    d. Oblique

12. Appreciation of size and shape of an object placed in hand is lost in the lesion of:
    a. Tactus gracilis
    b. Tractus cuneatus
    c. Spinothalamic tract
    d. Spinoreticular tract

13. Ablation of somatosensory area 1 of the cerebral leads to:
    a. Total loss of pain sensation
    b. Total loss of touch sensation
    c. Loss of tactile localization but not of 2 point discrimination
    d. Loss of tactile localization and 2 point discrimination

Answers

| 1. a | 2. c | 3. a | 4. b | 5. d | 6. c | 7. a |
| 8. b | 9. b | 10. c | 11. b | 12. b | 13. d | |

14. Perception of normal sensory stimulus as painful:
    a. Hyperalgesia
    b. Allodynia
    c. Hyperpathia
    d. Causalgia

15. Massage and application of liniments to painful areas in the body relieves pain due to:
    a. Stimulation of endogenous analgesic system
    b. Release of endorphins by the first order neuron in the brain stem
    c. Release of glutamate and substance P in the spinal cord
    d. Inhibition by large myelinated afferent fibre.

16. Pain sensitive intracranial structure:
    a. Pia mater
    b. Dura mater
    c. Pial vessels
    d. Brain matter

17. While doing a neurosurgery, the paracentral lobule was accidentally damaged, it will lead to which of the following?
    a. Hemiplegia
    b. Monoplegia
    c. Involvement of the perineum and lower limbs
    d. Quadriplegia

18. Setting a posture before planned movement:
    a. Premotor cortex
    b. Motor cortex
    c. Frontal cortex
    d. Supplementary motor area

19. UMN includes:
    a. Pyramidal cells
    b. Peripheral nerves
    c. Anterior horn cells
    d. Glial cells
    e. Schwann cells

20. Which of the following is not a medial pathway involved in the maintenance of posture?
    a. Reticulospinal tract
    b. Rubrospinal tract
    c. Vestibulospinal tract
    d. Tectospinal tract

21. According to Herrington classification the decerebrate rigidity is characterized by all except:
    a. Rigidity occurs in all the muscles of the body
    b. Increase in the rate of discharge of gamma motor neurons
    c. Increased excitability of the motor neuron pool
    d. Decerebration produces no phenomenon akin to spinal shock

22. True about experimental shame rage:
    a. Occurs in decorticate animals
    b. Is goal directed
    c. Is caused by removal of hypothalamus
    d. Appears slowly and goes slowly

23. The maintenance of posture in a normal human being depends upon:
    a. Integrity of reflex arc
    b. Muscle power
    c. Type of muscle fibre
    d. Joint movements in physiological range

24. The first reflex to occur after recovery of spinal shock:
    a. Stretch reflex
    b. Stepping reflex
    c. Flexor reflex
    d. Postural antigravity reflex

25. Cells present in the cerebellar cortex are all except:
    a. Purkinje
    b. Bipolar
    c. Granule
    d. Golgi

26. Purkinje fibres are inhibitory to:
    a. Deep cerebellar nuclei
    b. Climbing fibres
    c. Basket cells
    d. Spinocerebellar tract

27. Vestibulo-ocular reflex is concerned with:
    a. Paleocerebellum
    b. Neocerebellum
    c. Flocculonodular lobe
    d. Occipital lobe

28. The function of neocerebellum:
    a. Equilibrium maintenance
    b. Servo correction of voluntary movement
    c. Planning and programming of voluntary
    d. Maintenance of muscle tone

29. True about spinocerebellar tract:
    a. Equilibrium
    b. Smoothens and coordinates movement
    c. Learning induced by change in vestibulo-ocular reflex
    d. Planning and programming

30. Which of the following do not carry proprioceptive impulses:
    a. Olivo cerebellar tract
    b. Tecto cerebellar tract
    c. Spino cerebellar tract
    d. Cuneo cerebellar tract

Answers

14. b	15. d	16. b	17. c	18. a	19. a	20. b
21. a	22. a	23. a	24. c	25. b	26. a	27. c
28. c	29. b	30. b				

31. Lesion of the cerebellum cause all of the following *except:*
    a. Incoordination
    b. Intention tremor
    c. Resting tremor
    d. Ataxia

32. Globus pallidus, putamen are present in the:
    a. Pons
    b. Basal ganglia
    c. Cerebellum
    d. Thalamus

33. Glutamate as a neurotransmitter is synthesized in which part of basal ganglia?
    a. Globus pallidus interna
    b. Globus pallidus externa
    c. Subthalamic nucleus
    d. Putamen

34. Which of the following is most prone to hypoxic injury?
    a. Thalamus
    b. Hippocampus
    c. Caudate nucleus
    d. Cerebellum

35. Human brain is more intelligent than monkey's brain due to:
    a. Larger brain
    b. Increase convolutions
    c. Increased brain area compared to body surface area
    d. More blood supply

36. Neurophysiological defects in right lobe involvement all *except:*
    a. Visuospatial defect
    b. Anosognosia
    c. Dyscalculia
    d. Dysgraphia

37. Broca's area is concerned with:
    a. Word formation
    b. Comprehension
    c. Repetition
    d. Reading

38. The processing of short-term memory into long-term memory is done by:
    a. Hippocampus
    b. Neocortex
    c. Amygdala
    d. Prefrontal cortex

39. Striatum damage affects priming:
    a. Procedural memory
    b. Short-term memory
    c. Long-term memory
    d. Explicit memory

40. Associative learning:
    a. Associated with consciousness
    b. Includes skills and habits
    c. Relation of one stimulus with another
    d. Facilitation of recognition of words

41. Reward centre is:
    a. Insula
    b. Putamen
    c. Medial forebrain bundle
    d. Aqueduct of

42. The nucleus involved in Papez circuit:
    a. Pulvinar
    b. Intralaminar
    c. VPL nucleus
    d. Anterior nucleus of thalamus

43. Limbic system is involved in:
    a. Control of emotion
    b. Sexual behaviour
    c. Autonomic functions
    d. All of the above

44. Osmoreceptors are located in:
    a. Supra optic nuclei
    b. Paraventricular nuclei
    c. Anterior hypothalamus
    d. Lateral hypothalamus

45. The primary motor area for shivering:
    a. Cerebrum
    b. Red nucleus
    c. Ventromedial anterior hypothalamus
    d. Dorsomedial posterior hypothalamus

46. All of the following are known functions of hypothalamus *except:*
    a. Temperature regulation
    b. Food intake
    c. Increase in heart rate with exercise
    d. Hypophyseal control

47. Physiological effect in unacclimatized person suddenly exposed to cold:
    a. Tachycardia
    b. Shift of blood from shell to core
    c. Hypertension
    d. Nonshivering thermogenesis

48. In human being least physiological response to low temperature:
    a. Shivering
    b. Vasoconstriction
    c. Piloerection
    d. Release of thyroxine

49. When an individual is resting in a room temperature 21°C, and humidity 80%, the greatest amount of heat lost from body is:
    a. Elevation of body metabolism
    b. Respiration
    c. Radiation and conduction
    d. Vaporization of sweat

50. Under physiological conditions heat acclimatization is accomplished by all *except:*
    a. Decrease renal blood flow
    b. Increase sodium in urine
    c. Increase aldosterone
    d. Excessive sweating

Answers

31. c	32. b	33. c	34. b	35. a	36. c	37. a
38. a	39. a	40. c	41. c	42. d	43. d	44. c
45. d	46. c	47. b	48. c	49. c	50. b	

51. Injection of hypertonic saline in which region of hypothalamus induces thirst?
    a. Posterior region
    b. Paraventricular
    c. Preoptic
    d. Supraoptic

52. Appetite is stimulated by all except:
    a. AGRP
    b. MSH
    c. MCH
    d. Neuropeptide-y

53. Ghrelin false is:
    a. Secreted from oxyntic cells
    b. Increases fat deposition
    c. Stimulates appetite
    d. Secretion increased in anorexia

54. All are true about neuropeptide y except:
    a. Consists of 36 amino acids
    b. Decreases thermogenesis
    c. Decreased in starvation
    d. Same effect as melanocorticotropin

55. True regarding autonomic nervous system:
    a. High integration centre is medulla oblongata
    b. Conduction autonomic fibres is same as in somatic motor fibres
    c. Preganglionic parasympathetic fibres are more lengthy
    d. Ratio of preganglionic to postganglionic is 20:1

56. All are effects of sympathetic stimulation except:
    a. Increase conduction velocity
    b. Increase heart rate
    c. Increase in refractory period
    d. Increase in contractility of heart

57. During fight and fight reaction, which of the following is responsible for increase in local blood flow?
    a. Sympathetic nervous system mediated cholinergic release
    b. Local hormones
    c. Parasympathetic cholinergic
    d. Endocrine factors only

58. Nerve fibres innervating sweat gland secrete:
    a. Nor adrenaline
    b. Acetyl choline
    c. Dopamine
    d. Histamine

59. Cutaneous vasoconstriction is caused by:
    a. Sympathetic adrenergic
    b. Sympathetic cholinergic
    c. Parasympathetic cholinergic
    d. Somatic nerves

60. Vagal stimulation causes all the following except:
    a. Increase in intestinal secretion
    b. Constriction of intestinal musculature
    c. Relaxation of bronchial musculature
    d. Fall in blood pressure

61. Sleep waves in the hippocampal area are:
    a. Delta
    b. Beta
    c. Theta
    d. Alpha

62. Beta forms designate which of the following state of the patient?
    a. Deep anesthesia
    b. Surgical anesthesia
    c. Light, anesthesia, eyes closed, relaxed
    d. Awake/alert state

63. Alpha rhythm is seen in:
    a. Sleep with eyes closed with mind wandering
    b. Mental activity
    c. Awake with eyes open
    d. REM sleep

64. Slow wave sleep is associated with:
    a. Dreaming
    b. Atonia
    c. Sleep walking
    d. Irregular heart beat

65. Key regulators of sleep are located in:
    a. Hypothalamus
    b. Thalamus
    c. Putamen
    d. Limbic cortex

66. All are neuroglial cells except:
    a. Astrocytes
    b. Microglia
    c. Oligodendrocytes
    d. Troposomes

67. Arousal phenomenon is mediated by:
    a. Dorsal column
    b. RAS
    c. Spinothalamic tract
    d. Vestibulocerebellar tract

68. Blood brain barrier is present in all except:
    a. Hebenular nucleus
    b. Subfornical organ
    c. Cerebellum
    d. Pontine nucleus

69. CSF pressure is mainly regulated by:
    a. Rate of CSF formation
    b. Rate of CSF absorption
    c. Cerebral blood flow
    d. Venous pressure

70. Below what pressure CSF absorption stops?
    a. 60 mm
    b. 68 mm
    c. 50 mm
    d. 80 mm

Answers

51. b	52. b	53. b	54. c	55. c	56. c	57. a
58. b	59. a	60. c	61. c	62. d	63. a	64. c
65. a	66. d	67. b	68. b	69. b	70. b	

71. Substance P is increased in response to pain by which of the following?
   a. Mast cells
   b. Plasma cells
   c. Endothelium
   d. Nerve terminals

72. Excitatory neurotransmitter in CNS:
   a. Glycine
   b. Aspartate
   c. Glutamate
   d. Acetylcholine

73. Brain blood supply:
   a. 55 mL/100 gm tissue/min
   b. 400 mL/100 gm tissue/min
   c. 100 mL/100 gm/min
   d. 200 mL/100 gm/min

74. Cerebral blood flow is regulated by all *except:*
   a. Blood pressure
   b. Arterial PCO_2
   c. Potassium ion
   d. Cerebral metabolic rate

75. Increase intracranial pressure is not associated with:
   a. Deterioration of consciousness
   b. Tachycardia
   c. Respiratory depression
   d. Increase in BP

76. Which receptor is associated with mint cold?
   a. TRPM 8
   b. TRPV 1
   c. TRPV 4
   d. All of the above

77. Perception of normal sensory stimuli as painful is called:
   a. Hyperalgesia
   b. Allodynia
   c. Causalgia
   d. Secondary hyperalgesia

78. Bilateral damage to lateral hypothalamus causes:
   a. Hyperthermia
   b. Anorexia
   c. Hyperphagia
   d. Increased sexuality

79. Orexins are implicated in:
   a. Wakefulness
   b. Appetite
   c. Sexual behaviour
   d. Alzheimer's disease

80. Descending motor tract responsible for rapid skilled movements:
   a. Anterior corticospinal tract
   b. Rubrospinal tract
   c. Vestibulospinal tract
   d. Reticulospinal tract

81. Reciprocal inhibition is:
   a. Contraction of agonist with relaxation of antagonist
   b. Contraction of antagonist with relaxation of agonist
   c. Contraction of both agonist and antagonist
   d. Relaxation of both agonist and antagonist

82. Bruxism is associated with which phase of sleep:
   a. REM
   b. NREM 2
   c. NREM 3
   d. NREM 1

83. Assoiciative learning is:
   a. Associated with consciousness
   b. Includes skills and habits
   c. Procedural memory
   d. Facilitation of recognition of words

84. Skinners experiment is associated with:
   a. Unconditional learning
   b. Conditional learning
   c. Operant conditioning
   d. Habituation

85. Left lobe of the brain is mainly associated with:
   a. Agnosia
   b. Art and music
   c. Visuospatial relationship
   d. Written and spoken language

86. Gamma oscillations is EEG are associated with:
   a. Sleep
   b. Awake with eyes open
   c. Attention focused on something
   d. Lesion is brain

87. Function of nuclear bag fibre:
   a. Detect static response
   b. Detect change in transmission
   c. Detect dynamic length change
   d. To contract intrafusal muscle fibre

88. Phantom limb pain is best explained by:
   a. Golgi tendon organ
   b. Weber-Fechner law
   c. Law of projection
   d. Muller's law

89. Clasp-knife effect all are correct *except:*
   a. Hypertonia
   b. Golgi tendon organ
   c. Lengthening reaction
   d. Paccinian corpuscle

90. When a synapse is not facilitated by synaptic relationships between neighboring synapse it is called:
   a. Occlusion
   b. Summation
   c. Delay
   d. Post-tetanic potentiation

91. Itching is produced by:
   a. Type C unmyelinated nerve fibre
   b. Stimulation of paccinian corpuscles
   c. Histamine
   d. Calcitonin G related protein

Answers

71. d	72. c	73. a	74. b	75. b	76. a	77. b
78. b	79. b	80. b	81. a	82. b	83. a	84. c
85. d	86. c	87. c	88. c	89. d	90. a	91. c

92. Cerebellar glomeruli includes all the following *except:*
    a. Mossy fibres
    b. Climbing fibres
    c. Axons of golgi cell
    d. Dendrite of granule cell

93. The nucleus involved in Papez circuit:
    a. Pulvinar
    b. Intralaminar nuclei
    c. Anterior thalamic nuclei
    d. Reticular nuclei

94. EEG waves in the hippocampus:
    a. Alpha
    b. Beta
    c. Theta
    d. Delta

95. When toe is pressed on the ground, the reflex which causes simultaneous flexion and extension of limbs is:
    a. Righting reflexes
    b. Positive righting reflex
    c. Negative righting reflex
    d. Attitudinal reflex

96. Paralysis agitans is accompanied by imbalance of neurotransmitter contents in:
    a. Globus pallidus and substantia nigra
    b. Caudate nucleus and putamen
    c. Striatum and substantia nigra
    d. Caudate nucleus and subthalamic nuclei

97. Baragnosia is associated with lesion of:
    a. Spinothalamic tract
    b. Spinocerebellar tract
    c. Dorsal column
    d. Cuneocerebellar tract

98. Umami taste is due to the activation of _____ receptors:
    a. MGLUR4
    b. Gustducin
    c. HCN
    d. ENAC

99. The neurotransmitter involved in Renshaw cell inhibition:
    a. Glutamate
    b. Nor epinephrine
    c. GABA
    d. Glycine

100. The neurotransmitter used by granule cell in the olfactory bulb is:
    a. Glutamate
    b. GABA
    c. Glycine
    d. Acetyl choline

NEUROPATHOLOGY

101. Which is the marker of choice to characterise primary CNS lymphomas?
    a. CD 10
    b. CD 20
    c. CD 3
    d. Ki 67

102. Anaplastic astrocytoma is characterized by:
    a. Necrosis
    b. Microvascular proliferation
    c. Increased cellularity
    d. Increased mitotic activity

103. Oligodendrogliomas are characterized by all *except:*
    a. Perineuronal satellitosis
    b. Chicken wire calcification
    c. Fried egg appearance of cells
    d. IDH mutations

104. All of the following are embryonal tumors of the CNS *except:*
    a. Atypical teratoid/ rhabdoid tumor
    b. Medulloblastoma
    c. Primitive neuroectodermal tumor
    d. Dysembryoblastic neuroepithelial tumor

105. Criteria for calling a meningioma atypical includes all *except:*
    a. Mitotic activity >4 per 10 high power field
    b. Clear cell histology
    c. Bone invasion
    d. Small cell change

106. Molecular groups of medulloblastoma are classified on the basis of all of the following *except:*
    a. SHH pathway
    b. WNT pathway
    c. KRAS mutations
    d. N-MYC mutations

Answers

92. b	93. c	94. c	95. a	96. c	97. c	98. a
99. d	100. b	101. b	102. d	103. b	104. d	105. c
106. c						

107. Secondary glioblastoma is characterised by all *except*:
    a. Pre-existing low grade glial tumour
    b. P53 mutations
    c. PDGFR mutations
    d. EGFR mutations

108. To assess brain invasion in meningioma which of the following measures can be considered?
    a. Attachment to dura
    b. NF positive neurons
    c. Number of mitosis
    d. Evidence of necrosis

109. All of the following can be positive for GFAP *except*:
    a. Astrocytoma
    b. Ependymoma
    c. Medulloblastoma
    d. Oligodendroglioma

110. Dot-like positivity for epithelial membrane antigen is seen:
    a. Meningioma
    b. Metastatic carcinoma
    c. Ependymoma
    d. Medulloblastoma

111. Fibrous bodies are seen in:
    a. GH producing pituitary adenoma
    b. ACTH producing pituitary adenoma
    c. Prolactinoma
    d. All of the above

112. GNAS mutations are characteristically seen in:
    a. Medulloblastoma
    b. Malignant melanoma
    c. Pituitary adenoma
    d. Meningioma

113. The most common tumor in the posterior fossa is:
    a. Astrocytoma
    b. Medulloblastoma
    c. Oligodendroglioma
    d. Metastatic carcinoma

114. All of the following can present as small round blue cell tumors *except*:
    a. Medulloblastoma
    b. Retinoblastoma
    c. Atypical teratoid/ rhabdoid tumor
    d. Primitive neuroectodermal tumor

115. Soap bubble like appearance of brain parenchyma is seen in which CNS infection?
    a. Tuberculosis
    b. Toxoplasmosis
    c. Cryptococcosis
    d. Prion infections

116. Spongiform change is seen in all *except*:
    a. Creutzfeldt Jacob disease
    b. Fatal familial insomnia
    c. Kuru
    d. Mad cow disease

117. Most common CNS lymphoma is:
    a. Burkitt lymphoma
    b. Centroblastic lymphoma
    c. Immunoblastic lymphoma
    d. Diffuse large B cell lymphoma

118. All of the following can be positive in meningioma *except*:
    a. Progesterone receptor
    b. Vimentin
    c. Epithelial membrane antigen
    d. GFAP

119. Most common tumour to metastasize to brain is from:
    a. Lung
    b. Breast
    c. Skin
    d. Prostate

120. Mutation in which of the following allele predisposes the patient to early onset Alzheimer's disease?
    a. E2
    b. E3
    c. E4
    d. All of the above

121. Differential diagnosis of a cystic lesion in brain with a mural nodule include all of the following *except*:
    a. Hemangioblastoma
    b. Ganglioneuroma
    c. Pilocytic astrocytoma
    d. Medulloblastoma

122. All are true about Rosenthal fibres *except*:
    a. Found in pilocytic astrocytoma
    b. Found in long standing gliosis
    c. Are similar to Lafora bodies
    d. Found in periventricular areas in Alexander's disease

123. BRAF V600E mutations are seen in all *except*:
    a. Pilocytic astrocytoma
    b. Langerhans cell histiocytosis
    c. Hairy cell leukemia
    d. Malignant melanoma

Answers

107. d	108. b	109. c	110. c	111. a	112. c	113. a
114. c	115. c	116. b	117. c>d	118. d	119. a	120. c
121. d	122. c	123. b				

124. All of the following confer a good prognosis to the tumors they are mutated in *except:*
    a. IDH mutations
    b. CDKN2A
    c. P53
    d. 1p/19q codeletion

125. Mesenchymal type of glioblastoma is characterized by:
    a. TP53 mutations
    b. Deletions of NF1 gene
    c. NEFL mutations
    d. CDKN2A

126. Gliomatosis cerebri is considered to be which of the following grades according to WHO?
    a. I
    b. II
    c. III
    d. IV

127. Floating neurons are seen in:
    a. PNET
    b. DNET
    c. Hemangioblastoma
    d. Medulloblastoma

128. Lining of colloid cyst in brain is:
    a. Columnar
    b. Squamous
    c. Cuboidal
    d. Ciliated

129. Gangliogliomas present classically with:
    a. Increased intracranial pressure
    b. Seizures
    c. Visual abnormalities
    d. Cognitive changes

130. Tau proteins accumulation are seen in all:
    a. Alzheimer's disease
    b. Frontotemporal lobar degeneration
    c. Huntington's chorea
    d. Progressive supranuclear palsy

131. Red neurons are seen at what duration post injury?
    a. 4–12 hours
    b. 12–24 hours
    c. 24–48 hours
    d. 3–5 days

132. Neurofibrillary tangles are composed of:
    a. Tau protein
    b. A beta amyloid
    c. Alpha synuclein
    d. All of the above

133. Rosenthal fibres are seen characteristically in which tumor?
    a. Oligodendroglioma
    b. Pilocytic astrocytoma
    c. Medulloblastoma
    d. Glioblastoma

134. Epithelial membrane antigen may be positive in all *except:*
    a. Ependymoma
    b. Meningioma
    c. Metastatic carcinoma
    d. Oligodendroglioma

135. Ependymomas present characteristically with:
    a. Obstructive hydrocephalus
    b. Seizures
    c. Cognitive changes
    d. Behaviour changes

136. All are true about meningioma *except:*
    a. May increase in size with pregnancy
    b. Does not detach easily
    c. Most common site parasaggital convexity
    d. WHO divides them into 3 grades

137. Subependymal giant cell astrocytoma is associated with:
    a. Tuberous sclerosis
    b. Neurofibromatosis
    c. Sturge Weber syndrome
    d. von Hippel Lindau syndrome

138. Which special stain helps to highlight neurofibrillary tangles?
    a. Hematoxylin stain
    b. Bielschowsky stain
    c. Congo red stain
    d. PAS

139. Most common site of neuritic plaques is:
    a. Hippocampus
    b. Amygdala
    c. Entorhinal cortex
    d. Cerebellum

140. Atypical teratoid/rhabdoid tumor is characterized by all of the following *except:*
    a. INI-1 positivity
    b. Chromosome 22 mutations
    c. WHO grade IV
    d. Posterior fossa

Answers

124. c	125. b	126. c	127. b	128. c	129. b	130. c
131. b	132. a	133. b	134. d	135. a	136. b	137. a
138. b	139. a	140. a				

CHAPTER 3

Neurology

AN OVERVIEW OF "WHERE" AND "WHAT" OF THE LESIONS IN NEUROLOGY

THE LOCATION OF LESIONS

Lesions can be located in one or more of the following anatomic sites:
- **Muscles:** In muscle diseases, one sees weakness, sometimes with muscle atrophy. Deep tendon reflexes are usually depressed. Diseases of muscle include the dystrophies, which have specific genetic patterns and stages of onset and may preferentially involve certain muscle groups; and inflammatory disorders of muscle such as polymyositis. Diagnosis may be aided by measuring the level of enzymes (such as creatine phosphokinase) in the serum because damage to muscle fibers may lead to their release. Electromyography and muscle biopsy may help with diagnosis.
- **Motor end-plates:** Disorders of the motor end-plate include myasthenia gravis and the Lambert–Eaton myasthenic syndrome. In these disorders, there is weakness, sometimes accompanied by abnormal fatigability resulting from abnormal function (e.g., decreased effect of acetylcholine [ACh] on the post-junctional muscle or decreased release of ACh) at the neuromuscular junction. Weakness may involve the limbs or trunk or muscles involved in chewing, swallowing, or eye movements. In addition to the characteristic clinical pattern, electromyography may be helpful in diagnosis.
- **Peripheral nerves:** Peripheral nerve lesions may be differentiated from lesions of muscle or motor end-plate by clinical criteria, electrical tests, or biopsy. In many disorders of peripheral nerves, both motor (lower motor neuron) and sensory deficits are present, although in some cases motor or sensory function is impaired in a relatively pure way. In most peripheral neuropathies, functions subserved by the longest axons are impaired first, so that there is a "stocking-and-glove" pattern of sensory loss, together with loss of distal reflexes (such as the ankle jerks) and weakness of distal musculature (i.e., intrinsic muscles of the feet).
- **Roots:** A motor root lesion results in a precise segmental motor deficit, which in some cases (e.g., plexus lesions) is mediated through several nerves. A single sensory deficit may be difficult to diagnose because of the adjacent overlapping dermatomes. When a nerve root carrying axons mediating a deep tendon reflex is affected, the reflex may be depressed. Sensory root symptoms may include increased pain associated with the Valsalva maneuver, the forced expiratory effort caused by laughing, sneezing, or coughing.
- **Spinal cord:** The staggered pattern of decussation of the lateral corticospinal tract, dorsal column–medial lemniscal system, and spinothalamic tracts often permits localization of lesions within the spinal cord. Injury to the spinal cord, at a given level, may result in lower-motor-neuron signs and symptoms at that level, but will result in upper-motor-neuron abnormalities *below* the level of the lesion. Sensation may be impaired below the lesion; thus, the presence of a *sensory level* (i.e., a dermatomal level below which sensation is impaired) can alert the clinician to the possibility of injury to the spinal cord. The injury may be located at the sensory level or above it.
- **Brain stem:** Functional deficits in the long tracts that pass from the brain to the spinal cord or vice versa, together with cranial nerve signs and symptoms, suggest a lesion in the brain stem. As a result of the crowding of numerous fiber tracts and nuclei within the relatively compact brain stem, lesions at particular sites usually result in characteristic *syndromes.* Lesions in the medulla involve the last few cranial nerves, whereas lesions in the pons involve nerves V, VI, and VII, and lesions of the midbrain often involve nerve III and possibly nerve IV.
- **Cerebellum:** Lesions in the cerebellum or its peduncles result in characteristic abnormalities of motor integration. There is usually impaired coordination and decreased muscle tone *ipsilateral* to a lesion in the cerebellar hemisphere.
- **Diencephalon:** Hypothalamic lesions are often complex and can cause endocrinologic disturbances as well as visual abnormalities resulting from compression of neighboring optic tracts. Thalamic lesions often cause sensory dysfunction and

may produce motor deficits as a result of compression of the neighboring internal capsule. Subthalamic lesions may cause abnormal movements such as hemiballismus. Epithalamic lesions are most frequently pineal region tumors, which can compress the cerebral aqueduct, thereby producing hydrocephalus.

- **Subcortical white matter:** The presence of abnormal myelin (leukodystrophy, which is more common in infants and children than in adults) or the destruction of normal myelin (which can be caused by inflammatory disorders such as multiple sclerosis results in abnormal axonal conduction and deficits of function. Disease may be diffuse, focal, or multifocal with a parallel pattern of clinical involvement.
- **Subcortical gray matter (basal ganglia):** A variety of movement disorders, including Parkinson's disease and Huntington's disease, occur from involvement of the basal ganglia. Tremors and other abnormal movements, abnormalities of tone (e.g., cogwheel rigidity in Parkinson's disease), and slowed movements (bradykinesia) are often seen. These disorders often affect the basal ganglia bilaterally, but if there is unilateral disease, the movement disorder will affect the contralateral limbs.
- **Cerebral cortex:** Focal lesions may produce well-circumscribed deficits such as aphasia, the hemi-inattention and neglect syndromes, or Gerstmann's syndrome. In most patients, aphasia is due to the left hemisphere involvement. When the primary motor cortex is involved on one side, for example by a stroke or a tumor, there is usually a "crossed hemiparesis," that is, upper-motor-neuron weakness of the contralateral limbs. Irritative lesions of the cortex may result in seizures, which can be focal or generalized.
- **Meninges:** Hemorrhages in the subarachnoid, subdural, and epidural spaces have characteristic clinical and neuroradiologic features. Subarachnoid hemorrhage is often accompanied by severe headache ("worst headache of my life"). Subdural hemorrhages may occur acutely or chronically and can follow even trivial head injury, especially in elderly patients and young children. Epidural hemorrhages are often rapidly progressive and can produce sudden herniation of the brain. Infection of the subarachnoid space (meningitis) may present with signs of meningeal irritation (e.g., stiff neck) as well as other neurologic deficits, and the diagnosis can often be confirmed by lumbar puncture.
- **Skull, vertebral column, and associated structures:** Associated structures include the intervertebral disks, ligaments, and articulations. For example, metastatic tumors involving the vertebral column can produce spinal cord compression. Trauma often involves the skull and vertebral column as well as the brain and spinal cord.

The Nature of Lesions

The following is a common neuropathologic classification of disorders:

- **Vascular disorders:** Usually, with a sudden onset of signs and symptoms, cerebrovascular disease often occurs in the setting of hypertension. Stenosis or occlusion of the carotid artery in the neck may be responsible. Embolism, from ulcerated plaques in the carotid or from the heart (e.g., in patients with atrial fibrillation) can occlude more distal vessels such as the middle cerebral. Subarachnoid hemorrhage and intraparenchymal hemorrhage (often involving the basal ganglia, thalamus, pons, or cerebellum) occur in patients with hypertension. Subdural and epidural hemorrhages occur as a result of trauma, which can be trivial (and in many cases is not remembered) in the case of subdural hematoma.
- **Trauma:** As previously noted, epidural and subdural hematomas can develop as a result of head injury. In addition, penetrating injuries can directly destroy brain tissue, produce vascular lesions, or introduce infections. Injury to the spine is a common cause of paraplegia and quadriplegia.
- **Tumors:** Primary tumors of the brain and spinal cord, as well as metastases (e.g., from breast, lung, and prostate tumors) produce symptoms by direct invasion (and destruction) of neural tissue, compression of the brain and spinal cord, or compression of the ventricles and cerebral aqueduct, which can lead to hydrocephalus. Classically, tumors of the central nervous system produce subacutely or chronically progressive deterioration, which, in contrast to vascular disorders, progresses over weeks, months, or years. Signs of increased intracranial pressure (e.g., papilledema, sixth nerve palsy) may be present.
- **Infections and inflammations:** These disorders (e.g., meningitis, abscess formation, encephalitis, and granulomas) may be accompanied by fever, especially if the onset is acute. Most infections and inflammations have characteristic signs, symptoms, and causes.
- **Toxic, deficiency, and metabolic disorders:** A variety of intoxications, vitamin deficiencies (e.g., B_{12} deficiency), and enzyme defects leading to abnormal lipid storage in neurons are examples of this heterogeneous group of disorders. Various substances in different amounts (too much or too little) can cause selective lesions involving particular nuclei or tracts. Vitamin B12 deficiency, for example, causes degeneration of axons in the dorsal and lateral columns of the spinal cord.
- **Demyelinating diseases:** Multiple sclerosis is the prototype demyelinating disease. As expected for a disorder characterized by multiple lesions in the white matter, examination often provides evidence for involvement of several sites in the central nervous system. The cerebrospinal fluid (CSF) often shows characteristic abnormalities. Magnetic resonance imaging (MRI) scans are very useful in confirming the diagnosis.
- **Degenerative diseases:** This heterogeneous group of diseases for which the cause has not yet been determined includes spinal, cerebellar, subcortical, and cortical degenerative disorders that are often characterized by specific functional deficits.

- **Congenital malformations and perinatal disorders:** Exogenous factors (e.g., infection or radiation of the motor cortex) or genetic and chromosomal factors can cause abnormalities of the brain or spinal cord in newborn infants. Hydrocephalus, Chiari malformation, cortical lesions, cerebral palsy, neural tumors, vascular abnormalities, and other syndromes may become apparent after birth.
- **Neuromuscular disorders:** This group includes muscular dystrophies, congenital myopathies, neuromuscular junction disorders, transmitter deficiencies, and nerve lesions or neuropathies (inflammation, degeneration, and demyelination).

Clinical diagnosis in neurology requires several steps:
- Recognition of impaired function
- Identification of what site of the nervous system has been affected, that is, localization
- Definition of the most likely etiology, often resulting in a differential diagnostic list
- Use of ancillary procedures to determine which of the different possible etiologies is present in the given patient

SEIZURES AND EPILEPSY

A *seizure* is a paroxysmal event due to abnormal, excessive, hypersynchronous discharges from an aggregate of central nervous system (CNS) neurons.

Epilepsy describes a condition in which a person has *recurrent* seizures due to a chronic, underlying process. This definition implies that a person with a single seizure, or recurrent seizures due to correctable or avoidable circumstances, does not necessarily have epilepsy. Epilepsy refers to a clinical phenomenon rather than a single disease entity, since there are many forms and causes of epilepsy.

International League against Epilepsy (ILAE) Classification 1981

1. **Partial seizures**
    a. Simple partial seizures (with motor, sensory, autonomic, or psychic signs)
    b. Complex partial seizures
    c. Partial seizures with secondary generalization
2. **Primarily generalized seizures**
    a. Absence (petit mal)
    b. Tonic-clonic (grand mal)
    c. Tonic
    d. Atonic
    e. Myoclonic
3. **Unclassified seizures**
    a. Neonatal seizures
    b. Infantile spasms

Partial Seizures

- *Simple partial seizure*—consciousness is fully preserved
- *Complex partial seizure*—consciousness is impaired
- *Partial seizures with secondary generalization*—seizures that begin as partial seizures and then spread diffusely throughout the cortex

Simple Partial Seizures

Simple partial seizures cause motor, sensory, autonomic, or psychic symptoms without an obvious alteration in consciousness. These movements are typically clonic (i.e., repetitive, flexion/extension movements) at a frequency of ~2–3 Hz; pure tonic posturing may be seen as well. An ictal EEG may show abnormal discharges in a very limited region over the appropriate area of cerebral cortex if the seizure focus involves the cerebral convexity.

Features

- The abnormal motor movements may begin in a very restricted region such as the fingers and gradually progress (over seconds to minutes) to include a larger portion of the extremity. This phenomenon is known as a "Jacksonian march," represents the spread of seizure activity over a progressively larger region of motor cortex.
- Patients may experience a localized paresis (Todd's paralysis) for minutes to many hours in the involved region following the seizure.
- The seizure may continue for hours or days termed *epilepsia partialis continua*, is often refractory to medical therapy.

Complex Partial Seizures

Complex partial seizures are characterized by focal seizure activity accompanied by a transient impairment of the patient's ability to maintain normal contact with the environment. The seizures frequently begin with an aura (i.e., a simple partial seizure) that is stereotypic for the patient. The start of the ictal phase is often a sudden behavioral arrest or motionless stare, which marks the onset of the period of amnesia. The behavioral arrest is usually accompanied by *automatisms*, which are involuntary, automatic behaviors that have a wide range of manifestations. The routine interictal EEG in patients with complex partial seizures is often normal or may show brief discharges termed *epileptiform spikes*, or *sharp waves*.

Partial Seizures with Secondary Generalization

Partial seizures can spread to involve both cerebral hemispheres and produce a generalized seizure, usually of the tonic-clonic variety. Secondary generalization is observed frequently following simple partial seizures, especially those with a focus in the frontal lobe, but may also be associated with partial seizures occurring elsewhere in the brain.

Generalized Seizures

Absence Seizures (Petit Mal)

Absence seizures are characterized by sudden, brief lapses of consciousness without loss of postural control. The seizure typically lasts for only seconds, consciousness returns as suddenly as it was lost, and there is no postictal confusion. Absence seizures usually begin in childhood (ages 4–8) or early adolescence and are the main seizure type in 15–20% of children with epilepsy. TOC – ethosuximide followed by valproate.

The electrophysiologic hallmark of typical absence seizures is a generalized, symmetric, 3-Hz spike-and-wave discharge that begins and ends suddenly, superimposed on a normal EEG background.

Generalized, Tonic-Clonic Seizures (Grand Mal)

- The most common seizure type resulting from metabolic derangements and are therefore frequently encountered in many different clinical settings. The initial phase of the seizure is usually tonic contraction of muscles throughout the body, accounting for a number of the classic features of the event. Tonic contraction of the muscles of expiration and the larynx at the onset will produce a loud moan or "ictal cry". Contraction of the jaw muscles may cause biting of the tongue. A marked enhancement of sympathetic tone leads to increases in heart rate, bloodpressure, and pupillary size. After 10–20 s, the tonic phase of the seizure typically evolves into the clonic phase, produced by the superimposition of periods of muscle relaxation on the tonic muscle contraction. Bladder or bowel incontinence may occur at this point. Patients gradually regain consciousness over minutes to hours, and during this transition there is typically a period of postictal confusion.
- The EEG during the tonic phase of the seizure shows a progressive increase in generalized low-voltage fast activity, followed by generalized high-amplitude, polyspike discharges. In the clonic phase, the high-amplitude activity is typically interrupted by slow waves to create a spike-and-wave pattern. The postictal EEG shows diffuse slowing that gradually recovers as the patient awakens.

Atonic Seizures

Atonic seizures are characterized by sudden loss of postural muscle tone lasting 1–2 s. Consciousness is briefly impaired, but there is usually no postictal confusion. The EEG shows brief, generalized spike-and-wave discharges followed immediately by diffuse slow waves that correlate with the loss of muscle tone.

Myoclonic Seizures

- Myoclonus is a sudden and brief muscle contraction that may involve one part of the body or the entire body. Myoclonic seizures are considered to be true epileptic events since they are caused by cortical (versus subcortical or spinal) dysfunction. The EEG may show bilaterally synchronous spike-and-wave discharges synchronized with the myoclonus, although these can be obscured by movement artifact.
- Juvenile myoclonic epilepsy (JME) is a generalized seizure disorder of unknown cause that appears in early adolescence and is usually characterized by bilateral myoclonic jerks that may be single or repetitive. The myoclonic seizures are most frequent in the morning after awakening and can be provoked by sleep deprivation. Automatism is not a feature of JME.

Epilepsy Syndromes

- Autosomal dominant nocturnal frontal lobe epilepsy (ADNFLE)
- Benign familial neonatal convulsions (BFNC)
    - Autosomal dominant
        Voltage-dependent potassium channel *KCNQ2* (Chromosome 20)
    - Voltage-dependent potassium channel *KCNQ3* (Chromosome 8)
- Generalized epilepsy with febrile seizures plus (GEFS+)
    - Autosomal dominant

- Sodium channel *SCN1B* (chromosome 19)
- Sodium channel *SCN1A* (chromosome 2)
- Sodium channel *SCN2A*
- GABAA (chromosome 5)
- Autosomal dominant partial epilepsy with auditory features (ADPEAF)
  - *LGI1*, leucine-rich, glioma-inactivated 1 gene (Chromosome 10)
- Progressive myoclonus epilepsy (PME) (Unverricht-Lundborg disease)
- Progressive myoclonus epilepsy (Lafora's disease)

Lennox-Gastaut Syndrome
- Multiple seizure types (usually including generalized tonic-clonic, atonic, and atypical absence seizures)
- An EEG showing slow (<3 Hz) spike-and-wave discharges and a variety of other abnormalities
- Impaired cognitive function in most but not all cases.

Mesial Temporal Lobe Epilepsy Syndrome

Mesial temporal lobe epilepsy (MTLE) is the most common syndrome associated with complex partial seizures. Laboratory studies show Unilateral or bilateral anterior temporal spikes on EEG, Hypometabolism on interictal PET, Hypoperfusion on interictal SPECT and Material-specific memory deficits on intracranial amobarbital (Wada) test.
MRI show Small hippocampus with increased signal on T2-weighted sequences, Small temporal lobe with Enlarged temporal horn.

Localizing of seizure:

TLE: epigastric aura, followed by a quiet period of unresponsiveness with staring, oral automatisms like lip smacking, manual automatism like picking at sheets/ clothes, contralateral dystonic posturing, post ictal confusion and lethargy. If the origin of the seizure is from dominant hemisphere, there may be transient aphasia with delayed recovery of language

FLE: seizure will occur in sleep with n prior warning; patient will be restless and show prominent bilateral limb movements which will end quickly with immediate recovery; this can recur several times in the same night

OLE: often have visual aura and may progress into an FLE or TLE

PLE: least common; can have sensory aura, may mimic FLE

CAUSES OF SEIZURES

Neonates (<1 month)	Perinatal hypoxia and ischemia, Intracranial hemorrhage and trauma, Acute CNS infection, Metabolic disturbances (hypoglycemia, hypocalcemia, hypomagnesemia, pyridoxine deficiency), Drug withdrawal, Developmental disorders and Genetic disorders
Infants and children (>1 months and <12 years)	Febrile seizures, Genetic disorders (metabolic, degenerative, primary epilepsy syndromes), CNS infection, Developmental disorders and Trauma
Adolescents (12–18 years)	Trauma, Genetic disorders, Infection, Brain tumor and Illicit drug use
Young adults (18–35 years)	Trauma, Alcohol withdrawal, Illicit drug use, Brain tumor
Older adults (>35 years)	Cerebrovascular disease, Brain tumor, Alcohol withdrawal, Metabolic disorders (uremia, hepatic failure, electrolyte abnormalities, hypoglycemia), Alzheimer's disease and other degenerative CNS diseases

MECHANISMS OF SEIZURE INITIATION AND PROPAGATION

- *Seizure initiation* phase - characterized by two concurrent events in an aggregate of neurons:
  1. High-frequency bursts of action potentials and
  2. Hypersynchronization.
- *Seizure propagation* phase
  Epileptogenesis refers to the transformation of a normal neuronal network into one that is chronically hyperexcitable. There is often a delay of months to years between an initial CNS injury such as trauma, stroke, or infection and the first seizure. The injury appears to initiate a process that gradually lowers the seizure threshold in the affected region until a spontaneous seizure occurs.

Treatment
- Treatment of underlying conditions
- Avoidance of precipitating factors
- Antiepileptic drug therapy – discussed in the neuropharmacology section.

Refractory Epilepsy

Approximately 20–30% of patients with epilepsy are resistant to medical therapy despite efforts to find an effective combination of antiepileptic drugs. The most common surgical procedure for patients with temporal lobe epilepsy involves resection of the anteromedial temporal lobe (temporal lobectomy) or a more limited removal of the underlying hippocampus and amygdala (amygdalohippocampectomy). Focal seizures arising from extratemporal regions may be abolished by a focal neocortical resection with precise removal of an identified lesion (lesionectomy). Preliminary studies suggest that stereotactic radiosurgery may be effective in certain partial seizure disorders.

Status Epilepticus

Status epilepticus refers to continuous seizures or repetitive, discrete seizures with impaired consciousness in the interictal period. Status epilepticus has numerous subtypes, including generalized convulsive status epilepticus (GCSE) (e.g., persistent, generalized electrographic seizures, coma, and tonic-clonic movements), and nonconvulsive status epilepticus (e.g., persistent absence seizures or partial seizures, confusion or partially impaired consciousness, and minimal motor abnormalities). The duration of seizure activity sufficient to meet the definition of status epilepticus has traditionally been specified as 15–30 min. GCSE is an emergency and must be treated immediately.

Order followed for management of status epilepticus:

- Assess airway, breathing
- Give oxygen, establish i.v line, estimate blood glucose
- Specific therapy – Diazepam or Lorazepam i.v, repeat after 10 min if seizure continues
- Phenytoin or fosphenytoin i.v
- IV Phenobarbital
- IM paraldehyde
- Midazolam infusion
- Phenobarbital coma.

PARKINSON'S DISEASE

A group of progressive neurodegenerative disorders characterized by the clinical features of Parkinsonism, include bradykinesia (a paucity and slowness of movement), rest tremor, muscular rigidity, shuffling gait, and flexed posture. Nearly all forms of Parkinsonism result from a reduction of dopaminergic transmission within the basal ganglia.

GENETIC CONSIDERATIONS

Genetic factors play an important role in many forms of PD. Genes are involved in cellular processes that include protein ubiquitination and degradation via the proteasomal system, response to oxidative stress, mitochondrial function, protein phosphorylation, and protein folding. These genes that, when mutated, lead to dopaminergic cell loss. Eight genes have been clearly linked to familial forms of PD (PARK 1-8).

Locus	Gene	Protein	Function	Inheritance
PARK1	SNCA	Alpha synuclein	Uncertain;? vesicle trafficking	AD
PARK2	PRKN	Parkin	E3 ubiquitin ligase	AR
PARK4	SNCA	Alpha synuclein (Triplication or duplication)	Uncertain;? vesicle trafficking	AD
PARK5	UCH-L1	UCH-L1 (Ubiquitin carboxy-terminal hydroxylase L1)	Proteosomal processing	AD
PARK6	PINK1	PINK1	Mitochondrial kinase	AR
PARK7	DJ-1	DJ-1	Oxidative stress response	AR
PARK8	LRRK2	Dardarin	Cytosolic kinase	AD

Pathology

- Gross examination of the brain in PD reveals mild frontal atrophy with loss of the normal dark melanin pigment of the midbrain
- Microscopically there is degeneration of the dopaminergic cells with the presence of Lewy bodies (LBs) in the remaining neurons and processes of the substantia nigra pars compacta (SNpc); other brainstem nuclei; and regions such as the medial temporal, limbic, and frontal cortices
- LBs have a high concentration of alpha synuclein and are the pathologic hallmark of the disorder.

- Pathology appears first in the anterior olfactory nuclei and lower brainstem (glossopharyngeal and vagal nerve nuclei), with ascending brainstem involvement of the locus coeruleus, n. gigantocellularis, and the raphe, before extending to the magnocellular nuclei of the basal forebrain, the central nucleus of the amygdala, and the SNpc. Further progression extends to the thalamus and cerebral cortex.
- The biochemical consequence of dopaminergic cell loss in the SNpc is gradual denervation of the striatum, the main target projection for the SNpc neurons. Other target regions of these neurons include the intralaminar and parafascicular nuclei of the thalamus, the globus pallidus, and the subthalamic nucleus (STN). Symptoms develop when striatal dopamine depletion reaches 50–70% of normal.

Pathogenesis

- Nigral dopamine neurons and other cells die from a combination of factors.
    - Genetic vulnerability (e.g., abnormal processing or folding of alpha-synuclein)
    - Oxidative stress – by free radicals produced by the metabolism of dopamine and melanin.
    - Proteasomal dysfunction
    - Abnormal kinase activity
    - Environmental factors, most of which have yet to be identified.

Clinical Features

A diagnosis of PD can be made with at least two of the three cardinal signs—rest tremor, rigidity, and bradykinesia. A unilateral and gradual onset of symptoms further supports the diagnosis. Masked facies, decreased eye blinking, stooped posture, and decreased arm swing are associated.

- **Motor Features**
    - Bradykinesia—interferes with all aspects of daily living ; Fine motor control is also impaired, as evidenced by decreased manual dexterity and micrographia
    - Rest tremor—at a frequency of 4–6 Hz, typically appears unilaterally, first distally, involving the digits and wrist, where it may have a "pill-rolling" character.
    - Rigidity—felt as a uniform resistance to passive movement about a joint throughout the full range of motion, accompanied by a characteristic "plastic" quality to the movement. Brief, regular interruptions of resistance during passive movement, due to subclinical tremor, may give rise to a "cogwheeling" sensation
    - Gait disturbance—with shuffling short steps and a tendency to turn en bloc is a prominent feature of PD. Festinating gait, a classic sign of Parkinsonism, results from the combination of flexed posture and loss of postural reflexes, which cause the patient to accelerate in an effort to "catch up" with the body's center of gravity. Freezing of gait, a feature of more advanced PD, occurs commonly at the onset of locomotion (start hesitation), when attempting to change direction or turn around.
- **Non-Motor Features**
    - Non-motor aspects of PD include depression and anxiety, cognitive impairment, sleep disturbances, sensory abnormalities and pain, loss of smell (anosmia), and disturbances of autonomic function
    - Sensory symptoms often manifest as a distressing sensation of inner restlessness presumed to be a form of akathisia
    - Sleep disorders and impaired daytime alertness are common
    - Autonomic dysfunction can produce diverse manifestations, including orthostatic hypotension, constipation, urinary urgency and frequency, excessive sweating, and seborrhea
- **Neuropsychiatric Symptoms**
    - Changes in mood, cognition, and behavior are common accompaniments
    - Depression can occur at any phase of the illness
    - Mild or moderate cognitive abnormalities occur in the later stages of the illness and present as frontal lobe dysfunction.
    - Psychotic symptoms like visual illusions and formed visual hallucinations both with retained insight
    - Insidious behavioral disturbances referred to collectively as *impulse control disorders* (ICDs); include pathologic gambling, hypersexuality, compulsive shopping, and compulsive eating and are associated primarily with the use of dopaminergic agents.

DIFFERENTIAL DIAGNOSIS OF PARKINSONISM

Primary Parkinsonism

- Disorders associated with alpha-synuclein pathology
    - Multiple system atrophies—Striatonigral degeneration; Olivopontocerebellar atrophy; Shy-Drager syndrome
    - Dementia with Lewy bodies
- Disorders associated with primary tau pathology
    - Progressive supranuclear palsy; Frontotemporal dementia

- Disorders associated with primary amyloid pathology
  - Alzheimer's disease with parkinsonism
- Genetically mediated disorders with occasional Parkinsonian features
  - Wilson's disease
  - Chédiak-Higashi syndrome
  - X-linked dystonia-parkinsonism (DYT3)
  - Fragile X premutation associated ataxia-tremor-parkinsonism syndrome
  - Huntington's disease (Westphal variant)
- Miscellaneous
  - Vascular parkinsonism
  - Normal pressure hydrocephalus

Secondary Parkinsonism

- Repeated head trauma
- Infectious and postinfectious diseases Eg: Postencephalitic PD
- Metabolic conditions-Hypoparathyroidism or pseudohypoparathyroidism with basal ganglia calcifications
- Drugs-Neuroleptics, Dopamine-depleting agents, alpha-Methyldopa, etc.
- Toxins-1-Methyl-1,2,4,6 tetrahydropyridine (MPTP), Manganese, Cyanide, etc.

Treatment

See under Neuropharmacology section for drugs.

Neuroprotective Therapy

- Coenzyme Q_{10}, an antioxidant and a cofactor of complex I of the mitochondrial oxidative chain, has been shown to have neuroprotective effects.
- Other agents under study are nitric oxide synthetase inhibitors and antiapoptotic agents such as Jun N-terminal kinase inhibitors and desmethylselegiline

Surgical Treatments

- The most common indications for surgery in PD are intractable tremor and drug-induced motor fluctuations or dyskinesias. The best candidates are patients with clear levodopa-responsive parkinsonism who are free of significant dementia or psychiatric comorbidities.
- Deep brain stimulation (DBS) is most often performed bilaterally and simultaneously, but unilateral DBS can be highly effective for asymmetric cases.
- Basis for improvement appears to be the replacement of abnormal neural activity by a more tolerable pattern of activity.

Neurotransplantation

- Approaches are still purely investigational like fetal cell transplantation, using genetically engineered retinal epithelial cells in gelatin capsules to ensure their survival following implantation into the putamen and direct infusion of glial cell–derived neurotrophic factor (GDNF) to the putamen.

PARKINSONIAN DISORDERS

Multiple System Atrophy

Comprises a group of sporadic disorders characterized by varying degrees of Parkinsonism with cerebellar, corticospinal, and autonomic dysfunction. The unifying pathologic hallmark is the presence of alpha-synuclein-positive inclusions located in various brain regions. Disorders under MSA have now been reclassified as *striatonigral degeneration* (SND), *olivopontocerebellar atrophy* (OPCA), and *progressive autonomic failure* (PAF), either without parkinsonism or with parkinsonism (Shy-Drager syndrome).

- With disease progression, most of patients exhibit Parkinsonian signs and signs of autonomic failure; with upper motor neuron signs. Tremor is common, but unlike in PD, this and other Parkinsonian signs are more likely to present symmetrically. Parkinsonian symptoms are typically poorly responsive to dopaminergic therapy, although some patients may respond favorably for years.
- Corticospinal signs consist of spasticity, involving the legs more than the arms, and pseudobulbar palsy. This aspect of the illness may mimic primary lateral sclerosis with lower motor neurons being occasionally involved.

- Signs of autonomic failure include orthostatic hypotension, leg swelling not due to drug therapy, changes in sweating patterns, and autonomic storms with diaphoresis and flushing. Orthostatic hypotension can present with dizziness, faintness, or syncope
- In MSA LB's take the form of glial alpha-synuclein-positive intracytoplasmic inclusions in the substantia nigra, putamen, inferior olives, pontine nuclei, pigmented nuclei of the brainstem, intermediolateral nucleus of the spinal cord, and the cerebellum.

Progressive Supranuclear Palsy

A sporadic neurodegenerative disorder of unknown etiology associated with tau pathology which progresses more rapidly than PD, with death in 5–10 years. Risk factors include head trauma, vascular disease, dietary exposure to benzyl-tetrahydroisoquinolines (TIQ, reticuline), and beta-carbolines.
- Characterized by akinetic rigid parkinsonism, dizziness, unsteadiness, slowness, falls, and pseudobulbar dysarthria
- Supranuclear eye movement abnormalities affecting downgaze occur first, followed by variable limitations of upward and horizontal eye movement. The vestibular ocular reflex ("doll's eyes" maneuver) and the Bell's reflex remain intact.
- PSP is characterized by deposition of neurofibrillary tangles histochemically positive for tau (mostly 4-repeat tau) and negative for amyloid or alpha-synuclein. The deposits are associated with varying degrees of degeneration in the brainstem, basal ganglia, and cerebellum. There is loss of dopamine and dopamine receptors due to intrinsic striatal damage.
- Brain MRI reveals midbrain atrophy (superior colliculus), and PET studies show symmetric frontal and striatal hypometabolism.

Corticobasal Degeneration (CBD)

- It is a sporadic tauopathy which is less common but having a broader range of clinical presentations than PSP.
- The "alien limb" phenomenon, consisting of involuntary purposeful movements of a hand or limb, is a characteristic sign.
- The disorder progresses to become bilateral over 2–5 years, leading to total incapacity with, ultimately, paraplegia in flexion.
- Cases present with frontotemporal dementia or progressive aphasia, followed by asymmetric cortical sensory signs, including abnormalities of graphesthesia and astereognosis.
- CBD is a focal cortical degenerative process with asymmetric pathology and volume loss in the parietal and frontal regions. Histologically, gliosis and swollen (ballooned) achromatic neurons and neuronal loss are present in these cortical regions as well as in the nigra, caudate, putamen, and thalamus
- Brain MRI reveals focal cortical loss in the contralateral superior frontal and parietal lobes with corresponding hypometabolic changes on PET scan as well as hyperintense signal abnormalities in white matter and sometimes atrophy of the corpus callosum.

Drug-Induced Parkinsonism

Typically presents bilaterally with bradykinesia or tremor. It is commonly due to neuroleptics, some atypical antipsychotics, lithium carbonate, or antiemetic agents (especially metoclopramide). The severity of the Parkinsonian symptoms usually correlates with the dose or exposure to a medication or toxin. If due to medication, the symptoms tend to disappear within days to weeks after stopping the offending agent. It may respond to anticholinergic agents, amantadine, and levodopa.

Vascular Parkinsonism

Patients with vascular parkinsonism exhibit an akinetic-rigid syndrome with short mincing steps without tremor associated with upper motor neuron signs, pseudobulbar palsy, or dementia. Imaging studies are heterogeneous and may reveal basal ganglia lacunes or multiple infarcts. The hypertensive and diabetic microangiopathy and diffuse white matter disease are common causes.

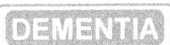

Dementia is a syndrome with many causes. It is defined as an acquired deterioration in cognitive abilities that impairs the successful performance of activities of daily living. Memory is the most common cognitive ability lost with dementia; 10% of persons >70 and 20–40% of individuals >85 have clinically identifiable memory loss. In addition to memory, other mental faculties are also affected in dementia; these include language, visuospatial ability, calculation, judgment, and problem solving. Neuropsychiatric and social deficits also develop in many dementia syndromes, resulting in depression, withdrawal, hallucinations, delusions, agitation, insomnia, and disinhibition. The most common forms of dementia are progressive, but some dementing illnesses are static and unchanging or fluctuate dramatically from day to day. Most diagnoses of dementia require some sort of memory deficit, although there are many dementias, such as frontotemporal dementia, where memory loss is not a presenting feature.

FUNCTIONAL ANATOMY OF THE DEMENTIAS

- Dementia results from the disruption of cerebral neuronal circuits; the quantity of neuronal loss and the location of affected regions are factors that combine to cause the specific disorder. Behavior and mood are modulated by noradrenergic, serotonergic, and dopaminergic pathways, while acetylcholine seems to be particularly important for memory. Therefore, the loss of cholinergic neurons in Alzheimer's disease (AD) may underlie the memory impairment, while in patients with non-AD dementias, the loss of serotonergic and glutaminergic neurons causes primarily behavioral symptoms, leaving memory relatively spared. Neurotrophins are also postulated to play a role in memory function, in part by preserving cholinergic neurons, and therefore represent a pharmacologic pathway toward slowing or reversing the effects of AD.
- Dementias have anatomically specific patterns of neuronal degeneration that dictate the clinical symptomatology. AD begins in the entorhinal cortex, spreads to the hippocampus, and then moves to posterior temporal and parietal neocortex, eventually causing a relatively diffuse degeneration throughout the cerebral cortex. *Multi-infarct dementia* is associated with focal damage in a random patchwork of cortical regions. Diffuse white matter damage may disrupt intracerebral connections and cause dementia syndromes similar to those associated with leukodystrophies, multiple sclerosis, and Binswanger's disease. Subcortical structures, including the caudate, putamen, thalamus, and substantia nigra, also modulate cognition and behavior in ways that are not yet well understood. The effect that these patterns of cortical degeneration have on disease symptomatology is clear: AD primarily presents as memory loss and is often associated with aphasia or other disturbances of language. In contrast, patients with frontal lobe or subcortical dementias such as *frontotemporal dementia* (FTD) or *Huntington's disease* (HD) are less likely to begin with memory problems and more likely to have difficulties with attention, judgment, awareness, and behavior.
- Lesions of specific cortical-subcortical pathways have equally specific effects on behavior. The dorsolateral prefrontal cortex has connections with dorsolateral caudate, globus pallidus, and thalamus. Lesions of these pathways result in poor organization and planning, decreased cognitive flexibility, and impaired judgment. The lateral orbital frontal cortex connects with the ventromedial caudate, globus pallidus, and thalamus. Lesions of these connections cause irritability, impulsiveness, and distractibility. The anterior cingulate cortex connects with the nucleus accumbens, globus pallidus, and thalamus. Interruption of these connections produces apathy and poverty of speech or even akinetic mutism.

THE CAUSES OF DEMENTIA

- AD is the most common cause of dementia in Western countries, representing more than half of demented patients.
- Vascular disease is the second most common cause of dementia.
- Dementia associated with Parkinson's disease (PD) is the next most common category, and in many instances these patients suffer from dementia with Lewy bodies (DLB). In patients under the age of 60, FTD rivals AD as the most common cause of dementia. Chronic intoxications, including those resulting from alcohol and prescription drugs, are an important and often treatable cause of dementia. The classification of dementing illnesses into two broad groups of reversible and irreversible disorders is a useful approach to the differential diagnosis of dementia.

GENERAL AND NEUROLOGIC EXAMINATION

- AD does not affect motor systems until later in the course.
- In contrast, FTD patients often develop axial rigidity, supranuclear gaze palsy.
- In DLB, initial symptoms may be the new onset of a Parkinsonian syndrome (resting tremor, cogwheel rigidity, bradykinesia, festinating gait) with the dementia following later, or vice versa.
- Corticobasal degeneration (CBD) is associated with dystonia, alien hand, and asymmetric extrapyramidal, pyramidal, or sensory deficits or myoclonus.
- Progressive supranuclear palsy (PSP) is associated with unexplained falls, axial rigidity, dysphagia, and vertical gaze deficits.
- CJD is suggested by the presence of diffuse rigidity, an akinetic state, and myoclonus.
- Hemiparesis or other focal neurologic deficits may occur in multi-infarct dementia or brain tumor. Dementia with a myelopathy and peripheral neuropathy suggests vitamin B_{12} deficiency. A peripheral neuropathy could also indicate an underlying vitamin deficiency or heavy metal intoxication. Dry, cool skin, hair loss, and bradycardia suggest hypothyroidism. Confusion associated with repetitive stereotyped movements may indicate ongoing seizure activity. Hearing impairment or visual loss may produce confusion and disorientation misinterpreted as dementia. Such sensory deficits are common in the elderly but can be a manifestation of mitochondrial disorders.

COGNITIVE AND NEUROPSYCHIATRIC EXAMINATION

- Brief screening tools such as the mini-mental state examination (MMSE) help to confirm the presence of cognitive impairment and to follow the progression of dementia. The MMSE, an easily administered 30-point test of cognitive function, contains tests of orientation, working memory (e.g., spell *world* backwards), episodic memory (orientation and recall), language comprehension, naming, and copying.
- Deficits in verbal or visual episodic memory are often the first neuropsychological abnormalities seen with AD, and tasks that require the patient to recall a long list of words or a series of pictures after a predetermined delay will demonstrate deficits in most AD patients. In FTD, the earliest deficits often involve frontal executive or language (speech or naming) function. DLB patients have more severe deficits in visuospatial function but do better on episodic memory tasks than patients with AD. Patients with vascular dementia often demonstrate a mixture of frontal executive and visuospatial deficits. In delirium, deficits tend to fall in the area of attention, working memory, and frontal function.

NEUROIMAGING STUDIES

- It will identify primary and secondary neoplasms, locate areas of infarction, diagnose subdural hematomas, and suggest NPH or diffuse white matter disease.
- They also lend support to the diagnosis of AD, especially if there is hippocampal atrophy in addition to diffuse cortical atrophy. Focal frontal and/or anterior temporal atrophy suggests FTD.
- The use of diffusion-weighted imaging with MRI will detect abnormalities in the cortical ribbon and basal ganglia in the vast majority of patients with CJD.
- Large white-matter abnormalities correlate with a vascular etiology for dementia.
- Single photon emission computed tomography (SPECT) and PET scanning will show temporal-parietal hypoperfusion or hypometabolism in AD and frontotemporal hypoperfusion or hypometabolism in FTD, but most of these changes reflect atrophy. Recently, amyloid imaging has shown promise for the diagnosis of AD.
- EEG is rarely helpful except to suggest CJD (repetitive bursts of diffuse high voltage sharp waves) or an underlying nonconvulsive seizure disorder (epileptiform discharges).
- Brain biopsy (including meninges) is not advised except to diagnose vasculitis, potentially treatable neoplasms, unusual infections, or systemic disorders such as vasculitis or sarcoid, or in young persons where the diagnosis is uncertain.
- Angiography should be considered when cerebral vasculitis is a possible cause of the dementia.

Disease	Symptoms	Mental status	Neuropsychiatry	Imaging
AD	Memory loss	Episodic memory loss	Initially normal	Entorhinal cortex and hippocampal atrophy
FTD	Apathy; poor judgment/ insight, speech/language; hyperorality	Frontal/executive, language	Apathy, disinhibition, hyperorality, euphoria, depression	Frontal and/or temporal atrophy; spares posterior parietal lobe
DLB	Visual hallucinations, REM sleep disorder, delirium, Capgras' syndrome, parkinsonism	Drawing and frontal/executive; spares memory	Visual hallucinations, depression, sleep disorder, delusions	Posterior parietal atrophy; hippocampi larger than in AD
CJD	Dementia, mood, anxiety, movement disorders	Variable, frontal/executive, focal cortical, memory	Depression, anxiety	Cortical ribboning and basal ganglia or thalamus hyperintensity on diffusion/flare MRI
Vascular	Often but not always sudden; variable; apathy, falls, focal weakness	Frontal/executive, cognitive slowing	Apathy, delusions, anxiety	Cortical and/or subcortical infarctions, confluent white matter disease

CLINICAL DIFFERENTIATION OF DEMENTIAS

Alzheimer's Disease

AD most often presents with subtle onset of memory loss followed by a slowly progressive dementia that has a course of several years. Pathologically, there is diffuse atrophy of the cerebral cortex with secondary enlargement of the ventricular system. Microscopically, there are neuritic plaques containing A-beta 42 amyloid, silver-staining neurofibrillary tangles (NFTs) in neuronal cytoplasm, and accumulation of A-beta 42 amyloid in arterial walls of cerebral blood vessels. The identification of four different susceptibility genes for AD has provided a foundation for rapid progress in understanding AD's biologic basis.

Clinical Manifestations
- The cognitive changes with AD tend to follow a characteristic pattern, beginning with memory impairment and spreading to language and visuospatial deficits.
- Some patients are unaware of these difficulties (*anosognosia*), while others have considerable insight. In the middle stages of AD, the patient is unable to work, is easily lost and confused, and requires daily supervision. Social graces, routine behavior, and superficial conversation may be surprisingly intact.
- Language becomes impaired—first naming, then comprehension, and finally fluency. In some patients, *aphasia* is an early and prominent feature. Word finding difficulties and circumlocution may be a problem even when formal testing demonstrates intact naming and fluency. *Apraxia* emerges, and patients have trouble performing sequential motor tasks. Visuospatial deficits begin to interfere with dressing, eating, solving simple puzzles, and copying geometric figures. Patients may be unable to do simple calculations or tell time.
- In the late stages of the disease, some persons remain ambulatory but wander aimlessly. Loss of judgment, reason, and cognitive abilities is inevitable. Delusions are common and usually simple in quality, such as delusions of theft, infidelity, or misidentification. Few of AD patients develop *Capgras' syndrome*, believing that a caregiver has been replaced by an impostor.

Differential Diagnosis
- Early in the disease course, other etiologies of dementia should be excluded. These include treatable entities such as thyroid disease, vitamin deficiencies, brain tumor, drug and medication intoxication, chronic infection, and severe depression (pseudodementia).
- Neuroimaging studies (CT and MRI) do not show a single specific pattern with AD and may be normal early in the course of the disease. As AD progresses, diffuse cortical atrophy becomes apparent, and MRI scans show atrophy of the hippocampus. Imaging helps to exclude other disorders, such as primary and secondary neoplasms, multi infarct dementia, diffuse white matter disease, and NPH; it also helps to distinguish AD from other degenerative disorders with distinctive imaging patterns such as FTD or CJD. Functional imaging studies in AD reveal hypoperfusion or hypometabolism in the posterior temporal-parietal cortex.
- The EEG in AD is normal or shows nonspecific slowing. Routine spinal fluid examination is also normal.

Pathology
- At autopsy, the most severe pathology is usually found in the hippocampus, temporal cortex, and nucleus basalis of Meynert (lateral septum).
- The most important microscopic findings are neuritic "senile" plaques and NFTs. These lesions accumulate in small numbers during normal aging of the brain but occur in excess in AD. There is increasing evidence to suggest that soluble amyloid fibrils called *oligomers* lead to the dysfunction of the cell and may be the first biochemical injury in AD. Misfolded A-beta 42 molecules may be the most toxic form of this protein. Accumulation of oligomers eventually leads to formation of neuritic plaques. The neuritic plaques contain a central core that includes A-beta amyloid, proteoglycans, Apo e4, antichymotrypsin, and other proteins.
- NFTs are silver staining, twisted neurofilaments in neuronal cytoplasm that represent abnormally phosphorylated TAU protein and appear as paired helical filaments by electron microscopy. Tau is a microtubule associated protein that may function to assemble and stabilize the microtubules that convey cell organelles, glycoproteins, and other important materials throughout the neuron.
- Biochemically, AD is associated with a decrease in the cerebral cortical levels of several proteins and neurotransmitters, especially acetylcholine, its synthetic enzyme choline acetyltransferase, and nicotinic cholinergic receptors. Reduction of acetylcholine may be related in part to degeneration of cholinergic neurons in the nucleus basalis of Meynert that project to many areas of cortex. There is also reduction in norepinephrine levels in brainstem nuclei such as the locus coeruleus.

Genetic Considerations
- Several genetic factors play important roles in the pathogenesis of at least some cases of AD. One is the *APP* gene on chromosome 21. Adults with trisomy 21 (Down syndrome) consistently develop the typical neuropathologic hallmarks of AD if they survive beyond age 40. Many develop a progressive dementia superimposed on their baseline mental retardation.
- Two additional AD genes, termed the *presenilins*. Presenilin-1 (*PS-1*) is on chromosome 14 and encodes a protein called S182. Mutations in this gene cause an early-onset AD (onset before age 60 and often before age 50) transmitted in an autosomal dominant, highly penetrant fashion. Presenilin-2 (*PS-2*) is on chromosome 1 and encodes a protein called STM2. Mutations in *PS-1* are much more common than those in *PS-2*.
- The *Apo e4* on chromosome 19 in the pathogenesis of late onset familial and sporadic forms of AD. *Apo e4* is involved in cholesterol transport and has three alleles: 2, 3, and 4. The *Apo e4* allele has a strong association with AD in the general population, including sporadic and late-onset familial cases.

Vascular Dementia
- Dementia associated with cerebral vascular disease can be divided into two general categories: multi-infarct dementia and diffuse white matter disease (also called *leukoaraiosis, subcortical arteriosclerotic encephalopathy* or *Binswanger's disease*).
- Individuals who have had several strokes may develop chronic cognitive deficits, commonly called *multi-infarct dementia*. The strokes may be large or small (sometimes lacunar) and usually involve several different brain regions. Physical examination usually shows focal neurologic deficits such as hemiparesis, a unilateral Babinski reflex, a visual field defect, or pseudobulbar palsy. Recurrent strokes result in a stepwise progression of disease.
- Neuroimaging studies show multiple areas of infarction. Thus, the history and neuroimaging findings differentiate this condition from AD. However, both AD and multiple infarctions are common and sometimes occur together. With normal aging, there is also an accumulation of amyloid in cerebral blood vessels, leading to a condition called *cerebral amyloid angiopathy of aging* (not associated with dementia), which predisposes older persons to hemorrhagic lobar stroke. AD patients with amyloid angiopathy may be at increased risk for cerebral infarction.
- Some individuals with dementia are discovered on MRI to have bilateral abnormalities of subcortical white matter, termed *diffuse white matter disease*, often occurring in association with lacunar infarctions.
- Other rare causes of white matter disease also present with dementia, such as adult metachromatic leukodystrophy (arylsulfatase A deficiency) and progressive multifocal leukoencephalopathy (papovavirus infection).
- A dominantly inherited form of diffuse white matter disease is known as *cerebral autosomal dominant arteriopathy with subcortical infarcts and leukoencephalopathy* (CADASIL). Clinically, there is a progressive dementia developing in the fifth to seventh decades in multiple family members who may also have a history of migraine and recurrent stroke without hypertension. Skin biopsy may show characteristic dense bodies in the media of arterioles. The disease is caused by mutations in the *notch 3* gene.
- Mitochondrial disorders can present with stroke like episodes and can selectively injure basal ganglia or cortex
- Treatment of vascular dementia must be focused on the underlying causes, such as hypertension, atherosclerosis, and diabetes. Recovery of lost cognitive function is not likely to occur, although fluctuations with periods of improvement are common. Anticholinesterase compounds are being studied as a treatment for vascular dementia.

Frontotemporal Dementia
- *Frontotemporal dementia* (FTD) often begins when the patient is in the fifth to seventh decades. *Unlike AD; behavioral symptoms predominate in the early stages of FTD.*
- The most common genetic mutations that cause an autosomal dominant form of FTD involve the *tau* or *progranulin* genes, both on chromosome 17. *Tau* mutations lead to a change in the alternate splicing of tau or cause loss of function in the tau molecule. With *progranulin*, a missense mutation in the coding sequence of the gene is the underlying cause for the neurodegeneration
- In FTD, early symptoms are divided among cognitive, behavioral, and sometimes motor abnormalities, reflecting degeneration of the anterior frontal and temporal regions, basal ganglia, and motor neurons. Patients with FTD often show an absence of insight into their condition. Common behavioral deficits include apathy, disinhibition, weight gain, food fetishes, compulsions, and euphoria.
- Asymmetric left-frontal cases present with nonfluent aphasias, while left anterior temporal degeneration is characterized by loss of words and concepts related to language (semantic dementia). Nonfluent patients quickly progress to mutism, while those with semantic dementia develop features of multimodality agnosia, losing the ability to recognize faces, objects, words, and the emotions of others. Memory and visuospatial skills are relatively spared in most FTD patients.
- The distinguishing anatomic hallmark of FTD is a marked lobar atrophy of temporal and/or frontal lobes, which can be visualized by neuroimaging. The atrophy is sometimes asymmetric and may involve the basal ganglia. Microscopic findings that are seen across all FTD cases include gliosis, neuronal loss, and spongiosus.
- *Pick's disease* has been described as a progressive degenerative disorder characterized clinically by selective involvement of the anterior frontal and temporal neocortex and pathologically by intracellular inclusions (*Pick bodies*). Classic Pick bodies stain positive with silver (argyrophilic) and tau, but many of the tau-positive inclusions in FTD cases are not labeled with silver stains.
- Treatment is symptomatic, and there are currently no therapies known to slow progression or improve cognitive symptoms.

Dementia with Lewy Bodies
- The Parkinsonian dementia syndromes are under increasing study, with many cases unified by the presence of Lewy bodies in both the substantia nigra and the cortex at pathology.
- The clinical syndrome is characterized by visual hallucinations, parkinsonism, fluctuating alertness, falls, and often REM sleep behavior disorder. Dementia can precede or follow the appearance of parkinsonism. DLB patients are highly susceptible to metabolic perturbations, and in some patients the first manifestation of illness is a delirium, often precipitated by an infection or other systemic disturbance.

- Cognitively, DLB patients tend to have relatively better memory but more severe visuospatial deficits than individuals with AD.
- The key neuropathologic feature is the presence of Lewy bodies throughout the cortex, amygdala, cingulate cortex, and substantia nigra. Lewy bodies are intraneuronal cytoplasmic inclusions that stain with periodic acid–Schiff (PAS) and ubiquitin. They are composed of straight neurofilaments 7–20 nm long with surrounding amorphous material. They contain epitopes recognized by antibodies against phosphorylated and nonphosphorylated neurofilament proteins, ubiquitin, and a presynaptic protein called alpha-synuclein. Lewy bodies are traditionally found in the substantia nigra of patients with idiopathic PD.
- A profound cholinergic deficit is present in many patients with DLB and may be a factor responsible for the fluctuations and visual hallucinations present in these patients. In patients without other pathologic features, the condition is referred to as *diffuse Lewy body disease*. In patients whose brains also contain excessive amounts of amyloid plaques and NFTs, the condition is called the *Lewy body variant of Alzheimer's disease*.

Other Causes of Dementia

Prion Disorders such as Creutzfeldt-Jakob Disease (CJD)
- CJD is a rapidly progressive disorder associated with dementia, focal cortical signs, rigidity, and myoclonus, causing death in <1 year from the first symptoms.
- The differential diagnosis for CJD usually includes other rapidly progressive dementing conditions such as viral or bacterial encephalitides, Hashimoto's encephalitis, CNS vasculitis, lymphoma, or paraneoplastic syndromes.
- The markedly abnormal periodic EEG discharges and cortical and basal ganglia abnormalities on diffusion-weighted MRI are unique diagnostic features of CJD.

Huntington's Disease (HD)
- It is an autosomal dominant, degenerative brain disorder. A DNA repeat expansion (CAG repeat) of the mutant gene on chromosome 4 forms the basis of a diagnostic blood test for the disease gene.
- The clinical hallmarks of the disease are chorea, behavioral disturbance, and frontal executive disorder.
- Memory is frequently not impaired until late in the disease, but attention, judgment, awareness, and executive functions may be seriously deficient at an early stage.
- Depression, apathy, social withdrawal, irritability, and intermittent disinhibition are common. Delusions and obsessive compulsive behavior may occur.

Normal-pressure Hydrocephalus (NPH)
- For NPH the clinical triad includes an abnormal gait (ataxic or apractic), dementia (usually mild to moderate), and urinary incontinence.
- Neuroimaging studies reveal enlarged lateral ventricles (hydrocephalus) with little or no cortical atrophy. This syndrome is a communicating hydrocephalus with a patent aqueduct of Sylvius, in contrast to congenital aqueductal stenosis, where the aqueduct is small.
- In many cases, periventricular edema is present. Lumbar puncture opening pressure is in the high normal range, and the CSF protein, sugar concentrations, and cell count are normal.
- NPH is presumed to be caused by obstruction to normal flow of CSF over the cerebral convexity and delayed absorption into the venous system.
- In contrast to AD, the NPH patient has an early and prominent gait disturbance and no evidence of cortical atrophy on CT or MRI. AD often masquerades as NPH, because the gait may be abnormal in AD and cortical atrophy sometimes is difficult to determine by CT or MRI early in the disease.
- Hippocampal atrophy on MRI is a clue favoring AD. Approximately 30–50% of patients identified by careful diagnosis as having NPH will show improvement with a ventricular shunting procedure. Gait may improve more than memory. Transient, short-lasting improvement is common. Patients should be carefully selected for this operation, because subdural hematoma and infection are known complications.

Other Causes

Dementia can accompany *chronic alcoholism*. This may be a result of associated malnutrition, especially of B vitamins and particularly thiamine. However, other poorly defined aspects of chronic alcohol ingestion may also produce cerebral damage. A rare idiopathic syndrome of dementia and seizures with degeneration of the corpus callosum is called Marchiafava-Bignami disease.
- *Thiamine (vitamin B_1) deficiency* causes Wernicke's encephalopathy. The clinical presentation is a triad of confusion, ataxia, and diplopia from ophthalmoplegia. Thiamine deficiency damages the thalamus, mammillary bodies, midline cerebellum, periaqueductal grey matter of the midbrain, and peripheral nerves. Damage to the dorsomedial thalamic region correlates most closely with the memory loss. Prompt administration of parenteral thiamine (100 mg intravenously for 3 days followed by daily oral dosage) may reverse the disease if given in the first days of symptom onset.

- In *Korsakoff's syndrome*, the patient is unable to recall new information despite normal immediate memory, attention span, and level of consciousness. Confabulation is common. There is no specific treatment because the previous thiamine deficiency has produced irreversible damage to the medial thalamic nuclei and mammillary bodies. Mammillary body atrophy may be visible on high-resolution MRI.
- *Vitamin B_{12} deficiency*—Neurologically, it most commonly produces a spinal cord syndrome (myelopathy) affecting the posterior columns (loss of position and vibratory sense) and corticospinal tracts (hyperactive tendon reflexes with Babinski responses); it also damages peripheral nerves, resulting in sensory loss with depressed tendon reflexes. Damage to cerebral myelinated fibers may also cause dementia. Treatment with parenteral vitamin B_{12} (1000 microg intramuscularly daily for a week, weekly for a month, and monthly for life for pernicious anemia) stops progression of the disease if instituted promptly, but reversal of advanced nervous system damage will not occur.
- A paraneoplastic syndrome of dementia associated with occult carcinoma (often small cell lung cancer) is termed *limbic encephalitis*. In this syndrome, confusion, agitation, seizures, poor memory, movement disorders, and frank dementia may occur in association with sensory neuropathy.
- *Isolated vasculitis of the CNS* (CNS granulomatous vasculitis) occasionally causes a chronic encephalopathy associated with confusion, disorientation, and cloudiness of consciousness.
- Recurrent head trauma in professional boxers may lead to a dementia sometimes called the "punch drunk" syndrome, or *dementia pugilistica*. Early in the condition, a personality change associated with social instability and sometimes paranoia and delusions occurs. Later, memory loss progresses to full dementia, often associated with Parkinsonian signs and ataxia or intention tremor.
- *Transient global amnesia* (TGA) is characterized by the sudden onset of a severe episodic memory deficit, usually occurring in persons >50. Often the memory loss occurs in the setting of an emotional stimulus or physical exertion. During the attack, the individual is alert and communicative, general cognition seems intact, and there are no other neurologic signs or symptoms. The patient may seem confused and repeatedly ask about present events. The ability to form new memories returns after a period of hours, and the individual returns to normal with no recall for the period of the attack.
- The *ALS/Parkinsonian/dementia complex of Guam* is a rare degenerative disease. Individuals may have any combination of Parkinsonian features, dementia, and motor neuron disease.
- *Psychiatric diseases* may mimic dementia. Severely depressed individuals may appear demented, a phenomenon called *pseudodementia*. Memory and language are usually intact when carefully tested in depressed persons, and a significant memory disturbance usually suggests an underlying dementia, even if the patient is depressed.

Treatment
- The major goals of management are to treat any correctable causes of the dementia and to provide comfort and support to the patient and caregivers. Treatment of underlying causes is the rule.
- The primary goal is to make the demented patient's life comfortable, uncomplicated, and safe.
- Agitation, hallucinations, delusions, and confusion are difficult to treat.
- Cholinesterase inhibitors are being used to treat AD, and other drugs, such as anti-inflammatory agents, are being investigated in the treatment or prevention of AD.

ATAXIAS AND MOVEMENT DISORDERS

ATAXIA
- Symptoms and signs of ataxia consist of gait impairment, unclear ("scanning") speech, and visual blurring due to nystagmus, hand incoordination, and tremor with movement. These result from the involvement of the cerebellum and its afferent and efferent pathways, including the spinocerebellar pathways, and the frontopontocerebellar pathway originating in the rostral frontal lobe.
- True cerebellar ataxia must be distinguished from ataxia associated with vestibular nerve or labyrinthine disease, as the latter results in a disorder of gait associated with a significant degree of dizziness, light-headedness, or the perception of movement. True cerebellar ataxia is devoid of vertiginous complaints and is clearly an unsteady gait due to imbalance.
- Sensory disturbances can also on occasion simulate the imbalance of cerebellar disease; with sensory ataxia, imbalance dramatically worsens when visual input is removed (Romberg sign).
- Rarely, weakness of proximal leg muscles mimics cerebellar disease.

SYMMETRIC ATAXIA
- Progressive and symmetric ataxia can be classified with respect to onset as acute (over hours or days), subacute (weeks or months), or chronic (months to years).

- Acute and reversible ataxias include those caused by intoxication with alcohol, phenytoin, lithium, barbiturates, and other drugs. Patients with a postinfectious syndrome (especially after varicella) may develop gait ataxia and mild dysarthria, both of which are reversible. Rare infectious causes of acquired ataxia include poliovirus, coxsackievirus, echovirus, Epstein-Barr virus, toxoplasmosis, *Legionella*, and Lyme disease
- The subacute development of ataxia of gait over weeks to months (degeneration of the cerebellar vermis) may be due to the combined effects of alcoholism and malnutrition, particularly with deficiencies of vitamins B_1 and B_{12}.
- Paraneoplastic cerebellar ataxia is associated with a number of different tumors (and autoantibodies) such as breast and ovarian cancers (anti-Yo), small-cell lung cancer (anti-PQ type voltage-gated calcium channel), and Hodgkin's disease (anti-Tr)
- Another immune-mediated progressive ataxia is associated with anti-gliadin (and anti-endomysium) antibodies and the HLA DQB1*0201 haplotype; in some affected patients, biopsy of the small intestine reveals villous atrophy consistent with gluten-sensitive enteropathy
- Chronic symmetric gait ataxia suggests an inherited ataxia, a metabolic disorder, or a chronic infection. Hypothyroidism must always be considered as a readily treatable and reversible form of gait ataxia. Infectious diseases that can present with ataxia are meningovascular syphilis and tabes dorsalis due to degeneration of the posterior columns and spinocerebellar pathways in the spinal cord.

FOCAL ATAXIA

- Acute focal ataxia commonly results from cerebrovascular disease, usually ischemic infarction, or cerebellar hemorrhage. These lesions typically produce cerebellar symptoms ipsilateral to the injured cerebellum and may be associated with an impaired level of consciousness due to brainstem compression and increased intracranial pressure; ipsilateral pontine signs, including sixth and seventh nerve palsies, may be present.
- Many of these lesions represent true neurologic emergencies, as sudden herniation, either rostrally through the tentorium or caudal herniation of cerebellar tonsils through the foramen magnum can occur and is usually devastating. Acute surgical decompression may be required
- Chronic etiologies of progressive ataxia include multiple sclerosis and congenital lesions such as a Chiari malformation or a congenital cyst of the posterior fossa (Dandy-Walker syndrome).

THE INHERITED ATAXIAS

- These may show autosomal dominant, autosomal recessive or maternal (mitochondrial) modes of inheritance.
- Although the clinical manifestations and neuropathologic findings of cerebellar disease dominate the clinical picture, there may also be characteristic changes in the basal ganglia, brainstem, spinal cord, optic nerves, retina, and peripheral nerves.

AUTOSOMAL DOMINANT ATAXIAS

The autosomal spinocerebellar ataxias (SCAs) include SCA types 1 through SCA28, dentatorubropallidoluysian atrophy (DRPLA), and episodic ataxia (EA) types 1 and 2.

SCA1, SCA2, SCA3 [Machado-Joseph disease (MJD)], SCA6, SCA7, and SCA17 are caused by CAG triplet repeat expansions in different genes. SCA8 is due to an untranslated CTG repeat expansion, SCA12 is linked to an untranslated CAG repeat, and SCA10 is caused by an untranslated pentanucleotide repeat. Expanded polyglutamine proteins, termed *ataxins* produce a toxic gain of function with autosomal dominant inheritance.

- SCA1—SCA1 was previously referred to as *olivopontocerebellar atrophy,* is characterized by the development in early or middle adult life of progressive cerebellar ataxia of the trunk and limbs, impairment of equilibrium and gait, slowness of voluntary movements, scanning speech, nystagmoid eye movements, and oscillatory tremor of the head and trunk. Cerebellar and brainstem atrophy are evident on MRI.
- SCA2—Although neuropathologic and clinical findings are compatible with a diagnosis of SCA1, including slow saccadic eye movements, ataxia, dysarthria, parkinsonian rigidity, optic disk pallor, mild spasticity, and retinal degeneration, SCA2 is a unique form of cerebellar degenerative disease.
- Machado-Joseph Disease/SCA3—MJD in most populations, is the most common autosomal dominant ataxia and has been classified into three clinical types. In type I MJD (amyotrophic lateral sclerosis–parkinsonism–dystonia type), neurologic deficits appear in the first two decades and involve weakness and spasticity of extremities, especially the legs, often with dystonia of the face, neck, trunk, and extremities. In type II MJD (ataxic type), true cerebellar deficits of dysarthria and gait and extremity ataxia begin in the second to fourth decades along with corticospinal and extrapyramidal deficits of spasticity, rigidity, and dystonia. Type II is the most common form of MJD. Type III MJD (ataxic-amyotrophic type) presents in the fifth to the seventh decades with a pancerebellar disorder that includes dysarthria and gait and extremity ataxia. Distal sensory loss

involving pain, touch, vibration, and position senses and distal atrophy are prominent, indicating the presence of peripheral neuropathy. The deep tendon reflexes are depressed to absent, and there are no corticospinal or extrapyramidal findings.
- SCA6—CAG repeat expansions result in late-onset progressive ataxia with cerebellar degeneration. Missense mutations in this gene result in familial hemiplegic migraine. Nonsense mutations resulting in termination of protein synthesis of the gene product yield hereditary paroxysmal cerebellar ataxia or EA. Some patients with familial hemiplegic migraine develop progressive ataxia and also have cerebellar atrophy.
- Dentatorubropallidoluysian Atrophy - DRPLA has a variable presentation that may include progressive ataxia, choreoathetosis, dystonia, seizures, myoclonus, and dementia. DRPLA is due to unstable CAG triplet repeats in the open reading frame of a gene named *atrophin* located on chromosome 12p12.
- Episodic Ataxia—EA types 1 and 2 are two rare dominantly inherited disorders that have been mapped to chromosomes 12p (a potassium channel gene) for type 1 and 19p for type 2. Patients with EA-1 have brief episodes of ataxia with myokymia and nystagmus that last only minutes. Startle, sudden change in posture, and exercise can induce episodes.

AUTOSOMAL RECESSIVE ATAXIAS

Friedreich's Ataxia

- This is the most common form of inherited ataxia, comprising one-half of all hereditary ataxias. It presents before 25 years of age with progressive staggering gait, frequent falling, and titubation. The lower extremities are more severely involved than the upper ones. Dysarthria occasionally is the presenting symptom; rarely, progressive scoliosis, foot deformity, nystagmus, or cardiopathy is the initial sign.
- The neurologic examination reveals nystagmus, loss of fast saccadic eye movements, truncal titubation, dysarthria, dysmetria, and ataxia of trunk and limb movements. Extensor plantar responses (with normal tone in trunk and extremities), absence of deep tendon reflexes, and weakness (greater distally than proximally) are usually found. Loss of vibratory and proprioceptive sensation occurs. The median age of death is 35 years. Women have a significantly better prognosis than men.
- Cardiac involvement occurs in 90% of patients. Cardiomegaly, symmetric hypertrophy, murmurs, and conduction defects are reported. Musculoskeletal deformities are common and include pes cavus, pes equinovarus, and scoliosis. MRI of the spinal cord shows atrophy.
- The primary sites of pathology are the spinal cord, dorsal root ganglion cells, and the peripheral nerves. Slight atrophy of the cerebellum and cerebral gyri may occur. Sclerosis and degeneration occur predominantly in the spinocerebellar tracts, lateral corticospinal tracts, and posterior columns.
- Cardiac pathology consists of myocytic hypertrophy and fibrosis, focal vascular fibromuscular dysplasia with subintimal or medial deposition of periodic acid–Schiff (PAS)–positive material, myocytopathy with unusual pleomorphic nuclei, and focal degeneration of nerves and cardiac ganglia.
- The classic form of Friedreich's ataxia has been mapped to 9q13, and the mutant gene, *frataxin*, contains expanded GAA triplet repeats in the first intron. Frataxin is a mitochondrial protein involved in iron homeostasis. Mitochondrial iron accumulation due to loss of the iron transporter coded by the mutant *frataxin* gene results in oxidized intramitochondrial iron. Excess oxidized iron results in turn in the oxidation of cellular components and irreversible cell injury.

Ataxia Telangiectasia

- Patients with ataxia telangiectasia (AT) present in the first decade of life with progressive telangiectatic lesions associated with deficits in cerebellar function and nystagmus. The neurologic manifestations correspond to those in Friedreich's disease, which should be included in the differential diagnosis. There is a high incidence of recurrent pulmonary infections and neoplasms of the lymphatic and reticuloendothelial system in patients with AT. Thymic hypoplasia with cellular and humoral (IgA and IgG2) immunodeficiencies, premature aging, and endocrine disorders such as type 1 diabetes mellitus are described.
- The most striking neuropathologic changes include loss of Purkinje, granule, and basket cells in the cerebellar cortex as well as of neurons in the deep cerebellar nuclei. The inferior olives of the medulla may also have neuronal loss.
- The gene for AT (the *ATM* gene) encodes a protein that is similar to several yeast and mammalian phosphatidylinositol-3'-kinases involved in mitogenic signal transduction, meiotic recombination, and cell cycle control. Defective DNA repair in AT fibroblasts exposed to ultraviolet light has been demonstrated.

Ataxic Disorders: Treatment

- The most important goal in management of patients with ataxia is to identify treatable disease entities. Mass lesions must be recognized promptly and treated appropriately. Ataxia with anti-gliadin antibodies and gluten-sensitive enteropathy may improve with a gluten-free diet.

- Malabsorption syndromes leading to vitamin E deficiency may lead to ataxia. The vitamin E deficiency form of Friedreich's ataxia must be considered, and serum vitamin E levels measured.
- The cerebrospinal fluid should be tested for a syphilitic infection in patients with progressive ataxia and other features of tabes dorsalis. Similarly, antibody titers for Lyme disease and *Legionella* should be measured and appropriate antibiotic therapy should be instituted in antibody-positive patients.
- There is no proven therapy for any of the autosomal dominant ataxias (SCA1 to -28). There is preliminary evidence that idebenone, a free-radical scavenger, can improve myocardial hypertrophy in patients with classic Friedreich ataxia. Acetazolamide can reduce the duration of symptoms of episodic ataxia.

HYPERKINETIC MOVEMENT DISORDERS

Disorders	Movement characteristics
Athetosis	Slow, distal, writhing, involuntary movements with a propensity to affect the arms and hands.
Chorea	Rapid, semipurposeful, graceful, dancelike, nonpatterned involuntary movements involving distal or proximal muscle groups.
Dystonia	Involuntary patterned sustained or repeated muscle contractions, often leading to twisting movements and abnormal posture.
Myoclonus	Sudden, brief (<100 ms), shock like, arrhythmic muscle twitches.
Tics	Brief, repeated, stereotyped muscle contractions that are often suppressible. Can be simple and involve a single muscle group or complex and affect a range of motor activities.
Tremor	Rhythmic oscillation of a body part due to intermittent muscle contractions.

Essential Tremor
- Essential tremor (ET) is the most common involuntary movement disorder. It is a progressive disorder which can present in childhood but dramatically increases in prevalence over the age of 70.
- ET is characterized by a high-frequency tremor (up to 11Hz) that predominantly affects the upper extremities. The tremor is most prominent when trying to maintain a posture (postural tremor) or perform an action such as touching the finger to an object (kinetic tremor). It is typically bilateral and symmetric, but one side can be predominantly affected. Tremor may also affect the head (horizontal or vertical), and speech may be tremulous.
- The specific etiology and pathophysiology of ET are not known. Approximately half of the cases have a positive family history with an autosomal dominant pattern of inheritance.
- The cerebellum and inferior olives have been implicated as possible sites of a "tremor pacemaker" based on the presence of cerebellar signs in some patients and findings of increased metabolic activity and blood flow in these regions.
- **Treatment:** Many cases are mild and require no treatment other than reassurance. Occasionally, tremor can be severe and interfere with eating, writing, and activities of daily living. Primidone and propranolol (20–80 mg/d) are the standard drug therapies. Surgical therapies targeting the VIM nucleus of the thalamus can be very effective in severe and drug-resistant cases.
- **Resting tremor:** Appears at rest and vanishes during movement; etiology: Parkinson and Parkinson plus syndrome
- **Treatment:** Dopamine agonists, levodopa, amantidine
- **Postural tremor:** Appears in a static state during anxiety; treatment: propranolol and clonazepam

Dystonia
- Dystonia consists of sustained or repetitive involuntary muscle contractions, frequently causing twisting movements with abnormal postures. Dystonia can range from minor contractions in an individual muscle group to severe and disabling involvement of multiple muscle groups.
- Dystonia can be classified based on age of onset (childhood vs. adult), distribution (focal, multifocal, segmental, or generalized), or etiology (primary or secondary).

Primary Dystonias
- Idiopathic torsion dystonia (ITD), or Oppenheim's dystonia, is predominantly a childhood-onset form of dystonia with an autosomal dominant pattern of inheritance. dystonia typically begins in a foot or arm and can progress to involve the other limbs as well as the head and neck. Most cases are linked to a mutation in the *DYT1* gene located on chromosome 9q34, which results in a trinucleotide GAG deletion.
- Dopa responsive dystonia (DRD) is a dominantly inherited form of childhood-onset dystonia due to a mutation in the gene that encodes for guanosine triphosphate (GTP) cyclohydrolase I, the rate-limiting enzyme for the synthesis of tetrahydrobiopterin.
- **Focal Dystonias**—These are the most common forms of dystonia. They typically present in the fourth to sixth decades and affect women more than men. The major types are:

- *Blepharospasm*: Dystonic contractions of the eyelids with increased blinking that can interfere with reading, watching TV, and driving.
- *Oromandibular dystonia* (OMD): Contractions of muscles of the lower face, lips, tongue, and jaw (opening or closing). Meige's syndrome is a combination of OMD and blepharospasm that predominantly affects women over the age of 60 years.
- *Spasmodic dysphonia*: Dystonic contractions of the vocal cords during phonation, causing impaired speech. Most cases affect the adductor muscles and cause speech to have a choking or strained quality. Less commonly, the abductors are affected, leading to speech with a breathy or whispering quality.
- *Cervical dystonia*: Dystonic contractions of neck muscles, causing the head to deviate to one side (*torticollis*), in a forward direction (*anterocollis*), or in a backward direction (*retrocollis*). Muscle contractions can be painful and associated with dystonic tremor and a secondary cervical radiculopathy.
- *Limb dystonias*: These can be present in either arms or legs and are often brought out by task-specific activities such as handwriting (writer's cramp) or playing a musical instrument (musician's cramp).

Secondary Dystonias

- These occur as a consequence of drugs or other neurologic problems. Drug-induced dystonia is most commonly seen with neuroleptic drugs or after chronic levodopa treatment in PD patients
- Secondary dystonia can also be observed following discrete lesions in the striatum, pallidum, thalamus, cortex, and brainstem due to infarction, anoxia, trauma, tumor, infection, toxins such as manganese, or carbon monoxide
- Dystonia-Plus Syndromes—Dystonia may occur as a part of neurodegenerative conditions such as Huntington's disease (HD), PD, Wilson's disease, corticobasal degeneration, progressive supranuclear palsy, the Lubag form of dystonia-parkinsonism (DYT3), and mitochondrial encephalopathies.

Treatment

- Treatment is symptomatic for the most part, except in rare cases where treatment of a primary underlying condition is available.
- Oral baclofen (25–120 mg) may be helpful, but benefits are usually modest, and side effects of sedation, weakness, and memory loss can be problematic. Intrathecal infusion of baclofen is more likely to be helpful, particularly with leg and trunk dystonia, but benefits are frequently not sustained and complications can be serious, including infection, seizures, and coma.
- Tetrabenazine may be helpful. In general, dystonic patients are not satisfactorily controlled with drug therapies, particularly if they have a generalized dystonia.
- Botulinum toxin can be of great benefit for patients with focal dystonia, particularly if involvement is limited to small muscle groups such as in blepharospasm, torticollis, and spasmodic dysphonia. Botulinum toxin acts by blocking the release of acetylcholine at the neuromuscular junction, leading to muscle weakness and reduced dystonia.
- Surgical therapy is an alternative for patients with severe dystonia who are not responsive to other treatments. Peripheral procedures such as rhizotomy and myotomy were used in the past to treat cervical dystonia but have been rarely employed since the introduction of botulinum toxin therapy. Bilateral deep brain stimulation (DBS) of the pallidum can provide dramatic benefits for patients with primary (DYT1) dystonia.

CHOREAS

Huntington's Disease

- HD is a progressive, fatal, autosomal dominant disorder characterized by motor, behavioral, and cognitive dysfunction. Onset is typically between the ages of 25 and 45 years.
- HD is characterized by rapid, nonpatterned, semipurposeful, involuntary choreiform movements. In the early stages the chorea tends to be focal or segmental, but it progresses over time to involve multiple body regions. Dysarthria, gait disturbance, and oculomotor abnormalities are common features. With advancing disease, there is a reduction in the chorea and emergence of dystonia, rigidity, bradykinesia, myoclonus, and spasticity.
- HD can present as an akinetic-rigid or Parkinsonian syndrome (Westphall variant).
- A clinical diagnosis of HD can be strongly suspected in cases of chorea with a positive family history. Neuropathologically, the disease predominantly strikes the striatum. Atrophy of the caudate nuclei, which form the lateral margins of the lateral ventricles, can be visualized on neuroimaging studies in the middle and late stages of the disease.
- HD is caused by an increase in the number of polyglutamine (CAG) repeats (>40) in the coding sequence of the Huntington gene located on the short arm of chromosome 4. The larger the number of repeats, the earlier the disease is manifest. Anticipation occurs, particularly in males, with subsequent generations having larger numbers of repeats and earlier age of disease onset. The gene encodes the highly conserved cytoplasmic protein huntingtin, which is widely distributed in neurons throughout the CNS, but whose function is not known.

- **Treatment:** Treatment involves a multidisciplinary approach with medical, neuropsychiatric, social, and genetic counseling for patients and their families. A neuroprotective therapy that slows or stops disease progression is the major unmet medical need in HD.

Other Choreas

- Sydenham's chorea (originally called Saint Vitus' dance) is more common in females and is typically seen in childhood (5– 15 years). It often develops in association with prior exposure to a group A streptococcal infection and is thought to be the result of an autoimmune-mediated inflammatory disorder.
- Chorea may recur in later life, particularly in association with pregnancy (chorea gravidarum) or treatment with sex hormones.
- Neuroacanthocytosis is a progressive and typically fatal autosomal recessive disorder that is characterized by chorea coupled with red cell abnormalities on peripheral blood smear (acanthocytes). A phenotypically similar X-linked form of the disorder has been described in older individuals who have reactivity with Kell blood group antigens (McLeod syndrome).
- Systemic lupus erythematosus is the most common systemic disorder that causes chorea; the chorea can last for days to years. Choreas can also be seen in patients with hyperthyroidism, various autoimmune disorders, infections including HIV, metabolic alterations, polycythemia rubra vera, following open heart surgery in the pediatric population, and in association with a wide variety of medications (especially anticonvulsants, cocaine, CNS stimulants, estrogens, and lithium).
- **Treatment**—Diagnosis and treatment of the underlying condition, where possible, is the first priority. Tetrabenazine, neuroleptics, dopamine-blocking agents, propranolol, clonazepam, and baclofen may be helpful. Treatment is not indicated if the condition is mild and self-limited.

Hemiballismus

- Hemiballismus is a violent form of chorea that comprises wild, flinging, large-amplitude movements on one side of the body. Proximal limb muscles tend to be predominantly affected. The movements may be so severe as to cause exhaustion, dehydration, local injury, and, in extreme cases, death.
- The most common cause is a partial lesion (infarct or hemorrhage) in the Subthalamic Nucleus of Luys, but cases can also be seen with lesions in the putamen. It is usually self-limiting and tends to resolve spontaneously after weeks or months.

Tourette Syndrome (TS)

- TS is a neurobehavioral disorder named after Gilles de la Tourette. It predominantly affects males. TS is characterized by multiple motor tics and vocalizations. Motor tics can be "simple," with movement only affecting an individual muscle group (e.g., blinking, twitching of the nose, jerking of the neck), or "complex," with coordinated involvement of multiple muscle groups [e.g., jumping, sniffing, head banging, and echopraxia (mimicking movements)]. Vocal tics can also be simple (e.g., grunting) or complex [e.g., echolalia (repeating other peoples words), palilalia (repeating your own words), and coprolalia (expression of obscene words)]. Patients may also experience sensory tics, consisting of unpleasant focal sensations in the face, head, or neck. Patients may experience an irresistible urge to express tics but characteristically can voluntarily suppress them for short periods of time.
- **Treatment**—Patients with mild disease often only require education and counseling (for themselves and family members). Therapy is generally initiated with the alpha agonist clonidine, starting at low doses and gradually increasing the dose and frequency until satisfactory control is achieved.
- Atypical neuroleptics are preferred as they are associated with a reduced risk of extrapyramidal side effects. If they are not effective, classical neuroleptics such as haloperidol, fluphenazine, or pimozide can be tried. Botulinum toxin injections can be effective in controlling focal tics that involve small muscle groups.

Myoclonus

- Myoclonus is a brief, rapid (<100 ms), shocklike, jerky movement consisting of single or repetitive muscle discharges. Myoclonic jerks can be focal, multifocal, segmental, or generalized and can occur spontaneously, in association with voluntary movement (action myoclonus), or in response to an external stimulus (reflex or startle myoclonus).
- Negative myoclonus consists of a twitch due to a brief loss of muscle activity (e.g., asterixis in hepatic failure).
- They can be seen in association with pathology in cortical, subcortical, or spinal cord regions, associated with hypoxic damage (especially following cardiac arrest), encephalopathy, and neurodegenerative disorders. Reversible myoclonus can be seen with metabolic disturbances (renal failure, electrolyte imbalance, hypocalcemia), toxins, and many medications.
- **Treatment**—Treatment primarily consists of treating the underlying condition or removing an offending agent. Pharmacologic therapy involves one or a combination of GABAergic agents. Levetiracetam may be particularly effective.

Drug-Induced Movement Disorders

- This important group of movement disorders is primarily associated with drugs that block dopamine receptors (neuroleptics) or central dopaminergic transmission. Hyperkinetic movement disorders secondary to neuroleptic drugs can be divided into those which present acutely, subacutely, or after prolonged exposure (tardive syndromes).
- *Dopamine*-blocking drugs can also be associated with a reversible Parkinsonian syndrome for which anticholinergics are often concomitantly prescribed, but there is concern that this may increase the risk of developing a tardive syndrome.
- Acute Dystonia is the most common acute hyperkinetic drug reaction. It is typically generalized in children and focal (e.g., blepharospasm, torticollis, or oromandibular dystonia) in adults. The reaction can develop within minutes of exposure and can be successfully treated in most cases with parenteral administration of anticholinergics (benztropine or diphenhydramine) or benzodiazepines (lorazepam or diazepam).
- *Subacute*—Akathisia is the commonest reaction in this category. It consists of motor restlessness with a need to move that is alleviated by movement. Therapy consists of removing the offending agent(s).
- *Tardive Syndromes*—These disorders develop months to years after initiation of neuroleptic treatment. Tardive dyskinesia (TD) is the commonest and typically comprises choreiform movements involving the mouth, lips, and tongue. In severe cases the trunk, limbs, and respiratory muscles may be affected. Atypical antipsychotics (e.g., clozapine, risperidone, olanzapine, quetiapine, ziprasidone, and aripiprazole) are associated with a significantly lower risk of TD in comparison to traditional antipsychotics. Treatment primarily consists of stopping the antipsychotic.
- Neuroleptic medications can also be associated with a neuroleptic malignant syndrome (NMS). NMS is characterized by muscle rigidity, elevated temperature, altered mental status, hyperthermia, tachycardia, labile blood pressure, and renal failure. Symptoms typically evolve within days or weeks after initiating the drug. NMS can also be precipitated by the abrupt withdrawal of antiparkinsonian medications in PD patients. Treatment involves immediate cessation of the offending antipsychotic drug and the introduction of a dopaminergic agent (e.g., dopamine agonists, levodopa), dantrolene, or benzodiazepines.

Clinicopathological Correlations of Movement Disorders

Symptoms	Correlations
Unilateral plastic rigidity with rest tremor	Contralateral substantia nigra
Unilatral hemiballismus and hemichorea	Contralateral subthalamic nucleus of Luys or luysial–pallidal connections
Chronic chorea	Caudate nucleus and putamen
Athetosis and dystonia	Contralateral striatum
Cerebellar incoordination, intention tremor, and hypotonia	Ipsilateral cerebellar hemisphere; ipsilateral middle or inferior cerebellar peduncle;
Decerebrate rigidity	Usually bilateral in tegmentum of upper brainstem at level of red nucleus or between red and vestibular nuclei
Palatal and facial myoclonus	Ipsilateral central tegmental tract with denervation of inferior olivary nucleus and nucleus ambiguus
Diffuse myoclonus	Neuronal degeneration

DEMYELINATING DISORDERS

Demyelinating disorders are characterized by inflammation and selective destruction of central nervous system (CNS) myelin. The peripheral nervous system (PNS) is usually spared.

MULTIPLE SCLEROSIS

Clinical Manifestations

- The onset of MS may be abrupt or insidious. *Weakness of the limbs* may manifest as loss of strength or dexterity, fatigue, or a disturbance of gait. Exercise-induced weakness is a characteristic symptom of MS. The weakness is of the upper motor neuron type and is usually accompanied by other pyramidal signs such as spasticity, hyperreflexia and Babinski signs. Occasionally a tendon reflex may be lost (simulating a lower motor neuron lesion) if an MS lesion disrupts the afferent reflex fibers in the spinal cord. *Spasticity* is often associated with spontaneous and movement-induced muscle spasms, interfering with ambulation, work, or self-care. *Optic neuritis* (ON) presents as diminished visual acuity, dimness, or decreased color perception (desaturation) in the central field of vision. Visual symptoms are generally monocular but may be bilateral. An afferent pupillary defect is usually present. Funduscopic examination may be normal or reveal optic disc swelling (papillitis). Pallor of the optic disc (optic atrophy) commonly follows ON.

- *Diplopia* may result from internuclear ophthalmoplegia (INO) or from palsy of the sixth cranial nerve (rarely the third or fourth). An INO consists of impaired adduction of one eye due to a lesion in the ipsilateral medial longitudinal fasciculus. Prominent nystagmus is often observed in the abducting eye, along with a small skew deviation. A bilateral INO is particularly suggestive of MS. Other common gaze disturbances in MS include (1) a horizontal gaze palsy, (2) a "one and a half" syndrome (horizontal gaze palsy plus an INO), and (3) acquired pendular nystagmus.
- *Sensory symptoms* are varied and include both paresthesias (e.g., tingling, prickling sensations, formications, "pins and needles," or painful burning) and hypesthesia (e.g., reduced sensation, numbness, or a "dead" feeling). It is often accompanied by a bandlike sensation of tightness around the torso. *Ataxia* usually manifests as cerebellar tremors Ataxia may also involve the head and trunk or the voice, producing a characteristic cerebellar dysarthria (scanning speech).
- *Bladder dysfunction* is present in >90% of MS patients, and in a third of patients, dysfunction results in weekly or more frequent episodes of incontinence.
- *Cognitive dysfunction* can include memory loss, impaired attention, difficulties in problem solving, slowed information processing, and problems shifting between cognitive tasks.
- *Ancillary Symptoms - Heat sensitivity* refers to neurologic symptoms produced by an elevation of the body's core temperature. For example, unilateral visual blurring may occur during a hot shower or with physical exercise (*Uhthoff's symptom*). *Lhermitte's symptom* is an electric shocklike sensation (typically induced by flexion or other movements of the neck) that radiates down the back into the legs. Rarely, it radiates into the arms. *Paroxysmal symptoms* are distinguished by their brief duration (10 s to 2 min), high frequency (5–40 episodes per day), lack of any alteration of consciousness or change in background electroencephalogram during episodes, and a self-limited course (generally lasting weeks to months). *Trigeminal neuralgia, hemifacial spasm,* and *glossopharyngeal neuralgia* can occur when the demyelinating lesion involves the root entry (or exit) zone of the fifth, seventh, and ninth cranial nerve, respectively. *Facial myokymia* consists of either persistent rapid flickering contractions of the facial musculature (especially the lower portion of the orbicularis oculus) or a contraction that slowly spreads across the face. It results from lesions of the corticobulbar tracts or brainstem course of the facial nerve.
- Pregnant MS patients experience fewer attacks than expected during gestation (especially in the last trimester), but more attacks than expected in the first 3 months postpartum. Disease-modifying therapy is generally discontinued during pregnancy, although the actual risk from the interferons and glatiramer acetate appears to be low.

Clinical Types of MS
- *Relapsing/remitting MS* (RRMS) accounts for 85% of MS cases at onset and is characterized by discrete attacks that generally evolve over days to weeks (rarely over hours). There is often complete recovery over the ensuing weeks to months
- *Secondary progressive MS* (SPMS) always begins as RRMS. At some point, however, the clinical course changes so that the patient experiences a steady deterioration in function unassociated with acute attacks (which may continue or cease during the progressive phase).
- *Primary progressive MS* (PPMS) accounts for ~15% of cases. These patients do not experience attacks but only a steady functional decline from disease onset
- *Progressive/relapsing MS* (PRMS) overlaps PPMS and SPMS and accounts for ~5% of MS patients. Patients experience a steady deterioration in their condition from disease onset with occasional attacks superimposed upon their progressive course.

Diagnosis and Treatment
- There is no definitive diagnostic test for MS. Diagnostic criteria for clinically definite MS require documentation of two or more episodes of symptoms and two or more signs that reflect pathology in anatomically noncontiguous white matter tracts of the CNS
- **Diagnostic Criteria for MS**
    - Examination must reveal *objective* abnormalities of the CNS.
    - Involvement must reflect predominantly disease of white matter long tracts, usually including (a) pyramidal pathways, (b) cerebellar pathways, (c) medial longitudinal fasciculus, (d) optic nerve, and (e) posterior columns.
    - Examination or history must implicate involvement of two or more areas of the CNS.
    - A confirmatory MRI must have either four lesions involving the white matter or three lesions if one is periventricular in location. Acceptable lesions must be >3 mm in diameter. For patients older than 50 years, two of the following criteria must also be met: (a) lesion size >5 mm, (b) lesions adjacent to the bodies of the lateral ventricles, and (c) lesion(s) present in the posterior fossa
    - The clinical pattern must consist of (a) two or more separate episodes of worsening involving different sites of the CNS, each lasting at least 24 h and occurring at least 1 month apart, or (b) gradual or stepwise progression over at least 6 months if accompanied by increased IgG synthesis or two or more oligoclonal bands.

- The patient's neurologic condition could not better be attributed to another disease.
    1. *Definite MS:* All five criteria fulfilled.
    2. *Probable MS:* All five criteria fulfilled except (a) only one objective abnormality despite two symptomatic episodes or (b) only one symptomatic episode despite two or more objective abnormalities.
    3. *At risk for MS:* Criteria 1, 2, 3, and 5 fulfilled; patient has only one symptomatic episode and one objective abnormality.
- MRI has revolutionized the diagnosis and management of MS. An increase in vascular permeability from a breakdown of the BBB is detected by leakage of intravenous gadolinium (Gd) into the parenchyma. Such leakage occurs early in the development of an MS lesion and serves as a useful marker of inflammation. Lesions are frequently oriented perpendicular to the ventricular surface, corresponding to the pathologic pattern of perivenous demyelination (Dawson's fingers). Approximately one-third of T2-weighted lesions appear as hypointense lesions (black holes) on T1-weighted imaging. Black holes may be a marker of irreversible demyelination and axonal loss. Newer MRI measures such as magnetization transfer ratio (MTR) imaging and proton magnetic resonance spectroscopic imaging (MRSI) may ultimately serve as surrogate markers of clinical disability.
- *Evoked potentials:* EP testing assesses function in afferent (visual, auditory, and somatosensory) or efferent (motor) CNS pathways. EPs use computer averaging to measure CNS electric potentials evoked by repetitive stimulation of selected peripheral nerves or of the brain. These tests provide the most information when the pathways studied are clinically uninvolved.
- *Cerebrospinal fluid:* CSF abnormalities found in MS include a mononuclear cell pleocytosis and an increased level of intrathecally synthesized IgG. The total CSF protein is usually normal or slightly elevated. The measurement of oligoclonal banding (OCB) in the CSF also assesses intrathecal production of IgG.
- **Therapy for MS can be divided into several categories:**
    - Treatment of acute attacks as they occur,
    - Treatment with disease-modifying agents that reduce the biological activity of MS, and
    - Symptomatic therapy. Treatments that promote remyelination or neural repair do not currently exist but would be highly desirable.
- The Kurtzke Expanded Disability Status Score (EDSS) is a useful measure of neurologic impairment in MS.
- Glucocorticoids are used to manage either first attacks or acute exacerbations. They provide short-term clinical benefit by reducing the severity and shortening the duration of attacks.
- Plasma exchange (seven exchanges: 40–60 mL/kg per exchange, every other day for 14 days) may benefit patients with fulminant attacks of demyelination that are unresponsive to glucocorticoids.
- Interferon beta is a class I interferon originally identified by its antiviral properties. Efficacy in MS probably results from immunomodulatory properties including:
    - Downregulating expression of MHC molecules on antigen-presenting cells,
    - Inhibiting proinflammatory and increasing regulatory cytokine levels,
    - Inhibition of T cell proliferation, and
    - Limiting the trafficking of inflammatory cells in the CNS.
- Glatiramer acetate is a synthetic, random polypeptide composed of four amino acids (L-glutamic acid, L-lysine, L-alanine, and L-tyrosine). Its mechanism of action may include:
    - Induction of antigen-specific suppressor T cells;
    - Binding to MHC molecules, thereby displacing bound MBP; or
    - Altering the balance between proinflammatory and regulatory cytokines.
- Natalizumab is a humanized monoclonal antibody, a cellular adhesion molecule expressed on the surface of lymphocytes. It prevents lymphocytes from binding to endothelial cells, thereby preventing lymphocytes from penetrating the BBB and entering the CNS.
- Mitoxantrone (Novantrone), an anthracenedione, exerts its antineoplastic action by
    - Intercalating into DNA and producing both strand breaks and interstrand cross-links,
    - Interfering with RNA synthesis, and
    - Inhibiting topoisomerase II (involved in DNA repair).
- *Symptomatic Therapy:* Potassium channel blockers may be helpful for *weakness*, especially for heat-sensitive symptoms. *Ataxia/tremor* is often intractable. *Spasticity* and *spasms* may improve with physical therapy, regular exercise, and stretching. *Pain* is treated with anticonvulsants, antidepressants or antiarrhythmics. If these approaches fail, patients should be referred to a comprehensive pain management program. *Bladder dysfunction* management is best guided by urodynamic testing. *Cognitive problems* may respond to the cholinesterase inhibitors.

Variants of MS

- *Neuromyelitis optica* (NMO), or Devic's syndrome, consists of separate attacks of acute ON and myelitis. ON may be unilateral or bilateral and precede or follow an attack of myelitis by days, months, or years. In contrast to MS, patients with NMO do not experience brainstem, cerebellar, and cognitive involvement, and the brain MRI is typically normal.
- *Acute MS (Marburg's variant)* is a fulminant demyelinating process that in some cases progresses inexorably to death within 1–2 years. Typically, there are no remissions. Does not follow infection/vaccination

Acute Disseminated Encephalomyelitis (ADEM)

- ADEM has a monophasic course and is frequently associated with antecedent immunization (postvaccinal encephalomyelitis) or infection (postinfectious encephalomyelitis). The hallmark of ADEM is the presence of widely scattered small foci of perivenular inflammation and demyelination.
- In severe cases, onset is abrupt and progression rapid (hours to days). In postinfectious ADEM, the neurologic syndrome generally begins late in the course of the viral illness as the exanthem is fading. Fever reappears, and headache, meningismus, and lethargy progressing to coma may develop. Seizures are common. Signs of disseminated neurologic disease are consistently present (e.g., hemiparesis or quadriparesis, extensor plantar responses, lost or hyperactive tendon reflexes, sensory loss and brainstem involvement).
- MRI findings that may support a diagnosis of ADEM include extensive and relatively symmetric white matter abnormalities and Gd enhancement of all abnormal areas, indicating active disease and a monophasic course.
- **Treatment**—Initial treatment is with high-dose glucocorticoids as for exacerbations of MS; depending on the response, treatment may need to be continued for 4–8 weeks. Patients who fail to respond within a few days may benefit from a course of plasma exchange or intravenous immunoglobulin.

MOTOR NEURON DISEASES (MND)

Causes of MND

- Upper and lower motor neurons
  - Amyotrophic lateral sclerosis
- Predominantly upper motor neurons
  - Primary lateral sclerosis
- Predominantly lower motor neurons
  - Multifocal motor neuropathy with conduction block
  - Motor neuropathy with paraproteinemia or cancer
  - Motor-predominant peripheral neuropathies
- *Acute causes:* Poliomyelitis, Herpes zoster and Coxsackie virus infections.

AMYOTROPHIC LATERAL SCLEROSIS

ALS is the most common form of progressive motor neuron disease. It is a prime example of a neurodegenerative disease.

Pathophysiology

- The pathologic hallmark of motor neuron degenerative disorders is death of lower motor neurons (consisting of anterior horn cells in the spinal cord and their brainstem homologues innervating bulbar muscles) and upper, or corticospinal, motor neurons (originating in layer five of the motor cortex and descending via the pyramidal tract to synapse with lower motor neurons, either directly or indirectly via interneurons)
- Focal enlargements are frequent in proximal motor axons; ultrastructurally, these "spheroids" are composed of accumulations of neurofilaments and other proteins. Also seen is proliferation of astroglia and microglia, the inevitable accompaniment of all degenerative processes in the central nervous system (CNS). The death of the peripheral motor neurons in the brainstem and spinal cord leads to denervation and consequent atrophy of the corresponding muscle fibers.
- As denervation progresses, muscle atrophy is readily recognized in muscle biopsies and on clinical examination. This is the basis for the term *amyotrophy*. The loss of cortical motor neurons results in thinning of the corticospinal tracts that travel via the internal capsule and brainstem to the lateral and anterior white matter columns of the spinal cord. The loss of fibers in the lateral columns and resulting fibrillary gliosis impart a particular firmness (*lateral sclerosis*). A remarkable feature of the disease is the selectivity of neuronal cell death.

- Within the motor system, there is some selectivity of involvement. Thus, motor neurons required for ocular motility remain unaffected, as do the parasympathetic neurons in the sacral spinal cord (the nucleus of Onufrowicz, or Onuf) that innervate the sphincters of the bowel and bladder.

Clinical Manifestations
- The manifestations of ALS are somewhat variable depending on whether corticospinal neurons or lower motor neurons in the brainstem and spinal cord are more prominently involved. With lower motor neuron dysfunction and early denervation, typically the first evidence of the disease is insidiously developing asymmetric weakness, usually first evident distally in one of the limbs. Weakness caused by denervation is associated with progressive wasting and atrophy of muscles and, particularly early in the illness, spontaneous twitching of motor units, or fasciculations. In the hands, a preponderance of extensor over flexor weakness is common.
- When the initial denervation involves bulbar rather than limb muscles, the problem at onset is difficulty with chewing, swallowing, and movements of the face and tongue. Early involvement of the muscles of respiration may lead to death before the disease is far advanced elsewhere. Degeneration of the corticobulbar projections innervating the brainstem results in dysarthria and exaggeration of the motor expressions of emotion which leads to involuntary excess in weeping or laughing (pseudobulbar affect).
- It is characteristic of ALS that, regardless of whether the initial disease involves upper or lower motor neurons, both will eventually be implicated.

Treatment
- No treatment arrests the underlying pathologic process in ALS. The drug riluzole (100 mg/d) was approved for ALS because it produces a modest lengthening of survival.
- In the absence of a primary therapy for ALS, a variety of rehabilitative aids may substantially assist ALS patients. Foot-drop splints facilitate ambulation by obviating the need for excessive hip flexion and by preventing tripping on a floppy foot. Finger extension splints can potentiate grip. Respiratory support may be life-sustaining. For patients electing against long-term ventilation by tracheostomy, positive-pressure ventilation by mouth or nose provides transient (several weeks) relief from hypercarbia and hypoxia.

OTHER MOTOR NEURON DISEASES

X-Linked Spinobulbar Muscular Atrophy (Kennedy's Disease)
This is an X-linked lower motor neuron disorder in which progressive weakness and wasting of limb and bulbar muscles begins in males in mid-adult life and is conjoined with androgen insensitivity manifested by gynecomastia and reduced fertility. The underlying molecular defect is an expanded trinucleotide repeat (-CAG-) in the first exon of the androgen receptor gene on the X chromosome.

Adult Tay-Sach's Disease
These tend to be distinguishable from ALS because they are very slowly progressive; dysarthria and radiographically evident cerebellar atrophy may be prominent.

Spinal Muscular Atrophy
- The SMAs are a family of selective lower motor neuron diseases of early onset. The defect in the majority of families with SMA maps to a locus on chromosome 5 encoding a putative motor neuron survival protein (SMN, for survival motor neuron) that is important in the formation and trafficking of RNA complexes across the nuclear membrane. Neuropathologically these disorders are characterized by extensive loss of large motor neurons; muscle biopsy reveals evidence of denervation atrophy.
- *Infantile SMA* (SMA I, Werdnig-Hoffmann disease) has the earliest onset and most rapidly fatal course. In some instances it is apparent even before birth, as indicated by decreased fetal movements late in the third trimester. Though alert, afflicted infants are weak and floppy (hypotonic) and lack muscle stretch reflexes. Death generally ensues within the first year of life.
- *Chronic childhood SMA* (SMA II) begins later in childhood and evolves with a more slowly progressive course.
- *Juvenile SMA* (SMA III, Kugelberg-Welander disease) manifests during late childhood and runs a slow, indolent course. Unlike most denervating diseases, in this chronic disorder weakness is greatest in the proximal muscles; indeed, the pattern of clinical weakness can suggest a primary myopathy such as limb-girdle dystrophy. Electrophysiologic and muscle biopsy evidence of denervation distinguish SMA III from the myopathic syndromes.

Multifocal Motor Neuropathy with Conduction Block

In this disorder lower motor neuron function is regionally and chronically disrupted by remarkably focal blocks in conduction. MMCB is not typically associated with corticospinal signs. In contrast with ALS, MMCB may respond dramatically to therapy such as IV immunoglobulin or chemotherapy.

Disorders of the Upper Motor Neuron

Primary Lateral Sclerosis

- PLS is characterized by progressive spastic weakness of the limbs, preceded or followed by spastic dysarthria and dysphagia, indicating combined involvement of the corticospinal and corticobulbar tracts. Fasciculations, amyotrophy, and sensory changes are absent; neither electromyography nor muscle biopsy shows denervation. On neuropathologic examination there is selective loss of the large pyramidal cells in the precentral gyrus and degeneration of the corticospinal and corticobulbar projections.
- Early in its course, PLS raises the question of multiple sclerosis or other demyelinating diseases such as adrenoleukodystrophy as diagnostic considerations.

Familial Spastic Paraplegia

- FSP is usually transmitted as an autosomal trait; most adult-onset cases are dominantly inherited. Symptoms usually begin in the third or fourth decade, presenting as progressive spastic weakness beginning in the distal lower extremities; however, there are variants with onset so early that the differential diagnosis includes cerebral palsy. Neuropathologically, in FSP there is degeneration of the corticospinal tracts, which appear nearly normal in the brainstem but show increasing atrophy at more caudal levels in the spinal cord; in effect, the pathologic picture is of a dying-back or distal axonopathy of long neuronal fibers within the CNS.
- An infantile-onset form of X-linked, recessive FSP arises from mutations in the gene for myelin proteolipid protein. This is an example of rather striking allelic variation, as they cause Pelizaeus-Merzbacher disease, a widespread disorder of CNS myelin. Another recessive variant is caused by defects in the *paraplegin* gene.

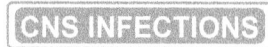

ACUTE BACTERIAL MENINGITIS

- *Bacterial meningitis* is an acute purulent infection within the subarachnoid space. It is associated with a CNS inflammatory reaction that may result in decreased consciousness, seizures, raised intracranial pressure (ICP), and stroke.
- *S. pneumoniae* is the most common cause of meningitis in adults. There are a number of predisposing conditions that increase the risk of pneumococcal meningitis, the most important of which is pneumococcal pneumonia. *N. meningitidis* accounts up to 60% of cases in children and young adults between the ages of 2 and 20. The presence of petechial or purpuric skin lesions can provide an important clue to the diagnosis of meningococcal infection. Enteric gram-negative bacilli are an increasingly common cause of meningitis in individuals with chronic and debilitating diseases such as diabetes, cirrhosis, or alcoholism and in those with chronic urinary tract infections. Group B streptococcus, or *S. agalactiae* are responsible for meningitis predominantly in neonates. *L. monocytogenes* has become an increasingly important cause of meningitis in neonates (<1 month of age), pregnant women, individuals >60 years, and immunocompromised individuals of all ages. *H. influenzae* causes meningitis in unvaccinated children and adults. *Staphylococcus aureus* and coagulase-negative staphylococci are important causes of meningitis that occurs following invasive neurosurgical procedures, particularly shunting procedures for hydrocephalus.

Clinical Presentation and Diagnosis

- Meningitis can present as either an acute fulminant illness that progresses rapidly in a few hours or as a subacute infection that progressively worsens over several days. The classic clinical triad of meningitis is fever, headache, and nuchal rigidity. Focal seizures are usually due to focal arterial ischemia or infarction, cortical venous thrombosis with hemorrhage, or focal edema. Generalized seizure activity and status epilepticus may be due to hyponatremia, cerebral anoxia.
- Raised ICP is an expected complication of bacterial meningitis and the major cause of obtundation and coma in this disease. Signs of increased ICP include a deteriorating or reduced level of consciousness, papilledema, dilated poorly reactive pupils, sixth nerve palsies, decerebrate posturing, and the Cushing reflex (bradycardia, hypertension, and irregular respirations).
- When bacterial meningitis is suspected, blood cultures should be immediately obtained and empirical antimicrobial therapy initiated. The diagnosis of bacterial meningitis is made by examination of the CSF. The classic CSF abnormalities in bacterial meningitis are:

- Polymorphonuclear (PMN) leukocytosis (>100 cells/microL),
- Decreased glucose concentration [<2.2 mmol/L (<40 mg/dL),
- Increased protein concentration [>0.45 g/L (>45 mg/dL)],
- Increased opening pressure (>180 mmH$_2$O).

- The CSF glucose concentration is low when the CSF/serum glucose ratio is <0.6. A CSF/serum glucose ratio <0.4 is highly suggestive of bacterial meningitis.
- A broad-range PCR can detect small numbers of viable and nonviable organisms in CSF. The latex agglutination (LA) test for the detection of bacterial antigens of *S. pneumoniae, N. meningitidis, H. influenzae* type b, group B streptococcus, and *E. coli* K1 strains in the CSF has been useful for making a diagnosis of bacterial meningitis but is being replaced by the CSF bacterial PCR assay.
- Neuroimaging studies should be performed during the course of their illness. MRI is preferred over CT because of its superiority in demonstrating areas of cerebral edema and ischemia. Diffuse meningeal enhancement is often seen after the administration of gadolinium.
- A number of noninfectious CNS disorders can mimic bacterial meningitis like subarachnoid hemorrhage.

Treatment

Specific Therapy

- The goal is to begin antibiotic therapy within 60 min of a patient's arrival in the emergency room. Empirical therapy of community-acquired suspected bacterial meningitis in children and adults should include a combination of dexamethasone, a third-generation cephalosporin (e.g., ceftriaxone or cefotaxime) and vancomycin.
- Ceftriaxone or cefotaxime provide good coverage for susceptible *S. pneumoniae*, group B streptococci, and *H. influenzae* and adequate coverage for *N. meningitidis*. Ampicillin should be added to the empirical regimen for coverage of *L. monocytogenes* in individuals <3 months of age, those >55, or those with suspected impaired cell-mediated immunity because of chronic illness, organ transplantation, pregnancy, malignancy, or immunosuppressive therapy.
- Meningococcal meningitis—penicillin G remains the antibiotic of choice for meningococcal meningitis caused by susceptible strains. CSF isolates of *N. meningitidis* should be tested for penicillin and ampicillin susceptibility, and if resistance is found, cefotaxime or ceftriaxone should be substituted for penicillin. A 7-day course of intravenous antibiotic therapy is adequate for uncomplicated meningococcal meningitis.
- Pneumococcal meningitis—Therapy of pneumococcal meningitis is initiated with a cephalosporin (ceftriaxone, cefotaxime, or cefepime) and vancomycin. A 2-week course of intravenous antimicrobial therapy is recommended for pneumococcal meningitis.
- Listeria meningitis—Meningitis due to *L. monocytogenes* is treated with ampicillin for at least 3 weeks. Gentamicin is often added.
- Staphylococcal meningitis—Vancomycin is the drug of choice for methicillin-resistant staphylococci and for patients allergic to penicillin.
- Gram-Negative bacillary meningitis—The third-generation cephalosporins—cefotaxime, ceftriaxone, and ceftazidime—are equally efficacious for the treatment of gram-negative bacillary meningitis, with the exception of meningitis due to *P. aeruginosa*, which should be treated with ceftazidime, cefepime, or meropenem.

Supportive Therapy

- Dexamethasone exerts its beneficial effect by inhibiting the synthesis of IL-1 and TNF at the level of mRNA, decreasing CSF outflow resistance, and stabilizing the blood-brain barrier.
- Emergency treatment of increased ICP includes elevation of the patient's head to 30–45°, intubation and hyperventilation (PaCO$_2$ 25–30 mm Hg), and mannitol.

Acute Viral Meningitis

- Patients with viral meningitis usually present with headache, fever, and signs of meningeal irritation coupled with an inflammatory CSF profile. The headache of viral meningitis is usually frontal or retroorbital and is often associated with photophobia and pain on moving the eyes. Nuchal rigidity is present in most cases but may be mild and present only near the limit of neck anteflexion.
- Seizures or focal neurologic signs or symptoms or neuroimaging abnormalities indicative of brain parenchymal involvement are not typical of viral meningitis and suggest the presence of encephalitis or another CNS infectious or inflammatory process.
- The most important agents are enteroviruses, HSV type 2 (HSV-2), and arboviruses.
- The most important laboratory test in the diagnosis of viral meningitis is examination of the CSF. The typical profile is a lymphocytic pleocytosis (25–500 cells/microL), a normal or slightly elevated protein concentration [0.2–0.8 g/L (20–80 mg/dL)], a normal glucose concentration, and a normal or mildly elevated opening pressure (100–350 mmH$_2$O).
- Organisms are *not* seen on Gram's or acid-fast stained smears or India ink preparations of CSF. The total CSF cell count in viral meningitis is typically 25–500/mL. The CSF glucose concentration is typically normal in viral infections.

- Amplification of viral-specific DNA or RNA from CSF using PCR amplification has become the single most important method for diagnosing CNS viral infections. For some viruses like arboviruses, serologic studies remain a crucial diagnostic tool. For viruses with low seroprevalence rates, diagnosis of acute viral infection can be made by documenting seroconversion between acute-phase and convalescent sera (typically obtained after 2–4 weeks) or by demonstrating the presence of virus-specific IgM antibodies.
- All patients with suspected viral meningitis should have a complete blood count and differential, liver and renal function tests, erythrocyte sedimentation rate (ESR) and C-reactive protein, electrolytes, glucose, creatine kinase, aldolase, amylase, and lipase.
- *Enteroviruses* are the most common cause of viral meningitis. CSF reverse transcriptase PCR (RT-PCR) is the diagnostic procedure of choice. The physical examination show stigmata of enterovirus infection, like exanthemata, hand-foot-mouth disease, herpangina, pleurodynia, myopericarditis, and hemorrhagic conjunctivitis.
- *HSV-2 meningitis* is recognized as a major cause of viral meningitis in adults. Diagnosis of HSV meningitis is usually by HSV CSF PCR as cultures may be negative, especially in patients with recurrent meningitis. Demonstration of intrathecal synthesis of HSV-specific antibody may also be useful in diagnosis. Most cases of recurrent viral or "aseptic" meningitis, including Mollaret's meningitis, are likely due to HSV. *VZV meningitis* should be suspected in the presence of concurrent chickenpox or shingles. *EBV infections* may also produce aseptic meningitis, with or without associated infectious mononucleosis. The presence of atypical lymphocytes in the CSF or peripheral blood is suggestive of EBV infection.
- *HIV meningitis* should be suspected in any patient presenting with viral meningitis with known or suspected risk factors for HIV infection. Meningitis may occur following primary infection with HIV or at later stages of illness. Cranial nerve palsies, most commonly involving cranial nerves V, VII, or VIII, are more common in HIV meningitis than in other viral infections.

Treatment

- Treatment of almost all cases of viral meningitis is primarily symptomatic. Fluid and electrolyte status should be monitored. Oral or intravenous acyclovir may be of benefit in patients with meningitis caused by HSV-1 or -2 and in cases of severe EBV or VZV infection. Patients with HIV meningitis should receive highly active antiretroviral therapy.
- Vaccination is an effective method of preventing the development of meningitis and other neurologic complications associated with poliovirus, mumps, and measles infection.

CSF Findings in Different Types of Meningitis

Condition	Cells	Protein	Glucose
Bacterial infection	WBC >50/mm³, often greatly increased	100–250 mg%	20–50 mg%; lower than half of blood glucose level
Viral, fungal, spirochetal infection	WBC 10–100/mm³	50–200 mg%	Normal or slightly reduced
Tuberculous infection	WBC >25/mm³	100–1,000 mg%	<50, markedly reduced

Viral Encephalitis

- In contrast to meningitis, where the infectious process and associated inflammatory response are limited largely to the meninges, in encephalitis the brain parenchyma is also involved usually with associated meningitis (meningoencephalitis) and, in some cases, involvement of the spinal cord or nerve roots (encephalomyelitis, encephalomyeloradiculitis).
- In addition to the acute febrile illness with evidence of meningeal involvement characteristic of meningitis, the patient with encephalitis commonly has an altered level of consciousness (confusion, behavioral abnormalities), or a depressed level of consciousness, ranging from mild lethargy to coma, and evidence of either focal or diffuse neurologic signs and symptoms. The most commonly encountered focal findings are aphasia, ataxia, upper or lower motor neuron patterns of weakness, involuntary movements (e.g., myoclonic jerks, tremor), and cranial nerve deficits (e.g., ocular palsies, facial weakness).
- The most important viruses causing sporadic cases of encephalitis in immunocompetent adults are herpesviruses (HSV, VZV, EBV). Epidemics of encephalitis are caused by arboviruses, [*Alphaviruses Flaviviruses* and *Bunyaviruses*].
- The characteristic CSF profile is indistinguishable from that of viral meningitis and typically consists of a lymphocytic pleocytosis, a mildly elevated protein concentration, and a normal glucose concentration. Patients who are severely immunocompromised by HIV infection, glucocorticoid or other immunosuppressant drugs, chemotherapy, or lymphoreticular malignancies may fail to mount a CSF inflammatory response. A decreased CSF glucose concentration is unusual in viral encephalitis and should suggest the possibility of bacterial, fungal, tuberculous, parasitic, leptospiral, syphilitic, sarcoid, or neoplastic meningitis.
- CSF PCR has become the primary diagnostic test for CNS infections caused by CMV, EBV, VZV, HHV-6, and enteroviruses. The basic approach to the serodiagnosis of viral encephalitis is identical to that discussed earlier for viral meningitis. In patients with HSV encephalitis, both antibodies to HSV-1 glycoproteins and glycoprotein antigens have been detected in the CSF.
- Patients with suspected encephalitis almost invariably undergo neuroimaging studies and often EEG. These tests help identify or exclude alternative diagnoses and assist in the differentiation between a focal, as opposed to a diffuse, encephalitic process.
- Patients with VZV encephalitis may show multifocal areas of hemorrhagic and ischemic infarction reflecting the tendency of this virus to produce a CNS vasculopathy rather than true encephalitis.

- Infection caused by the ameba *Naegleria fowleri* can also cause acute meningoencephalitis (primary amebic meningoencephalitis), whereas that caused by *Acanthamoeba* and *Balamuthia* more typically produces subacute or chronic granulomatous amebic meningoencephalitis. Infection has typically occurred in immunocompetent children with a history of swimming in potentially infected water. The CSF, in contrast to the typical profile seen in viral encephalitis, often resembles that of bacterial meningitis with a neutrophilic pleocytosis and hypoglycorrhachia. Motile trophozoites can be seen in a wet mount of warm, fresh CSF.

Treatment

- Basic management and supportive therapy should include careful monitoring of ICP, fluid restriction, avoidance of hypotonic intravenous solutions, and suppression of fever. Specific antiviral therapy should be initiated when appropriate. Acyclovir is of benefit in the treatment of HSV and should be started empirically in patients with suspected viral encephalitis, especially if focal features are present, while awaiting viral diagnostic studies. Oral antiviral drugs with efficacy against HSV, VZV, and EBV, including acyclovir, famciclovir, and valacyclovir.
- Ganciclovir and foscarnet, either alone or in combination, are often utilized in the treatment of CMV-related CNS infections. Cidofovir may provide an alternative in patients who fail to respond to ganciclovir and foscarnet.

Subacute Meningitis

- Common causative organisms include *M. tuberculosis*, *C. neoformans*, *H. capsulatum*, *C. immitis*, and *T. pallidum*.
- Initial infection with *M. tuberculosis* is acquired by inhalation of aerosolized droplet nuclei. Tuberculous meningitis in adults does not develop acutely from hematogenous spread of tubercle bacilli to the meninges. Rather, millet seed–size (miliary) tubercles form in the parenchyma of the brain during hematogenous dissemination of tubercle bacilli in the course of primary infection. These tubercles enlarge and are usually caseating. Fungal infections are typically acquired by the inhalation of airborne fungal spores. The most common pathogen causing fungal meningitis is *C. neoformans*. This fungus is found worldwide in soil and bird excreta. Syphilis is a sexually transmitted disease that is manifest by the appearance of a painless chancre at the site of inoculation. *T. pallidum* invades the CNS early in the course of syphilis.
- The classic CSF abnormalities in tuberculous meningitis are as follows:
  - Elevated opening pressure,
  - Lymphocytic pleocytosis (10–500 cells/microL),
  - Elevated protein concentration in the range of 1–5 g/L (10–500 mg/dL), and
  - Decreased glucose concentration in the range of 1.1–2.2 mmol/L (20–40 mg/dL).
- *The combination of unrelenting headache, stiff neck, fatigue, night sweats, and fever with a CSF lymphocytic pleocytosis and a mildly decreased glucose concentration is highly suspicious for tuberculous meningitis.*
- Cultures of CSF take 4–8 weeks to identify the organism and are positive in ~50% of adults. Culture remains the "gold standard" to make the diagnosis of tuberculous meningitis.
- The characteristic CSF abnormalities in fungal meningitis are a mononuclear or lymphocytic pleocytosis, an increased protein concentration, and a decreased glucose concentration. The cryptococcal polysaccharide antigen test is a highly sensitive and specific test for cryptococcal meningitis.
- The diagnosis of syphilitic meningitis is made when a reactive serum treponemal test [fluorescent treponemal antibody absorption test (FTA-ABS) or microhemagglutination-*T. pallidum* (MHA-TP)] is associated with a CSF lymphocytic or mononuclear pleocytosis and an elevated protein concentration. A negative CSF FTA-ABS or MHA-TP rules out neurosyphilis.

Treatment

- A 6-month course of Anti-tubercular therapy is acceptable, but therapy should be prolonged for 9–12 months in patients who have an inadequate resolution of symptoms of meningitis or who have positive mycobacterial cultures of CSF during the course of therapy. Dexamethasone therapy is recommended for patients who develop hydrocephalus.
- Meningitis due to *C. neoformans* is treated with amphotericin B (0.7 mg/kg IV per day) for 2 weeks or until CSF culture is sterile. This treatment is followed by an 8–10-week course of fluconazole (400–800 mg/d PO). amphotericin B lipid complex (5 mg/kg per day) can be substituted for amphotericin B in patients who have or who develop significant renal dysfunction.
- Syphilitic meningitis is treated with aqueous penicillin G in a dose of 3–4 million units intravenously every 4 h for 10–14 days. An alternative regimen is 2.4 million units of procaine penicillin G intramuscularly daily with 500 mg of oral probenecid four times daily for 10–14 days.

Chronic Encephalitis

Progressive Multifocal Leukoencephalopathy

- Progressive multifocal leukoencephalopathy (PML) is a progressive disorder characterized pathologically by multifocal areas of demyelination of varying size distributed throughout the brain but sparing the spinal cord and optic nerves.

- Oligodendrocytes have enlarged, densely staining nuclei that contain viral inclusions formed by crystalline arrays of JC virus (JCV) particles. Almost all patients have an underlying immunosuppressive disorder.
- The CSF is typically normal, although mild elevation in protein and/or IgG may be found. PCR amplification of JCV DNA from CSF is an important diagnostic tool. Detection of JCV antigen or genomic material should only be considered diagnostic of PML if accompanied by characteristic pathologic changes.

Treatment

No effective therapy for PML is available. Some patients with HIV-associated PML have shown disease stabilization and improvement in their immune status following institution of HAART.

Subacute Sclerosing Panencephalitis (SSPE)

- SSPE is a chronic, progressive demyelinating disease of the CNS associated with a chronic infection of brain tissue with measles virus. Most patients give a history of primary measles infection at an early age (2 years), which is followed after a latent interval of 6–8 years by the development of progressive neurologic disorder. As the disease progresses, patients develop progressive intellectual deterioration, focal and/or generalized seizures, myoclonus, ataxia, and visual disturbances. In the late stage of the illness, patients are unresponsive, quadriparetic, and spastic with hyperactive tendon reflexes and extensor plantar responses.
- The EEG may initially show only nonspecific slowing, but with disease progression, patients develop a characteristic periodic pattern with bursts of high-voltage, sharp, slow waves every 3–8s, followed by periods of attenuated ("flat") background. The CSF is acellular with a normal or mildly elevated protein concentration and a markedly elevated gamma globulin level (>20% of total CSF protein).
- CSF antimeasles antibody levels are elevated and oligoclonal antimeasles antibodies are often present.
- No definitive therapy for SSPE is available. Treatment with isoprinosine (Inosiplex, 100 mg/kg per day), alone or in combination with intrathecal or intraventricular alpha interferon can be useful.

Brain Abscess

- A brain abscess is a focal, suppurative infection within the brain parenchyma, typically surrounded by a vascularized capsule. Predisposing conditions include otitis media and mastoiditis, paranasal sinusitis, pyogenic infections in the chest or other body sites, penetrating head trauma or neurosurgical procedures, and dental infections.
- In immunocompetent individuals the most important pathogens are *Streptococcus* spp., Enterobacteriaceae, anaerobes, and staphylococci. In immunocompromised hosts with underlying HIV infection, organ transplantation, cancer, or immunosuppressive therapy, most brain abscesses are caused by *Nocardia* spp., *Toxoplasma gondii*, *Aspergillus* spp., *Candida* spp., and *C. neoformans*.
- **A brain abscess may develop**
    - By direct spread from a contiguous cranial site of infection, such as paranasal sinusitis, otitis media, mastoiditis, or dental infection;
    - Following head trauma or a neurosurgical procedure; or
    - As a result of hematogenous spread from a remote site of infection.
- The classic clinical triad of headache, fever, and a focal neurologic deficit is present. The most common symptom in patients with a brain abscess is headache which is often characterized as a constant, dull, aching sensation, either hemicranial or generalized, and it becomes progressively more severe and refractory to therapy. The clinical presentation of a brain abscess depends on its location, the nature of the primary infection if present, and the level of the ICP.
- Hemiparesis is the most common localizing sign of a frontal lobe abscess. A temporal lobe abscess may present with a disturbance of language (dysphasia) or an upper homonymous quadrantanopia. Nystagmus and ataxia are signs of a cerebellar abscess
- Diagnosis is made by neuroimaging studies. MRI is better than CT for demonstrating abscesses in the early (cerebritis) stages and is superior to CT for identifying abscesses in the posterior fossa.
- Microbiologic diagnosis of the etiologic agent is most accurately determined by Gram's stain and culture of abscess material obtained by stereotactic needle aspiration. Aerobic and anaerobic bacterial cultures and mycobacterial and fungal cultures should be obtained.

Treatment

- Optimal therapy of brain abscesses involves a combination of high-dose parenteral antibiotics and neurosurgical drainage. In patients with penetrating head trauma or recent neurosurgical procedures, treatment should include ceftazidime as the third-generation cephalosporin to enhance coverage of *Pseudomonas* spp. and vancomycin for coverage of staphylococci.
- Aspiration and drainage of the abscess under stereotactic guidance are beneficial for both diagnosis and therapy. Complete excision of a bacterial abscess via craniotomy or craniectomy is generally reserved for multiloculated abscesses or those in which stereotactic aspiration is unsuccessful.

- In addition to surgical drainage and antibiotic therapy, patients should receive prophylactic anticonvulsant therapy. Anticonvulsant therapy is continued for at least 3 months after resolution of the abscess, and decisions regarding withdrawal are then based on the EEG.
- Intravenous dexamethasone therapy (10 mg every 6 h) is usually reserved for patients with substantial periabscess edema and associated mass effect and increased ICP.

Subdural Empyema

- A subdural empyema (SDE) is a collection of pus between the dura and arachnoid membranes. Sinusitis is the most common predisposing condition and typically involves the frontal sinuses, either alone or in combination with the ethmoid and maxillary sinuses. Secondary infection of a subdural effusion may also result in empyema.
- Aerobic and anaerobic streptococci, staphylococci, Enterobacteriaceae, and anaerobic bacteria are the most common causative organisms of sinusitis-associated SDE. Sinusitis-associated SDE develops as a result of either retrograde spread of infection from septic thrombophlebitis of the mucosal veins draining the sinuses or contiguous spread of infection to the brain from osteomyelitis in the posterior wall of the frontal or other sinuses.
- A patient with SDE typically presents with fever and a progressively worsening headache. As the infection progresses, focal neurologic deficits, seizures, nuchal rigidity, and signs of increased ICP commonly occur. Contralateral hemiparesis or hemiplegia is the most common focal neurologic deficit and can occur from the direct effects of the SDE on the cortex or as a consequence of venous infarction.
- MRI is superior to CT in identifying SDE and any associated intracranial infections. The administration of gadolinium greatly improves diagnosis by enhancing the rim of the empyema.

Treatment

- SDE is a medical emergency. Emergent neurosurgical evacuation of the empyema, either through burr-hole drainage or craniotomy, is the definitive step in the management of this infection. Parenteral antibiotic therapy should be continued for a minimum of 4 weeks. Specific diagnosis of the etiologic organisms is made based on Gram's stain and culture of fluid obtained via either burr holes or craniotomy.

Prion Diseases

Prions are infectious proteins that cause degeneration of the central nervous system (CNS). Prion diseases are disorders of protein conformation, the most common of which in humans is called Creutzfeldt-Jakob disease (CJD).
1. Prions are the only known infectious pathogens that are devoid of nucleic acid.
2. Prion diseases may be manifest as infectious, genetic, and sporadic disorders.
3. Prion diseases result from the accumulation of PrP^{Sc}, the conformation of which differs substantially from that of its precursor, PrP$_C$.
4. PrP^{Sc} can exist in a variety of different conformations, each of which seems to specify a particular disease phenotype.

The sporadic form of CJD is the most common prion disorder in humans. Sporadic CJD (sCJD) accounts for most of the cases of human prion disease. Familial CJD (fCJD), Gerstmann-Sträussler-Scheinker (GSS) disease, and fatal familial insomnia (FFI) are all dominantly inherited prion diseases that are caused by mutations in the PrP gene. Diseases of animals caused by prions are—Scrapie of sheep and goats, Mink encephalopathy, BSE, feline spongiform encephalopathy, and exotic ungulate encephalopathy.

A major feature that distinguishes prions from viruses is the finding that both PrP isoforms are encoded by a chromosomal gene. In humans, the PrP gene is designated *PRNP* and is located on the short arm of chromosome 20. Both the rods and the PrP amyloid filaments found in brain tissue exhibit similar ultrastructural morphology and green-gold birefringence after staining with Congo red dye.

Infectious Prion Diseases

Iatrogenic CJD

- Corneas from donors with inapparent CJD have been transplanted to apparently healthy recipients who developed CJD after prolonged incubation periods. Surgical procedures may have resulted in accidental inoculation of patients with prions, presumably because some instrument or apparatus in the operating theater became contaminated when a CJD patient underwent surgery.
- There is a possibility of transmission of CJD from contaminated human growth hormone (hGH) preparations derived from human pituitaries.
- Frequently the brains of patients with CJD have no recognizable abnormalities on gross examination. Patients who survive for several years have variable degrees of cerebral atrophy. On light microscopy, the pathologic hallmarks of CJD are spongiform degeneration and astrocytic gliosis.

- Amyloid plaques have been found in ~10% of CJD cases. Purified CJD prions from humans and animals exhibit the ultrastructural and histochemical characteristics of amyloid when treated with detergents during limited proteolysis. In vCJD, a characteristic feature is the presence of "florid plaques." These are composed of a central core of PrP amyloid, surrounded by vacuoles in a pattern suggesting petals on a flower.

Clinical Features and Diagnosis

- Nonspecific prodromal symptoms usually occur in patients with CJD and may include fatigue, sleep disturbance, weight loss, headache, malaise, and ill-defined pain. Most patients with CJD present with deficits in higher cortical function. These deficits almost always progress over weeks or months to a state of profound dementia characterized by memory loss, impaired judgment, and a decline in virtually all aspects of intellectual function.
- Most patients with CJD exhibit myoclonus that appears at various times throughout the illness. Unlike other involuntary movements, myoclonus persists during sleep. The constellation of dementia, myoclonus, and periodic electrical bursts in an afebrile 60-year-old patient generally indicates CJD.
- The conformation-dependent immunoassay (CDI) for diagnosis is based on immunoreactive epitopes that are exposed in PrP^C but buried in PrP^{Sc}. In humans, the diagnosis of CJD can be established by brain biopsy if PrP^{Sc} is detected. CT may be normal or show cortical atrophy. MRI is valuable for distinguishing sCJD from most other conditions. FLAIR sequences and diffusion-weighted imaging show increased intensity in the basal ganglia and cortical ribboning.
- CSF is nearly always normal but may show protein elevation and, rarely, mild pleocytosis.
- The EEG is often useful in the diagnosis of CJD. During the early phase of CJD, the EEG is usually normal or shows only scattered theta activity. In most advanced cases, repetitive, high-voltage, triphasic, and polyphasic sharp discharges are seen.

GSS

In GSS disease, ataxia is usually a prominent and presenting feature, with dementia occurring late in the disease course. GSS disease typically presents earlier than CJD and is typically more slowly progressive than CJD; death usually occurs within 5 years of onset.

Fatal Familial Insomnia

FFI is characterized by insomnia and dysautonomia; dementia occurs only in the terminal phase of the illness. Rare sporadic cases have been identified. The only specific diagnostic tests for CJD and other human prion diseases measure PrP^{Sc}.

Management

- Biosafety level 2 practices, containment equipment, and facilities are recommended by the Centers for Disease Control and Prevention and the National Institutes of Health. The primary problem in caring for patients with CJD is the inadvertent infection of health care workers by needle and stab wounds.
- Prions are extremely resistant to common inactivation procedures. Autoclaving at 134°C for 5 h or treatment with 2 N NaOH for several hours is recommended for sterilization of prions.
- There is no known effective therapy for preventing or treating CJD. The acridines and anti-PrP antibodies have been shown to eliminate PrP^{Sc} from cultured cells. Several drugs, including pentosan polysulfate and porphyrin derivatives, delay the onset of disease in animals inoculated intracerebrally with prions if the drugs are given intracerebrally beginning soon after inoculation.

CEREBROVASCULAR DISORDERS

Cerebrovascular disease is the most common cause of neurologic disability in adults and the third most common cause of death in our society. Cerebrovascular disease is usually classified into *ischemic* and *hemorrhagic* disorders.

As a result of its high metabolic rate and limited energy reserves, the central nervous system (CNS) is uniquely sensitive to ischemia. Ischemia results in rapid depletion of adenosine triphosphate (ATP) stores in the CNS. Because Na^+-K^+ ATPase function is impaired, K^+ accumulates in the extracellular space, which leads to neuronal depolarization. Transient ischemia, if brief enough, may produce reversible signs and symptoms of neuronal dysfunction. If ischemia is prolonged, however, death of neurons (infarction) occurs and is usually accompanied by persistent neurologic deficits.

Surrounding the area of infarction, there is often a penumbra, in which neurons have been metabolically compromised and are electrically silent but are not yet dead. Neurons within the penumbra may be salvageable, and various neuroprotective strategies that interfere with calcium influx are being experimentally studied.

CLASSIFICATION

- **Occlusive cerebrovascular disorders:** These result from arterial or venous thrombosis, or embolism, and can lead to infarction of well-defined parts of the brain. Because each artery irrigates a specific part of the brain, it is often possible, on the basis of the neurologic deficit, to identify the vessel that is occluded.
- Transient cerebral ischemia: Transient ischemia, if brief enough, can occur without infarction. Episodes of this type are termed transient ischemic attacks (TIAs). As with occlusive cerebrovascular disease, the neurologic abnormalities often permit the clinician to predict the vessel that is involved.
- **Hemorrhage:** The rupture of a blood vessel is often associated with hypertension or vascular malformations or with trauma.
- Vascular malformations and developmental abnormalities: These include aneurysms or arteriovenous malformations (AVMs), which can lead to hemorrhage. Hypoplasia or absence of vessels occurs in some brains.
- Degenerative diseases of the arteries: These can lead to occlusion or to hemorrhage.
- Inflammatory diseases of the arteries: Inflammatory diseases, including systemic lupus erythematosus, giant cell arteritis, and syphilitic arteritis, can result in occlusion of cerebral vessels, which, in turn, can produce infarction.

OCCLUSIVE CEREBROVASCULAR DISEASE

- Insufficient blood supply to portions of the brain leads to infarction and swelling with necrosis of brain tissue. Most infarcts are caused by atherosclerosis of the vessels, leading to narrowing, occlusion, or thrombosis; a cerebral embolism, that is, occlusion caused by an embolus (a plug of tissue or a foreign substance) from outside the brain; or other conditions such as prolonged hypotension, drug action, spasm, or inflammation of the vessels. Venous infarction may occur when a venous channel becomes occluded.
- The extent of an infarct depends on the presence or absence of adequate anastomotic channels. When arterial occlusion occurs proximal to the circle of Willis, *collateral circulation* through the anterior communicating artery and posterior communicating arteries may permit sufficient blood flow to prevent infarction. Although sudden occlusion can lead to irreparable damage, slowly developing local ischemia may be compensated for by increased flow through anastomoses involving one or more routes: the circle of Willis, the ophthalmic artery (whose branches communicate with external carotid vessels), or corticomeningeal anastomoses from meningeal vessels.

Atherosclerosis of the Brain

- The principal pathologic change in the arteries of the brain occurs in the vasculature of the neck and brain. Disturbances in metabolism, especially of fats, are believed to be a prominent associated change. Hypertension accelerates the progression of atherosclerosis and is a treatable risk factor for stroke.
- The muscularis is the main site of proliferation; the intima may be absent. The areas most often involved are near branchings or confluences of vessels. The most common and severe atherosclerotic lesions are in the carotid bifurcation.

Cerebral Embolism

- The sudden occlusion of a brain vessel by a blood clot, a piece of fat, a tumor, a clump of bacteria, or air abruptly interrupts the blood supply to a portion of the brain and can result in infarction. One of the most common causes of cerebral embolism is atrial fibrillation. Other common causes include endocarditis and mural thrombus after myocardial infarction.

TRANSIENT CEREBRAL ISCHEMIA

- Focal cerebral ischemic attacks, especially in middle- aged and older persons, can be caused by transient occlusion of an already narrow vessel. The cause is thought to be a vasospasm, a small embolus that is later carried away, or thrombosis of a diseased vessel (and subsequent anastomosis).
- TIAs are powerful forerunners of stroke. TIAs are short-lived episodes of acute, focal, nonconvulsive neurologic dysfunction presumably caused by reversible ischemia to an area of the retina or brain. Onset of symptoms is sudden and often unprovoked, reaching maximum intensity almost immediately. TIAs involving the anterior or carotid circulation should be separated from those involving the posterior or vertebrobasilar circulation. Most TIAs have an embolic ipsilateral carotid or cardiac source; hemodynamic mechanisms are less common.
- There is usually full recovery from a TIA in less than 24 hours (commonly within 30 minutes).

STROKE SYNDROMES

- They may arise from an infarct or a hemorrhage. An infarct is usually due to either thrombosis from atherosclerotic lesions or embolism from the heart, aorta, or extracranial/intracranial vasculature. Hemorrhage may be epidural, subdural, subarachnoid, intra-parenchymal, or intraventricular, and may have various etiologies, including arterial hypertension, saccular aneurysms, arteriovenous malformations, blood dyscrasias, vasculitis, sympathomimetic drugs, cerebral amyloid angiopathy, trauma, or neoplasms. Stroke in evolution or progressive stroke describes the temporal profile in which the neurologic deficit occurs in a stepwise or progressive fashion, culminating in a major deficit in the absence of treatment.

Carotid Artery Syndrome

- The only feature distinguishing the carotid artery syndrome from the MCA syndrome is amaurosis fugax or transient monocular blindness.
- Patients with amaurosis fugax often describe the sudden onset of transient painless monocular loss of vision sometimes described as a curtain or shade being pulled from the top or bottom of a visual field. The characteristics of the attacks of visual loss are often described as a blackout, dimming, blurring, graying, or fogging of vision.
- The length of visual loss is approximately 1 to 5 minutes; but rarely it may last 20 to 30 minutes. During attacks the pupil is amaurotic and the retinal vessels collapse. Amaurosis fugax often results from embolism from the carotid artery, heart, or aorta, hypoperfusion, hypercoagulable states, or vasospasm.
- Unilateral loss of vision in bright light (amaurosis) may occur in patients with high-grade stenosis or occlusion of the ipsilateral carotid artery.
- Atherothrombotic disease of the carotid system has a predilection for the bifurcation of the common carotid artery and the proximal ICA. Infarction of the homolateral hemisphere may occur when the collateral circulation is inadequate.
- Infarcts may involve the entire territory of the MCA (total), the areas of supply nearest the ICA or MCA (proximal), the border zone between the ACA and MCA (watershed), or only the white matter supplied by peripheral branches of the MCA (terminal).
- Patients may initially complain of localized or generalized headaches, and focal seizures may occur. Contralateral hemiplegia, hemianesthesia, homonymous hemianopia, and aphasia (if the dominant hemisphere is compromised) or apractagnosia (if the nondominant hemisphere is involved) may ensue.
- In most cases, patients present with uniform (proportionate) hemiparesis (face, shoulder, hand, hip, and foot), or faciobrachial weakness. Severe stenosis or occlusion of the ICA may cause progressive or episodic weakness of one lower extremity, often aggravated or precipitated by standing or walking.
- Other atypical carotid distribution transient ischemic manifestations include orthostatic TIAs, transient anosognosia, and transient loss of pitch perception. Infarcts of the genu of the internal capsule may cause contralateral facial and lingual paresis with dysarthria.

Anterior Choroidal Artery Syndrome

- Infarction in the AChA territory typically results in hemiparesis due to involvement of the pyramidal tract in the posterior limb of the internal capsule, hemisensory loss due to involvement of the superior thalamic radiations situated in the thalamolenticular portion of the posterior limb of the internal capsule, and homonymous hemianopia sparing the horizontal meridian. A relative afferent pupillary defect may be present in the eye contralateral to the side of the lesion (optic tract lesion).
- Clinical syndromes with AChA infarction include a pure motor syndrome, a sensorimotor syndrome, and ataxic hemiparesis. CT scan or MRI examination reveals abnormality in the posterior limb of the internal capsule, sparing the thalamus medially and encroaching on the tip of the globus pallidus laterally.
- Bilateral AChA infarction may result in bilateral capsular infarction, causing acute pseudobulbar mutism accompanied by varying degrees of facial diplegia, hemiparesis, hemisensory loss, lethargy, neglect, and affect changes.

Anterior Cerebral Artery Syndrome

- Infarction in the ACA territory causes damage primarily to the medial frontal area. Infarction in the territory of the hemispheric branches of the ACA often results in contralateral weakness involving primarily the lower extremity and, to a lesser extent, the arm (especially the shoulder).
- Patients may display lack of initiative or abulia. Paratonia (gegenhalten) is often present. With involvement of the anterior corpus callosum, they may have left arm apraxia (anterior disconnection syndrome). Sensory examination may show contralateral tactile sensory loss affecting primarily the lower extremity.
- Infarction in the territory of the medial lenticulostriate artery (artery of Heubner) results in contralateral weakness of the face and arm without accompanying sensory loss. Therefore, with proximal ACA infarction, severe contralateral hemiplegia may result, with paralysis of the face, tongue, and arm from damage to the anterior limb of the interior capsule and paralysis of the leg from paracentral damage.

- Infarction of the basal branches of the ACA cause transient memory disorders, anxiety, and agitation. Patients with occlusion of the pericallosal branches may show apraxia, agraphia, and tactile anomia of the left hand.

Middle Cerebral Artery Syndrome
- The MCA is the largest branch of the ICA and a continuation of this artery in the direction of the Sylvian fissure.
- Contralateral weakness affecting the face, the arm, and, to a lesser extent, the leg is a common manifestation of MCA territory infarction. With MCA territory infarction, there may be paresis and apraxia of conjugate gaze to the opposite side, with transient tonic deviation of the eyes and head toward the side of the lesion.
- Infarcts in the dominant hemisphere for language can be followed by Broca's, Wernicke's, conduction, or global aphasia, depending on the site and extent of involvement. Alexia with agraphia may occur with the involvement of the left angular gyrus.
- Complete MCA territory infarctions have a poor outcome and may result in severe hemiparesis, forced eye and head deviation, a progressive diminishing level of consciousness secondary to space-occupying ischemic brain edema, brain shifts, and subsequent herniation.

Posterior Cerebral Artery Syndrome
- The clinical picture of PCA territory infarction varies according to the site of occlusion and the availability of collaterals. Occlusion of the precommunal P1 segment causes midbrain, thalamic, and hemispheric infarction.
- Infarction in the distribution of the hemispheric branches of the PCA may produce contralateral homonymous hemianopia caused by infarction of the striate cortex, the optic radiations, or the lateral geniculate body. There is partial or complete macular sparing if the infarction does not reach the occipital pole. The visual field defect may be limited to a quadrantanopia.
- Infarction in the distribution of the callosal branches of the PCA involving the left occipital region and the splenium of the corpus callosum produces alexia without agraphia (pure word blindness). In this syndrome, patients can write, speak, and spell normally, but are unable to read words and sentences.
- Bilateral occipital or occipitoparietal infarctions may result in cortical blindness with preserved pupillary reflexes. Patients often deny or are unaware of their blindness (*Anton's syndrome*).

Vertebrobasilar Artery Syndromes of the Brainstem and Cerebellum
- Connected to the brainstem by three pairs of cerebellar peduncles, the main symptoms of cerebellar infarction include vertigo, dizziness, nausea, vomiting, gait unsteadiness, limb clumsiness, headache, dysarthria, diplopia, and decreased alertness.
- With a cerebellar pressure cone (tonsillar hernia) there is downward displacement of the cerebellar tonsils through the foramen magnum, resulting in hemorrhagic necrosis of the cerebellar tonsils and grooving of the ventral surface of the medulla oblongata. Clinical manifestations may include neck stiffness, cardiac and respiratory rhythm disturbances, and apnea.
- Although a PICA occlusion can be the cause of Wallenberg (lateral medullary) syndrome, this syndrome is more often caused by an intracranial vertebral artery occlusion.
- The anterior inferior cerebellar artery syndrome causes a ventral cerebellar infarction. The signs and symptoms include vertigo, nausea, vomiting, and nystagmus caused by involvement of the vestibular nuclei. Ipsilateral deafness and facial paralysis occurs because of the involvement of the lateral pontomedullary tegmentum. An ipsilateral Horner syndrome is present because of the compromise of the descending oculosympathetic fibers.
- The superior cerebellar artery vascularizes the superior half of the cerebellar hemisphere and vermis, dentate nucleus, and upper aspect of the pontine tegmentum. Infarction in the territory of the superior cerebellar artery produces a dorsal cerebellar syndrome. Vertigo, Nystagmus, ipsilateral Horner syndrome, Ipsilateral ataxia and asynergia and gait ataxia are caused.

Midbrain Syndromes
- *Weber's syndrome* is caused by infarction in the distribution of the penetrating branches of the PCA affecting the cerebral peduncle, especially medially, with damage to the fascicle of CN III and the pyramidal fibers. The resultant clinical findings are contralateral hemiparesis caused by corticospinal and corticobulbar tract involvement and ipsilateral oculomotor paresis, including a dilated pupil.
- *The midbrain syndrome of Foville* in which the supranuclear fibers for horizontal gaze are interrupted in the medial cerebral peduncle, causing a conjugate palsy to the opposite side. Dorsal pontine lesion; ipsilateral 6th and 7th nerve palsy with contralateral hemiplegia.
- *Benedikt's syndrome* is caused by a lesion affecting the mesencephalic tegmentum in its ventral portion, with the involvement of the red nucleus, brachium conjunctivum, and fascicle of CN III. This syndrome is caused by infarction in the distribution of the penetrating branches of the PCA to the midbrain. The clinical manifestations are an ipsilateral third nerve paresis, usually with pupillary dilation, and a contralateral hemitremor, hemiathetosis, or hemichorea.

- *Claude's syndrome* (featuring elements of both Benedikt's and Nothnagel's syndromes) is caused by lesions that are more dorsally placed in the midbrain tegmentum than in Benedikt's syndrome. There is injury to the dorsal red nucleus, which results in more prominent cerebellar signs (asynergia, ataxia, dysmetria, and dysdiadochokinesia) without the involuntary movements. Consists of ipsilateral 3rd nerve palsy and contralateral tremors and ataxia
- *Nothnagel's syndrome* is characterized by an ipsilateral third nerve paresis with contralateral cerebellar ataxia. Nothnagel's syndrome is caused by a lesion in the area of the superior cerebellar peduncle, in the distribution of the penetrating branches of the PCA to the midbrain, and may represent a variant of the dorsal midbrain syndrome.
- *Parinaud's (dorsal midbrain syndrome*, pretectal syndrome, Sylvian aqueduct syndrome, P1) syndrome can result from infarctions in the midbrain territory of the PCA penetrating branches (artery of Percheron) – lesion in the superior colliculus. This syndrome is characterized by supranuclear paralysis of vertical gaze, defective convergence, spasm/paresis of accommodation, convergence retraction nystagmus, light-near dissociation of the pupils, lid retraction (Collier's sign), and skew deviation.
- *Locked-in syndrome* (ventral pontine syndrome or de-efferented state) is the result of bilateral destruction usually at the level of the basis pontis involving the rostral and middle pontine segments interrupting the descending corticobulbar and corticospinal tracts, causing quadriplegia, aphonia, anarthria, and impairment of the horizontal eye movements. The patient can move his or her eyes vertically and can blink because the supranuclear ocular motor pathway lies more dorsally; 3rd nerve is normal.
- Occlusion of the anterior inferior cerebellar artery can lead to the lateral inferior pontine syndrome. Findings associated with this syndrome include ipsilateral facial paralysis, impaired facial sensation, and paralysis of conjugate gaze to the side of the lesion, deafness, tinnitus, and ataxia. Contralateral to the lesion, there is hemibody impairment to pain and temperature, which in some instances includes the face.
- The medial inferior pontine syndrome is caused by occlusion of a paramedian branch of the basilar artery. With this syndrome, there is ipsilateral paralysis of conjugate gaze to the side of the lesion, abducens nerve palsy, nystagmus, and ataxia. Contralateral to the lesion, there is hemibody impairment of tactile and proprioceptive sensation and paralysis of the face, arm, and leg.
- *The lateral medullary syndrome (Wallenberg syndrome)* is most often caused by atherosclerotic occlusion or dissection of the intracranial segment of the vertebral artery. Wallenberg syndrome consists of a constellation of signs and symptoms including
  - Ipsilateral limb and gait ataxia with a tendency to fall to the ipsilateral side (body lateropulsion) due to involvement of the restiform body and inferior surface of the cerebellar hemisphere
  - Ipsilateral facial hypalgesia and thermoanesthesia because of involvement of the descending tract and nucleus of the trigeminal nerve
  - Paresis of the pharyngeal muscles with palatal weakness, decreased gag reflex, dysphagia, and dysphonia due to ipsilateral vocal cord paresis caused by the involvement of the nucleus ambiguous
  - An ipsilateral Horner syndrome is present because of compromise of the descending oculosympathetic pathways
  - Contralateral trunk and extremity hypalgesia and thermoanesthesia occurs caused by involvement of the spinothalamic tract.
- The medial medullary syndrome (Dejerine's syndrome) is less common and may be caused by distal atherosclerotic vertebral artery occlusive disease The findings associated with this syndrome include an ipsilateral lower motor neuron paralysis of the tongue and contralateral paralysis of the arm and leg and ataxia. The face is often spared.
- The occlusion of the vertebral artery can lead to a total unilateral hemimedullary (Babinski-Nageotte) syndrome, which is a combination of the medial and lateral medullary syndrome.

Syndromes of Thalamic Infarction

- The thalamus is the largest subdivision of the diencephalon. The main thalamic blood supply originates from the posterior communicating arteries and the perimesencephalic segment of the PCA. Three common clinical syndromes may occur: pure sensory stroke, sensorimotor stroke, and the thalamic syndrome of Dejerine-Roussy.
- In the Dejerine-Roussy syndrome, the patient has contralateral sensory loss to all modalities, severe dysesthesias of the involved side (thalamic pain), vasomotor disturbances, transient contralateral hemiparesis, and choreoathetoid or ballistic movements.

Border Zone Ischemia

- Border zone ischemia is often explained by the combination of two frequently interrelated processes: hypoperfusion and embolization. Border zone ischemia may result in several characteristic syndromes:
- Ischemia in the border zone territory of all three major arterial systems (anterior, middle, and PCA) may result in bilateral parieto-occipital lesions.
- Ischemia between the anterior and middle cerebral arteries (bilateral) may result in bibrachial cortical sensorimotor impairment, initially affecting whole limbs but later confined to the hands and forearms.
- Ischemia of the border zone territory between the middle and PCA may result in bilateral parietotemporal lesions.
- Unilateral watershed infarcts may occur during episodes of systemic hypotension when there is preexisting ipsilateral vascular disease causing focal hypoperfusion in the most distal territory.

Lacunar Infarcts

- Lacuna refers to small necrotic/cystic lesions of the brain or brainstem associated with arterial hypertension. A lacunar syndrome is the clinical picture due to lacuna or lacune. However, lacunar syndromes may be associated with nonlacunar mechanisms of infarction, and may even be mimicked by subcortical and brainstem hemorrhages.
- Lacunes are small ischemic infarcts in the deep regions of the brain or brainstem that range in diameter from 0.5 to 15 mm resulting from occlusion of a single perforating vessel (e.g., AChA, MCA, posterior cerebral artery, or basilar artery). Lacunes usually occur in patients with lipohyalinosis of penetrating arteries or branches related to long-standing arterial hypertension.
- The most frequent sites of lacunes are the putamen, basis pontis, thalamus, posterior limb of the internal capsule, and caudate nucleus, in that order.

The four best recognized clinical syndromes related to lacunar strokes can be described as follows:

- Pure motor hemiparesis or pure motor stroke is often due to an internal capsule, corona radiata, or basis pontis lacune and is characterized by a unilateral motor deficit (hemiparesis or hemiplegia) involving the face, arm, and, to a lesser extent, the leg, accompanied by mild dysarthria, particularly at the onset of stroke.
- Pure sensory stroke, also known as pure paresthetic stroke or pure hemisensory stroke, is often due to a lacune involving the ventroposterolateral nucleus of the thalamus. It is characterized by numbness, paresthesias, and a unilateral hemisensory deficit involving the face, arm, trunk, and leg.
- Ataxic hemiparesis is often due to a lacune affecting either the contralateral posterior limb of the internal capsule or the contralateral basis pontis.
- Clumsy hand syndrome is often due to a lacune involving the depth of the basis pontis between its upper third and lower two-thirds and is characterized by supranuclear facial weakness, deviation of the protruded tongue, dysarthria, dysphagia, loss of fine motor control of the hand, and an extensor plantar response

Hemorrhage

The different types of intracerebral hemorrhage are explained in Neurosurgery.

Carotid-Cavernous Fistula

When symptomatic, this lesion is associated with the following:

- Ocular pain
- Pulsating exophthalmos (unilateral or bilateral)
- Cephalic or ocular bruit, which can be diminished by digital carotid compression in the neck
- Chemosis and redness of the conjunctiva
- Diplopia, caused either by cranial nerve palsy or mechanical restriction of the globe (abducens palsy is the most common cause)
- Decreased visual acuity due to pressure on the optic nerve, glaucoma, or retinal and optic nerve hypoxia

Management of Ischemic Stroke

The first goal is to prevent or reverse brain injury. Attend to the patient's airway, breathing, circulation, and treat hypoglycemia or hyperglycemia if identified. Perform an emergency noncontrast head CT scan in order to differentiate between ischemic stroke and hemorrhagic stroke; there are no reliable clinical findings that conclusively separate ischemia from hemorrhage, although a more depressed level of consciousness, higher initial blood pressure, or worsening of symptoms after onset favor hemorrhage, and a deficit that remits suggests ischemia.

MEDICAL SUPPORT

- When ischemic stroke occurs, the immediate goal is to optimize cerebral perfusion in the surrounding ischemic penumbra. Attention is also directed toward preventing the common complications of bedridden patients—infections (pneumonia, urinary tract, and skin) and deep venous thrombosis (DVT) with pulmonary embolism.
- The larger the infarct, the greater the likelihood that clinically significant edema will develop. Water restriction and IV mannitol may be used to raise the serum osmolarity, but hypovolemia should be avoided as this may contribute to hypotension and worsening infarction.
- Intravenous Thrombolysis with rtPA—The risk of intracranial hemorrhage appears to rise with larger strokes, longer times from onset of symptoms, and higher doses of rtPA administered. The established dose of 0.9 mg/kg administered IV within 3 h of stroke onset appears safe. The time of stroke onset is defined as the time the patient's symptoms began or the time the patient was last seen as normal.

ENDOVASCULAR TECHNIQUES

Occlusions in such large vessels [middle cerebral artery (MCA), internal carotid artery, and the basilar artery] generally involve a large clot volume and often fail to open with IV rtPA alone. Therefore, using thrombolytics via an intraarterial route to increase the concentration of drug at the clot and minimize systemic bleeding complications has been useful.

Antithrombotic Treatment

- Platelet Inhibition—Aspirin is the only antiplatelet agent that has been proven effective for the acute treatment of ischemic stroke.
- Anticoagulation—Heparin given SC affords no additional benefit over aspirin and increased bleeding rates.

Neuroprotection

Neuroprotection is the concept of providing a treatment that prolongs the brain's tolerance to ischemia. Hypothermia is a powerful neuroprotective treatment in patients with cardiac arrest, but it has not been adequately studied in patients with ischemic stroke.

STROKE CENTERS AND REHABILITATION

- Proper rehabilitation of the stroke patient includes early physical, occupational, and speech therapy.
- It is directed toward educating the patient and family about the patient's neurologic deficit, preventing the complications of immobility (e.g., pneumonia, DVT and pulmonary embolism, pressure sores of the skin, and muscle contractures), and providing encouragement and instruction in overcoming the deficit.

SPINAL CORD DISEASES

The common treatable spinal cord diseases include Compressive disorders, Vascular, Inflammatory, Infectious, Developmental and Metabolic disorders. The staggered pattern of decussation of the lateral corticospinal tract, dorsal column–medial lemniscal system, and spinothalamic tracts often permits localization of lesions within the spinal cord.

DETERMINING THE LEVEL OF THE LESION

- The presence of a horizontally defined level below which sensory, motor, and autonomic function is impaired is a hallmark of spinal cord disease. The sensory level indicates damage to the spinothalamic tract one to two segments above the perceived level of a unilateral spinal cord lesion and at the level of a bilateral lesion. That is the result of the ascent of second-order sensory fibers, which originate in the dorsal horn, proceed to cross anterior to the central canal while ascending to join the opposite spinothalamic tract. Lesions that transect the descending corticospinal and other motor tracts cause paraplegia or quadriplegia, with the evolution over time of increased muscle tone, heightened deep tendon reflexes, and Babinski signs (the upper motor neuron syndrome).
- The uppermost level of a spinal cord lesion can also be localized by attention to the *segmental signs* corresponding to disturbed motor or sensory innervation by an individual cord segment. A band of altered sensation (hyperalgesia or hyperpathia) at the upper end of the sensory disturbance, fasciculations or atrophy in muscles innervated by one or several segments, or a muted or absent deep tendon reflex may be noted at this level. With severe and acute transverse lesions, the limbs initially may be flaccid rather than spastic. This state of "spinal shock" lasts for several days, rarely for weeks, and should not be mistaken for extensive damage to many segments of the cord or for an acute polyneuropathy.
- Upper cervical cord lesions produce quadriplegia and weakness of the diaphragm. Lesions at C4-C5 produce quadriplegia; at C5-C6, there is loss of power and reflexes in the biceps; at C7 weakness is found only in finger and wrist extensors and triceps; and at C8, finger and wrist flexion are impaired. Horner's syndrome (miosis, ptosis, and facial hypohidrosis) may accompany a cervical cord lesion at any level.
- Lesions here are localized by the sensory level on the trunk and by the site of midline back pain if it accompanies the syndrome. Useful markers for localization are the nipples (T4) and umbilicus (T10). Leg weakness and disturbances of bladder and bowel function accompany the paralysis. Lesions at T9-T10 paralyze the lower—but not the upper—abdominal muscles, resulting in upward movement of the umbilicus when the abdominal wall contracts (*Beevor's sign*).
- Lesions at the L2-L4 spinal cord levels paralyze flexion and adduction of the thigh, weaken leg extension at the knee, and abolish the patellar reflex. Lesions at L5-S1 paralyze only movements of the foot and ankle, flexion at the knee, and extension of the thigh, and abolish the ankle jerks (S1).

- The conus medullaris is the tapered caudal termination of the spinal cord, comprising the lower sacral and single coccygeal segments. The conus syndrome is distinctive, consisting of bilateral saddle anesthesia (S3-S5), prominent bladder and bowel dysfunction (urinary retention and incontinence with lax anal tone), and impotence. The bulbocavernosus (S2-S4) and anal (S4-S5) reflexes are absent. Muscle strength is largely preserved.
- Lesions of the cauda equina, the cluster of nerve roots derived from the lower cord, are characterized by low back and radicular pain, asymmetric leg weakness and sensory loss, variable areflexia in the lower extremities, and relative sparing of bowel and bladder function. Mass lesions in the lower spinal canal often produce a mixed clinical picture in which elements of both cauda equina and conus medullaris syndromes coexist.

Spinal Cord Syndromes

Brown-Sequard Hemicord Syndrome

- This consists of ipsilateral weakness (corticospinal tract) and loss of joint position and vibratory sense (posterior column), ipsilateral plantar extensor and pyramidal tract features with contralateral loss of pain and temperature sense (spinothalamic tract) one or two levels below the lesion.
- Segmental signs, such as radicular pain, muscle atrophy, or loss of a deep tendon reflex, are unilateral.

Central Cord Syndrome

The central cord syndrome results from damage to the gray matter nerve cells and crossing spinothalamic tracts near the central canal. In the cervical cord, the central cord syndrome produces arm weakness out of proportion to leg weakness and a "dissociated" sensory loss, signifying a loss of pain and temperature sense in a cape distribution over the shoulders, lower neck, and upper trunk in contrast to preservation of light touch, joint position, and vibration sense in these regions. Trauma, syringomyelia, tumors, and anterior spinal artery ischemia (including from aortic dissection) are the main causes.

Anterior Spinal Artery Syndrome

Infarction of the cord is generally the result of occlusion or diminished flow in this artery. The result is extensive bilateral tissue destruction that spares the posterior columns. All spinal cord functions—motor, sensory, and autonomic—are lost below the level of the lesion, with the exception of retained vibration and position sensation.

Foramen Magnum Syndrome

Lesions in this area interrupt decussating pyramidal tract fibers destined for the legs, which cross caudal to those of the arms, resulting in weakness of the legs (*crural paresis*). Compressive lesions near the foramen magnum may produce weakness of the ipsilateral shoulder and arm followed by weakness of the ipsilateral leg, then the contralateral leg, and finally the contralateral arm, an "around the clock" pattern that may begin in any of the four limbs.

Intramedullary and Extramedullary Syndromes

- It is useful to differentiate *intramedullary* processes, arising within the substance of the cord, from *extramedullary* ones that compress the spinal cord or its vascular supply.
- With extramedullary lesions, radicular pain is often prominent, and there is early sacral sensory loss (lateral spinothalamic tract) and spastic weakness in the legs (corticospinal tract) due to the superficial location of leg fibers in the corticospinal tract.
- Intramedullary lesions tend to produce poorly localized burning pain rather than radicular pain and spare sensation in the perineal and sacral areas ("sacral sparing"), reflecting the laminated configuration of the spinothalamic tract with sacral fibers outermost; corticospinal tract signs appear later.

ACUTE AND SUBACUTE SPINAL CORD DISEASES

- The initial symptoms of disease that evolve over days or weeks are focal neck or back pain, followed by various combinations of paresthesias, sensory loss, motor weakness, and sphincter disturbance evolving over hours to several days.
- There may be only mild sensory symptoms or a devastating functional transection of the cord. Partial lesions selectively involve the posterior columns or anterior spinothalamic tracts or are limited to one side of the cord. Paresthesias or numbness typically begins in the feet and ascends symmetrically or asymmetrically. These symptoms initially simulate Guillain-Barré syndrome, but involvement of the trunk with a sharply demarcated spinal cord level indicates the myelopathic nature of the process.
- In severe and abrupt cases, areflexia reflecting spinal shock may be present, but hyperreflexia supervenes over days or weeks; persistent areflexic paralysis with a sensory level indicates necrosis over multiple segments of the spinal cord.

COMPRESSIVE AND NONCOMPRESSIVE MYELOPATHY

- A treatable compression of the cord is commonly caused by a mass. The common causes are tumor, epidural abscess or hematoma, herniated disc, or vertebral pathology. Epidural compression due to malignancy or abscess often causes warning signs of neck or back pain, bladder disturbances, and sensory symptoms that precede the development of paralysis. Spinal subluxation, hemorrhage, and noncompressive etiologies such as infarction are more likely to produce myelopathy without antecedent symptoms.
- Noncompressive causes of acute myelopathy that are intrinsic to the cord are primarily vascular, inflammatory, and infectious etiologies.

COMPRESSIVE MYELOPATHIES

- In adults, most neoplasms are epidural in origin, resulting from metastases to the adjacent spinal bones. The propensity of solid tumors to metastasize to the vertebral column probably reflects the high proportion of bone marrow located in the axial skeleton. Almost any malignant tumor can metastasize to the spinal column, with breast, lung, prostate, kidney, lymphoma, and plasma cell dyscrasia being particularly frequent. The thoracic cord is most commonly involved; exceptions are metastases from prostate and ovarian cancer, which occur disproportionately in the sacral and lumbar vertebrae, probably resulting from spread through Batson's plexus, a network of veins along the anterior epidural space.
- Pain is usually the initial symptom; it may be aching and localized or sharp and radiating in quality. This spinal ache typically worsens with movement, coughing, or sneezing and characteristically awakens patients at night. A recent onset of persistent back pain, particularly if in the thoracic spine (which is uncommonly involved by spondylosis), should prompt consideration of vertebral metastasis.
- MRI provides excellent anatomic resolution of the extent of spinal tumors and is able to distinguish between malignant lesions and other masses—epidural abscess, tuberculoma, or epidural hemorrhage, among others—that present in a similar fashion. Vertebral metastases are usually hypointense relative to a normal bone marrow signal on T1-weighted MRI scans.
- If spinal cord compression is suspected, imaging should be obtained promptly. If there are radicular symptoms but no evidence of myelopathy, it is usually safe, if necessary, to defer imaging for 24–48 h. With back or neck pain only, imaging studies may be obtained within a few days.
- *Treatment*—Management of cord compression includes glucocorticoids to reduce cord edema, local radiotherapy (initiated as early as possible) to the symptomatic lesion, and specific therapy for the underlying tumor type. Radiotherapy appears to be as effective as surgery, even for most classically radioresistant metastases. Surgery, either decompression by laminectomy or vertebral body resection, should be considered when signs of cord compression worsen despite radiotherapy, when the maximum tolerated dose of radiotherapy has been delivered previously to the site, or when a vertebral compression fracture or spinal instability contributes to cord compression.
- Meningiomas are often located posterior to the thoracic cord or near the foramen magnum, although they can arise from the meninges anywhere along the spinal canal. Symptoms usually begin with radicular sensory symptoms followed by an asymmetric, progressive spinal cord syndrome. Therapy is by surgical resection.
- Primary intramedullary tumors of the spinal cord are uncommon. They present as central cord or hemicord syndromes, often in the cervical region; there may be poorly localized burning pain in the extremities and sparing of sacral sensation. In adults, these lesions are ependymomas, hemangioblastomas, or low-grade astrocytomas. Complete resection of an intramedullary ependymoma is often possible with microsurgical techniques. Debulking of an intramedullary astrocytoma can also be helpful, as these are often slowly growing lesions; the value of adjunctive radiotherapy and chemotherapy is uncertain. Secondary (metastatic) intramedullary tumors are also common, especially in patients with advanced metastatic disease.

Spinal Epidural Abscess

- Spinal epidural abscess presents as a clinical triad of midline dorsal pain, fever, and progressive limb weakness. Aching pain is almost always present, either over the spine or in a radicular pattern. Fever is usual, accompanied by elevated white blood cell count and sedimentation rate. As the abscess expands, further spinal cord damage results from venous congestion and thrombosis. Two-thirds of epidural infections result from hematogenous spread of bacteria from the skin (furunculosis), soft tissue (pharyngeal or dental abscesses), or deep viscera (bacterial endocarditis). Most cases are due to *Staphylococcus aureus*; gram-negative bacilli, *Streptococcus*, anaerobes, and fungi can also cause epidural abscesses. Tuberculosis from an adjacent vertebral source, Pott's disease, remains an important cause in the underdeveloped world.
- MRI scans localize the abscess and exclude other causes of myelopathy. Lumbar puncture is only required if encephalopathy or other clinical signs raise the question of associated meningitis. The level of the puncture should be planned to minimize the risk of meningitis due to passage of the needle through infected tissue or herniation due to decompression below an area of obstruction to the flow of cerebrospinal fluid (CSF). A high cervical tap is often the safest approach. CSF abnormalities in subdural abscess consist of pleocytosis with a preponderance of polymorphonuclear cells, an elevated protein level, and a reduced glucose level, but the responsible organism is not cultured unless there is associated meningitis.

- ***Treatment***—Treatment is by decompressive laminectomy with debridement combined with long-term antibiotic treatment. Surgical evacuation prevents development of paralysis and may improve or reverse paralysis in evolution, but it is unlikely to improve deficits of more than several days duration. If surgery is contraindicated, long-term administration of systemic and oral antibiotics can be used; in such cases, the choice of antibiotics may be guided by results of blood cultures.

Spinal Epidural Hematoma

Hemorrhage into the epidural (or subdural) space causes acute focal or radicular pain followed by variable signs of a spinal cord or conus medullaris disorder. Therapeutic anticoagulation, trauma, tumor, or blood dyscrasia are predisposing conditions. Treatment consists of prompt reversal of any underlying clotting disorder and surgical decompression.

Hematomyelia

Hemorrhage into the substance of the spinal cord is a rare result of trauma, intraparenchymal vascular malformation, vasculitis due to polyarteritis nodosa or systemic lupus erythematosus (SLE), bleeding disorders, or a spinal cord neoplasm. Hematomyelia presents as an acute painful transverse myelopathy. With large lesions, extension into the subarachnoid space may occur, resulting in subarachnoid hemorrhage.

Noncompressive Myelopathies

The most frequent causes of noncompressive acute transverse myelopathy are spinal cord infarction; systemic inflammatory disorders, including SLE and sarcoidosis; demyelinating diseases, including multiple sclerosis (MS) and neuromyelitis optica; postinfectious or idiopathic transverse myelitis, which is presumed to be an immune condition related to acute disseminated encephalomyelitis and infectious (primarily viral) causes.

Spinal Cord Infarction

- Spinal cord ischemia can occur at any level; however, the presence of the artery of Adamkiewicz creates a watershed of marginal blood flow in the upper thoracic segments. With systemic hypotension, cord infarction occurs at the level of greatest ischemic risk, usually T3-T4, and also at boundary zones between the anterior and posterior spinal artery territories. The latter may result in a rapidly progressive syndrome over hours of weakness and spasticity with little sensory change.
- Acute infarction in the territory of the *anterior spinal artery* produces paraplegia or quadriplegia, dissociated sensory loss affecting pain and temperature sense but sparing vibration and position sense, and loss of sphincter control ("anterior cord syndrome"). Less common is infarction in the territory of the *posterior spinal arteries*, resulting in loss of posterior column function.
- Spinal cord infarction results from aortic atherosclerosis, dissecting aortic aneurysm (manifest as chest or back pain with diminished pulses in legs), vertebral artery occlusion or dissection in the neck, or profound hypotension from any cause. Cardiogenic emboli, vasculitis related to collagen vascular disease (particularly SLE and the antiphospholipid antibody syndrome, and surgical interruption of aortic aneurysms are other causative conditions). In cord infarction due to presumed thromboembolism, acute anticoagulation is probably not indicated, with the exception of the unusual transient ischemic attack or incomplete infarction with a stuttering or progressive course.

Inflammatory and Immune Myelopathies (Myelitis)

- This category includes MS and postinfectious myelitis, both of which are demyelinating in nature, as well as connective tissue disease. In approximately one-quarter of cases of myelitis, no underlying cause can be identified. Some will later manifest additional symptoms of a systemic immune-mediated disease such as SLE or, more often, MS.
- ***Systemic Inflammatory Disorders***—Myelitis occurs in a small number of patients with SLE, many cases of which are associated with antiphospholipid antibodies. The CSF is usually normal or shows a mild lymphocytic pleocytosis; oligoclonal bands are a variable finding.
- ***Demyelinating Myelopathies***—Multiple sclerosis may present with myelitis, causes a complete transverse myelopathy (i.e., acute bilateral signs), but it is among the most common causes of a partial syndrome. Neuromyelitis optica is a demyelinating syndrome consisting of a severe myelopathy associated with optic neuritis; the optic neuritis is often bilateral and may precede or follow myelitis by weeks or months.
- ***Postinfectious Myelitis***—Many cases of myelitis, termed *postinfectious* or *postvaccinal*, follow an infection or vaccination. Numerous organisms have been implicated, including Epstein-Barr virus (EBV), cytomegalovirus (CMV), mycoplasma, influenza, measles, varicella, rubeola, and mumps. Treatment is usually with glucocorticoids or, in fulminant cases, plasma exchange.
- ***Acute Infectious Myelitis***—Herpes zoster is the best characterized viral myelitis, but HSV types 1 and 2, EBV, CMV, and rabies virus are other well-described causes. HSV-2 (and less commonly HSV-1) produces a distinctive syndrome of recurrent sacral myelitis in association with outbreaks of genital herpes mimicking MS.

CHRONIC MYELOPATHIES

Spondylitic Myelopathy

- Spondylitic myelopathy is one of the most common causes of gait difficulty in the elderly. Neck and shoulder pain with stiffness are early symptoms; impingement of bone and soft tissue overgrowth on nerve roots results in radicular arm pain, most often in a C5 or C6 distribution. Compression of the cervical cord, which occurs in fewer than one-third of cases, produces a slowly progressive spastic paraparesis, at times asymmetric and often accompanied by paresthesias in the feet and hands. Vibratory sense is diminished in the legs, there is a Romberg sign, and occasionally there is a sensory level for vibration on the upper thorax. In individual cases, radicular, myelopathic, or combined signs may predominate.
- Extrinsic cord compression and deformation is appreciated on axial MRI views, and T2-weighted sequences may reveal areas of high signal intensity within the cord adjacent to the site of compression.
- A cervical collar may be helpful in milder cases, but definitive therapy consists of surgical decompression. Posterior laminectomy or an anterior approach with resection of the protruded disc and bony material may be required.

Vascular Malformations of the Cord and Dura

- True arteriovenous malformations (AVMs) are located posteriorly along the surface of the cord or within the dura, where they are more properly classified as fistulas. Most are at or below the midthoracic level. The typical presentation is a middle-aged man with a progressive myelopathy that worsens slowly or intermittently and may have periods of apparent remission resembling MS. The motor disorder may predominate and produce a mixture of upper and restricted lower motor neuron signs, simulating amyotrophic lateral sclerosis (ALS).
- A rare AVM process presents as a progressive thoracic myelopathy with paraparesis developing over weeks or several months, characterized pathologically by abnormally thick, hyalinized vessels within the cord (Foix-Alajouanine syndrome).
- High-resolution MRI with contrast administration detects many but not all AVMs. Definitive diagnosis requires selective spinal angiography, which defines the feeding vessels and the extent of the malformation. Endovascular embolization of the major feeding vessels may stabilize a progressive neurologic deficit or allow for gradual recovery.

Retrovirus-Associated Myelopathies

The myelopathy associated with the human T cell lymphotropic virus type I (HTLV-I), formerly called tropical spastic paraparesis, is a slowly progressive spastic syndrome with variable sensory and bladder disturbance. The neurologic signs may be asymmetric, often lacking a well-defined sensory level; the only sign in the arms may be hyperreflexia after several years of illness. Diagnosis is made by demonstration of HTLV-I–specific antibody in serum by enzyme-linked immunosorbent assay (ELISA), confirmed by radioimmunoprecipitation or western blot analysis. There is no effective treatment, but symptomatic therapy for spasticity and bladder symptoms may be helpful.

Syringomyelia

- Syringomyelia is a developmental cavitary expansion of the cervical cord that is prone to enlarge and produce progressive myelopathy.
- More than half of all cases are associated with Chiari type 1 malformations in which the cerebellar tonsils protrude through the foramen magnum and into the cervical spinal canal. Acquired cavitations of the cord in areas of necrosis are also termed *syrinx cavities*; these follow trauma, myelitis, necrotic spinal cord tumors, and chronic arachnoiditis due to tuberculosis.
- The classic presentation is a central cord syndrome consisting of a dissociated sensory loss and areflexic weakness in the upper limbs. The sensory deficit is recognizable by loss of pain and temperature sensation with sparing of touch and vibration in a distribution that is "suspended" over the nape of the neck, shoulders, and upper arms (cape distribution) or in the hands.
- Muscle wasting in the lower neck, shoulders, arms, and hands with asymmetric or absent reflexes in the arms reflects expansion of the cavity into the gray matter of the cord. As the cavity enlarges and further compresses the long tracts, spasticity and weakness of the legs, bladder and bowel dysfunction, and a Horner's syndrome appear.
- Extension of the syrinx into the medulla, syringobulbia, causes palatal or vocal cord paralysis, dysarthria, horizontal or vertical nystagmus, episodic dizziness, and tongue weakness.
- MRI scans accurately identify developmental and acquired syrinx cavities and their associated spinal cord enlargement.
- ***Treatment***—Treatment of syringomyelia is generally unsatisfactory. The Chiari tonsillar herniation is usually decompressed, generally by suboccipital craniectomy, upper cervical laminectomy, and placement of a dural graft. Obstruction of fourth ventricular outflow is reestablished by this procedure. With Chiari malformations, shunting of hydrocephalus should generally precede any attempt to correct the syrinx. Syringomyelia secondary to trauma or infection is treated with a decompression and drainage procedure in which a small shunt is inserted between the syrinx cavity and the subarachnoid space; alternatively, the cavity can be fenestrated. Cases due to intramedullary spinal cord tumor are generally managed by resection of the tumor.

Subacute Combined Degeneration (Vitamin B_{12} Deficiency)

- This myelopathy presents with subacute paresthesias in the hands and feet, loss of vibration and position sensation, and a progressive spastic and ataxic weakness. Loss of reflexes due to an associated peripheral neuropathy in a patient who also has Babinski signs, is an important diagnostic clue. Optic atrophy and irritability or other mental changes may be prominent in advanced cases and are rarely the presenting symptoms.
- The myelopathy of subacute combined degeneration tends to be diffuse rather than focal; signs are generally symmetric and reflect predominant involvement of the posterior and lateral tracts, including Romberg's sign.
- The diagnosis is confirmed by the finding of macrocytic red blood cells, a low serum B_{12} concentration, elevated serum levels of homocysteine and methylmalonic acid, and in uncertain cases a positive Schilling test.
- Treatment is by replacement therapy, beginning with 1000 microg of intramuscular vitamin B_{12} repeated at regular intervals or by subsequent oral treatment.

Tabes Dorsalis

- The classic syndromes of tabes dorsalis and meningovascular syphilis of the spinal cord are now less frequent than in the past but must be considered in the differential diagnosis of spinal cord disorders. The characteristic symptoms of tabes are fleeting and repetitive lancinating pains, primarily in the legs or less often in the back, thorax, abdomen, arms, and face. Ataxia of the legs and gait due to loss of position sense occurs in half of patients.
- The cardinal signs of tabes are loss of reflexes in the legs; impaired position and vibratory sense; Romberg's sign; and, in almost all cases, bilateral Argyll Robertson pupils, which fail to constrict to light but accommodate.

Adrenomyeloneuropathy

- This X-linked disorder is a variant of adrenoleukodystrophy. Affected males usually have a history of adrenal insufficiency beginning in childhood and then develop a progressive spastic (or ataxic) paraparesis beginning in early adulthood; some patients also have a mild peripheral neuropathy. The responsible gene encodes ADLP, a peroxisomal membrane transporter that is a member of the ATP-binding cassette (ABC) family.
- Steroid replacement is indicated if hypoadrenalism is present, and bone marrow transplantation and nutritional supplements have been attempted for this condition without clear evidence of efficacy.

DISEASES OF THE NEUROMUSCULAR JUNCTION

MYASTHENIA GRAVIS (MG)

- It is a neuromuscular disorder characterized by weakness and fatigability of skeletal muscles. The underlying defect is a decrease in the number of available acetylcholine receptors (AChRs) at neuromuscular junctions due to an antibody-mediated autoimmune attack.
- In the neuromuscular junction, acetylcholine (ACh) is synthesized in the motor nerve terminal and stored in vesicles. When an action potential travels down a motor nerve and reaches the nerve terminal, ACh from 150–200 vesicles is released and combines with AChRs that are densely packed at the peaks of postsynaptic folds. When ACh combines with the binding sites on the alpha subunits of the AChR, the channel in the AChR opens, permitting the rapid entry of cations, chiefly sodium, which produces depolarization at the end-plate region of the muscle fiber. If the depolarization is sufficiently large, it initiates an action potential that is propagated along the muscle fiber, triggering muscle contraction. This process is rapidly terminated by hydrolysis of ACh by acetylcholinesterase (AChE), which is present within the synaptic folds, and by diffusion of ACh away from the receptor
- In MG, the fundamental defect is a decrease in the number of available AChRs at the postsynaptic muscle membrane. These changes result in decreased efficiency of neuromuscular transmission. Therefore, although ACh is released normally, it produces small end-plate potentials that may fail to trigger muscle action potentials. Failure of transmission at many neuromuscular junctions results in weakness of muscle contraction.
- The amount of ACh released per impulse normally declines on repeated activity (termed *presynaptic rundown*). In the myasthenic patient, the decreased efficiency of neuromuscular transmission combined with the normal rundown results in the activation of fewer and fewer muscle fibers by successive nerve impulses and hence increasing weakness, or *myasthenic fatigue*.
- The neuromuscular abnormalities in MG are brought about by an autoimmune response mediated by specific anti-AChR antibodies. The anti-AChR antibodies reduce the number of available AChRs at neuromuscular junctions by three distinct mechanisms:
    - Accelerated turnover of AChRs by a mechanism involving cross-linking and rapid endocytosis of the receptors;
    - Blockade of the active site of the AChR, i.e., the site that normally binds ACh; and
    - Damage to the postsynaptic muscle membrane by the antibody in collaboration with complement.

- An immune response to muscle-specific kinase (MuSK) can also result in myasthenia gravis, possibly by interfering with AChR clustering. The pathogenic antibodies are IgG and are T cell dependent. Thus, immunotherapeutic strategies directed against T cells are effective in this antibody-mediated disease.

Clinical Features
- MG affects individuals in all age groups, but peaks of incidence occur in women in their twenties and thirties and in men in their fifties and sixties. The cardinal features are *weakness* and *fatigability* of muscles. The weakness increases during repeated use (fatigue) and may improve following rest or sleep.
- The distribution of muscle weakness often has a characteristic pattern. The cranial muscles, particularly the lids and extraocular muscles, are often involved early in the course of MG, and diplopia and ptosis are common initial complaints. Difficulty in swallowing may occur as a result of weakness of the palate, tongue, or pharynx, giving rise to nasal regurgitation or aspiration of liquids or food.
- Bulbar weakness is especially prominent in MuSK antibody–positive MG. The limb weakness in MG is often proximal and may be asymmetric. Despite the muscle weakness, deep tendon reflexes are preserved. If weakness of respiration becomes so severe as to require respiratory assistance, the patient is said to be in *crisis*.

Diagnosis
- The diagnosis is suspected on the basis of weakness and fatigability in the typical distribution described above, without loss of reflexes or impairment of sensation or other neurologic function.
- **Antibodies to AChR or MuSK**—The presence of anti-AChR antibodies is virtually diagnostic of MG, but a negative test does not exclude the disease. The measured level of anti-AChR antibody does not correspond well with the severity of MG in different patients. MuSK antibodies are rarely present in AChR antibody-positive patients or in patients with MG limited to ocular muscles.
- **Electrodiagnostic Testing**—Repetitive nerve stimulation often provides helpful diagnostic evidence of MG. in myasthenic patients there is a rapid reduction of >10–15% in the amplitude of the evoked responses.
- **Anticholinesterase Test**—Edrophonium is used most commonly for diagnostic testing because of the rapid onset (30 s) and short duration (~5 min) of its effect. An initial IV dose of 2 mg of edrophonium is given. If definite improvement occurs, the test is considered positive and is terminated. If there is no change, the patient is given an additional 8 mg IV. False-positive tests occur in occasional patients with other neurologic disorders, such as amyotrophic lateral sclerosis, and in placebo-reactors. The edrophonium test is now reserved for patients with clinical findings that are suggestive of MG but who have negative antibody and electrodiagnostic test results.
- Myasthenic patients have an increased incidence of several associated disorders. Thymic abnormalities occur in 75% of patients. Neoplastic change (thymoma) may produce enlargement of the thymus, which is detected by CT or MRI scanning of the anterior mediastinum. A thymic shadow on CT scan may normally be present through young adulthood, but enlargement of the thymus in a patient >40 years old is highly suspicious of thymoma.

Inherited Myasthenic Syndromes
- The congenital myasthenic syndromes (CMS) comprise a heterogeneous group of disorders of the neuromuscular junction that are not autoimmune but rather are due to genetic mutations in which virtually any component of the neuromuscular junction may be affected.
- These disorders share many of the clinical features of autoimmune MG, including weakness and fatigability of skeletal muscles, in some cases involving extraocular muscles (EOMs), lids, and proximal muscles, similar to the distribution in autoimmune MG. CMS should be suspected when symptoms of myasthenia have begun in infancy or childhood and AChR antibody tests are consistently negative.

Lambert-Eaton Myasthenic Syndrome (LEMS)
- LEMS is a presynaptic disorder of the neuromuscular junction that can cause weakness similar to that of MG. The proximal muscles of the lower limbs are most commonly affected, but other muscles may be involved as well. Cranial nerve findings, including ptosis of the eyelids and diplopia, occur in up to 70% of patients and resemble features of MG.
- However, the two conditions are readily distinguished, since patients with LEMS have depressed or absent reflexes, experience autonomic changes such as dry mouth and impotence, and have incremental rather than decremental responses on repetitive nerve stimulation.
- LEMS is caused by autoantibodies directed against P/Q type calcium channels at the motor nerve terminals. These autoantibodies result in impaired release of ACh from nerve terminals. Most patients with LEMS have an associated malignancy, most commonly small cell carcinoma of the lung, which may express calcium channels that stimulate the autoimmune response.
- Treatment of LEMS involves plasmapheresis and immunosuppression, as for MG.

Treatment
- The most useful treatments for MG include anticholinesterase medications, immunosuppressive agents, thymectomy, and plasmapheresis or intravenous immunoglobulin (IVIg)
- *Anticholinesterase Medications*—Pyridostigmine is the most widely used anticholinesterase drug. Long-acting pyridostigmine may occasionally be useful to get the patient through the night but should never be used for daytime medication because of variable absorption. The maximum useful dose of pyridostigmine rarely exceeds 120 mg every 3–6 h during daytime.
- *Thymectomy*—Surgical removal of a thymoma is necessary because of the possibility of local tumor spread, although most thymomas are histologically benign. The advantage of thymectomy is that it offers the possibility of long-term benefit, in some cases diminishing or eliminating the need for continuing medical treatment. However patients with MuSK antibody– positive MG may not respond to thymectomy.
- *Immunosuppression*—Immunosuppression using glucocorticoids, azathioprine, and other drugs is effective in nearly all patients with MG. The choice of drugs or other immunomodulatory treatments should be guided by the relative benefits and risks for the individual patient and the urgency of treatment. The beneficial effects of azathioprine and mycophenolate mofetil usually begin after many months (up to a year), but these drugs have advantages for the long-term treatment of patients with MG. Glucocorticoids produce improvement in myasthenic weakness in the great majority of patients. Mycophenolate mofetil has become one of the most widely used drugs in the treatment of MG because of its effectiveness and relative lack of side effects.
- *Plasmapheresis*—Plasmapheresis has been used therapeutically in MG. Plasma, which contains the pathogenic antibodies, is mechanically separated from the blood cells, which are returned to the patient. A course of five exchanges (3–4 L per exchange) is generally administered over a 10- to 14-day period. Plasmapheresis produces a short-term reduction in anti-AChR antibodies, with clinical improvement in many patients.
- *Intravenous Immunoglobulin*—The indications for the use of IVIg are to produce rapid improvement to help the patient through a difficult period of myasthenic weakness or prior to surgery. The usual dose is 2 g/kg, which is typically administered over 5 days (400 mg/kg per day). If tolerated, the course of IVIg can be shortened to administer the entire dose over a 3-day period.
- *Management of Myasthenic Crisis*—Myasthenic crisis is defined as an exacerbation of weakness sufficient to endanger life; it usually consists of respiratory failure caused by diaphragmatic and intercostal muscle weakness. The most common cause of crisis is intercurrent infection. This should be treated immediately, because the mechanical and immunologic defenses of the patient can be assumed to be compromised. Early and effective antibiotic therapy, respiratory assistance, and pulmonary physiotherapy are essentials of the treatment program.
- *Drugs to Avoid in Myasthenic Patients*—Many drugs have been reported to have adverse effects in patients with MG [Commonly asked in entrance exam. A very important list]
    1. **Antibiotics:** Aminoglycosides, Quinolones, Macrolides
    2. **Nondepolarizing muscle relaxants for surgery:** D-Tubocurarine (curare), pancuronium, vecuronium, atracurium
    3. **Beta-blocking agents:** Propranalol, atenolol, metoprolol
    4. **Local anesthetics and related agents:** Procaine, xylocaine in large amounts; Procainamide (for arrhythmias)
    5. **Botulinum toxin:** Botox exacerbates weakness
    6. **Quinine derivatives**—Quinine, quinidine, chloroquine, mefloquine
    7. Magnesium
    8. Penicillamine

MUSCULAR DYSTROPHIES

- Skeletal muscle diseases, or myopathies, are disorders with structural changes or functional impairment of muscle. These conditions can be differentiated from other diseases of the motor unit (e.g., lower motor neuron or neuromuscular junction pathologies) by characteristic clinical and laboratory findings.
- The most common clinical findings of a myopathy are proximal, symmetric limb weakness (arms or legs) with preserved reflexes and sensation. An associated sensory loss suggests injury to peripheral nerve or the central nervous system (CNS) rather than myopathy.
- Symptoms of muscle weakness can be either intermittent or persistent. Disorders causing *intermittent weakness* include myasthenia gravis, periodic paralyses (hypokalemic, hyperkalemic, and paramyotonia congenita), and metabolic energy deficiencies of glycolysis (especially myophosphorylase deficiency) and fatty acid utilization (carnitine palmitoyltransferase deficiency and some mitochondrial myopathies).
- Most muscle disorders cause *persistent weakness*. In the majority of these, including most types of muscular dystrophy, polymyositis, and dermatomyositis, the proximal muscles are weaker than the distal and are symmetrically affected, and the facial muscles are spared, a pattern referred to as *limb-girdle*.

- Facial weakness (difficulty with eye closure and impaired smile) and scapular are characteristic of facioscapulohumeral dystrophy. Facial and distal limb weakness associated with hand grip myotonia is virtually diagnostic of myotonic dystrophy. A pathognomonic pattern characteristic of inclusion body myositis is atrophy and weakness of the flexor forearm (e.g., wrist and finger flexors) and quadriceps muscles that is often asymmetric.
- Any disorder causing muscle weakness may be accompanied by *fatigue*, referring to an inability to maintain or sustain a force (pathologic fatigability). Pathologic fatigability occurs in disorders of neuromuscular transmission and in disorders altering energy production, including defects in glycolysis, lipid metabolism, or mitochondrial energy production. Pathologic fatigability also occurs in chronic myopathies because of difficulty accomplishing a task with less muscle.
- Muscle pain can be associated with cramps, spasms, contractures, and stiff or rigid muscles. In distinction, true myalgia (muscle aching), which can be localized or generalized, may be accompanied by weakness, tenderness to palpation, or swelling. A *muscle cramp* or *spasm* is a painful, involuntary, localized, muscle contraction with a visible or palpable hardening of the muscle. Cramps are abrupt in onset, short in duration, and may cause abnormal posturing of the joint. A *muscle contracture* is different from a muscle cramp. In both conditions, the muscle becomes hard, but a contracture is associated with energy failure in glycolytic disorders. The muscle is unable to relax after an active muscle contraction.
- In *neuromyotonia (Isaacs' syndrome)* there is hyperexcitability of the peripheral nerves manifesting as continuous muscle fiber activity. *Myokymia* (groups of fasciculations associated with continuous undulations of muscle) and impaired muscle relaxation are the result. Muscles of the leg are stiff, and the constant contractions of the muscle cause increased sweating of the extremities. *Myotonia* is a condition of prolonged muscle contraction followed by slow muscle relaxation. It always follows muscle activation (action myotonia), usually voluntary, but may be elicited by mechanical stimulation (percussion myotonia) of the muscle.
- In many limb-girdle muscular dystrophies (dystrophinopathies) enlarged calf muscles are typical. The calf muscles remain very strong even late in the course of these disorders. Muscle enlargement can also result from infiltration by sarcoid granulomas, amyloid deposits, bacterial and parasitic infections, and focal myositis. In contrast, muscle atrophy is characteristic of other myopathies. Atrophy of the humeral muscles is characteristic of facioscapulohumeral muscular dystrophy.
- CK is the preferred muscle enzyme to measure in the evaluation of myopathies. Damage to muscle causes the CK to leak from the muscle fiber to the serum. The MM isoenzyme predominates in skeletal muscle, while CK-MB is the marker for cardiac muscle.
- *Electrodiagnostic Studies*—EMG, repetitive nerve stimulation, and nerve conduction studies are essential methods for evaluation of the patient with suspected muscle disease. In combination they provide the information necessary to differentiate myopathies from neuropathies and neuromuscular junction diseases.
- *Muscle Biopsy*—Muscle biopsy is an important step in establishing the diagnosis of a suspected myopathy. The biopsy is usually obtained from a quadriceps or biceps brachii muscle, less commonly from a deltoid muscle.

DUCHENNE MUSCULAR DYSTROPHY

- This is an X-linked recessive disorder, sometimes also called *pseudohypertrophic muscular dystrophy*.
- Duchenne dystrophy is caused by a mutation of the gene that encodes dystrophin, a 427-kDa protein localized to the inner surface of the sarcolemma of the muscle fiber. It is localized to the short arm of the X chromosome at Xp21. The most common gene mutation is a deletion. The size varies but does not correlate with disease severity. Less often, Duchenne dystrophy is caused by a gene duplication or point mutation.

Clinical Features

- Duchenne dystrophy is present at birth, but the disorder usually becomes apparent between ages 3 and 5. On getting up from the floor, the patient uses his hands to climb up himself called the Gowers' maneuver. Contractures of the heel cords and iliotibial bands become apparent by age 6, when toe walking is associated with a lordotic posture.
- Loss of muscle strength is progressive, with predilection for proximal limb muscles and the neck flexors; leg involvement is more severe than arm involvement. Between ages 8 and 10 walking may require the use of braces; joint contractures and limitations of hip flexion, knee, elbow, and wrist extension are made worse by prolonged sitting. By age 12, most patients are wheelchair dependent. Contractures become fixed, and a progressive scoliosis often develops that may be associated with pain. The chest deformity with scoliosis impairs pulmonary function, which is already diminished by muscle weakness. By age 16 to 18, patients are predisposed to serious, sometimes fatal pulmonary infections.
- A cardiac cause of death is uncommon despite the presence of a cardiomyopathy in almost all patients.

Diagnosis

- Serum CK levels are invariably elevated to between 20 and 100 times normal. The levels are abnormal at birth but decline late in the disease because of inactivity and loss of muscle mass. EMG demonstrates features typical of myopathy. The muscle biopsy shows muscle fibers of varying size as well as small groups of necrotic and regenerating fibers. Connective tissue and fat replace lost muscle fibers.
- A definitive diagnosis of Duchenne dystrophy can be established on the basis of dystrophin deficiency in a biopsy of muscle tissue or mutation analysis on peripheral blood leukocytes.
- A diagnosis of Duchenne dystrophy can also be made by Western blot analysis of muscle biopsy specimens, revealing abnormalities on the quantity and molecular weight of dystrophin protein. In addition, immunocytochemical staining of muscle with dystrophin antibodies can be used to demonstrate absence or deficiency of dystrophin localizing to the sarcolemmal membrane.

Treatment—Glucocorticoids, administered as prednisone in a dose of 0.75 mg/kg per day, significantly slow progression of Duchenne dystrophy for up to 3 years. Duchenne disease may benefit from novel therapies that either replace the defective gene or missing protein.

BECKER MUSCULAR DYSTROPHY

- This form of X-linked recessive muscular dystrophy results from allelic defects of the same gene responsible for Duchenne dystrophy.
- In Becker dystrophy, the DNA deletion does not alter the translational reading frame of messenger RNA. These "in-frame" mutations allow for production of some dystrophin, which accounts for the presence of altered rather than absent dystrophin.

Clinical Features

- The pattern of muscle wasting in Becker muscular dystrophy closely resembles that seen in Duchenne. Proximal muscles, especially of the lower extremities, are prominently involved. As the disease progresses, weakness becomes more generalized. Hypertrophy of muscles, particularly in the calves, is an early and prominent finding.
- Most patients with Becker dystrophy first experience difficulties between ages 5 and 15 years, although onset in the third or fourth decade or even later can occur. By definition, patients with Becker dystrophy walk beyond age 15, while patients with Duchenne dystrophy are typically in a wheelchair by the age of 12. Patients with Becker dystrophy have a reduced life expectancy, but most survive into the fourth or fifth decade.
- Cardiac involvement occurs in Becker dystrophy and may result in heart failure.

Diagnosis

Serum CK levels, results of EMG, and muscle biopsy findings closely resemble those in Duchenne dystrophy. The diagnosis of Becker muscular dystrophy requires Western blot analysis of muscle biopsy samples demonstrating a reduced amount or abnormal size of dystrophin or mutation analysis of DNA from peripheral blood leukocytes.

LIMB-GIRDLE MUSCULAR DYSTROPHY

- In the syndrome of limb-girdle muscular dystrophy (LGMD) both males and females are affected, with onset ranging from late in the first decade to the fourth decade. The LGMDs typically manifest with progressive weakness of pelvic and shoulder girdle musculature. Respiratory insufficiency from weakness of the diaphragm may occur, as may cardiomyopathy.
- Presently there are 5 autosomal dominant and 10 autosomal recessive disorders, under the syndrome of LGMD.

EMERY-DREIFUSS MUSCULAR DYSTROPHY

- There are two genetically distinct forms of Emery-Dreifuss muscular dystrophy (EDMD). One is inherited as an X-linked disorder, while the other is autosomal dominant.
- Prominent contractures can be recognized in early childhood and teenage years, often preceding muscle weakness. The contractures persist throughout the course of the disease and are present at the elbows, ankles, and neck. Muscle weakness affects humeral and peroneal muscles at first and later spreads to a limb-girdle distribution.
- The cardiomyopathy is potentially life threatening and may result in sudden death.
- Serum CK may be elevated two- to tenfold. EMG is myopathic. Muscle biopsy shows nonspecific dystrophic features. Immunohistochemistry reveals absent emerin staining of myonuclei in X-lined EDMD.

MYOTONIC DYSTROPHY

- Myotonic dystrophy is also known as *dystrophia myotonica* (DM). The condition is composed of at least two clinical disorders with overlapping phenotypes and distinct molecular genetic defects: myotonic dystrophy type 1 (DM1) and myotonic dystrophy type 2 (DM2), also called *proximal myotonic myopathy* (PROMM).
- The clinical expression of myotonic dystrophy varies widely and involves many systems other than muscle. Affected patients have a typical "hatchet-faced" appearance due to temporalis, masseter, and facial muscle atrophy and weakness. Frontal baldness is also characteristic of the disease. Neck muscles, including flexors and sternocleidomastoids, and distal limb muscles are involved early.
- Myotonia, which usually appears by age 5 years, is demonstrable by percussion of the thenar eminence, the tongue, and wrist extensor muscles. Myotonia causes a slow relaxation of hand grip after a forced voluntary closure.
- Cardiac disturbances occur commonly in patients with DM1. ECG abnormalities include first-degree heart block and more extensive conduction system involvement. Complete heart block and sudden death can occur.
- DM2, or PROMM, has a distinct pattern of muscle weakness affecting mainly proximal muscles. Other features of the disease overlap with DM1, including cataracts, testicular atrophy, insulin resistance, constipation, hypersomnia, and cognitive defects.
- The diagnosis of myotonic dystrophy can usually be made on the basis of clinical findings. Serum CK levels may be normal or mildly elevated. EMG evidence of myotonia is present in most cases of DM1 but may be more patchy in DM2. Muscle biopsy shows muscle atrophy. Typically, numerous internalized nuclei can be seen in individual muscle fibers as well as atrophic fibers with pyknotic nuclear clumps in both DM1 and DM2.

Treatment—Phenytoin and mexiletine are the preferred agents for the occasional patient who requires an antimyotonia drug. A cardiac pacemaker should be considered for patients with unexplained syncope, advanced conduction system abnormalities with evidence of second-degree heart block, or trifascicular conduction disturbances with marked prolongation of the PR interval.

FACIOSCAPULOHUMERAL (FSH) MUSCULAR DYSTROPHY

- FSH dystrophy is caused by deletions of tandem 3.3-kb repeats at 4q35.
- The condition typically has an onset in childhood or young adulthood. In most cases, facial weakness is the initial manifestation, appearing as an inability to smile, whistle, or fully close the eyes. Weakness of the shoulder girdles, rather than the facial muscles, usually brings the patient to medical attention. Scapular winging becomes apparent with attempts at abduction and forward movement of the arms. Biceps and triceps muscles may be severely affected, with relative sparing of the deltoid muscles. In most patients, the weakness remains restricted to facial, upper extremity, and distal lower extremity muscles.
- Characteristically, patients with FSH dystrophy do not have involvement of other organ systems
- The serum CK level may be normal or mildly elevated. EMG usually indicates a myopathic pattern. The muscle biopsy shows nonspecific features of a myopathy. A prominent inflammatory infiltrate, which is often multifocal in distribution, is present in some biopsy samples.

DISTAL MYOPATHIES

- A group of muscle diseases, the distal myopathies, are notable for their preferential distal distribution of muscle weakness in contrast to most muscle conditions associated with proximal weakness.
- *Welander, Udd,* and *Markesbery-Griggs distal myopathies* are all late-onset, dominantly inherited disorders of distal limb muscles, usually beginning after age 40 years.
- Welander distal myopathy preferentially involves the wrist and finger extensors, whereas the others are associated with anterior tibial weakness leading to progressive footdrop. *Nonaka distal myopathy* and *Miyoshi myopathy* are distinguished by autosomal recessive inheritance and onset in the late teens or twenties.
- Serum CK level is particularly helpful in diagnosing Miyoshi myopathy since it is very elevated. In the other conditions serum CK is only slightly increased. EMGs are myopathic.
- Occupational therapy is offered for loss of hand function; ankle-foot orthoses can support distal lower limb muscles.

MITOCHONDRIAL MYOPATHIES

- Mitochondria play a key role in energy production. Oxidation of the major nutrients derived from carbohydrate, fat, and protein leads to the generation of reducing equivalents. The latter are transported through the respiratory chain in the process known as *oxidative phosphorylation*. The energy generated by the oxidation-reduction reactions of the respiratory chain is stored in an electrochemical gradient coupled to ATP synthesis.

- The genetics of mitochondrial diseases differ from the genetics of chromosomal disorders. The DNA of mitochondria is directly inherited from the cytoplasm of the gametes, mainly from the oocyte. The sperm contributes very little of its mitochondria to the offspring at the time of fertilization. Thus, mitochondrial genes are derived almost exclusively from the mother, accounting for maternal inheritance of some mitochondrial disorders.

Kearns-Sayre Syndrome (KSS)
- KSS is a widespread multiorgan system disorder with a defined triad of clinical findings: onset before age 20, Chronic progressive external ophthalmoplegia, and pigmentary retinopathy plus one or more of the following features: complete heart block, cerebrospinal fluid (CSF) protein > 1.0 g/L (100 mg/dL), or cerebellar ataxia.
- The cardiac disease includes syncopal attacks and cardiac arrest related to the abnormalities in the cardiac conduction system: prolonged intraventricular conduction time, bundle branch block, and complete atrioventricular block.
- Serum CK levels are normal or slightly elevated. Serum lactate and pyruvate levels may be elevated. EMG is myopathic. Nerve conduction studies may be abnormal related to an associated neuropathy. Muscle biopsies reveal ragged red fibers, highlighted in oxidative enzyme stains, many showing defects in cytochrome oxidase. By electron microscopy there are increased numbers of mitochondria that often appear enlarged and contain paracrystalline inclusions.

Progressive External Ophthalmoplegia (PEO)
- This condition is caused by nuclear DNA mutations affecting mtDNA copy number and integrity and is thus inherited in a Mendelian fashion. The neurologic examination confirms the ptosis and ophthalmoplegia, usually asymmetric in distribution.
- Serum CK is normal or mildly elevated. The resting lactate level is normal or slightly elevated but may rise excessively after exercise. CSF protein is normal. The EMG is myopathic, and nerve conduction studies are usually normal. Ragged red fibers are prominently displayed in the muscle biopsy.
- This autosomal dominant form of CPEO has been linked to loci on three chromosomes: 4q35, 10q24, and 15q22-26. Autosomal recessive PEO has also been described with mutations in the *POLG* gene.

Myoclonic Epilepsy with Ragged Red Fibers (MERRF)
- The onset of MERRF is variable, ranging from late childhood to middle adult life. Characteristic features include myoclonic epilepsy, cerebellar ataxia, and progressive muscle weakness. The seizure disorder is an integral part of the disease and may be the initial symptom. The third major feature of the disease is muscle weakness in a limb-girdle distribution.
- Serum CK levels are normal or slightly increased. The serum lactate may be elevated. EMG is myopathic, and in some patients nerve conduction studies show a neuropathy. The electroencephalogram is abnormal, corroborating clinical findings of epilepsy. Typical ragged red fibers are seen on muscle biopsy.

Mitochondrial Myopathy, Encephalopathy, Lactic Acidosis, and Stroke-Like Episodes (MELAS)
- MELAS is caused by maternally inherited point mutations of mitochondrial tRNA genes.
- MELAS is the most common mitochondrial encephalomyopathy. The term *stroke-like* is appropriate because the cerebral lesions do not conform to a strictly vascular distribution. Seizures, usually partial motor or generalized, are common and may represent the first clearly recognizable sign of disease. The cerebral insults that resemble strokes cause hemiparesis, hemianopia, and cortical blindness.
- Serum lactic acid is typically elevated. Muscle biopsies show ragged red fibers. Neuroimaging demonstrates basal ganglia calcification in a high percentage of cases. Focal lesions that mimic infarction are present predominantly in the occipital and parietal lobes.

CHANNELOPATHIES

Hypokalemic Periodic Paralysis (HypoKPP)
- HypoKPP is caused by mutations in either of two genes. HypoKPP type 1, the most common form, is inherited as an autosomal dominant disorder with incomplete penetrance. These patients have mutations in the voltage-sensitive, skeletal muscle calcium channel gene, *CALCL1A3*. Approximately 10% of cases are HypoKPP type 2, arising from mutations in the voltage-sensitive sodium channel gene (*SCN4A*).
- Onset occurs at adolescence. Attacks are often provoked by meals high in carbohydrates or sodium and may accompany rest following prolonged exercise. Weakness usually affects proximal limb muscles more than distal. Ocular and bulbar muscles are less likely to be affected. Respiratory muscles are usually spared but when they are involved, the condition may prove fatal.

- Attacks of thyrotoxic periodic paralysis resemble those of primary HypoKPP. Despite a higher incidence of thyrotoxicosis in women, men are more likely to manifest this complication. Attacks abate with treatment of the underlying thyroid condition.
- A low serum potassium level during an attack, excluding secondary causes, establishes the diagnosis. Interattack muscle biopsies show the presence of single or multiple centrally placed vacuoles or tubular aggregates. Provocative tests with glucose and insulin to establish a diagnosis are usually not necessary and are potentially hazardous. In the midst of an attack of weakness, motor conduction studies may demonstrate reduced amplitudes, whereas EMG may show electrical silence in severely weak muscles. In between attacks, the EMG and nerve conduction studies are normal, with the exception that myopathic motor unit action potentials may be seen in patients with fixed weakness.

Treatment

- The acute paralysis improves after the administration of potassium. Muscle strength and ECG should be monitored. Oral KCl (0.2–0.4 mmol/kg) should be given every 30 min. Only rarely is IV therapy necessary (e.g., when swallowing problems or vomiting is present). Mannitol is the preferred vehicle for administration of IV potassium.
- Prophylactic administration of acetazolamide (125–1000 mg/d in divided doses) reduces or may abolish attacks in HypoKPP type 1.

Hyperkalemic Periodic Paralysis (HyperKPP)

- HyperKPP is inherited as autosomal dominant disorders. Mutations of the voltage-gated sodium channel *SCN4A* gene cause this condition.
- The term *hyperkalemic* is misleading since patients are often normokalemic during attacks. The fact that attacks are precipitated by potassium administration best defines the disease. Weakness affects proximal muscles, sparing bulbar muscles. Attacks are precipitated by rest following exercise and fasting. The symptoms are aggravated by cold, and myotonia makes the muscles stiff and painful.
- Potassium may be slightly elevated but may also be normal during an attack. As in HypoKPP, nerve conduction studies in HyperKPP muscle may demonstrate reduced motor amplitudes and the EMG may be silent in very weak muscles. In between attacks of weakness, the conduction studies are normal. The EMG will often demonstrate myotonic discharges during and between attacks. The muscle biopsy shows vacuoles that are smaller, less numerous, and more peripheral compared to the hypokalemic form or tubular aggregates.

Paramyotonia Congenita

- It is inherited as an autosomal dominant condition; voltage-gated sodium channel mutations are responsible and thus this disorder is allelic with HyperKPP and potassium-aggravated myotonia.
- In paramyotonia congenita (PC) the attacks of weakness are cold-induced or occur spontaneously and are mild. Myotonia is a prominent feature but worsens with muscle activity (paradoxical myotonia).
- Serum CK is usually mildly elevated. Routine sensory and motor nerve conduction studies are normal. Cooling of the muscle often dramatically reduces the amplitude of the compound muscle action potentials. EMG reveals diffuse myotonic potentials in PC. Upon local cooling of the muscle the myotonic discharges disappear as the patient becomes unable to activate motor unit action potentials.
- Oral administration of glucose or other carbohydrates hastens recovery. Since interattack weakness may develop after repeated episodes, prophylactic treatment is usually indicated. Thiazide diuretics and mexiletine are reported to be helpful. Potassium Channel Disorders

Andersen-Tawil Syndrome

- The disease is caused by mutations of the inwardly rectifying potassium channel (*Kir 2.1*) gene.
- This rare disease is characterized by episodic weakness, cardiac arrhythmias, and dysmorphic features (short stature, scoliosis, clinodactyly, hypertelorism, small or prominent low set ears, micrognathia, and broad forehead).
- The cardiac arrhythmias are potentially serious and life threatening. They include long QT, ventricular ectopy, bidirectional ventricular arrhythmias, and tachycardia.

Cloride Channelopathies

- Two forms of this disorder, autosomal dominant (*Thomsen's disease*) and autosomal recessive (*Becker's disease*) are related to the same gene abnormality. The disease is inherited as dominant or recessive and is caused by mutations of the chloride channel gene.

- Myotonia is worsened by cold and improved by activity. The gait may appear slow and labored at first but improves with walking.
- In Thomsen's disease muscle strength is normal, but in Becker's, which is usually more severe, there may be muscle weakness. Muscle hypertrophy is usually present. Myotonic discharges are prominently displayed by EMG recordings. Serum CK is normal or mildly elevated. The muscle biopsy shows hypertrophied fibers.

THE INFLAMMATORY MYOPATHIES

- They are classified into three major groups: polymyositis (PM), dermatomyositis (DM), and inclusion body myositis (IBM).
- These disorders present as progressive and symmetric muscle weakness except for IBM, which can have an asymmetric pattern. Patients usually report increasing difficulty with everyday tasks requiring the use of proximal muscles. Fine-motor movements that depend on the strength of distal muscles are affected only late in the course of PM and DM, but fairly early in IBM. Falling is common in IBM because of early involvement of the quadriceps muscle with buckling of the knees.
- Ocular muscles are spared, even in advanced, untreated cases. Facial muscles are unaffected in PM and DM, but mild facial muscle weakness is common in patients with IBM. In all forms of inflammatory myopathy, pharyngeal and neck-flexor muscles are often involved, causing dysphagia or difficulty in holding up the head (*head drop*).

Polymyositis

It is a subacute inflammatory myopathy affecting adults, and rarely children, who *do not have* any of the following: rash, involvement of the extraocular and facial muscles, family history of a neuromuscular disease, history of exposure to myotoxic drugs or toxins, endocrinopathy, neurogenic disease, muscular dystrophy, biochemical muscle disorder (deficiency of a muscle enzyme), or IBM as excluded by muscle biopsy analysis. PM is a diagnosis of exclusion.

Dermatomyositis

- Dermatomyositis is a distinctive entity identified by a characteristic rash accompanying, or more often preceding, muscle weakness. The rash may consist of a blue-purple discoloration on the upper eyelids with edema (heliotrope rash), a flat red rash on the face and upper trunk, and erythema of the knuckles with a raised violaceous scaly eruption (*Gottron's sign*). The erythematous rash can also occur on other body surfaces, including the knees, elbows, malleoli, neck and anterior chest (often in a *V sign*), or back and shoulders (*shawl sign*), and may worsen after sun exposure.
- In some patients the rash is pruritic, especially on the scalp, chest, and back. Dilated capillary loops at the base of the fingernails are also characteristic. The cuticles may be irregular, thickened, and distorted, and the lateral and palmar areas of the fingers may become rough and cracked, with irregular, "dirty" horizontal lines, resembling *mechanic's hands*.

Inclusion Body Myositis

- Weakness and atrophy of the distal muscles, especially foot extensors and deep finger flexors, occur in almost all cases of IBM and may be a clue to early diagnosis. Dysphagia is common, occurring in up to 60% of IBM patients, and may lead to episodes of choking. The pattern of distal weakness, which superficially resembles motor neuron or peripheral nerve disease, results from the myopathic process affecting distal muscles selectively.
- IBM is usually associated with systemic autoimmune or connective tissue diseases. Males are more commonly affected.
- IBM has the least favorable prognosis of the inflammatory myopathies. Muscle biopsy shoes vacuolated fibres and they are resistant to immunosuppressive therapies. Most patients will require the use of an assistive device such as a cane, walker, or wheelchair within 5–10 years of onset.

Extramuscular Manifestations of Inflammatory Myopathies

- *Systemic symptoms,* such as fever, malaise, weight loss, arthralgia, and Raynaud's phenomenon, especially when inflammatory myopathy is associated with a connective tissue disorder.
- *Joint contractures,* mostly in DM and especially in children.
- *Dysphagia and gastrointestinal symptoms,* due to involvement of oropharyngeal striated muscles and upper esophagus, especially in DM and IBM.
- *Cardiac disturbances,* including atrioventricular conduction defects, tachyarrhythmias, dilated cardiomyopathy, a low ejection fraction, and congestive heart failure, may rarely occur, either from the disease itself or from hypertension associated with long-term use of glucocorticoids.
- *Pulmonary dysfunction,* due to weakness of the thoracic muscles, interstitial lung disease, or drug-induced pneumonitis (e.g., from methotrexate), which may cause dyspnea, nonproductive cough, and aspiration pneumonia. Interstitial lung disease may precede myopathy or occur early in the disease and develops in up to 10% of patients with PM or DM, most of whom have antibodies to t-RNA synthetases.

- *Subcutaneous calcifications,* in DM, sometimes extruding on the skin and causing ulcerations and infections.
- *Arthralgias,* synovitis, or deforming arthropathy with subluxation in the interphalangeal joints can occur in some patients with DM and PM who have the antibody directed against the histidyl-transfer RNA synthetase, called *anti-Jo-1* Jo-1 antibodies.

Diagnosis
- The most sensitive enzyme is CK, which in active disease can be elevated as much as 50-fold. Although the CK level usually parallels disease activity, it can be normal in some patients with active IBM or DM, especially when associated with a connective tissue disease. The CK is always elevated in patients with active PM.
- Needle EMG shows myopathic potentials characterized by short-duration, low-amplitude polyphasic units on voluntary activation and increased spontaneous activity with fibrillations, complex repetitive discharges, and positive sharp waves. Mixed potentials (polyphasic units of short and long duration) indicating a chronic process and muscle fiber regeneration are often present in IBM. These EMG findings are not diagnostic of an inflammatory myopathy but are useful to identify the presence of active or chronic myopathy and to exclude neurogenic disorders.
- Muscle biopsy is the definitive test for establishing the diagnosis of inflammatory myopathy and for excluding other neuromuscular diseases. Inflammation is the histologic hallmark for these diseases; however, additional features are characteristic of each subtype

Treatment
- The goal of therapy is to improve muscle strength, thereby improving function in activities of daily living, and ameliorate the extramuscular manifestations (rash, dysphagia, dyspnea, fever).
- *Glucocorticoids*—Oral prednisone is the initial treatment of choice. High-dose prednisone, at least 1 mg/kg per day, is initiated as early in the disease as possible. After 3–4 weeks, prednisone is tapered slowly over a period of 10 weeks to 1 mg/kg every other day. If prednisone provides no objective benefit after 3 months of high-dose therapy, the disease is probably unresponsive to the drug and tapering should be accelerated while the next-in-line immunosuppressive drug is started. The long-term use of prednisone may cause increased weakness associated with a normal or unchanged CK level; this effect is referred to as *steroid myopathy.*
- *Immunosuppressive* drugs—They are given when a patient fails to respond adequately to glucocorticoids after a 3-month trial, the patient becomes glucocorticoid-resistant, glucocorticoid-related side effects appear, attempts to lower the prednisone dose repeatedly result in a new relapse, or rapidly progressive disease with evolving severe weakness and respiratory failure develops. *Azathioprine* is well tolerated, has few side effects, and appears to be as effective for long-term therapy as other drugs. The dose is up to 3 mg/kg daily. *Methotrexate* and *Mycophenolate mofetil* have a faster onset of action than azathioprine. Monoclonal anti-CD20 (rituximab) has been shown to benefit patients with DM..
- *Immunomodulation*—intravenous immunoglobulin (IVIg) improves not only strength and rash but also the underlying immunopathology. The benefit is often short-lived; repeated infusions every 6–8 weeks are generally required to maintain improvement. A dose of 2 g/kg divided over 2–5 days per course is recommended.

PERIPHERAL NEUROPATHIES

PERIPHERAL NEUROPATHY

Peripheral neuropathy describes disorders of peripheral nerves, including the dorsal or ventral nerve roots; dorsal root ganglia; brachial or lumbosacral plexus; cranial nerves (except I and II); and other sensory, motor, autonomic, or mixed nerves.

Mononeuropathy
- It refers to disease or damage of a single nerve. The most common causes are compression, entrapment, and trauma. Extrinsic compression usually occurs when a limb is maintained in a fixed position that produces sustained pressure on the nerve. The neuropathy is often reversible if the position is changed. Common entrapment neuropathies include the median nerve at the wrist (carpal tunnel), ulnar nerve at the cubital tunnel or in the ulnar groove, lower trunk of the brachial plexus at the thoracic outlet, common peroneal nerve at the fibular head, posterior tibial nerve at the tarsal tunnel, and lateral femoral cutaneous nerve at the inguinal ligament.
- Histologic changes of subacute compression consist of a mixture of segmental demyelination and Wallerian degeneration reflecting retrograde axonal injury.
- Sensory symptoms may include numbness, pins and needles, tingling, prickling, burning, or electric shock sensations. Light touch is often more affected than pinprick, and subtle sensory abnormalities may be revealed by measuring two-point discrimination. Aching and nondescript pain can also occur proximal to the site of nerve compression. Sensory testing may occasionally provoke paresthesias. Reflexes are generally unaffected since most entrapped nerves are distal to the deep tendon reflexes typically examined.

- Percussion of the nerve at the affected site may induce paresthesias (Tinel's sign). Placing the limb in a posture known to aggravate the compression may accentuate symptoms (e.g., Phalen's sign evoked by flexing the wrist for carpal tunnel syndrome).
- Electrodiagnostic studies confirm the clinical diagnosis and provide information about location, severity, and prognosis. Focal demyelination is detected as a focally reduced nerve conduction velocity along the length of the sensory and/or motor fibers. Wallerian degeneration is reflected in a reduction of distal amplitudes and as denervation potentials.
- Treatment for acute and subacute compressive neuropathies consists of identifying and removing extrinsic contributors and the use of splints to avoid further compression. In patients with chronic compressive neuropathies, exacerbating factors should be identified and treated before surgical correction is considered. Surgical treatment may be required for management of chronic compressive neuropathies when conservative measures have failed and the site of entrapment is clearly delineated.

Mononeuropathy Multiplex

- *Mononeuropathy multiplex* refers to the multifocal involvement of individual peripheral nerves. Among the causes, systemic vasculitides such as polyarteritis nodosa, rheumatoid arthritis, systemic lupus erythematosus (SLE), Churg-Strauss syndrome, Wegener's granulomatosis, and hypersensitivity vasculitis should be considered which are often associated with constitutional symptoms such as fever and weight loss.
- ***Treatment***—Therapy of the necrotizing systemic vasculitides can stabilize and in some cases improve the neuropathy. Glucocorticoids [prednisone (1.5 mg/kg per day)] plus a cytotoxic agent (usually oral cyclophosphamide at 2 mg/kg per day) is the treatment of choice. Therapy of hypersensitivity vasculitis is focused primarily upon removal of the offending antigen trigger.

POLYNEUROPATHIES

Diabetic Neuropathy

- Diabetes mellitus is associated with various neuropathy syndromes which can be broadly divided into symmetric and asymmetric types.
- Symmetric neuropathies may present as small-fiber involvement (e.g., dysesthesias in the feet) or autonomic dysfunction (e.g., sexual impotence), but often both occur together.
- The asymmetric neuropathies are divided into those with acute onset and those with gradual onset. Asymmetric abrupt-onset neuropathies include diabetic truncal radiculoneuropathy (DTRN), diabetic lumbosacral radiculoplexus neuropathy (DLSRPN), and oculomotor (third or sixth nerve) neuropathy.
- Neuropathies of more gradual onset are usually caused by entrapment or compression and include median neuropathy at the wrist, ulnar neuropathy at the elbow, peroneal neuropathy at the fibular head, and lateral cutaneous neuropathy at the thigh at the inguinal ligament *(meralgia paresthetica)*.

Symmetric Diabetic Neuropathy

- Diabetic sensorimotor polyneuropathy (DSPN) is a mixed neuropathy with small- and large-fiber sensory, autonomic, and motor nerve involvement in various combinations, although sensory and autonomic symptoms are more prominent than motor ones. Proposed criteria for the diagnosis of DSPN are two or more of the following: symptoms or signs of neuropathy, abnormal EDx studies, quantitative sensation test abnormalities, heart rate decrease with deep breathing or Valsalva maneuver.
- Initial symptoms may consist of numbness, tingling, buzzing, burning, or prickling sensation affecting the toes and feet. Paresthesias ascend up to the legs and then hands in a stocking-glove distribution. Ankle reflexes are invariably reduced or absent. The length-dependent pattern of neuropathy is evident in the stocking-glove sensory loss. Autonomic symptoms including impotence, nocturnal diarrhea, difficulty voiding, abnormalities of sweating, and abnormal fullness after eating and orthostatic hypotension may be present.
- A glucose tolerance test is indicated in all patients presenting with neuropathy. EDx studies show mixed findings of axonal loss and demyelination in a length-dependent pattern. Nerve biopsy and lumbar puncture are not necessary unless alternative diagnoses are being considered.
- Treatment consists of strict glucose control, which prevents the neuropathy from worsening; established neuropathy does not usually reverse. Aldose reductase inhibitors sorbinol and tolrestat are found to improve electrophysiologic or morphometric markers of DSPN. Alpha lipoic acid (thioctic acid), an antioxidant, has been shown to improve diabetic neuropathy. Glycemic control is essential for the prevention of diabetic autonomic neuropathy.

Asymmetric Diabetic Neuropathy

Cranial Neuropathies

- The oculomotor nerves (in decreasing order of frequency the sixth, third, and rarely fourth nerves) are most often affected. Abducens (sixth) nerve palsy manifests as the sudden onset of painless double vision, and examination shows paralysis of abduction on the affected side.

- Unlike compressive etiologies (e.g., aneurysms of the superior cerebellar or posterior communicating arteries), which present with an enlarged pupil, the pupil is nearly always spared in diabetic third nerve palsy. This is due to the fact that pupillomotor fibers are present on the outer layers of the third nerve fascicle, and an ischemic lesion tends to involve the center of the fascicle.

Limb Mononeuropathies

- Diabetics are also susceptible to entrapment neuropathies, including median neuropathy at the wrist (carpal tunnel syndrome), ulnar neuropathy at the elbow, fibular (peroneal) neuropathy at the fibular head, and lateral cutaneous neuropathy at the inguinal ligament (meralgia paresthetica).
- The special susceptibility of diabetic nerves may be related to endoneurial edema and vascular factors.
- Decompressive surgery may be needed if there is associated weakness, numbness, or pain in the distribution of the affected nerves and if no reversible extrinsic source of compression (position/habits) can be identified.

Radiculopathies and Plexopathies

- *Diabetic truncal radiculoneuropathy* occurs in diabetics in middle or later life, usually in association with underlying DSPN. Patients present with an abrupt onset, typically over days to weeks, of severe pain in the thoracic spine, flank, rib cage, or upper abdomen. The pain is described as burning, stabbing, or belt-like.
- A needle EMG of the affected muscles may confirm denervation in the abdominal or intercostal muscles; the paraspinal muscles may be spared. This finding, and a reduced fiber density measured by skin biopsy from symptomatic regions, suggests that the injury in diabetic truncal radiculoneuropathy is at, or distal to, the sensory ganglion.
- Pain management may be difficult and includes topical capsaicin and narcotics.

Diabetic Amyotrophy (Femoral Neuropathy; Proximal Diabetic Neuropathy)

- It occurs in older patients, usually with type 2 diabetes. Patients present with the abrupt onset of severe pain affecting the anterior thigh. The pain is worse at night and is described as burning. Weakness and wasting in the thigh muscles leads to difficulty climbing stairs and walking.
- Examination shows prominent wasting of the quadriceps muscle unilaterally with weakness of the knee extensor and hip flexor and, variably, ankle dorsiflexor, accompanied by sensory loss in the thigh and leg in the distribution of the femoral nerve, and a reduced knee jerk on the affected side.
- EDx studies show findings of radiculopathy (L2-4), lumbar plexopathy, or femoral neuropathy along with a distal sensorimotor neuropathy. An MRI of the lumbosacral spine and plexus is indicated to exclude a compressive cause. Cerebrospinal fluid (CSF) examination and nerve biopsy should be considered whenever the diagnosis is uncertain.
- Treatment with high-dose glucocorticoids or intravenous immunoglobulin (IVIg) has been effective in case reports, although controlled trials have not shown clear benefit. Physiotherapy and orthotic devices are helpful.

Toxic Neuropathies

- Most toxic neuropathies are distal axonal degenerations that develop gradually over time. The causes are varied, including drugs, heavy metals, and industrial and environmental substances. Novel anticancer drugs and antiretroviral agents are the most common drugs implicated, to cause neuropathy.
- The neuropathy may first manifest or may continue to progress after discontinuing the substance; a phenomenon known as *coasting*, is seen with the platinum cancer drugs, hexacarbons, nucleoside analogue reverse transcriptase inhibitors, and pyridoxine.
- Nerve biopsy occasionally demonstrates pathognomonic features such as osmiophilic Schwann cell inclusions in amiodarone, perhexiline and chloroquine neuropathies, and paranodal giant axonal swellings in hexacarbon neuropathies.
- An acute onset of neuropathy occurs with drugs such as paclitaxel, suramin, and vacor, and with biologic agents such as ciguatera, puffer fish (tetrodotoxin), and buckthorn.
    - The neuropathy may be predominantly motor—with lead, inorganic mercury, organophosphates, buckthorn, dapsone, and vincristine
    - Small-fiber sensory—with DMAPN, thallium, nucleoside analogue reverse transcriptase inhibitors (dideoxycytidine ddC, dideoxyinosine ddI, stavudine d4T), ethionamide, metronidazole, and taxane
    - Large-fiber sensory—with cisplatin, high doses of taxol, pyridoxine, or acrylamide. Autonomic dysfunction can occur with vincristine, vacor, perhexiline, high dose-pyridoxine, and platinum.
- *Treatment*—Removal of the toxic substance is the most important step. Treatment for heavy metal toxicity includes chelation therapy: penicillamine or calcium-EDTA for lead toxicity; penicillamine or British anti-Lewisite (BAL) for arsenic toxicity; and potassium chloride or Prussian blue for thallium toxicity.

Nutritional Neuropathies

Thiamine (Vitamin B_1) (Dry Beriberi)

- Thiamine deficiency can be a result of inadequate intake, as may occur in alcoholism, anorexia, intentional dieting, starvation, or bulimia. Protracted vomiting, e.g., in patients receiving chemotherapy or in pregnant women with hyperemesis gravidarum, may also cause thiamine deficiency.
- Neuropathy from thiamine deficiency presents as the acute or subacute onset of paresthesias, dysesthesias, and mild weakness in the legs. On examination a stocking-glove sensory loss, distal weakness in the legs, and loss of ankle jerks is typical.
- Nerve conduction tests and sural nerve biopsies show axonal degeneration. Erythrocyte transketolase activity is reduced in the blood.
- Treatment consists of oral thiamine replacement, 100 mg/d.

Pyridoxine (Vitamin B_6)

- A subacute length-dependent axonal neuropathy occurs as a result of pyridoxine deficiency. Causes include dietary deficiency and drugs such as isoniazid, cycloserine, and penicillamine, which act as pyridoxine antagonists by combining to the aldehyde moiety of the vitamin.
- Measurement of xanthurenic acid after tryptophan loading can help confirm the diagnosis.
- Treatment consists of oral pyridoxine, 30 mg/d. Pyridoxine supplements are recommended for prophylaxis during pregnancy and for patients taking isoniazid.

Vitamin B_{12} (Cobalamin)

- Peripheral neuropathy is a minor part of the vitamin B_{12} deficiency syndrome; subacute combined degeneration of the spinal cord is more prominent.
- Distal sensory loss predominantly involving large-fiber modalities, dysequilibrium, Lhermitte's sign, and the combination of an absent ankle jerk and upgoing toe may be present.
- Diagnosis of vitamin B_{12} deficiency is made by low serum cobalamin levels and raised levels of methylmalonic acid and homocysteine. Autoantibodies to intrinsic factor and gastric parietal cells are present in pernicious anemia.
- Treatment is with parenteral administration of cobalamin (vitamin B_{12})

Riboflavin, Nicotinic Acid and Other B-Group Vitamins

- Riboflavin and nicotinic acid deficiencies have been incriminated in neuropathies, usually in association with deficiencies of other water-soluble vitamins. Peripheral neuropathy may be accompanied by dermatitis, diarrhea, and dementia (pellagra).
- *Strachan's syndrome* is characterized by a painful sensory neuropathy associated with orogenital dermatitis, amblyopia, and deafness. Distal sensory loss with hyporeflexia at the ankles (peripheral nerve lesion), combined with hyperreflexia at the knees and an ataxic gait (spinal cord involvement), indicate the combined peripheral and central axonal loss that is characteristic of this deficiency state.

Infections and Peripheral Neuropathy

HIV Infection

- HIV infection is associated with polyradiculopathies, distal symmetric polyneuropathies, inflammatory demyelinating polyneuropathies, multifocal mononeuropathies, cranial neuropathies.
- Lumbosacral polyradiculopathies are usually due to CMV infection and occur with advanced HIV/AIDS. These present with pain, incontinence, and rapidly progressive asymmetric lower extremity weakness leading to paraplegia. Saddle anesthesia is always present. Deep tendon reflexes are often preserved. EMG reveals findings of both peripheral neuropathy and lumbosacral radiculopathy.
- A toxic neuropathy follows exposure to specific dideoxynucleosides (d4T, ddI, and especially ddC), particularly in advanced HIV disease. Sural nerve biopsy shows severe axonal destruction, most prominently in unmyelinated fibers, along with mitochondrial abnormalities.
- **Treatment**—Treatment consists of discontinuing the offending dideoxynucleoside and changing the highly active antiretroviral therapy (HAART) regimen, provided that there is another regimen to offer.

Leprous Neuritis

- *Mycobacterium leprae* causes mononeuropathy multiplex affecting peripheral nerves in cooler regions of the body, reflecting the predilection for this bacterium to thrive at cooler temperatures.
- Leprosy is classified into tuberculoid, lepromatous, and borderline types; peripheral nerves may be affected in all three types, and involved nerves are often palpably thickened.

Inherited Neuropathies

Charcot-Marie-Tooth Disease

- CMT neuropathy is the most common heritable neuromuscular disorder. It is a chronic distal sensory and motor neuropathy presenting as longstanding gait difficulty with frequent tripping. Wasting and weakness of the distal muscles of the legs (inverted champagne bottle appearance) with hammer toes and high arched feet (pes cavus) are commonly present, along with steppage gait, distal sensory loss, and distal loss of reflexes.
- Pes cavus and hammer toes indicate that the neuropathy dates from early life. An inability to walk on the heels or perform tandem gait is often present.
- Demyelinating forms of CMT are classified as CMT1, and axonal forms as CMT2. Patients with nerve conduction velocities (NCVs) intermediate between CMT1 and CMT2 are classified as having "intermediate CMT," and most of these cases are X-linked. CMT is usually transmitted as an autosomal dominant trait.
- EDx studies show a pattern of generalized demyelination with NCVs that are uniformly and proportionately slowed in distal, intermediate, and proximal segments of the same nerve on the opposite side, and in adjacent nerves. Findings suggestive of heterogeneous demyelination, such as conduction block or dispersion, are not seen. Proliferation of Schwann cells occurs in an attempt to remyelinate; the supernumerary Schwann cells are concentrically arranged around demyelinated and remyelinated axons, giving a characteristic "onion bulb" appearance.

Hereditary Motor Neuropathies (HMN)

The distal HMNs present with distal motor weakness with sparing of sensory fibers. The common HMNs present as footdrop with severe wasting and weakness distally. Some variants may manifest with predominantly upper limb involvement, vocal cord paralysis, or with upper motor neuron signs mimicking amyotrophic lateral sclerosis.

Hereditary Sensory Neuropathies (HSN)

HSNs, also called *hereditary sensory and autonomic neuropathies* (HSANs), are a heterogeneous group of disorders affecting the sensory and/or autonomic neurons. The predominant clinical presentation is of progressive distal sensory loss, although some weakness and wasting is also observed. HSN 3 (HSAN 3), also called *Riley-Day syndrome*, has prominent dysautonomia.

Refsum Disease

- This is an autosomal recessive hypertrophic neuropathy caused by defective oxidation of phytanic acid, a branched-chain fatty acid found in dairy products, beef, lamb, and fish.
- Shows a slowly progressive course of a sensorimotor demyelinating neuropathy with sensorineural deafness, cerebellar ataxia, and anosmia. Retinitis pigmentosa presenting as night blindness often precedes the onset of neuropathy.

Tangier Disease (TD)

- This syndrome is caused by a severe deficiency of high-density lipoproteins (HDL) in plasma. Peripheral neuropathy is the most disabling feature of TD. Mononeuropathies involving the oculomotor nerve, long thoracic nerve, or any of the limb nerves may occur.
- The syringomyelic presentation includes wasting of hand muscles, loss of pain and temperature sensation, and facial diplegia. There is no treatment available; a low-cholesterol diet or other dietary changes do not modify the natural history.

Porphyric Neuropathy

- Peripheral neuropathy accompanies the inherited hepatic porphyrias. The triad of acute neuropathy, psychiatric symptoms, and abdominal involvement are similar in all hepatic porphyrias. Abdominal pain, constipation, vomiting, and mental changes frequently herald the attacks.
- Peripheral neuropathy has an acute onset and may be preceded or accompanied by autonomic manifestations such as tachycardia, hypertension, and postural hypotension.
- Measuring 24-h urinary excretion of porphobilinogen and aminolevulinic acid and 24-h fecal excretion of protoporphyrin and coproporphyrin during a symptomatic period is the most helpful method of determining whether symptoms are due to acute porphyria.
- Treatment is largely supportive during the acute crisis and includes fluid management, ventilatory support, management of heart rate and blood pressure (autonomic dysfunction), and avoidance of medications that are known to precipitate an acute attack. Oral and IV glucose and heme arginate are the mainstays of treatment. Recovery from an acute attack may take several months.

Autonomic Neuropathy

- Symptoms may include orthostatic hypotension (syncope, light headedness, dizziness, fatigue, and lethargy), heat intolerance, abnormal (reduced or increased) sweating, constipation, diarrhea, incontinence, sexual dysfunction, dry eyes, dry mouth, or visual blurriness.
- Autonomic neuropathy is usually a manifestation of a more generalized polyneuropathy, as in diabetes, GBS, and alcoholic polyneuropathy, but occasionally syndromes of pure pandysautonomia are encountered.

Plexopathy

- This refers to disorders of either the brachial or the lumbosacral plexus. *Brachial plexopathy* is a broad term used to define any injury, traumatic or otherwise, to the brachial plexus. Causes include birth injury, trauma, neoplasm, radiation, and familial and immune-mediated processes.
- Brachial plexus lesions demonstrate characteristic motor and sensory signs. When the upper parts of the brachial plexus (cervical roots 5–7) are affected, weakness and atrophy of shoulder girdle and upper arm muscles occurs. Injuries to the lower brachial plexus (C8-T1 roots) produce distal arm weakness, atrophy, and focal sensory deficits in the forearm and hand.
- The *lumbosacral plexus* is formed by the ventral primary rami of L1–S4. Although often considered as a single entity, it can be divided into a lumbar plexus (ventral rami of L1–L4) and a sacral plexus (lumbosacral trunk L4 and L5 and ventral rami of S1–S4). Most patients present with varying degrees of pain, sensory deficits, and weakness in the lower limbs, generally in an asymmetric distribution.

Peripheral Nerve Injury

- Physical damage to peripheral nerves may result from sudden compression, crush, transection, or stretching of a nerve. The mildest form of nerve injury results when a stretch or pressure injury distorts the myelin overlying the nodes of Ranvier and produces focal conduction block.
- This type of injury with conduction block but without Wallerian degeneration, is referred to as *neurapraxia,* or *class 1 injury*. This results in a transient sensation of numbness in an extremity, as occurs after lying or sitting in a certain position.
- Nerve injury that interrupts the axon's continuity and results in Wallerian degeneration of the nerve distal to the lesion is considered moderate or severe. If the endoneurium is preserved, the lesion is considered moderate and is called *axonotmesis*, or *class 2 injury*. If the endoneurium is destroyed, the lesion is considered severe and is called *neurotmesis*.
- The appearance of an advancing Tinel's sign in the distribution of the injured nerve indicates that the nerve is in continuity and justifies postponement of surgery.

Guillain-Barré Syndrome

- Guillain-Barré syndrome (GBS) is an acute and fulminant polyradiculoneuropathy that is autoimmune in nature.
- GBS manifests as rapidly evolving areflexic motor paralysis with or without sensory disturbance. The usual pattern is an ascending paralysis that may be first noticed as rubbery legs. Weakness typically evolves over hours to a few days and is frequently accompanied by tingling dysesthesias in the extremities.
- The lower cranial nerves are also frequently involved, causing bulbar weakness with difficulty handling secretions and maintaining an airway. Most patients require hospitalization and require ventilatory assistance at some time during the illness.
- Autonomic involvement is common and may occur even in patients whose GBS is otherwise mild.
- Several subtypes of GBS are recognized, as determined primarily by electrodiagnostic and pathologic distinctions. These include the axonal variants, which are often clinically severe—either acute motor axonal neuropathy (AMAN – anti GD1a antibodies) or acute motor sensory axonal neuropathy (AMSAN). The Miller Fisher syndrome presents as rapidly evolving ataxia and areflexia of limbs without weakness, and ophthalmoplegia, often with pupillary paralysis.
- Approximately 70% of cases of GBS occur 1–3 weeks after an acute infectious process, usually respiratory or gastrointestinal, commonly caused by Campylobactor *jejuni*. GBS also occurs more frequently in patients with lymphoma (including Hodgkin's disease), in HIV-seropositive individuals, and in patients with systemic lupus erythematosus (SLE).
- Anti-GQ1b IgG antibodies are found in >90% of patients with MFS, and titers of IgG are highest early in the course. Anti-GQ1b antibodies are not found in other forms of GBS unless there is extraocular motor nerve involvement.
- In the demyelinating forms of GBS, the basis for flaccid paralysis and sensory disturbance is conduction block. This finding, demonstrable electrophysiologically, implies that the axonal connections remain intact. When a severe primary axonal pattern is encountered electrophysiologically, the implication is that axons have degenerated and become disconnected from their targets, specifically the neuromuscular junctions, and must therefore regenerate for recovery to take place.

Diagnosis
- CSF findings are distinctive, consisting of an elevated CSF protein level [1–10 g/L (100–1000 mg/dL)] without accompanying pleocytosis.
- Electrodiagnostic features are mild or absent in the early stages of GBS and lag behind the clinical evolution. In cases with demyelination, prolonged distal latencies, conduction velocity slowing, evidence of conduction block, and temporal dispersion of compound action potential are the usual features.

Treatment
- IVIg is often the initial therapy chosen because of its ease of administration and good safety record. IVIg is administered as five daily infusions for a total dose of 2 g/kg body weight.
- A course of plasmapheresis usually consists of ~40–50 mL/kg plasma exchange (PE) four times over a week.
- Glucocorticoids have not been found to be effective in GBS.
- 30% of patients with GBS require ventilatory assistance, sometimes for prolonged periods of time (several weeks or longer). Approximately 85% of patients with GBS achieve a full functional recovery within several months to a year. Few patients with typical GBS have one or more late relapses; such cases are then classified as chronic inflammatory demyelinating polyneuropathy (CIDP).

Chronic Inflammatory Demyelinating Polyneuropathy
- CIDP is distinguished from GBS by its chronic course. This neuropathy shares many features with the common demyelinating form of GBS, including elevated CSF protein levels and the electrodiagnostic findings of acquired demyelination.
- The diagnosis rests on characteristic clinical, CSF, and electrophysiologic findings. The CSF is usually acellular with an elevated protein level, sometimes several times normal. Electrodiagnostically, variable degrees of conduction slowing, prolonged distal latencies, temporal dispersion of compound action potentials, and conduction block are the principal features
- **Treatment**—Treatment with glucocorticoids (60–80 mg prednisone PO daily for 1–2 months, followed by a gradual dose reduction of 10 mg per month as tolerated),is effective. Patients who fail therapy with IVIg and glucocorticoids may benefit from treatment with immunosuppressive agents such as azathioprine, methotrexate, cyclosporine, and cyclophosphamide, either alone or as adjunctive therapy.

Multiple Myeloma
- Clinically overt polyneuropathy occurs in few patients with the commonly encountered type of multiple myeloma, which exhibits either lytic or diffuse osteoporotic bone lesions.
- These neuropathies are sensorimotor, are usually mild and slowly progressive but may be severe, and generally do not reverse with successful suppression of the myeloma. Electrodiagnostic and pathologic features are consistent with a process of axonal degeneration.
- In contrast, myeloma with osteosclerotic features, is associated with polyneuropathy in one-half of cases. These neuropathies, which may also occur with solitary plasmacytoma, are distinct because they
  1. Are usually demyelinating in nature;
  2. Often respond to radiation therapy or removal of the primary lesion;
  3. Are associated with different monoclonal proteins and light chains (almost always lambda as opposed to primarily kappa in the lytic type of multiple myeloma);
  4. May occur in association with other systemic findings including thickening of the skin, hyperpigmentation, hypertrichosis, organomegaly, endocrinopathy, anasarca, and clubbing of fingers. These are features of the POEMS syndrome (*poly*-neuropathy, *o*rganomegaly, *e*ndocrinopathy, *M* protein, and *s*kin changes).
- Therapy with chlorambucil, or cyclophosphamide combined with glucocorticoids, often results in improvement of the neuropathy associated with a prolonged reduction in the levels in the circulating paraprotein.

Vasculitic Neuropathy
- Peripheral nerve involvement is common in polyarteritis nodosa (PAN). The most common pattern is multifocal (asymmetric) motor-sensory neuropathy (mononeuropathy multiplex) due to ischemic lesions of nerve trunks and roots.
- The electrodiagnostic findings are those of an axonal process. A high frequency of neuropathy occurs in allergic angiitis and granulomatosis (Churg-Strauss syndrome).
- Diagnosis of suspected vasculitic neuropathy is made by a combined nerve and muscle biopsy, with serial section or skip-serial techniques.
- Vasculitic neuropathy may also be seen as part of the vasculitis syndrome occurring in the course of other connective tissue disorders like rheumatoid arthritis, but ischemic neuropathy due to involvement of vasa nervorum may also occur in mixed cryoglobulinemia, Sjögren's syndrome, Wegener's granulomatosis, hypersensitivity angiitis, and progressive systemic sclerosis.

Anti-Hu Paraneoplastic Neuropathy

- This immune-mediated disorder manifests as a sensory neuronopathy (i.e., selective damage to sensory nerve bodies in dorsal root ganglia).
- The onset is often asymmetric with dysesthesias and sensory loss in the limbs that soon progress to affect all limbs, the torso, and face. Marked sensory ataxia, pseudoathetosis, and inability to walk, stand, or even sit unsupported are frequent features and are secondary to the extensive deafferentation.
- Diagnosis of the underlying SCLC requires awareness of the association, paraneoplastic testing, and often PET scanning for the tumor.
- The target antigens are a family of RNA binding proteins (HuD, HuC, and Hel-N1) that in normal tissues are only expressed by neurons. An encephalomyelitis may accompany the sensory neuronopathy.
- Most cases are unresponsive to treatment with glucocorticoids, IVIg, PE, or immunosuppressant drugs.

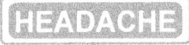

The key structures involved in primary headache, those in which headache and its associated features are the disorder in itself appear to be:
- The large intracranial vessels and dura mater
- The peripheral terminals of the trigeminal nerve that innervate these structures
- The caudal portion of the trigeminal nucleus, which extends into the dorsal horns of the upper cervical spinal cord and receives input from the first and second cervical nerve roots (the trigeminocervical complex)
- The pain modulatory systems in the brain that receive input from trigeminal nociceptors

PRIMARY HEADACHE SYNDROMES

Migraine Headache

- Migraine is usually an episodic headache that is associated with certain features such as sensitivity to light, sound, or movement; nausea and vomiting often accompany the headache. Migraine can often be recognized by its activators, referred to as *triggers*. The brain of the migraine patient is particularly sensitive to environmental and sensory stimuli; migraine-prone patients do not habituate easily to sensory stimuli. This sensitivity is amplified in females during the menstrual cycle. Headache can be initiated or amplified by various triggers, including glare, bright lights, sounds, or other afferent stimulation; hunger; excess stress; physical exertion; stormy weather or barometric pressure changes; hormonal fluctuations during menses; lack of or excess sleep; and alcohol or other chemical stimulation.
- The sensory sensitivity that is characteristic of migraine is probably due to dysfunction of monoaminergic sensory control systems located in the brainstem and thalamus
- Pharmacologic and other data point to the involvement of the neurotransmitter 5-hydroxytryptamine (5-HT; also known as serotonin) in migraine
- Migraine genes identified by studying families with familial hemiplegic migraine (FHM) reveal involvement of ion channels, suggesting that alterations in membrane excitability can predispose to migraine. Mutations involving the Ca2.1 (P/Q) type voltage-gated calcium channel *CACNA1A* gene are now known to cause FHM 1. Functional neuroimaging has suggested that brainstem regions in migraine and the posterior hypothalamic gray matter region close to the human circadian pacemaker cells of the suprachiasmatic nucleus in cluster headache.
- *Types:*
  - Classical migraine–migraine with aura; Common migraine – migraine without aura
  - Acephalgic migraine – migraine without headache or mild headache
  - Brainstem migraine – migraine with prominent brainstem symptoms

Diagnosis and Clinical Features

- A high index of suspicion is required to diagnose migraine: the migraine aura, consisting of visual disturbances with flashing lights or zigzag lines moving across the visual field or of other neurologic symptoms
- Migraine must be differentiated from tension-type headache, the most common primary headache syndrome seen in clinical practice. Migraine at its most basic level is headache with associated features, and tension-type headache is headache that is featureless. Most patients with disabling headache probably have migraine.

Diagnostic Criteria for Migraine

Repeated attacks of headache lasting 4–72 h in patients with a normal physical examination, no other reasonable cause for the headache, and:

At least 2 of the following features: Unilateral pain, Throbbing pain, Aggravation by movement, Moderate or severe intensity

Plus at least 1 of the following features: Nausea/vomiting, Photophobia and phonophobia

Treatment

Nonpharmacologic Management

- Migraine can often be managed to some degree by a variety of nonpharmacologic approaches. Most patients benefit by the identification and avoidance of specific headache triggers. A regulated lifestyle is helpful, including a healthful diet, regular exercise, regular sleep patterns, avoidance of excess caffeine and alcohol, and avoidance of acute changes in stress levels.
- Nonpharmacologic measures are unlikely to prevent all migraine attacks. When these measures fail to prevent an attack, pharmacologic approaches are then needed to abort an attack.

Acute Attack Therapies for Migraine

- Mild migraine attacks can usually be managed by oral agents. Severe migraine attacks may require parenteral therapy. Most drugs effective in the treatment of migraine are members of one of three major pharmacologic classes: anti-inflammatory agents, $5HT_{1B/1D}$ receptor agonists, and dopamine receptor antagonists.
- Nonsteroidal Anti-Inflammatory Drugs (NSAIDs) - Both the severity and duration of a migraine attack can be reduced significantly by anti-inflammatory agents. The combination of acetaminophen, aspirin, and caffeine has been approved for use by the U.S. Food and Drug Administration (FDA) for the treatment of mild to moderate migraine. The combination of aspirin and metoclopramide has been shown to be equivalent to a single dose of sumatriptan.
- $5\text{-}HT_1$ Agonists–
  - *Oral:* Stimulation of $5\text{-}HT_{1B/1D}$ receptors can stop an acute migraine attack. Ergotamine and dihydroergotamine are nonselective receptor agonists, while the triptans are selective $5\text{-}HT_{1B/1D}$ receptor agonists. A variety of triptans (e.g., naratriptan, rizatriptan, eletriptan, sumatriptan, zolmitriptan, almotriptan, frovatriptan) are now available for the treatment of migraine. Rizatriptan and eletriptan are the most efficacious of the triptans.
  - *Nasal:* The fastest-acting nonparenteral antimigraine therapies that can be self-administered include nasal formulations of dihydroergotamine, zolmitriptan, or sumatriptan. The nasal sprays result in substantial blood levels within 30–60 min.
  - *Parenteral:* Parenteral administration of drugs such as dihydroergotamine and sumatriptan is approved by the FDA for the rapid relief of a migraine attack. Peak plasma levels of dihydroergotamine are achieved 3 min after intravenous dosing, 30 min after intramuscular dosing, and 45 min after subcutaneous dosing.
- Triptans are not effective in migraine with aura unless given after the aura is completed and the headache initiated. Side effects are common though often mild and transient. $5\text{-}HT_{1B/1D}$ agonists are contraindicated in individuals with a history of cardiovascular and cerebrovascular disease.
- Ergotamine preparations offer a nonselective means of stimulating $5\text{-}HT_1$ receptors. In general, ergotamine appears to have a much higher incidence of nausea than triptans, but less headache recurrence.
- **Medication-Overuse Headache**—Acute attack medications, particularly codeine or barbiturate-containing compound analgesics, have a propensity to aggravate headache frequency and induce a state of refractory daily or near-daily headache called *medication-overuse headache*.

Preventive Treatments for Migraine

- Patients with an increasing frequency of migraine attacks, or with attacks that are either unresponsive or poorly responsive to abortive treatments, are good candidates for preventive agents. In general, a preventive medication should be considered in the subset of patients with five or more attacks a month.
- The drugs that have been approved by the FDA for the prophylactic treatment of migraine include propranolol, timolol, sodium valproate, topiramate, and methysergide though, a number of other drugs appear to display prophylactic efficacy like amitriptyline, nortriptyline, flunarizine, phenelzine, gabapentin, topiramate, and cyproheptadine.

Tension-Type Headache

- The term *tension-type headache* (TTH) is commonly used to describe a chronic head-pain syndrome characterized by bilateral tight, bandlike discomfort. The pain typically builds slowly, fluctuates in severity, and may persist more or less continuously for many days. The headache may be episodic or chronic (present >15 days per month).

- A useful clinical approach is to diagnose TTH in patients whose headaches are completely without accompanying features such as nausea, vomiting, photophobia, phonophobia, osmophobia, throbbing, and aggravation with movement – featureless headache.
- The name *tension-type headache* implies that pain is a product of *nervous tension*. Headache > 15 days/month – chronic tension type headache
- ***Treatment***—The pain of TTH can generally be managed with simple analgesics such as acetaminophen, aspirin, or NSAIDs. Behavioral approaches including relaxation can also be effective. For chronic TTH, amitriptyline is the only proven treatment.

Trigeminal Autonomic Cephalalgias

- The trigeminal autonomic cephalalgias (TACs) are a group of primary headaches that includes cluster headache, paroxysmal hemicrania, hemicrania continua and SUNCT (*s*hort-lasting *u*nilateral *n*euralgiform headache attacks with *c*onjunctival injection and *t*earing). It is associated with pituitary tumours and has migrainous headache features.
- TACs are characterized by relatively short-lasting attacks of head pain associated with cranial autonomic symptoms, such as lacrimation, conjunctival injection, or nasal congestion. Pain is usually severe and may occur more than once a day.
- TACs must be differentiated from short-lasting headaches that do not have prominent cranial autonomic syndromes, notably trigeminal neuralgia, primary stabbing headache, and hypnic headache.

Cluster Headache

- In Cluster headache the pain is deep, usually retroorbital, often excruciating in intensity, nonfluctuating, and explosive in quality.
- A core feature of cluster headache is periodicity. At least one of the daily attacks of pain recurs at about the same hour each day for the duration of a cluster bout. The typical cluster headache patient has daily bouts of one to two attacks of relatively short-duration unilateral pain for 8–10 weeks a year; this is usually followed by a pain-free interval that averages 1 year.
- Onset is nocturnal in most of patients, and men are affected three times more often than women.
- Cluster headache is associated with ipsilateral symptoms of cranial parasympathetic autonomic activation: conjunctival injection or lacrimation, rhinorrhea or nasal congestion, or cranial sympathetic dysfunction such as ptosis. Cluster headache is likely to be a disorder involving central pacemaker neurons in the region of the posterior hypothalamus.

Treatment

- During acute attacks, many patients with acute cluster headache respond very well to oxygen inhalation. This should be given as 100% oxygen at 10–12 L/min for 15–20 min. Sumatriptan 6 mg subcutaneously is rapid in onset and will usually shorten an attack to 10–15 min. Oral sumatriptan is not effective for prevention or for acute treatment of cluster headache.
- **Preventive Treatments**—For patients with relatively short bouts, limited courses of oral glucocorticoids or methysergide can be very useful. A 10-day course of prednisone, beginning at 60 mg daily for 7 days and followed by a rapid taper, may interrupt the pain bout for many patients.
- When medical therapies fail in chronic cluster headache, neurostimulation therapy strategies can be employed. Deep-brain stimulation of the region of the posterior hypothalamic gray matter has proven successful in a substantial proportion of patients.

SUNCT

- SUNCT is a rare primary headache syndrome characterized by severe, unilateral orbital or temporal pain that is stabbing or throbbing in quality. Diagnosis requires at least 20 attacks, lasting for 5–240 s; ipsilateral conjunctival injection and lacrimation should be present.
- The pain of SUNCT is unilateral and may be located anywhere in the head. Three basic patterns can be seen: single stabs, which are usually short-lived; groups of stabs; or a longer attack comprising many stabs between which the pain does not completely resolve, thus giving a "saw-tooth" phenomenon with attacks lasting many minutes.
- Characteristics that lead to a suspected diagnosis of SUNCT are the cutaneous (or other) trigger ability of attacks, a lack of refractory period to triggering between attacks, and the lack of a response to indomethacin. SUNCT can be seen with posterior fossa or pituitary lesions. All patients with SUNCT should be evaluated with pituitary function tests and a brain MRI with pituitary views.

Treatment

Long-term prevention to minimize disability and hospitalization is the goal of treatment. The most effective treatment for prevention is lamotrigine, 200–400 mg/d. Topiramate and gabapentin may also be effective.

Common Headache Types

Type	Site	Age and sex	Clinical characteristics	Diurnal pattern	Provoking factors
Migraine	Frontotemporal	Adolescents, young to middle-aged adults,	Throbbing (pulsatile); worse behind one eye or ear	Upon awakening or later in day	Bright light, noise, tension, alcohol
	Uni- or bilateral	Sometimes children, more common in women	Becomes dull ache and generalized	Duration: 4–24 h in most cases, sometimes longer	Relieved by darkness and sleep
			Scalp sensitive		Alcohol in some
Cluster (histamine headache, migrainous neuralgia)	Orbitotemporal	Adolescent and adult males (90%)	Intense, nonthrobbing	Usually nocturnal, 1–2 h after falling asleep	
	Unilateral			Occasionally diurnal	
Tension headaches	Generalized	Mainly adults, both sexes, more common in women	Pressure (nonthrobbing), tightness, aching	Continuous, variable intensity, for days, weeks, or months	Fatigue and nervous strain

Post-Traumatic Headache

- A traumatic event can trigger a headache process that lasts for many months or years after the event. Complaints of dizziness, vertigo, and impaired memory can accompany the headache. Symptoms may remit after several weeks or persist for months and even years after the injury.
- Typically the neurologic examination is normal and CT or MRI studies are unrevealing. Chronic subdural hematoma may on occasion mimic this disorder.
- Post-traumatic headache may also be seen after carotid dissection and subarachnoid hemorrhage, and following intracranial surgery.

Trigeminal Neuralgia (Tic Douloureux)

- The trigeminal (fifth cranial) nerve supplies sensation to the skin of the face and anterior half of the head.
- Trigeminal neuralgia is characterized by excruciating paroxysms of pain in the lips, gums, cheek, or chin and, very rarely, in the distribution of the ophthalmic division of the fifth nerve. The pain seldom lasts more than a few seconds or a minute or two but may be so intense that the patient winces, hence the term *tic*.
- Characteristic feature is the presence of trigger zones, typically on the face, lips, or tongue, that provoke attacks; patients may report that tactile stimuli—e.g. washing the face, brushing the teeth, or exposure to a draft of air—generate excruciating pain.
- *An essential feature of trigeminal neuralgia is that objective signs of sensory loss cannot be demonstrated on examination.*
- Symptoms result from ectopic generation of action potentials in pain-sensitive afferent fibers of the fifth cranial nerve root just before it enters the lateral surface of the pons. Compression of the trigeminal nerve root by a blood vessel, most often the superior cerebellar artery or on occasion a tortuous vein, is the source of trigeminal neuralgia in a substantial proportion of patients.
- Trigeminal neuralgia must be distinguished from other causes of face and head pain arising from diseases of the jaw, teeth, or sinuses. Pain from migraine or cluster headache tends to be deep-seated and steady, unlike the superficial stabbing quality of trigeminal neuralgia; rarely, cluster headache is associated with trigeminal neuralgia, a syndrome known as *cluster-tic*. In temporal arteritis, superficial facial pain is present but is not typically shocklike, the patient frequently complains of myalgias and other systemic symptoms, and an elevated erythrocyte sedimentation rate (ESR) is usually present.

Treatment

Medical

- Drug therapy with carbamazepine is effective in most of the patients. Carbamazepine should be started as a single daily dose of 100 mg taken with food and increased gradually (by 100 mg daily every 1–2 days) until substantial pain relief is achieved. Most patients require a maintenance dose of 200 mg qid.
- If carbamazepine is not well tolerated or is ineffective, phenytoin, 300–400 mg daily, can be tried; other anticonvulsants may also be effective. Baclofen may also be administered, either alone or in combination with carbamazepine or phenytoin.

Surgical

- If drug treatment fails, surgical therapy should be offered. The most widely applied procedure creates a heat lesion of the trigeminal (gasserian) ganglion or nerve, a method termed *radiofrequency thermal rhizotomy*.
- Gamma knife radiosurgery is also utilized for treatment and results in complete pain relief in more than two-thirds of patients; the response is often long-lasting. Compared with thermal rhizotomy, gamma knife surgery appears to be somewhat less effective but has a lower risk of serious complications.
- A third surgical treatment, microvascular decompression to relieve pressure on the trigeminal nerve as it exits the pons, requires a suboccipital craniotomy.

Migraine Headache

- Migraine is usually an episodic headache that is associated with certain features such as sensitivity to light, sound, or movement; nausea and vomiting often accompany the headache. Migraine can often be recognized by its activators, referred to as *triggers*. The brain of the migraine patient is particularly sensitive to environmental and sensory stimuli; migraine-prone patients do not habituate easily to sensory stimuli. This sensitivity is amplified in females during the menstrual cycle. Headache can be initiated or amplified by various triggers, including glare, bright lights, sounds, or other afferent stimulation; hunger; excess stress; physical exertion; stormy weather or barometric pressure changes; hormonal fluctuations during menses; lack of or excess sleep; and alcohol or other chemical stimulation.
- The sensory sensitivity that is characteristic of migraine is probably due to dysfunction of monoaminergic sensory control systems located in the brainstem and thalamus.
- Pharmacologic and other data point to the involvement of the neurotransmitter 5-hydroxytryptamine (5-HT; also known as serotonin) in migraine.
- Migraine genes identified by studying families with familial hemiplegic migraine (FHM) reveal involvement of ion channels, suggesting that alterations in membrane excitability can predispose to migraine. Mutations involving the Ca2.1 (P/Q) type voltage-gated calcium channel *CACNA1A* gene are now known to cause FHM 1. Functional neuroimaging has suggested that brainstem regions in migraine and the posterior hypothalamic gray matter region close to the human circadian pacemaker cells of the suprachiasmatic nucleus in cluster headache.

Types

- Classical migraine–migraine with aura
- Common migraine–migraine without aura
- Acephalgic migraine–migraine without headache or mild headache
- Brainstem migraine–migraine with prominent brainstem symptoms

Diagnosis and Clinical Features

- A high index of suspicion is required to diagnose migraine: the migraine aura, consisting of visual disturbances with flashing lights or zigzag lines moving across the visual field or of other neurologic symptoms
- Migraine must be differentiated from tension-type headache, the most common primary headache syndrome seen in clinical practice. Migraine at its most basic level is headache with associated features, and tension-type headache is headache that is featureless. Most patients with disabling headache probably have migraine.
- Activators of migraine–triggers
- **Common triggers**:
  - Glare, bright lights, loud sounds or other afferent stimuli
  - Physical exertion, stress
  - Stormy weather, barometric pressure changes
  - Lack/excess of sleep, alcohol, hormone changes during menses

Diagnostic Criteria for Migraine

Repeated attacks of headache lasting 4–72 h in patients with a normal physical examination, no other reasonable cause for the headache, and:
  At least 2 of the following features: Unilateral pain, Throbbing pain, Aggravation by movement, Moderate or severe intensity
  Plus at least 1 of the following features: Nausea/vomiting, Photophobia and phonophobia

Treatment

Nonpharmacologic Management

- Migraine can often be managed to some degree by a variety of nonpharmacologic approaches. Most patients benefit by the identification and avoidance of specific headache triggers. A regulated lifestyle is helpful, including a healthful diet, regular exercise, regular sleep patterns, avoidance of excess caffeine and alcohol, and avoidance of acute changes in stress levels.
- Nonpharmacologic measures are unlikely to prevent all migraine attacks. When these measures fail to prevent an attack, pharmacologic approaches are then needed to abort an attack.

Acute Attack Therapies for Migraine

- Mild migraine attacks can usually be managed by oral agents. Severe migraine attacks may require parenteral therapy. Most drugs effective in the treatment of migraine are members of one of three major pharmacologic classes: anti-inflammatory agents, $5HT_{1B/1D}$ receptor agonists, and dopamine receptor antagonists.

- **Nonsteroidal Anti-Inflammatory Drugs (NSAIDs)**—Both the severity and duration of a migraine attack can be reduced significantly by anti-inflammatory agents. The combination of acetaminophen, aspirin, and caffeine has been approved for use by the U.S. Food and Drug Administration (FDA) for the treatment of mild to moderate migraine. The combination of aspirin and metoclopramide has been shown to be equivalent to a single dose of sumatriptan
- 5-HT1 Agonists:
    - *Oral*—Stimulation of $5\text{-HT}_{1B/1D}$ receptors can stop an acute migraine attack. Ergotamine and dihydroergotamine are nonselective receptor agonists, while the triptans are selective $5\text{-HT}_{1B/1D}$ receptor agonists. A variety of triptans (e.g., naratriptan, rizatriptan, eletriptan, sumatriptan, zolmitriptan, almotriptan, frovatriptan) are now available for the treatment of migraine. Rizatriptan and eletriptan are the most efficacious of the triptans.
    - *Nasal*—The fastest-acting nonparenteral antimigraine therapies that can be self-administered include nasal formulations of dihydroergotamine, zolmitriptan, or sumatriptan. The nasal sprays result in substantial blood levels within 30–60 min.
    - *Parenteral*—Parenteral administration of drugs such as dihydroergotamine and sumatriptan is approved by the FDA for the rapid relief of a migraine attack. Peak plasma levels of dihydroergotamine are achieved 3 min after intravenous dosing, 30 min after intramuscular dosing, and 45 min after subcutaneous dosing.
- Triptans are not effective in migraine with aura unless given after the aura is completed and the headache initiated. Side effects are common though often mild and transient. $5\text{-HT}_{1B/1D}$ agonists are contraindicated in individuals with a history of cardiovascular and cerebrovascular disease.
- Ergotamine preparations offer a nonselective means of stimulating 5-HT_1 receptors. In general, ergotamine appears to have a much higher incidence of nausea than triptans, but less headache recurrence.
- **Medication-Overuse Headache**—Acute attack medications, particularly codeine or barbiturate-containing compound analgesics, have a propensity to aggravate headache frequency and induce a state of refractory daily or near-daily headache called *medication-overuse headache*.

Preventive Treatments for Migraine

- Patients with an increasing frequency of migraine attacks, or with attacks that are either unresponsive or poorly responsive to abortive treatments, are good candidates for preventive agents. In general, a preventive medication should be considered in the subset of patients with five or more attacks a month.
- The drugs that have been approved by the FDA for the prophylactic treatment of migraine include propranolol, timolol, sodium valproate, topiramate, and methysergide though, a number of other drugs appear to display prophylactic efficacy like amitriptyline, nortriptyline, flunarizine, phenelzine, gabapentin, topiramate, and cyproheptadine.

Tension-Type Headache

Most common type of primary headache – 90% of headaches; 3% of population has TTH
- The term *tension-type headache* (TTH) is commonly used to describe a chronic head-pain syndrome characterized by bilateral tight, bandlike discomfort. The pain typically builds slowly, fluctuates in severity, and may persist more or less continuously for many days. The headache may be episodic or chronic (present >15 days per month).
- Pain can radiate from the neck back eyes
- A useful clinical approach is to diagnose TTH in patients whose headaches are completely without accompanying features such as nausea, vomiting, photophobia, phonophobia, osmophobia, throbbing, and aggravation with movement – featureless headace.
- The name *tension-type headache* implies that pain is a product of *nervous tension*. Headache > 15 days/month– chronic tension type headache
- *Treatment:*
    - The pain of TTH can generally be managed with simple analgesics such as acetaminophen, aspirin, or NSAIDs.
    - Behavioral approaches including relaxation can also be effective.
    - For chronic TTH, amitriptyline is the only proven treatment.

Trigeminal Autonomic Cephalalgias

- The trigeminal autonomic cephalalgias (TACs) are a group of primary headaches that includes cluster headache, paroxysmal hemicrania, hemicrania continua and SUNCT (*s*hort-lasting *u*nilateral *n*euralgiform headache attacks with *c*onjunctival injection and *t*earing).
- It is associated with pituitary tumours and has migrainous headache features
- TACs are characterized by relatively short-lasting attacks of head pain associated with cranial autonomic symptoms, such as lacrimation, conjunctival injection, or nasal congestion. Pain is usually severe and may occur more than once a day.
- TACs must be differentiated from short-lasting headaches that do not have prominent cranial autonomic syndromes, notably trigeminal neuralgia, primary stabbing headache, and hypnic headache.

Cluster Headache

- In Cluster headache the pain is deep, usually retroorbital, often excruciating in intensity, nonfluctuating, and explosive in quality. It is associated with unilateral photophobia and phonophobia
- A core feature of cluster headache is periodicity. At least one of the daily attacks of pain recurs at about the same hour each day for the duration of a cluster bout.
- The typical cluster headache patient has daily bouts of one to two attacks of relatively short-duration unilateral pain for 8–10 weeks a year; this is usually followed by a pain-free interval that averages 1 year.
- Onset is nocturnal in most of patients, and men are affected three times more often than women.
- Cluster headache is associated with ipsilateral symptoms of cranial parasympathetic autonomic activation: conjunctival injection or lacrimation, rhinorrhea or nasal congestion, or cranial sympathetic dysfunction such as ptosis.
- Cluster headache is likely to be a disorder involving central pacemaker neurons in the region of the posterior hypothalamus.

Treatment

- During acute attacks, many patients with acute cluster headache respond very well to oxygen inhalation. This should be given as 100% oxygen at 10–12 L/min for 15–20 min.
- Sumatriptan 6 mg subcutaneously is rapid in onset and will usually shorten an attack to 10–15 min. Oral sumatriptan is not effective for prevention or for acute treatment of cluster headache.
- ***Preventive treatments***: For patients with relatively short bouts, limited courses of oral glucocorticoids or methysergide can be very useful. A 10-day course of prednisone, beginning at 60 mg daily for 7 days and followed by a rapid taper, may interrupt the pain bout for many patients.
- When medical therapies fail in chronic cluster headache, neurostimulation therapy strategies can be employed.
- Deep-brain stimulation of the region of the posterior hypothalamic gray matter has proven successful in a substantial proportion of patients.

Lennox-Gastaut Syndrome

- Multiple seizure types (usually including generalized tonic-clonic, atonic, and atypical absence seizures)
- An EEG showing slow (<3 Hz) spike-and-wave discharges and a variety of other abnormalities
- Impaired cognitive function in most but not all cases.
- ***Drugs effective in Lennox-Gastaut syndrome:***
  - Lamotrigine
  - Topiramate
  - Clobazam
  - Felbamate
  - Rufinamide
- ***Reflex epilepsy:*** Seizures induced by highly specific stimuli such as video game monitor, music or an individuals voice
- ***Febrile seizures:***
  - Seizures associated with fever but with no evidence of CNS infection or other defined cause
  - A simple febrile seizure is a single isolated event, brief and symmetric in appearance
  - More likely to occur during the rising phase of the temperature curve ie during the first day than well into the illness
  - Peak incidence: 18–24 months
  - MC seizures occurring during late infancy and early childhood – febrile seizures
- ***Complex febrile seizures:***
  - Repeated seizure activity
  - lasts for more than 15 minutes
  - Features of focal seizures
- ***Risk factors associated with recurrent seizures:***
  - Seizures that present as status epilepticus
  - Seizures associated with post ictal Todds paralysis
  - Strong family history of seizures
  - Abnormal neurological examination
  - Abnormal EEG

Mesial Temporal Lobe Epilepsy Syndrome

Mesial temporal lobe epilepsy (MTLE) is the most common syndrome associated with complex partial seizures.
- Highly selective loss of specific cell populations within hippocampus
- Characteristics:

- History of:
  - Febrile seizures
  - Rare generalized seizures
  - Early onset intractable seizures
  - Family history of epilepsy
  - Remitting relapsing seizures
- Clinical:
  - Aura – common
  - Post ictal disorientation
  - Behavioral arrest/stare
  - Memory loss
  - Complex automatisms
  - Dysphasia
  - Unilateral posturing
- Laboratory studies:
  - EEG – U/L or B/L anterior temporal spikes
  - PET – hypometabolism on inter ictal PET
  - SPECT – hypoperfusion on inter ictal SPECT
  - Wada test (intracranial amobarbital test) – material specific memory deficits
  - MRI findings: hippocampal sclerosis – characteristic
  - Small hippocampus with increased signal on T2 weighted sequences
  - Small temporal lobe
  - Enlarged temporal horn
- Pregnancy and epilepsy:
- Potential harm of uncontrolled epilepsy on pregnant women is more than that of anticonvulsants, it is recommended that they are maintained on lowest effective dose preferably monotherapy especially during first trimester
- As the antifolate effects of anticonvulsants are thought to play a role in the teratogenic neural tube defects during pregnancy, intake of folate (1-4 mg/d) by the pregnant mothers is recommended
- Enzyme inducing drugs like phenytoin, carbamazepine, oxcarbazepine, topiramate, Phenobarbital, primodone cause a transient reversible deficiency of vitamin K dependant clotting factors in 50% newborn infants although neonatal hemorrhage is uncommon, mothers should be given oral vitamin K (20 mg/d) in the last two weeks of pregnancy and infants should receive intra muscular injection vitamin K(1 mg) at birth.
- **Fabry disease:**
  - X-linked disorder – men are more commonly and severely affected
  - Results from mutations in alpha galactosidase A gene
- **Clinical presentation:**
  - Angiokeratoma – telangiectatic skin lesions
  - Hypohidrosis
  - Corneal/lenticular opacities
  - Acroparesthesia
  - Progressive small vessel disease of kidney, heart and brain
- **Angiokeratoma**:
  - Symmetric
  - Dark blue or black
  - Flat or slightly raised
  - Do not blanch with pressure
  - Tend to increase in size and number with age
  - Usually more dense between umbilicus and knees – bathing suit area
- **Acroparesthesia**: Debilitating episodic burning pain of the hands, feet and promixal extremities – lasting for minutes to days, precipitated by changes in temperature, exercise, fatigue, fever. phenytoin and carbamazepine diminish episodic and chronic acroparesthesia
  - Proteinuria, isosthenuria and progressive renal dysfunction occur in 2nd to 4th decades
  - Death is due to renal failure/cardiovascular/cerebrovascular disease in untreated males

Myelopathy–Sarcoidosis

- Sarcoidosis is an important cause of acute or subacute myelopathy
- Presents with slowly progressive weakness or a relapsing – remitting course
- Sarcoid myelopathy—concomitant sensory loss with weakness
- MRI—diffuse edema of spinal cord with gadolinium enhancement in active lesions
- Nodular enhancement of the adjacent surface of the spinal cord is seen – disease affects various levels of the spinal cord
- Lumbar puncture—lymphocyte predominant cell count with mildly elevated CSF protein
- Examination for evidence of multi system disease:
  - CXR
  - Serum calcium levels
  - ECG
  - Slit lamp eye examination
- Presence of noncaseating granuloma on biopsy during pathologic examination is definitive diagnosis
- *Treatment:* High dose glucocorticoids (decrease swelling and stimulate regression of the granulomatous lesions) or alternative immunosuppresants

Vogt-Koyanangi-Harada Syndrome:

- Meningitis
- Uveitis
- Tinnitus
- Hearing loss

Progressive Multifocal Leukoencephalopathy

- Progressive multifocal leukoencephalopathy (PML) is a progressive disorder characterized pathologically by multifocal areas of demyelination of varying size distributed throughout the brain but sparing the spinal cord and optic nerves.
- Occurs in natalizumab treated Multiple Sclerosis patients
- Homonymous hemianopia is the most common clinical feature.
- Mirtazapine prolongs the survival
- Oligodendrocytes have enlarged, densely staining nuclei that contain viral inclusions formed by crystalline arrays of JC virus (JCV) particles. Almost all patients have an underlying immunosuppressive disorder.
- The CSF is typically normal, although mild elevation in protein and/or IgG may be found. PCR amplification of JCV DNA from CSF is an important diagnostic tool. Detection of JCV antigen or genomic material should only be considered diagnostic of PML if accompanied by characteristic pathologic changes.

Treatment

No effective therapy for PML is available. Some patients with HIV-associated PML have shown disease stabilization and improvement in their immune status following institution of HAART

Multiple System Atrophy

Comprises a group of sporadic disorders characterized by varying degrees of Parkinsonism with cerebellar, corticospinal, and autonomic dysfunction. The unifying pathologic hallmark is the presence of alpha-synuclein-positive inclusions located in various brain regions. Disorders under MSA have now been reclassified as *striatonigral degeneration* (SND), *olivopontocerebellar atrophy* (OPCA), and *progressive autonomic failure* (PAF), either without parkinsonism or with parkinsonism (Shy-Drager syndrome).

- They can be divided into MSA –p (predominantly Parkinsonian form) and MSA-c (predominantly cerebellar form)
- With disease progression, most of patients exhibit Parkinsonian signs and signs of autonomic failure; with upper motor neuron signs. Tremor is common, but unlike in PD, this and other Parkinsonian signs are more likely to present symmetrically. Parkinsonian symptoms are typically poorly responsive to dopaminergic therapy, although some patients may respond favorably for years.
- Corticospinal signs consist of spasticity, involving the legs more than the arms, and pseudobulbar palsy. This aspect of the illness may mimic primary lateral sclerosis with lower motor neurons being occasionally involved.
- Signs of autonomic failure include orthostatic hypotension, leg swelling not due to drug therapy, changes in sweating patterns, and autonomic storms with diaphoresis and flushing. Orthostatic hypotension can present with dizziness, faintness, or syncope
- In MSA LB's take the form of glial alpha-synuclein-positive intracytoplasmic inclusions in the substantia nigra, putamen, inferior olives, pontine nuclei, pigmented nuclei of the brainstem, intermediolateral nucleus of the spinal cord, and the cerebellum.

- MRI shows
  - Pathological iron accumulation in the striatum
  - High signal change in the region of the external surface of the putamen (putaminal rim) – MSA-p
  - Cerebellar and brainstem atrophy (pontine hot cross buns) – MSA-c
- Mutations in coq2 gene–familial and sporadic MSA

Foster Kennedy Syndrome
- Olfactory groove meningioma
- Characterized by ipsilateral optic atrophy, loss of vision and contralateral disc edema due to increased cranial pressure

Gerstmann Syndrome: Components
- Alexia
- Acalculia
- Dysgraphia
- Finger agnosia
- Right left confusion

P1 syndromes
- Webers syndrome
- Benedikts syndrome
- Nothangles syndrome
- Claudes syndrome
- Parinauds syndrome
- Thalamic Dejerine-Roussy syndrome
- Millard-Gubler syndrome
- Consists of 6th and 7th nerve palsy with contralateral hemiplegia

Metachromatic Leukodystrophy
- Lysosomal storage disease–progressive, inherited, neurodegenerative disorders 4 types (vary with onset and course)
  - Late infantile
  - Early juvenile
  - Late juvenile
  - Adult.
- All forms involve a progressive deterioration of motor and neurocognitive function
- Presence of white matter abnormalities on brain images is characteristic
- *Pathophysiology:* Inability to degrade sulfated glycolipidis (galactosyl-3-sulfate ceramides)
- A deficiency in the lysosomal enzyme sulfatide sulfatase (arylsulfatase A)

Peripheral Neuropathy
Demyelinating causes
- GBS
- CIDP
- Amiodarone
- Hereditary sensorimotor neuropathies (HSMN) type I

Axonal pathology
- Alcohol
- Diabetes mellitus
- Vitamin b12 deficiency
- HSMN type II

Predominantly motor loss
- GBS
- Porphyria
- Lead poisoning
- CIDP
- Diphtheria

Predominantly sensory loss
- Diabetes
- Uremia
- Leprosy
- Alcoholism
- Amyloidosis
- Vitamin b12 deficiency

UMN vs LMN lesion

Feature	UMN Lesion	LMN Lesion
Function	Inhibitory effect on muscle stretch reflex	Motor component of muscle reflex
Type of paralysis	Spastic	Flaccid
DTR	Hyper reflexia	Hyper reflexia
Muscle tone	• Hypertonic • Decorticate rigidity – lesion above midbrain • Decerebrate rigidity – lesion below midbrain	Hypertonic
Muscle mass	Disuse atrophy	Wasting atrophy
Fasciculations	No	Present
Babinski sign	Positive	No
Other reflexes	Abdominal and cremasteric lost	—
Voluntary movement	Decreased speed	Lost
Area of body involved	Large area	Small area

- ***Carpopedal Spasm:*** Spasm of hand or foot seen in tetany
- Painful, involuntary muscle contraction (spasm) in hands and feet
- Causes:
  - Hypocalcemia
  - Hypomagnesemia
  - Parkinsons disease
  - Huntingtons disease
  - Multiple sclerosis
  - Thyroid dysfunction
  - Drugs–estrogen, loop diuretics, anti-biotics, bisphosphonates, anti-epileptic drugs

Hypocalcemia: Presentation
- **Acute** – syncope, CHF, angina
- **Neuromuscular symptoms:**
  - Numbness and tingling sensation—peri-oral area, fingers, toes
  - Muscle cramps—back and lower extremities
  - Bronchospasm—wheezing
  - Laryngospasm—voice change
  - Dysphagia

- **Neurological symptoms:**
  - Irritability, depression, personality changes
  - Fatigues, seizures, uncontrolled movements
- **Dermatological manifestation:**
  - Course hair, brittle nails, psoriasis, dry skin, chronic pruritis, poor dentition, cataract

Internal Capsule

Fibres

Part	Descending tracts	Ascending tracts
1. Anterior limb	Frontopontine fibres (a part of the corticoponto-cerebellar pathway)	Anterior thalamic radiation (fibres from anterior and medial nuclei of thalamus)
2. Genu	Corticonuclear fibres (a part of the pyramidal tract going to motor nuclei of cranial nerves and forming their supranuclear pathway)	Anterior part of the superior thalamic radiation (fibres from posterior ventral nucleus of thalamus)
3. Posterior limb	• Corticospinal tract (pyramidal tract for the upper limb, trunk and lower limb) • Corticopontine fibres • Corticorubral fibres	1. Superior thalamic radiation 2. Fibres from globus pallidus to subthalamic nucleus
4. Retrolentiform part	• Parietopontine and occipitopontine fibres • Fibres from occipital cortex to superior colliculus and pretectal region	Posterior thalamic radiation made up of: • Mainly by optic radiation • Partly by fibres connecting the parietal and occipital lobes to the thalamus (posterior part)
5. Sublentiform part	• Parietopontine and temporopontine fibres • Interconnections between temporal lobe and thalamus	Auditory radiation

Locked in Syndrome

- Condition in which patient is aware but cannot move or communicate verbally due to complete paralysis of nearly all voluntary muscles (Quadriplegia and paralysis of cranial nerves) in the body except those responsible for vertical eye movements
- Vertical movements are intact as they are under the control of interstitial nucleus of cajal and MLF situated in tegmentum of midbrain—usually spared in locked in syndrome
- **Site of lesion:**
  - Lateral 2/3rd of cerebral peduncle laterally
  - Ventral aspect of medulla and basis pontis bilaterally sparing tegmentum
- **Etiology:**
  - Lacunar infarcts
  - Demyelination (central pontine myelinosis)
  - Hemorrhage
  - Trauma
  - Tumours
- *Features*
  - Patient is conscious awake and alert (ARAS intact) and blinking movements of eyes preserved hence communication– telegraphic method
- *Pseudo locked in states*
  - GBS
  - Acute polyneuritis
  - Myasthenia gravis
  - Poliomyelitis
- *Ramsay Hunt syndrome*
  - Pain and vesicles – external auditory canal
  - Loss of taste sensation – anterior 2/3rd of tongue
  - Ipsilateral facial palsy
- *Etiology*
  - Herpes zoster of geniculate ganglion – sensory branch of facial nerve involved
  - Often 8th cranial nerve is also affected

- *Arsenic neuropathy*
  - Arsenic is a heavy metal that causes a toxic sensory polyneuropathy
  - Manifests 5-10 days after ingestion of arsenic – progresses for several weeks; mimics GBS
- *Symptoms and signs*
  - Abrupt onset of abdominal discomfort, nausea, vomiting, pain and diarrhea
  - Burning pain in feet and hands
  - Skin changes
    - Loss of superficial epidermal layer – patchy regions of increased or decreased pigmentation after acute/chronic ingestion
    - Mees lines: not specific for arsenic toxicity; can also occur in thallium poisoning
    - Transverse lines at the base of finger nails and toe nails; evident only after 1–2 months of ingestion
  - Arsenic is rapidly cleared from blood; arsenic levels are raised in urine, hair and fingernails of those exposed – useful in diagnosing
  - Anemia with stippling of erythrocytes, pancytopenia, aplastic anemia

Hypertensive ICH

- *MC locations of hypertensive ICH*
  - Basal ganglia (putamen and caudate)
  - Thalamus
  - Pons
  - Cerebellum
- *Signs and symptoms depend on location affected*
  - Putamen—MC site for hypertensive ICH (35%)
  - Headache nausea vomiting
  - Contralateral hemiparesis and hemi-sensory loss
  - Dysarthria
  - Eyes deviate towards side of lesion
  - Depending on size of lesion—depressed level of consciousness/brainstem signs/death
- *Neurocsyticercosis*
  - MC parasitic disease of the CNS
- *Source and transmitter of infection*
  - Ingestion of food contaminated with the eggs of T. solium—undercooked pork/drinking water or food contaminated by human feces. Perpetuation is due to poor hygiene/sanitation
  - T. gondii—ingestion of undercooked meat/handling cat feces

Clinical Manifestation

- There is a variable time difference between point of infection and onset of symptoms
- Varies based on location and number of cysticerci and associated inflammatory response
  - *Neurological manifestations*—MC; seizures (generalized/focal/jacksonian) associated with inflammation surrounding cysticerci in parenchyma
  - *Hydrocephalus*—CSF outflow obstruction due to arachnoiditis or cysticerci
  - *Signs of increased ICP*—headache, nausea, vomiting, changes in vision, dizziness, ataxia, confusion

Pathology

- *Escobars pathological changes*
  - *Vesicular:* Viable parasite with intact membrane – no host reaction
  - *Colloidal vesicular:* Parasite dies within 4-5 years – cyst fluid becomes turbid – membrane becomes leaky – edema surrounds the cyst – most symptomatic stage
  - *Granular nodular:* Edema decreases as the cyst retracts further – enhancement persists
  - *Nodular calcifies:* End stage calcified quiescent cyst remnant; no edema
- *Location:*
  - Subarachnoid space – cysts can be very large (up to 9 cm)
  - MC located brain parenchyma – small cysts (1 cm)
  - 2nd MC – grey and white matter junction basal cisterns – grape like race mose
- *SIADH:* (Syndrome of inappropriate antidiuretic hormone secretion)

- Inappropriate, continued secretion or action of ADH results in hyponatremia or hypoosmolality despite normal or increased plasma volume resulting in impaired water excretion.
- **Features**
    - Hyponatremia (dilutional hyponatremia with Na <135 mmol/L)
    - Decreased plasma osmolality (<280 mOsm/kg)with inappropriately increased urine osmolality > 150 mOsm)
    - Urine sodium > 20 mEq/L
    - Low blood urea nitrogen (high BUN suggests a volume contracted state and excludes a diagnosis of SIADH)
    - Hypouricemia (< 4 mg/dL)
    - Absence of cardiac, liver, renal disease/ normal thyroid and adrenal function

Sheehan's Syndrome

- HYPOPITUITARISM results from destructive processes that involve the adenohypophysis (anterior or pituitary)
    - These processes may be acute (sudden) or chronic. Sheehan's syndrome, also known as postpartum pituitary necrosis results from the sudden infarction of the anterior lobe of the pituitary This can occur with obstetric complications such as hemorrhage or shock
- Pituitary gland normally doubles in size during pregnancy, hypovolemia during delivery decreases blood flow and may result in infarction of the anterior pituitary. Sheehan's syndrome produces symptoms of hypopituitarism. The initial sign is cessation of lactation, which may be followed by secondary amenorrhoea due to loss of gonadotropins.
- Other signs of hypopituitarism include hypothyroidism and decreased functioning of the adrenal gland. Acute destruction of the pituitary is also associated with DIC and thrombosis of the cavernous sinus
- Chronic causes of hypopituitarism include nonsecretory chromophobe pituitary adenomas adenomas, empty sella syndrome and suprasellar hypothalamic tumours
- Nonsecretory chromophobe adenomas present as space-occupying lesions that cause decreased hormone production.
- Gonadotropins are lost first, which results in signs of hypogonadism
    - Types of chromophobe adenomas Include null cell adenomas (no cytoplasmic granules), chromophobes (sparse granules) and oncocytic adenomas (increased cytoplasmic mitochondria). The term pituitary apoplexy refers to spontaneous hemorrhage into a pituitary tumor, while the empty sella syndrome is caused by a defective diaphragm sellae, which permits CSF from the third ventricle to enter the sella
- It may also be secondary to Infarction or necrosis. A CT scan reveals the sella to be enlarged or to appear empty

Opisthotonus Posture

- Opisthotonus is a state of extreme hyperextension and spasticity of the head, neck and spinal column
- It is most often caused by tetanus but may also result from Strychnine poisoning(in the presence of risus sardonicus), Spinal meningitis, as a side effect of treatment with neuroleptics or as a hysterical manifestation. In jaundiced neonates it may be a manifestation of kernicterus
- Is seen in some cases of severe cerebral palsy and traumatic brain injury or as a result of severe muscular spasms associated with tetanus. It can be a feature of severe acute hydrocephalus. It can also be seen in lithium intoxication
- Hyperextension occurs due to facilitation of the anterior reticulospinal tract caused by the inactivation of inhibitory cortico reticular fibres which normally act upon the pons reticular formation
- Opisthotonus in the neonate may be a sign of tetanus, meningitis, severe kernicterus or maple syrup urine disease
- Marked extensor tone can cause infants to rear backwards and stiffen out as the mother or nurse attempts to feed them; A similar tonic posturing may be seen in Sandifer syndrome. It can be induced by any attempt at movement such as smiling, feeding, vocalization. Individuals with opisthotonus are quite challenging to position, especially in wheelchairs and car seats
- It is also described as a potential CNS symptom of heat stroke along with bizarre behavior, hallucinations, decerebrate rigidity, oculogyric crisis and cerebellar dysfunction.
- It is seen with drowning victims—called the "Opisthotonic Death Pose"

Syphilitic Meningitis

- **General:** Peak incidence 1-2 years after infection; often with cranial nerve involvement (most common in CN VI, VIII followed by II, III, IV and then V)
- This is the least common neurosyphilitic manifestation.

Meningovascular Syphilis

- **General:** Peak incidence 5-7 years after infection; usually presents as focal neurologic deficits secondary to comprised cerebral circulation

- Can be seen in about 10% of cases diagnosed with CNS involvement
- *Gross:* Diffuse or localized to the base of the brain
- Hydrocephalus secondary to meningeal fibrosis is frequent.
- *Histology:* Perivascular lymphoplasmocytic infiltration around small blood vessels in the thickened meninges (periarthritis)
- Involvement of cranial nerves (particularly CN II and causes optic nerve atrophy) and spinal nerves are common.
- *Heubner's arteritis:* Inflammation of arteries within the circle of Willis secondary to chronic basal meningitis from tubercle bacillusor a fungus such as Cryplococcus, Histop/asma, or Coccidioides
- Heubner's arteritis consists of crescentic endarteritis obliterans and corresponding thining of the media.
- The elastic lamina remains intact.
- Vasa vasorum are cuffed by lymphoplasmocytic cells
- *Posterior spinal cord syndrome:*
  - Lesions of posterior column—loss of vibration and position sense below level of lesion
  - Larger lesions—encroachment on the lateral corticospinal tracts causing UMN type weakness
  - MC cause—Diabetes mellitus, neurosyphilis
  - Other causes—trauma, MS, extrinsic compression from posteriorly located tumours
- *Anterior spinal cord syndrome:*
  - Infarction of the cord is the result of occlusion or diminished flow in the artery resulting in extensive B/L tissue destruction sparing the posterior columns
  - All spinal cord functions are lost below the level of lesion only retaining vibration and position sensation
  - In anterior cord syndrome results in damage to anterolateral pathways causing loss of pain and temperature sensations below level of lesion as well as damage to anterior horn cells producing LMN type of weakness at the level of lesion; with larger lesions, the corticospinal tract may also be involved causing UMN signs. Incontinence is common because descending pathways controlling sphincter function tend to be ventrally located. Causes: trauma, MS and anterior spinal artery infarct

Limbic Encephalitis

- Tumours which can result in limbic encephalitis:
- Small cell carcinoma of the lung, testicular germ cell tumour, thymic tumours, breast cancer, ovarian carcinoma, hematologic malignancies, gastrointestinal malignancies
- *Clinical presentation:* is variable; but typically causes short term memory loss and mental status changes. Seizures and psychosis have also been reported

Radiographic Features

- *MRI:* High T2 signal without enhancement. Appearance is similar to herpes simplex encephalitis and changes are most evident in the mesial temporal lobes. Bilateral involvement is most common (60%)
- *PET scan:* Increased FDG uptake

DD

- Herpes simplex encephalitis – acute time course, fever
- Status epilepticus, low grade astrocytoma, gliomatosis cerebri

Intracranial Calcifications

- Physiologic
- Posttraumatic and dystrophic
- Subdural/epidural hematoma
- Radiation/chemotherapy
- Ischemia/infarct

Congenital Disorders (phakomatoses)

- Neurofibromatosis I and II
- Tuberous sclerosis
- Basal cell nevus syndrome
- Sturge-Weber syndrome

Vascular Disorders
- *Vascular malformations:* AVM/AVF, cavernous angioma, venous angioma, and capillary telangiectasia
- Aneurysm
- Intracranial atherosclerosis
- Ischemia/infarct
- Vein of Galen malformation

Infections
- *Congenital:* CMV toxoplasmosis, HIV, herpes
- *Acquired:* Cysticercosis, tuberculosis, HIV, cryptococcosis

Inflammatory Disorders
- Sarcoidosis
- Systemic lupus erythematosus
- Tumors
- *Intra-axial:* Astrocytomas, oligodendroglioma, medulloblastoma, ganglioglioma, DNET, metastases
- *Extra-axial:* Meningioma, pineal tumors, pituitary tumors, craniopharyngioma, epidermoid/dermoid teratoma, colloid cyst, lipoma, metastases
- *Intraventricular:* Ependymoma, choroid plexus tumors, central neurocytoma, metastases

Metabolic
- Hyperparathyroidism
- Hypoparathyroidism
- Hypothyroidism
- Fahr disease
- MELAS syndrome

Intracranial calcifications are common in certain locations and often do not lead to any clinical concern. These could be grouped in
- *Normal intracranial calcifications:* For all age-related physiologic and neurodegenerative calcification
- Intracranial arteries atherosclerosis.
- *Distal ICA:* Especially in the cavernous sinus; intradural vertebral arteries; basilar artery
- Concerning calcification is much less common and occurs in a variety of settings such as:
  - *Infection:* Neurocysticercosis; Cerebral toxoplasmosis; TORCH infection
  - *Metabolic:* Hypoparathyroidism; Pseudohypoparathyroidism; Fahr disease
  - *Previous cerebral insult:* Healed cerebral abscess; Healed infarct; Healed hematoma
  - *Vascular malformation*: Cerebral AVM; Sturge-Weber syndrome; von Hippel-Lindau syndrome
  - *Radiation:* Mineralising microangiopathy

Dyspraxia
- Partial loss of ability to coordinate and perform skilled purposeful movements
- In dyspraxia, gross and fine motor skills may be affected along with motor planning and organization, speech and language and activities of daily living
- It often coexists with ADHD< aspergers syndrome, PDD, dyslexia

Frontal Gait Disorder
- Shuffling freezing gait with imbalance and other signs of cerebellar dysfunction
- Difficulty in gait initiation – slipping clutch syndrome
- Strength is usually preserved
- MC cause – vascular disease, subcortical small vessel disease
- Lesions MC seen in deep frontal white matter and foramen ovale.

Multiple Choice Questions

1. A female aged 30, presents with episodic throbbing headache for past 4 years. It usually involves one half of the face and is associated with nausea and vomiting. There is no aura. Most likely diagnosis is:
   a. Classic migraine
   b. Common migraine
   c. Acephalgic migraine
   d. Brainstem migraine

2. Which of the following is most common cause of secondary headache?
   a. Systemic infection
   b. Vascular disorders
   c. Subarachnoid hemorrhage
   d. Brain tumor

3. Migraine activators include all *except:*
   a. Excess of sleep
   b. Hunger
   c. Pregnancy
   d. Lack of sleep

4. Which of the following is least prominent, in acephalgic migraine?
   a. Nausea
   b. Vomiting
   c. Headache
   d. Vertigo

5. Which of the following is true regarding Tension type Headache?
   a. It may be associated with nausea, vomiting
   b. Amitriptyline is the only approved drug for episodic tension type headache
   c. Tension is not an etiology
   d. It is called as chronic when it occurs on daily or near daily basis

6. Which of the following is false regarding trigeminal autonomic cephalgias?
   a. It consist of Hemicrania continua, cluster headache paroxysmal hemicrania
   b. It is associated with pituitary tumors
   c. Not associated with photophobia, phonophobia
   d. It includes SUNCT and SUNA

7. Which of the following is false about cluster headache?
   a. Central pacemaker neurons in the hypothalamus are involved in pathology
   b. Associated with bilateral photophobia and phonophobia
   c. Periodicity is core feature, at least one of the daily attacks of pain recurs at about the same hour each day
   d. Associated with ipsilateral symptoms of cranial parasympathetic autonomic activation.

8. Which of the following is TRUE regarding Kernohan-Woltman syndrome?
   a. Contralateral pupillary dilatation
   b. Waxing and waning of levels of consciousness
   c. Compression of posterior cerebral artery
   d. Ipsilateral pupil constriction

9. Ocular bobbing is diagnostic of:
   a. Bilateral occipital infarct
   b. Bilateral pontine damage
   c. Bilateral temporal lobe infarct
   d. Cerebellar damage

10. All of the following are true regarding "FEBRILE SEIZURES" *except:*
    a. Febrile seizures is likely to occur during peak of the temperature
    b. Febrile seizures have peak incidence between 18 and 24 months
    c. Most common seizures arising in late infancy and early childhood are febrile seizures
    d. Febrile seizures are seizures associated with fevers but without evidence of CNS infection or other defined cause

11. Characteristics of complex febrile seizures are all *except:*
    a. Repeated seizure activity
    b. Symmetric in appearance
    c. Duration more than 15 mins
    d. Features of focal seizures

Answers

| 1. b | 2. a | 3. c | 4. c | 5. c | 6. c | 7. b |
| 8. c | 9. b | 10. a | 11. b | | | |

12. All of the following are characteristics of MESIAL TEMPORAL LOBE EPILEPSY except:
    a. Usually family history of epilepsy is absent
    b. Aura is common
    c. MRI shows enlarged temporal horn
    d. MRI shows hippocampal sclerosis

13. All of the following are risk factors associated with recurrent seizures except:
    a. Seizures presenting as a status epilepticus
    b. Seizures associated with postictal confusion
    c. Seizures associated with Postictal Todd's paralysis
    d. Strong family history of seizures

14. A 24-year-old married female is a known case of focal seizure with dyscognitive features. She is taking carbamazepine regularly and her seizures are well controlled. Now she comes to OPD with positive HCG urine test. What will be your treatment plan?
    a. Change the drug carbamazepine with safest drug in pregnancy Lamotrigine
    b. Add lamotrigine and gradually taper carbamazepine
    c. Continue only CBZ and treat the mother with oral vitamin k in last 2 weeks and infant with intramuscular vitamin K at birth
    d. Add lamotrigine, continue CBZ and lamotrigine combination in lowest dose for first trimester then taper CBZ

15. A 22-year-old male who is a known case of GTCS and taking lamotrigine regularly is having Generalized Convulsive Status Epilepticus since 45 minutes. Initially injection lorazepam 0.1 mg/kg followed by injection phenytoin was given: Still seizures are uncontrolled. What should be next plan of treatment?
    a. Inj Midazolam 0.2 mg/kg
    b. Inj phenobarbital
    c. Inj Ketamine
    d. Inj Propofol 2 mg/kg followed by 2–10 mg/kg/hr

16. Initial bursting activity (Paroxysmal depolarization shift) in seizure is caused by:
    a. Influx of extracellular calcium channels
    b. Opening of voltage dependent sodium channels
    c. Closure of potassium channels
    d. Closure of GABA mediated chloride channels

17. Antiepileptic drug that acts by inhibiting voltage gated calcium channels is:
    a. Phenytoin
    b. Lamotrigine
    c. Levetericetam
    d. Topiramate

18. Which of the following sentence is false about EEG:
    a. The presence of electrographic seizure activity during the clinically evident event clearly establishes the diagnosis
    b. EEG cannot be used for assessing prognosis of seizure disorder
    c. The absence of electrographic seizure activity does not exclude a seizure disorder
    d. The EEG is always abnormal during generalized tonic-clonic seizures

19. Reflex epilepsy best relates to:
    a. Sleep deprivation
    b. An individual's voice
    c. Alcohol
    d. Physical exertion

20. A child presents with short episodes of vacant stare several times a day. The vacant episode begins abruptly and the child remains unresponsive during the episode. These episodes were not followed by postictal confusion. The drug of choice for this patient is:
    a. Lamotrigine
    b. Valproate
    c. Ethosuximide
    d. Carbamazepine

21. A 5-year-old boy has the onset of episodes of loss of body tone, with associated falls as well as generalized tonic-conic seizures. His cognitive function has been deteriorating. EEG shows 1.5 to 2 HZ spike and wave discharge. All of the following the antiepileptic drugs are effective in this case except:
    a. Carbamazepine
    b. Clobazam
    c. Felbamate
    d. Rufinamide

22. A 30-year-old female brought by her relative with chief complaints of abnormal jerky movements of body associated with decreased response, bladder incontinence, uprolling of eyeballs and frothing at mouth. You observe her head turning vigorously side to side with large-amplitude limb shaking a upward thrusting of the pelvis. Which of the following sentence is correct regarding blood investigation of this patient?
    a. A normal creatine kinase level within 30 minutes of the episode
    b. A normal prolactin level within 30 minutes of the episode
    c. An elevated creatine kinase within 30 minutes of the episode
    d. An elevated prolactin level within 30 minutes of the episode

Answers

12. a	13. b	14. c	15. d	16. a	17. a	18. b
19. b	20. c	21. a	22. b			

23. A 38-year-old man with a history of seizure disorder presents with generalized convulsive status epilepticus. He had been having persistent seizure activity for 20 minutes when emergency medical services were activated. He was given lorazepam 8 mg intravenously (IV). His initial temperature is 39.2°C with blood pressure of 182/92 mm Hg, heart rate of 158 bpm, respiratory rate of 38 breaths/min.
What is the next step in the management of this patient?
   a. Isoflurane anesthesia
   b. Fosphenytoin 20 mg/kg IV
   c. Pentobarbital 5 mg/kg bolus followed by an infusion at 1 mg/kg/hr
   d. Propofol 2 mg/kg bolus followed by an infusion at 2 mg/kg/hr

24. A 26-year-old woman has throbbing right-sided headaches that are centered around her right eye. They are worse with movement and aggravated by loud noises. There are no premonitory warnings. Triggers for the headaches include lack of sleep, stress, and red wine. A mild attack can be treated by ibuprofen, but nonsteroidal anti-matory drugs have no effect on more severe pain. which of the following best characterizes about the pathogenesis of the patient's headache syndrome?
   a. Diffuse muscular contraction of the neck and scalp
   b. Disinhibition of the central pacemaker neurons in the posterior hypothalamic region
   c. Dysfunction of monoaminergic sensory control systems in brainstem and hypothalamus
   d. Focal cerebral vasodilation in the region of the brain that is the focus of the pain

25. A 32-year-old man presents to the emergency department with progressive lower extremity weakness that has been present for the past month. It has now progressed to the point that he is unable to bear weight. He also has been experiencing loss of sensation and aching pains in his mid-back and a sensation of incomplete voiding with mild urinary incontinence. Today, he also had incontinence of stool.
Physical examination confirms lower extremity paresis with strength of only 3/5 and decreased deep tendon reflexes. Sensation to light tough and pinprick is absent in the lower extremities. He develops sensory perception at the umbilicus. An MRI shows multilevel enhancement of the spinal cord consistent with edema. It has predominance in the mid- thoracic spinal cord. Gadolinium administration shows enhancement in a nodular fashion of the surface of the cord. Lumbar puncture is performed. There are 32 white blood cells (WBC)/L (90% lymphocytes). The cerebrospinal fluid protein level is 75 mg/dL. The glucose level is normal. A chest radiograph demonstrates enlargement of the hilar lymph nodes without pulmonary infiltrates. On chest CT, bilateral hilar, subcarinal, and precarinal lymphadenopathy is observed with the largest lymph node measuring 2 × 1.8 cm. Serum calcium is 12.5 mg/dL. A biopsy of the hilar lymph nodes is planned. What is the most likely finding on biopsy?
   a. Abundant atypical lymphocytes that demonstrate clonality on flow cytometry
   b. Caseating granulomatous inflammation
   c. Noncaseating granulomatous inflammation
   d. Nonspecific chronic inflammatory changes

26. You are evaluating a 50-year-old diabetic woman for complaints of tingling, burning in her lower extremities. All of the following questions are important for the history and physical examination *except:*
   a. What is the nature of sensory involvement?
   b. What is the temporal evolution?
   c. What does the electromyogram and nerve conduction study demonstrate?
   d. What is the distribution of the weakness?

27. All of the following are true about Charcot-Marie-Tooth (CMT) disease *except:*
   a. CMT is the most common type of hereditary neuropathy
   b. Autosomal dominant
   c. Nerve biopsy is required for diagnosis
   d. It presents with distal leg weakness (Foot drop)

28. A 19-year-old hypertensive male presented with burning pain in hands and feet. On examination there are reddish- purple maculopapular lesions (size 1–3 mm) present around the umbilicus, scrotum and inguinal region. What is the probable diagnosis?
   a. Fabry disease   b. Adrenoleukodystrophy
   c. Refsum disease   d. Tangier disease

29. A 26-year-old male, known case of rheumatic heart disease with atrial fibrillation presents with acute onset weakness of side of body (both upper and lower limb) which recovered in 20 hours. CT scan brain showed ischemic changes in right internal capsule. The most likely diagnosis is:
   a. Embolic stroke
   b. Thrombotic stroke
   c. Transient ischemic attack
   d. Hemorrhagic stroke

Answers

23. b   24. c   25. c   26. c   27. c   28. a   29. a

30. When cerebral blood flow falls to <16 to 18 min/100 gm per min, how long it will take for brain infarction?
    a. 1 hour
    b. 2 hours
    c. 4 to 10 mins
    d. 1 min

31. A woman has moderate bilateral headache that worsens with emotional stress. She has two children, both doing badly in school. Headache attack is throbbing and associated with vomiting which lasts for 4 to 5 hours. Diagnosis is:
    a. Migraine
    b. Cluster headache
    c. Tension headache
    d. Trigeminal neuralgia

32. Patient is having impaired comprehension and naming but normal repetition and fluency. What is the probable diagnosis?
    a. Anterior transcortical aphasia
    b. Posterior transcortical aphasia
    c. Isolation aphasia
    d. Broca's aphasia

33. A 40-year-old female is brought to emergency room after being unresponsive following a sudden bout of severe headache at work. On examination her BP is 180/110 and her respiration is irregular and of cheyne stokes type. She is agitated and doesn't follow commands, but moves her extremities spontaneously most likely diagnosis is:
    a. SAH
    b. ICH
    c. SDH
    d. TIA

34. Vogt-Koyanagi-Harada syndrome refers to?
    a. Drug induced hypersensitivity meningitis
    b. Carcinomatous meningitis
    c. Meningitis associated with sarcoid
    d. Uveomeningitic syndrome

35. A 50-year-old male known case of type 2 Diabetes, now with fever headache decreased level of consciousness. On examination neck stiffness is positive. CT scan brain is normal. Routine investigations of blood are Hb-12, sugar-133, AST-25, ALT-20, CSF analysis showing WBC-1200, protein-100, Sugar 40. What is probable diagnosis?
    a. Viral meningitis
    b. Bacterial meningitis
    c. Fungal meningitis
    d. Tuberculosis meningitis

36. In CSF analysis, lymhocyticpelocytosis with low glucose concentration should suggest which of the following:
    a. Tuberculous meningitis
    b. Fungal meningitis
    c. Listerial meningitis
    d. All of the above

37. Regarding Kennedy's disease which of the following is false:
    a. X-linked spinomuscular atrophy
    b. LMN disorder
    c. Expanded CTG repeats
    d. Gynaecomastia and reduced fertility

38. Which of the following is associated with anticipation?
    a. DRPLA
    b. BMD
    c. DMD
    d. None

39. A 36-year-old male coming with severe suboccipital pain radiating to neck, shoulder which increases on sneezing, coughing, straining. Patient also complaints of weakness of right upper limb which was gradually progressed to right lower limb then left lower limb then left upper limb. What is probable diagnosis?
    a. Intramedullary compressive myelopathy at foramen magnum
    b. Extramedullary intradural compressive myelopathy at foramen magnum
    c. Extramedullary extradural compressive myelopathy at foramen magnum
    d. Noncompressive myelopathy

40. A 45-year-old male presents with recurrent falls. MRI brain shows atrophy of mid-brain what is probable diagnosis?
    a. Multiple system atrophy
    b. Progressive supranuclear palsy
    c. Lewy body dementia
    d. Shy dragger syndrome

41. Anterior choroidal artery is a branch of:
    a. ICA distal to posterior communicating artery
    b. ICA proximal to posterior communicating artery
    c. PCA distal to posterior communicating artery
    d. PCA proxima to posterior communicating artery

42. A 5-year-old boy has the onset of episodes of loss of body tone, with associated falls as well as generalized tonic-conic seizures. His cognitive function has been deteriorating. EEG shows 1.5 to 2 HZ spike and ware discharge. The most likely diagnosis is:
    a. Juvenile myoclonic epilepsy
    b. Lennox-Gastaust syndrome
    c. Mesial temporal lobe epilepsy
    d. Unclassified seizure

Answers

| 30. a | 31. a | 32. b | 33. a | 34. d | 35. b | 36. d |
| 37. c | 38. a | 39. c | 40. b | 41. a | 42. b | |

43. About 3 weeks after diarrhea, 18-year-old boy complains of weakness of his lower limbs. Over several days, weakness progress to include his upper limbs also. On physical examination he has weakness in all 4 limbs, absent reflexes CSF examination showed increase in protein only most likely diagnosis is:
    a. ATM
    b. GBS
    c. Bell's palsy
    d. NMO

44. A 46-year-old patient complaining of severe bursting headache on examination he was found to be conscious but restless neck stiffness and drooping of right eyelid were observed. Clinical diagnosis is:
    a. Cerebral embolism
    b. Posterior communicating artery aneurysm with SAH
    c. Anterior communicating artery aneurysm with SAH
    d. Cavernous sinus thrombosis

45. Which of the following feature differentiate ADEM from MS:
    a. CSF Oligoclonal banding
    b. Optic nerve involvement
    c. Abnormal MRI
    d. Polysymptomatic

46. Distinguishing point for acute transverse myelitis in shock stage from GBS is:
    a. Decreased DTR
    b. Decreased superficial reflexes
    c. Hypotonia
    d. Exact level of sensory loss

47. Triad of normal pressure hydrocephalus includes:
    a. Tremors, aphasia, dementia
    b. Ataxia, aphasia, gait disorder
    c. Ataxia, urinary incontinence, dementia
    d. Ataxia, urinary incontinence, dysarthria

48. Which of the following is not K+ ion channelopathy?
    a. Episodic ataxia type 1
    b. EA-2
    c. Benign neonatal familial convulsion
    d. Jervell Lange-Nielsen syndrome

49. Which of the following clinical feature is least common in friedreich ataxia:
    a. Cardiomyopathy
    b. DM
    c. Scoliosis
    d. Mental retardation

50. In progressive multifocal leucoencephalopathy, which of the following is not involved?
    a. Frontal cortex
    b. Cerebellum
    c. Mid-brain
    d. Spinal cord

51. All of the following are Non-motor features of Parkinson's disease, *except*:
    a. Sleep disturbances
    b. Cognitive impairment
    c. Loss of taste
    d. Loss of smell

52. A 60-year-old male patient having miosis, ptosis, anhydrosis on left side and difficulty in walking. Patient also gives complaints of dysphagia, dysarthria. On examination, you found that pain and temperature lost on right side of the body and left side of face. What is probable diagnosis?
    a. Left medial medullary syndrome
    b. Left lateral medullary syndrome
    c. Right lateral medullary syndrome
    d. Right medial medullary syndrome

53. A 24-year-old male awakens with bilateral lower limb weakness and numbness, urinary retention, blurring of vision. On examination, you found that all modalities of sensations are lost up to the level nipple. MRI brain is normal. CSF analysis showed pleocytosis. What is likely diagnosis?
    a. Multiple sclerosis
    b. Neuromyelitis optica
    c. Acute disseminated encephalomyelitis
    d. GBS

54. Factors linked to reduced incidence of Parkinson's disease include all *except*:
    a. Coffee drinking
    b. Smoking
    c. NSAIDS use
    d. Alcohol use

55. All of the following are true about Multiple System Atrophy (MSA) *except*:
    a. It manifests as a combination of Parkinsonian, cerebellar and autonomic features
    b. Degeneration of the substantia nigra pars compacta, striatum cerebellum and inferior olivary nuclei
    c. Accumulation of ubiquitin in neurons
    d. Pontine HOT CROSS BUNS SIGN is characteristic MRI feature

56. All of the following are true about Gradenigo's syndrome *except*:
    a. It is due to cavernous sinus thrombosis
    b. Associated with otitis media
    c. 6th nerve palsy
    d. Facial pain present

57. Most common symptom of brain abscess is:
    a. Headache
    b. Fever
    c. Seizure
    d. Focal neurologic deficit

Answers

43. b	44. b	45. d	46. d	47. c	48. b	49. d
50. d	51. c	52. b	53. b	54. d	55. c	56. a
57. a						

58. Which of the following drug is used in treatment of SSPE?
    a. Acyclovir
    b. Mirtazapine
    c. Isoprinosine
    d. Foscarnet

59. Oligoclonal bands are found in all except:
    a. Multiple sclerosis
    b. Syphilis
    c. Lyme borreliosis
    d. Neuromyelitis optica

60. Which of the following is a calcium channelopathy?
    a. Hypokalemic periodic paralysis
    b. Hyperkalemic periodic paralysis
    c. Paramyotonia congenita
    d. Andersen-Tawil syndrome

61. Werdnig-Hoffman disease is the name given to:
    a. SMA-1
    b. SMA-II
    c. SMA-III
    d. Kennedy's disease

62. All of the following are acute sporadic motor neuron diseases except:
    a. Polio
    b. Primary lateral sclerosis
    c. Herpes zoster
    d. Coxsackie virus

63. All of the following are included in diagnostic criteria of chronic fatigue syndrome:
    a. Fatigue last for at least 6 months
    b. Fatigue is of new or definite onset
    c. Fatigue is not the result of an organic disease or of continuing exertion
    d. Fatigue is alleviated by rest

64. A 20-year-old heroin addict has been using a street version of artificial heroin. Neurological syndrome for which he is at risk is clinically indistinguishable from which of the following:
    a. Huntington's disease
    b. Friedreich disease
    c. Sydenham's chorea
    d. Parkinson's disease

65. A 70-year-old male coming with left sided weakness of body which recovered completely within 18 hours. On examination blood pressure was 150/80. Patient is a known case of hypertension and diabetes. Which of the following is correct regarding this patient?
    a. ABCD2 score is 7 and risk of stroke is 22%
    b. ABCD2 score is 4 and risk of stroke is 8%
    c. ABCD2 score is 2 and risk of stroke is 3%
    d. ABCD2 score is 6 and risk of stroke is 17%

66. Abulia is due to obstruction of:
    a. M1 segment of MCA
    b. M2 segment of MCA
    c. A1 segment of ACA
    d. A2 segment of ACA

67. Cortical blindness, amnesia and thalamic pain are associated with occlusion of:
    a. Anterior cerebral artery
    b. Basilar artery
    c. Middle cerebral artery
    d. Posterior cerebral artery

68. Which of the following is contraindication for thrombolysis in a patient of ischemic stroke?
    a. BP >185/100
    b. Blood glucose <100
    c. CT scan showing edema<1/3" of MCA
    d. Platelet count < 1 lac

69. A 76-year-old male came with left sided weakness of body which recovered completely within 18 hours. On examination pulse was irregularly irregular and blood pressure was 150/80. Patient is a known case of hypertension and diabetes. 2DECHO is done which shows no evidence of rheumatic heart disease. Which of the following is true regarding management?
    a. Start aspirin only
    b. Start aspirin plus warfarin
    c. Start warfarin only
    d. Start aspirin plus clopidogrel

70. All of the following are risk factors associated with recurrent seizure except:
    a. Patient presenting as a status epilepticus
    b. Abnormal neurological examination
    c. Abnormal MRI brain
    d. Abnormal EEG

71. All of the following statements about treatment of migraine are true, except:
    a. Naratriptan has slower onset and longer t1/2 than sumatriptan
    b. Rizatriptan is more efficacious than sumatriptan
    c. Sumatriptan is a selective 5-HT 1B/1D agonist
    d. Sumatriptan is used for chronic migraine

72. A child presents with short episodes of vacant stare several times a day. The vacant episode begins abruptly and the child remains unresponsive during the episode followed by postictal confusion. There is no associated history of aura and the child is otherwise normal. The likely diagnosis is:
    a. Atypical absence seizures
    b. Typical absence seizures
    c. Focal seizure with dyscognitive features
    d. Day dreaming

Answers

58. c	59. d	60. a	61. a	62. b	63. d	64. d
65. a	66. d	67. d	68. d	69. c	70. c	71. d
72. c						

73. All of the following are features of juvenile myoclonic epilepsy, *except:*
    a. Myoclonus on awakening
    b. Generalized tonic-clonic seizures
    c. Automatism
    d. Consciousness is preserved

74. The drug of choice for absence seizure:
    a. Valproate
    b. Gabapentin
    c. Carbamezapine
    d. Phenytoin

75. All of the following drugs are used for managing status epilepticus *except:*
    a. Pregabalin
    b. Topiramate
    c. Thiopentone sodium
    d. Carbamazepine

76. Generalized tonic clonic status epilepticus, treatment of choice:
    a. Ethosuximide
    b. Sodium valproate
    c. Lamotrigine
    d. Lorazepam

77. A 15-year-old boy with epilepsy on treatment with combination of valproate and phenytoin has good control of seizures. Levels of both drugs are in the therapeutic range. All of the following adverse effects can be attributed to valproate *except:*
    a. Weight gain of 5 kg
    b. Serum alanine aminotransaminase 150 IU/L
    c. Rise in serum ammonia level by 20uE/du
    d. Lymphadenopathy

78. A 24-year-old man awakens with bilateral leg weakness and numbness, urinary retention. On enquiry he also gives history of blurring of vision. On examination, abdominal reflex absent in lower quadrant of abdomen, bicep and tricep reflexes are normally present bilaterally, knee and ankle reflex absent bilaterally. MRI brain and spinal cord is normal. What is the probable diagnosis?
    a. Multiple sclerosis
    b. Neuromyelitis optica
    c. Acute disseminated encephalomyelitis
    d. Central pontine myelinolysis

79. Which of the following is most common antecedent infection associated with Acute Disseminated Encephalomyelitis?
    a. Measles
    b. Varicella
    c. EBV
    d. Campylobacter jejuni

80. Which of the following sentence is correct regarding Neuromyelitis optica:
    a. Males are more commonly affected than females
    b. Symptoms are progressive in nature
    c. It is astrocytopathy
    d. Oligoclonal band is a common finding

81. All of the following sentences are correct regarding acute disseminated encephalomyelitis *except:*
    a. It is abrupt in onset and rapidly progressive in nature
    b. CSF shows lymphocytic pleocytosis
    c. Glucocorticoid is the treatment
    d. Optic nerve is generally spared

82. Mitoxantrone is indicated in all of the following conditions *except:*
    a. Acute neurologic change in relapsing remitting multiple sclerosis
    b. Secondary progressive MS
    c. Progressive relapsing MS
    d. Worsening relapsing remitting MS

83. All of the following sentences are correct regarding Marburg's variant *except:*
    a. It is clinical variant of multiple sclerosis
    b. It follows infection or vaccination
    c. It is acute in nature
    d. Progresses to death within 1 to 2 years

84. All of the following drugs are approved for relapsing remitting multiple sclerosis *except:*
    a. Mycophenolate mofetil
    b. Mitoxantrone
    c. Teriflunomide
    d. Alemtuzumab

85. A 22-year-old female patient presents with sudden onset blurring of vision, diminished visual acuity and periorbital pain which increases on movement. You are suspecting the diagnosis of multiple sclerosis first attack. Which of the following is required to prove the diagnosis of MS?
    a. Simultaneous presence of asymptomatic gadolinium enhancing and non-enhancing lesions at anytime
    b. More than 1 T2 lesion in at least 2 out of 4 MS-typical regions of the CNS AND simultaneous presence of asymptomatic gadolinium-enhancing and non enhancing lesions at anytime
    c. More than 1 T2 lesion on MRI in at least 2 out of 4 MS-typical regions of the CNS
    d. Positive CSF (isoelectric focusing evidence of oligoclonal bands)

86. All of the following are included in diagnostic criteria of primary progressive multiple sclerosis *except:*
    a. 1 year of disease progression
    b. Evidence for dissemination in space in the brain based on 1 T2+ lesions in the MS-characteristic periventricular juxtacortical or infratentorial regions
    c. Positive CSF (isoelectric focusing evidence of oligoclonal bands and/or elevated IgG index)
    d. Await a second clinical attack

Answers

| 73. c | 74. a | 75. d | 76. d | 77. d | 78. b | 79. a |
| 80. c | 81. d | 82. a | 83. b | 84. a | 85. b | 86. d |

87. Which of the following is false about one and half syndrome?
    a. Contralateral abductor palsy
    b. Ipsilateral abductor palsy
    c. Ipsilateral adductor palsy
    d. Lesion is in MLF and 6 h nerve nucleus

88. Uthoff's symptoms in multiple sclerosis like visual blurring:
    a. Increased redistribution of potassium channel along the naked axon
    b. Increased redistribution of sodium channel along the naked axon
    c. Increased redistribution of calcium channel along the naked axon
    d. Increased redistribution of chloride channel along the naked axon

89. Which of the following is false regarding inter nuclear ophthalmoplegia?
    a. Ipsilateral nystagmus
    b. Lesion is in MLR
    c. Ipsilateral adductor palsy
    d. Diplopia

90. A 64-year-old woman is evaluated for weakness. She has had several weeks of difficulty brushing her teeth, combing her hair, climbing steps. She has also noted a rash on her face. Examination is notable for erthyematous flat topped papules on interphalangeal joints. Serum creatinine kinase (CK) is elevated. What is the probable diagnosis?
    a. Polymyositis
    b. Dermatomyositis
    c. Inclusion body myositis D
    d. Myaesthenia Gravis

91. A 64-year-old woman is evaluated for weakness. She has had several weeks of difficulty brushing her teeth, combing her hair, climbing steps. She has also noted a rash on her face. Examination is notable for erthyematous flat topped papules on interphalangeal joints. Serum creatinine kinase (CK) is elevated. Initially treatment started with high dose prednisone but it was not effective. What will be your next step in management?
    a. Mycophenolate
    b. Intravenous immunoglobulin
    c. Rituximab
    d. Plasmapheresis

92. All of the following are true regarding inclusion body myositis (IBM) *except:*
    a. Males are more commonly affected than females
    b. Pharyngeal muscles are affected
    c. Muscle biopsy shows perifascicular inflammation
    d. IBM is resistant to immunosuppressive therapies

93. A 50-year-old male coming with fever, headache, decreased level of consciousness. On examination neck stiffness is positive. CT scan brain is normal. Routine investigations of blood are Hb-12, AST 25, ALT-20, CSF analysis showing WBC-1000 (NEUTROPHIL predominant), protein=100, Sugar-20. What is probable diagnosis?
    a. Viral meningitis
    b. Bacterial meningitis
    c. Fungal meningitis
    d. Tuberculoses meningitis

94. A 50-year-old male coming with fever, headache, decreased level of consciousness. On examination neck stiffness is positive. CT scan brain is normal. Routine investigations of blood are Hb-12, AST-25, ALT-20, CSF analysis showing WBC 75 (lymphocyte predominant), protein-150, Sugar-20. What is probable diagnosis?
    a. Viral meningitis
    b. Bacterial meningitis
    c. Fungal meningitis
    d. Tuberculous meningitis

95. A 50-year-old male coming with fever, headache, decreased level of consciousness. On examination neck stiffness is positive. CT scan brain is normal. Routine investigations of blood are Hb-12, AST-25, ALT-20, CSF analysis showing WBC-400 (lymphocyte predominant), protein 40, Sugar-60. What is probable diagnosis?
    a. Viral meningitis
    b. Bacterial meningitis
    c. Fungal meningitis
    d. Tuberculous meningitis

96. A 50-year-old male coming with fever, headache, decreased level of consciousness. On examination neck stiffness is positive. CT scan brain is normal. Routine investigations of blood are Hb-12, AST -25, ALT-20, CSF analysis showing WBC-550 (lymphocyte predominant), protein-200 mg/dl, Sugar 50 mg/dl. What is probable diagnosis?
    a. Viral meningitis
    b. Bacterial meningitis
    c. Fungal meningitis
    d. Tuberculous meningitis

97. A 50-year-old male, coming with fever, headache and decreased level of consciousness. On examination neck rigidity is present. CT scan brain is normal. What is your next step in the management?
    a. Intravenous ceftriaxone + vancomycin
    b. Intravenous ceftriaxone + vancomycin + ampicillin
    c. Intravenous dexamethasone
    d. Intravenous ampicillin + gentamycin

Answers

87. a	88. b	89. a	90. b	91. a	92. c	93. b
94. d	95. a	96. c	97. c			

98. A 50-year-old male, coming with fever, headache and decreased level of consciousness. On examination neck rigidity is present. CT scan brain is normal. Routine investigations of blood are Hb-12, AST-25, ALT-20, CSF analysis showing, WBC=1000 (NEUTROPHIL predominant), protein-100, Sugar-20. What is your next step in management?
    a. Intravenous ceftriaxone + vancomycin
    b. Intravenous ceftriaxone + vancomycin + ampicillin
    c. Intravenous ceftriaxone + ampicillin + gentamycin
    d. Intravenous ampicillin + gentamycin

99. A 60-year-old alcoholic male, coming with fever, headache and decreased level of consciousness. On examination neck rigidity is present. CT scan brain is normal. Routine investigations of blood are Hb-12, AST -25, ALT-20, CSF analysis showing WBC-1000 (NEUTROPHIL predominant) protein-100, Sugar-20. What is your next step in management?
    a. Intravenous ceftriaxone + vancomycin
    b. Intravenous ceftriaxone + vancomycin + ampicillin
    c. Intravenous ceftriaxone ampicillin + gentamycin
    d. Intravenous ampicillin + gentamycin

100. Classic triad of meningitis consists of all of the following except:
    a. Headache
    c. Irregular respiration
    b. Fever
    d. Neck stiffness

101. Cushing reflex in raised ICP relates to all of the following except:
    a. Bradycardia
    b. Hypertension
    c. Irregular respiration
    d. Hypotension

102. Diagnostic procedure of choice for viral meningitis caused by enterovirus is:
    a. PCR from CSF
    b. RTPCR from CSF
    c. IgM antibody from CSF
    d. Gene expert

103. Mollaret's meningitis is due to?
    a. HIV
    b. HSV
    c. EBV
    d. CMV

104. Which of the following is not seen in tubercular meningitis?
    a. Low sugar
    b. High protein
    c. Low opening pressure
    d. Lymphocytic pleocytosis

105. Acyclovir is used in all of the following viral meningitis except:
    a. HSV
    b. EBV
    c. VZV
    d. Enterovirus

106. All of the following are correct regarding Friedreich ataxia except:
    a. It is most common hereditary ataxia with autosomal recessive pattern
    b. Increased GAA repeats in chromosome 9
    c. First pathological change is seen in posterior column
    d. It is associated with optic atrophy

107. All of the following are categories of symptomatic neurosyphilis except:
    a. General paresis
    b. Meningoencephalitis
    c. Tabes dorsalis
    d. Meningovascular

108. Which of the following Motor neuron disease involves only upper motor neuron:
    a. Amyotrophic lateral sclerosis
    b. Primary lateral sclerosis
    c. Adult Tay-Sachs disease
    d. Kennedy's disease

109. All of the following are motor neuron diseases involving predominantly lower motor neuron except:
    a. Multifocal motor neuropathy with conduction block
    b. Adult Tay-Sachs disease
    c. Kennedy's disease
    d. Familial spastic paraplegia

110. Amyotrophic lateral sclerosis can be diagnosed by all of the following except:
    a. Wasting of muscle
    b. Exaggerated deep tendon reflexes
    c. Absent deep tendon reflexes
    d. Dementia

111. All of the following are never involved structures in MND except:
    a. Bladder
    b. Nuclei of cranial nerves
    c. Dementia
    d. Cognition

112. All of the following are true about Kennedy's disease except:
    a. It is X linked spinobulbar muscular atrophy
    b. Androgen insensitivity
    c. Expanded CTG repeats
    d. Lower motor neuron disorder

Answers

98. a	99. b	100. c	101. d	102. b	103. b	104. c
105. d	106. c	107. b	108. b	109. d	110. d	111. b
112. c						

113. Dorsal column may be involved in which of the following motor neuron disease:
    a. Primary lateral sclerosis
    b. Familial spastic paraplegia
    c. Amyotrophic lateral sclerosis
    d. Kugelberg-Welander disease

114. About 3 weeks after diarrhea, 18-year-old boy complains of weakness of his both lower limbs. Over several days, weakness progress to include his upper limbs also. On examination he has weakness in all 4 limbs, absent reflexes CSF examination showed increase in protein only most likely diagnosis is:
    a. Amyotrophic lateral sclerosis
    b. Guillain–Barré syndrome
    c. Bell's palsy
    d. Multiple sclerosis

115. Which of the following is not found in Miller Fisher syndrome?
    a. Ataxia
    b. Areflexia of limbs
    c. Weakness of limbs
    d. Ophthalmoplegia

116. Miller-Fisher syndrome (MFS) is strongly associated with which of the following antibodies?
    a. GQ1a
    b. GQ1b
    c. GQ1c
    d. GQ1d

117. Which of the following statements about Guillain-Barré syndrome (GBS) is false?
    a. Bladder involvement occurs in severe cases
    b. Anti GD1a antibodies are found in patients of acute Motor axonal neuropathy (AMAN) subtype of GBS
    c. Glucocorticoids are effective in GBS
    d. Facial diparesis found in 50% of cases

118. Lewis-Sumner syndrome is:
    a. Multifocal acquired demyelinating sensory and motor neuropathy
    b. Multifocal motor neuropathy
    c. Distal acquired demyelinating symmetric neuropathy
    d. Motor neuron disease

119. Treatment of choice for GBS:
    a. Intravenous immunoglobulin
    b. Intravenous methylprednisolone
    c. Intravenous cyclophosphamide
    d. Rituximab

120. Intravenous immune globulin has been established to be efficacious in all of the following except:?
    a. Corticosteroid-resistant dermatomyositis
    b. Kawasaki's syndrome
    c. Guillain–Barré syndrome
    d. Inclusion body myositis

121. Kearns-Sayre syndrome consists of all of the following except:
    a. CSF protein less than 100 mg/dL
    b. Onset before age 20 years
    c. Chronic progressive external ophthalmoplegia
    d. Pigmentary retinopathy

122. In progressive multifocal leukoencephalopathy, which of the following is not involved?
    a. Frontal cortex
    b. Cerebellum
    c. Midbrain
    d. Spinal cord

123. Which of the following is false about progressive multifocal leukoencephalopathy?
    a. Occurs in Natalizumab treated multiple sclerosis patients
    b. It is due to JC virus infection
    c. Isoprinosine prolongs the survival
    d. Homonymous hemianopia is most common clinical feature

124. Which of the following is not a manifestation of subacute sclerosing panencephalitis?
    a. Fever
    b. Poor school performance
    c. Focal or generalized or myoclonic seizures
    d. Visual disturbance

125. Which of the following drugs is used in the treatment of subacute sclerosing panencephalitis (SSPE)?
    a. Acyclovir
    b. Isoprinosine
    c. Mirtazapine
    d. Praziquantel

126. Most common parasitic disease of the CNS worldwide is?
    a. Neurocysticercosis
    b. Toxoplasmosis
    c. Schistosomiasis
    d. Amebiasis

127. CNS toxoplasmosis is treated with:
    a. Combination of sulfadiazine plus pyrimethamine
    b. Combination of albendazole plus praziquantel
    c. Combination of sulfadiazine plus clindamycin
    d. Combination of clindamycin plus pyrimethamine

128. Which of the following is most common predisposing condition for subdural empyema (Collection of pus between dura and arachnoid membrane)?
    a. Sinusitis
    b. Head trauma
    c. Secondary infection of subdural hematoma
    d. Neurosurgery

Answers

113. b	114. b	115. c	116. b	117. c	118. a	119. a
120. d	121. a	122. d	123. c	124. a	125. b	126. a
127. a	128. a					

129. Which of the following sentence is false regarding anterior choroidal artery syndrome?
    a. Contralateral hemiplegia
    b. Contralateral hemianesthesia
    c. Anterior limb of internal capsule is involved
    d. Contralateral homonymous hemianopia

130. Lenticulostriate arteries arises from:
    a. M1 segment of middle cerebral artery
    b. M2 segment superior division of middle cerebral artery
    c. M2 segment inferior division of middle cerebral artery
    d. Posterior cerebral artery

131. All of the following are branches of superior division of middle cerebral artery *except:*
    a. Anterior parietal
    b. Posterior parietal
    c. Rolandic
    d. Orbitofrontal

132. All of the following are branches of inferior division of middle cerebral artery *except:*
    a. Anterior temporal
    b. Posterior temporal
    c. Anterior parietal
    d. Posterior parietal

133. A 26-year-old male known case of rheumatic heart disease came with sudden onset weakness of right side of body involving both upper limb and lower limb. He is also having difficulty in talking. On evaluation you found that comprehension is normal, naming is impaired, repetition is impaired and fluency is severely decreased. Which of the following artery is most probably blocked?
    a. M1 segment of middle cerebral artery
    b. M2 segment superior division of middle cerebral artery
    c. M2 segment inferior division of middle cerebral artery
    d. Lenticulostriate branch of middle cerebral artery

134. Facial weakness with language dysfunction in the form of normal comprehension, impaired naming, impaired repetition and severely decreased fluency with or without arm weakness is called as:
    a. Brachial syndrome
    b. Frontal opercular syndrome
    c. Clumsy hand dysarthria lacunar syndrome
    d. Anterior choroidal artery syndrome

135. All of the following are P1 syndromes *except:*
    a. Anton's syndrome
    b. Weber's syndrome
    c. Benedict's syndrome
    d. Nothnagel syndrome

136. Patient is having anterograde auditory amnesia with right homonymous hemianopia with macular sparing which of the following artery is blocked?
    a. Left anterior cerebral artery
    b. Left middle cerebral artery
    c. Left posterior cerebral artery
    d. Right posterior cerebral artery

137. Alexia without agraphia is due to lesion of:
    a. Splenium of corpus callosum in dominant cerebral hemisphere
    b. Splenium of corpus callosum in nondominant cerebral hemisphere
    c. Bilateral visual association area
    d. Angular gyrus of dominant hemisphere

138. Anton's syndrome is due to:
    a. Unilateral distal posterior cerebral artery occlusion
    b. Bilateral distal posterior cerebral artery occlusion
    c. Bilateral visual association area lesion
    d. Lesion of splenium of corpus callosum in nondominant cerebral hemisphere

139. All of the following are true regarding Anton's syndrome *except:*
    a. Bilateral distal posterior distal cerebral artery occlusion
    b. Patient is unaware of his blindness
    c. Optic ataxia
    d. Tiny islands of vision persists

140. All of the following are characteristics of Balint's syndrome *except:*
    a. Palinopsia
    b. Asimultagnosia
    c. Oculomotor apraxia
    d. Patient is unaware of his blindness

141. Experiencing persistence of a visual image for several minutes despite of gazing at another scene is called as:
    a. Optic ataxia
    b. Ocular ataxia
    c. Simultagnosia
    d. Palinopsia

142. All of the following are true regarding Foster Kennedy syndrome *except:*
    a. It is due to olfactory groove meningioma
    b. Ipsilateral optic atrophy
    c. Contralateral disc edema due to increased intracranial pressure
    d. Contralateral loss of vision

143. Blood supply of paracentral lobule is:
    a. Anterior cerebral artery
    b. Anterior choroidal artery
    c. Anterior communicating artery
    d. Middle cerebral artery

144. A lesion in paracentral lobule causes:
    a. Contralateral foot weakness
    b. Seizures
    c. Migraine
    d. Cognitive loss

Answers

129. c	130. a	131. b	132. c	133. b	134. b	135. a
136. c	137. a	138. b	139. c	140. d	141. d	142. d
143. a	144. a					

145. Antisocial behaviour is a feature of damage to:
    a. Prefrontal area of frontal lobe
    b. Primary frontal area of frontal lobe
    c. Premotor area of frontal lobe
    d. Paracentral lobule of frontal lobe

146. All of the following are components of Gerstmann syndrome *except:*
    a. Dysgraphia
    b. Acalculia
    c. Finger agnosia
    d. Astereognosis

147. Lesion of left temporal lobe produces all of the following *except:*
    a. Aphasia
    b. Quadrantanopia
    c. Anterograde amnesia
    d. Apraxia

148. Patient is having impaired comprehension only for reading but normal comprehension for spoken language. Naming, repetition of spoken words and fluency are normal.
    What is the probable diagnosis?
    a. Posterior transcortical aphasia
    b. Pure alexia without agraphia
    c. Pure alexia with agraphia
    d. Isolation aphasia

149. Patient is having impaired comprehension only for reading but normal comprehension for spoken language Naming, repetition of spoken words and fluency are normal.
    Where is the lesion?
    a. Splenium of dominant hemisphere
    b. Angular gyrus of dominant hemisphere
    c. Inferior parietal lobule
    d. Hippocampus

150. A 50-year-old patient came with sudden onset weakness of right side of body involving upper and lower limb. On examination left eye is deviated to down and out with pupil dilated. What is probable diagnosis?
    a. Weber syndrome
    b. Benedikt's syndrome
    c. Nothnagel's syndrome
    d. Parinaud syndrome

151. Benedikt's syndrome is a midbrain syndrome which consists of:
    a. Ipsilateral 3'd nerve palsy contralateral tremors
    b. Ipsilateral 3'd nerve palsy contralateral ataxia
    c. Ipsilateral 3'd nerve palsy contralateral hemiplegia
    d. Ipsilateral 3'd nerve palsy Ipsilateral tremors

152. Nothnagel syndrome is a midbrain syndrome which consists of:
    a. Ipsilateral 3"t nerve palsy contralateral tremors
    b. Ipsilateral 3'd nerve palsy contralateral ataxia
    c. Ipsilateral 3"d nerve palsy contralateral hemiplegia
    d. Ipsilateral 3rd nerve palsy Ipsilateral tremors

153. Claude's syndrome is a midbrain syndrome which consists:
    a. Ipsilateral 3"d nerve palsy contralateral tremors plus contralateral ataxia
    b. Ipsilateral 3d nerve palsy ipsilateral tremors plus contralateral ataxia
    c. Ipsilateral 3d nerve palsy contralateral tremors plus ipsilateral ataxia
    d. Ipsilateral 3d nerve palsy ipsilateral tremors plus ipsilateral ataxia

154. Which of the following is false regarding Parinaud syndrome:
    a. It is P1 syndrome
    b. Lesion is in superior colliculus of mid brain
    c. Obstruction of thalamogeniculate branch of posterior cerebral artery
    d. Upward gaze palsy

155. Which of the following is false regarding Locked in syndrome?
    a. Bilateral ventral pontine lesion
    b. Bilateral dorsal pontine lesion
    c. Quadriplegia
    d. 3rd nerve is normal

156. Which of the following is false regarding Millard Gubler syndrome?
    a. 6th nerve palsy
    b. 7th nerve palsy
    c. Contralateral hemiplegia
    d. Horizontal gaze palsy

157. Which of the following is false regarding Foville syndrome?
    a. Dorsal pontine lesion
    b. Ipsilateral 6th nerve palsy
    c. Ipsilateral 7th nerve palsy
    d. No weakness

158. A 60-year-old female coming with right side hemiplegia with deviation of tongue to left side. Facial nerve examination is normal. What is the probable diagnosis?
    a. Millard-Gubler syndrome
    b. Left medial medullary syndrome
    c. Left lateral medullary syndrome
    d. Right medial medullary syndrome

Answers

| 145. a | 146. d | 147. d | 148. b | 149. a | 150. a | 151. a |
| 152. b | 153. a | 154. c | 155. b | 156. d | 157. d | 158. b |

159. All of the following are indications for thrombolysis in case of acute ischemic stroke *except:*
    a. Clinical diagnosis of stroke
    b. CT scan brain showing edema more than one third of middle cerebral artery territory
    c. Onset of symptoms to drug administration time less than 4.5 hours
    d. Age more than 18 years

160. All of the following are contraindications for thrombolysis in case of acute ischemic stroke *except:*
    a. Sustained BP 185/110 mm Hg despite of treatment
    b. Glucose > 400 mg/dL
    c. Rapidly improving symptoms
    d. Platelets< 200,000

161. A young female presents with severe headache and neck stiffness of abrupt onset followed by progressive III cranial nerve palsy. She says, she has never had such severe headache before. She also complains of associated nausea and photophobia. Likely diagnosis is:
    a. Subarachnoid hemorrhage (SAH)
    b. Migraine
    c. Viral encephalitis
    d. Hydrocephalus

162. Hunt and Hess scale is used for grading of:
    a. Subarachnoid hemorrhage
    b. Intracranial hemorrhage
    c. Subdural hemorrhage
    d. Extradural hemorrhage

163. 3H therapy for treatment of subarachnoid hemorrhage consists of all of the following *except:*
    a. Hypertension
    b. Hemodilution
    c. Hypervolumia
    d. Hyponatremia

164. A 63-year-old male presented with history of progressive right side weakness of 1 month duration. Patient is also having speech difficulty. Fundus examination showed papilloedema. 2 months ago he also had fall in his bathroom and stuck his head against a wall. The most likely diagnosis is:
    a. Intracerebral hemorrhage
    b. Subdural hemorrhage
    c. Extradural hemorrhage
    d. Diffuse axonal injury

165. Which of the following is false regarding TIC DOULOUREUX?
    a. It is more common in female
    b. Ophthalmic division of trigeminal is commonly involved
    c. Tactile stimuli acts as trigger for pain
    d. Carbamazepine is drug of choice

166. CLUSTER TIC means:
    a. Cluster headache associated with Tics like jerking of head etc.
    b. Cluster headache associated with trigeminal neuralgia
    c. Tics associated with trigeminal neuralgia
    d. Multiple types of tics associated with vocalization

167. Facial nerve palsy is associated with all of the following *except:*
    a. Bell's palsy
    b. Ramsay-Hunt syndrome
    c. Melkersson Rosenthal syndrome
    d. Todd's paralysis

168. Melkersson Rosenthal syndrome is:
    a. Recurrent facial nerve palsy plus permanent facial edema
    b. Recurrent facial edema with permanent facial nerve palsy
    c. 7th nerve palsy plus 8th nerve palsy plus vesicular eruptions in external auditory canal
    d. Lower motor neuron lesion of facial nerve

169. Which muscles are spared in upper motor neuron lesion of facial nerve?
    a. Frontalis and orbicularis oculi
    b. Frontalis and buccinator
    c. Frontalis and orbicularis oris
    d. Frontalis and zygomaticus

170. All of the following are true about Lurching gait *except:*
    a. Patient lurch on normal (non-paralysed) side
    b. It is due to unilateral weakness of gluteus medius
    c. Fall of pelvis on non-paralysed (contralateral) side
    d. Seen in polio

171. A 12-year-old boy presents to the outpatient department with history of progressively increasing difficulty in walking and frequent falls. Physical examination reveals an ataxic gait. All deep tendon reflexes were observed to be absent while the plantar response was 'extensor. Blood investigations showed high sugar level. What is the most likely diagnosis?
    a. Friedreich's ataxia
    b. Subacute combined degeneration of cord (SACD)
    c. Becker's muscular dystrophy
    d. Tabes dorsalis

172. All of the following are true regarding scissoring gait *except:*
    a. Seen in cerebral palsy
    b. Adduction and internal rotation of hip
    c. Extension at knee
    d. Plantar flexion at ankle

Answers

159. b	160. d	161. a	162. a	163. d	164. b	165. b
166. b	167. d	168. a	169. a	170. a	171. a	172. c

173. Lesions of the lateral cerebellum cause all of the following except:
    a. Incoordination
    b. Intention tremor
    c. Resting tremor
    d. Ataxia

174. Flapping tremors may be associated with all of the following, except:
    a. Hepatic encephalopathy
    b. Uremia
    c. CO_2 narcosis
    d. Thyrotoxicosis

175. A 12-year-old girl with tremors and emotional liability has golden brown discolouration in Descemet's membrane. The most likely diagnosis is:
    a. Fabry's disease
    b. Wilson's disease
    c. Glycogen storage disease
    d. Acute rheumatic fever

176. Which of the following is false regarding essential tremors?
    a. It is commonest movement disorder
    b. Manifest as postural or action tremor
    c. Treatment is propanolol
    d. Frequency is 4 to 6 H2

177. All are true about Huntington's disease except:
    a. Chorea
    b. Increased CAG repeats
    c. Early onset of memory loss
    d. Seizure

178. Which of the following is false regarding hyperkinetic movement disorders?
    a. Chorea is due to lesion in caudate nucleus
    b. Hemiballismus is due to lesion in subthalamic nucleus
    c. Dystonia is due to lesion in putamen
    d. Athetosis is due to lesion in globus pallidus

179. A patient with traumatic paraplegia due to injury of the thoracic cord of T3 level' is observed to have a blood pressure of 210/110. What should be the initial management?
    a. Subcutaneous LMWH   b. Steroids
    c. Nifedipine   d. Normal saline

180. Subacute combined degeneration due to Vit B12 deficiency involves all of the following except:
    a. Peripheral nerve   b. Corticospinal tract
    c. Posterior column   d. Spinothalamic tract

181. Features of syringomyelia include all of the following, except:
    a. Dissociative sensory loss
    b. Early sacral involvement
    c. Suspended sensory loss
    d. Wasting of small muscles of hand

182. All of the following are core symptoms for diagnosis of Restless leg syndrome except:
    a. Unpleasant sensations on the legs
    b. Symptoms begins with the rest
    c. Symptoms improved by alcohol
    d. Symptoms becomes worse in the evening or night

183. Which of the following statements about Prions is true?
    a. Kuru is inherited prion disease
    b. They affect only nervous system
    c. They have rich nuclear material
    d. They causes abnormal stimulation of immune system

184. Which one of the following is not a human prion disease?
    a. Scrapie
    b. Kuru
    c. Creutzfeldt-Jakob disease
    d. Gerstmann-Straussler Scheinker disease

185. In spinal cord sacral fibers are placed laterally in all except:
    a. Lateral spinothalamic tract
    b. Lateral corticospinal tract
    c. Ventral spinothalamic
    d. Dorsal column

186. Bulbar paralysis refers to:
    a. UMN Paralysis of cranial nerve III to XII
    b. UMN Paralysis of cranial nerve IX to XII
    c. LMN Paralysis of cranial nerve IX to XIII
    d. LMN Paralysis of cranial nerve III to XII

187. Pseudobulbar paralysis refers to:
    a. UMN Paralysis of cranial nerve III to XII
    b. UMN Paralysis of cranial nerve IX to XII
    c. LMN Paralysis of cranial nerve IX to XI
    d. LMN Paralysis of cranial nerve III to XII

188. Which of the following represents the site of lesion in motor neuron disease:
    a. Anterior horn cells   b. Peripheral nerve
    c. Spinothalamic tract   d. Spinocerebellar tract

Answers

173. c	174. d	175. b	176. d	177. c	178. c	179. c
180. d	181. b	182. c	183. b	184. a	185. d	186. c
187. b	188. a					

189. All of the following are features of Amyotrophic lateral sclerosis *except:*
    a. More common in male than female
    b. Death of posterior horn cell neurons
    c. Death of neurons in motor cortex in cerebral hemisphere
    d. Bladder is not involved

190. A middle aged man presents with dysphagia, dysarthria, progressive atrophy and weakness of right hand and forearm. On examination he is found to have slight spasticity of the left leg with exaggerated knee and ankle reflex on left side. MRI of brain and spinal cord report is awaited. The most likely clinical diagnosis is:
    a. Definite amyotrophic lateral sclerosis
    b. Possible amyotrophic lateral sclerosis
    c. Probable amyotrophic lateral sclerosis
    d. Absolute amyotrophic lateral sclerosis

191. All of the following are true about Brown-Sequard syndrome, *except:*
    a. Ipsilateral pyramidal tract features
    b. Contralateral spinothalamic tract features
    c. Contralateral posterior column features
    d. Ipsilateral plantar extensor

192. Which of the following statements about Brown Sequard syndrome is true?
    a. Ipsilateral loss of temperature
    b. Contralateral loss of pain
    c. Contralateral loss of vibration
    d. Contralateral plantar extensor

193. Which of the following is not a feature of extramedullary tumour?
    a. Early corticospinal signs and paralysis
    b. Root pain or midline back pain
    c. Asymmetric weakness
    d. Sacral sparing

194. Clinical features of Conus medullaris syndrome include all of the following *except:*
    a. Plantar extensor response
    b. Absent knee and ankle jerks
    c. Sacral anesthesia
    d. Lower sacral and coccygeal segments involvement

195. Early loss of bladder control is seen in:
    a. Conus medullaris syndrome
    b. Cauda equina syndrome
    c. Guillain-Barrè syndrome
    d. Amyotrophic lateral sclerosis

196. Spinal shock is characterized by all of the following *except:*
    a. Wasting
    b. Sensory loss
    c. Urinary retention
    d. Areflexia

197. Spastic paraplegia is caused by all, *except:*
    a. Vitamin B12 deficiency
    b. Cervical spondylosis
    c. Lead poisoning
    d. Motor neuron disease

198. All of the following are causes of acute motor neuron disease *except:*
    a. Polio
    b. West nile
    c. Herpes
    d. Amyotrophic lateral sclerosis

199. A patient involved in a road traffic accident presents with quadriparesis, sphincter disturbance, sensory level up to the upper border of sternum and breathing difficulty. The likely level of lesion is:
    a. C1-C2
    b. C4-C5
    c. T1-T2
    d. T3-T4

200. Anterior spinal artery thrombosis is characterized by all, *except:*
    a. Loss of pain and touch
    b. Loss of vibration sense
    c. Loss of power in lower limb
    d. Sphincter dysfunction

201. Cognitive changes of Alzheimer's disease characteristically begin with:
    a. Memory impairment
    b. Language deficit
    c. Visuospatial deficit
    d. Apraxia

202. Coma results due to damage in reticular activating system (RAS) at the level of:
    a. Medulla oblongata
    b. Pons
    c. Lower midbrain
    d. Upper midbrain

203. "Waxy flexibility" is a feature of which of the following?
    a. Abulia
    b. Akinetic mutism
    c. Catatonia
    d. Locked-in state

Answers

189. b	190. a	191. c	192. b	193. d	194. b	195. a
196. a	197. c	198. d	199. b	200. b	201. a	202. d
203. c						

204. **Bilaterally dilated and unreactive pupils indicate?**
   a. Severe cortical damage
   b. Severe thalamic damage
   c. Severe midbrain damage
   d. Severe pontine damage

205. **All of the following are risk factors for Alzheimer's disease** *except:*
   a. Old age
   b. Positive family history
   c. APO E2 gene
   d. Female gender

206. **A ß peptide results from cleavage of amyloid precursor protein (APP) by:**
   a. β secretase
   b. ß secretase
   c. and secretase
   d. a secretase

207. **Neurofibrillary tangles (NFTs) in Alzheimer's disease is characterized by all** *except:*
   a. Found in neuronal cytoplasm
   b. Twisted neurofilaments
   c. Represent abnormally phosphorylated tau protein
   d. Gold staining

208. **Which of the following statements about Frontotemporal dementia (FTD) is false?**
   a. Begins in fifth to seventh decade
   b. More common in men than women
   c. Behavioral symptoms predominate in early states
   d. Memory and visuospatial skills are severely affected

209. **"Alien hand" phenomenon is a feature of:**
   a. Progressive supranuclear palsy
   b. Lewy body dementia
   c. Corticobasal degeneration
   d. Alzheimer's dementia

210. **Which of the following degenerates in Marchiafava-Bignami disease?**
   a. Caudate nucleus
   b. Thalamus
   c. Corpus callosum
   d. Substantia nigra

211. **Orthostatic hypotension is defined as:**
   a. Sustained drop in systolic blood pressure more than or equal to 30 mm Hg after 2-3 mins of standing
   b. Sustained drop in systolic blood pressure more than or equal to 20 mm Hg after 1 min of standing
   c. Sustained drop in diastolic blood pressure more than on equal to 10 mm Hg after 2-3 mins of standing
   d. Sustained drop in diastolic blood pressure more than or equal to 10 mm Hg after 1 min of standing

212. **All of the following clinical features can present in cervical myelopathy** *except:*
   a. Facial sensory loss
   b. Brisk jaw jerk
   c. Urinary bladder dysfunction
   d. Horner's syndrome

213. **A 63-year-old female presented to the emergency room with an acute aneurismal subarachnoid hemorrhage (SAH) and underwent a clipping procedure on admission. She has since been recovering in the intensive care unit. On the tenth postoperative day she was noted to have slurred speech worsening right facial droop and right arm weakness. She was more difficult to rouse. Non-contrast head computed tomography and four vessel angiogram showed ischemia in MCA territory. Which of the following is best treatment for her condition?**
   a. Intravenous rtPA
   b. Intra-arterial calcium channel blocker
   c. VP shunt
   d. Intravenous fosphenytoin

214. **Which of the following sentence is false regarding BOTULISM?**
   a. Blurring of vision and diplopia are initial neural symptoms of disease and recovery first occurs in ocular movements
   b. Pupils are reactive to light
   c. Severe constipation is characteristic of botulism
   d. Consciousness is retained throughout the illness unless severe degrees of anoxia develop as a result of respiratory failure

215. **All of the following are neurological events in HIV patient in advance stage (CD4 count less than 200)** *except:*
   a. Mononeuritis multiplex
   b. Cryptococcal meningitis
   c. Cerebral toxoplasmosis
   d. Primary CNS lymphoma

216. **Which type of spinocerebellar ataxia occurs due to a pentanucleotide repeat expansion?**
   a. Spinocerebellar ataxia type 2
   b. Spinocerebellar ataxia type 6
   c. Spinocerebellar ataxia type 10
   d. Spinocerebellar ataxia type 3

217. **Which of the following viral meningitis can show predominant neutrophils in CSF analysis?**
   a. West nile virus
   b. Herpes simplex virus 2
   c. Epstein-Barr virus
   d. Human herpes virus 6

Answers

| 204. c | 205. d | 206. a | 207. d | 208. d | 209. c | 210. c |
| 211. c | 212. b | 213. b | 214. b | 215. a | 216. c | 217. a |

218. Which of the following clinical sign is demonstrated in the image?
    a. Caudate nucleus
    b. Thalamus
    c. Corpus callosum
    d. Substantia nigra

219. Which of the following sentence is incorrect regarding Machado Joseph Disease (MJD):
    a. It is the most common form of inherited autosomal dominant ataxia
    b. Mean age is 25 years
    c. Type 2 MJD is called as Ataxic-Amyotrophic type MJD
    d. Intellectual function is normal in MJD

220. Miller Fisher test is used for:
    a. Evaluating cognition in NPH
    b. Severity of paralysis in Miller-Fisher syndrome
    c. Grading muscle involvement in ALS
    d. Measuring disability in multiple sclerosis

221. Brighton criteria for diagnosis of Miller-Fischer syndrome consists of all of the following *except:*
    a. Monophasic pattern of limb weakness
    b. No alteration in consciousness
    c. Cytoalbuminological dissociation in CSF analysis
    d. Nerve conduction study may be normal

222. Clinical grading system used for grading myasthenia gravis:
    a. Brackmann grading system
    b. EDSS
    c. Hunt and Hess scale
    d. Osserman staging

223. Which of the following sentence is false regarding subacute combined degeneration (SACD)?
    a. It is most common form of metabolic myelopathy
    b. Most severely affected tract is lateral corticospinal tract at cervical and upper thoracic level
    c. It is associated with optic atrophy
    d. The classic syndrome of folate deficiency is similar to SACD

224. Micturation reflex center is present in:
    a. Paracentral lobule in medial frontal lobe
    b. Nucleus of onuf in anterior horn of spinal cord at S2-S3-S4 level
    c. Anterior horn of spinal cord at T12-L1 level
    d. Barrington's nucleus in Pons

225. Which of the following sentence is incorrect regarding Hirayama disease?
    a. Most common presentation is slowly progressive painless weakness and atrophy in one hand
    b. The cranial nerves may be involved
    c. Pyramidal tract and the autonomic nervous system are normal
    d. UMN signs are absent

226. Which of the following sentence is incorrect regarding Decerebrate rigidity?
    a. Fingers are flexed at metacarpophalangeal joints and extended at interphalangeal joints
    b. Decerebrate rigidity is an exaggeration of normal standing position
    c. Increased tone in antigravity muscles
    d. Opisthotonos is extreme decerebrate rigidity

227. Which of the following motor neurons in anterior horn of spinal cord are placed anteriorly?
    a. Proximal
    b. Distal
    c. Flexors
    d. Extensors

228. Which of the following test is used to check parasympathetic autonomic nervous system?
    a. Heart rate variation with deep breathing
    b. Orthostatic hypotension
    c. Thermoregulatory sweat test
    d. Quantitative sudomotor axon reflex test

229. which of the following sentence is incorrect regarding Anderson Tawil syndrome?
    a. It is potassium channelopathy
    b. It is autosomal recessive in inheritance
    c. Usually age of onset is early childhood
    d. It is associated with cardiac arrhythmias

230. Hyperpathia is a broad term that encompasses all of the following *except:*
    a. Hyperesthesia
    b. Allodynia
    c. Hyperalgesia
    d. Hypoesthesia

231. Hyperesthesia means:
    a. Pain in response to touch
    b. Non-painful stimulus is experienced as painful
    c. Severe pain in response to mildly noxious stimulus
    d. Sensations that are perceived without an apparent stimulus

232. Detrusor-sphincter dyssynergia occurs when lesion is present in:
    a. Pons
    b. Spinal cord at T12-L1 level
    c. Spinal cord at S2S3S4 level
    d. Frontal lobe

233. All of the following constituents are found in higher concentration in CSF than in blood *except:*
    a. Magnesium
    b. Sugar
    c. Chloride
    d. Lactate

Answers

218. b	219. c	220. a	221. a	222. d	223. b	224. d
225. b	226. a	227. d	228. a	229. b	230. d	231. a
232. a	233. b					

234. In the tests to confirm brain death, "hollow-skull sign" is a finding in which of the following?
    a. EEG
    b. Dynamic radionuclide brain scan
    c. Cerebral angiography
    d. Transcranial Doppler measurements

235. Cingulate gyrus is likely to be involved in which of the following herniations?
    a. Temporal transtentorial herniation
    b. Central transtentorial herniation
    c. Transfalcial herniation
    d. Foraminal herniation

236. Cerebellar tonsils are likely to be involved in which of the following brain herniations?
    a. Temporal transtentorial herniation
    b. Central transtentorial herniation
    c. Transfalcial herniation
    d. Foraminal herniation

237. "Ocular dipping" is diagnostic of?
    a. Diffuse cortical anoxic damage
    b. ICSOL
    c. SAH
    d. Tubercular meningitis

238. Which of the following is not a function of dominant parietal lobe?
    a. Comprehension
    b. Logic
    c. Spatial orientation
    d. Calculation

239. Horner's syndrome is characterized by all of the following except:
    a. Miosis
    b. Enophthalmos
    c. Ptosis
    d. Cycloplegia

240. The most sensitive test for the diagnosis of generalised myasthenia gravis is:
    a. Elevated serum Ach-receptor binding antibodies
    b. Repetitive nerve stimulation test
    c. Positive edrophonium test
    d. Single fibre electromyography

241. Duchenne muscular dystrophy is a disease of:
    a. Neuromuscular junction
    b. Sarcolemmal proteins
    c. Muscle contractile proteins
    d. Disuse atrophy due to muscle weakness

242. Following are the features of cortiospinal tract involvement except:
    a. Cog-wheel rigidity
    b. Spasticity
    c. Plantar extensor response
    d. Exaggerated deep tendon reflexes

243. A chromosomal anomaly associated with Alzheimer's dementia is:
    a. Trisomy 18
    b. Patau syndrome
    c. Trisomy 21
    d. Turner syndrome

Answers

| 234. b | 235. c | 236. d | 237. a | 238. c | 239. d | 240. d |
| 241. b | 242. a | 243. c | | | | |

CHAPTER 4

Neuropharmacology

SEDATIVES

Sedatives are commonly prescribed for the treatment of Insomnia. The cause of insomnia should be established before administering hypnotic drugs. Common causes include alcohol or other drug misuse and physical or psychiatric disorder (especially depression). Drugs used against anxiety can also be classified in this group.

The main groups of drugs are as follows:
- Benzodiazepines: Diazepam is the prototype. Others are flurazepam, nitrazepam, flunitrazepam, triazolam, midazolam, lorazepam, clonazepam and chlordiazepoxide.
- Newer sedatives: Zopiclone, Zolpidem—non-benzodiazepine sedative.
- Barbiturates: Phenobarbitone is long acting. Thiopentone and Methohexitone are ultra short acting.
- Miscellaneous other drugs (e.g. chloral hydrate, meprobamate and methaqualone)—no longer recommended.
- Sedative antihistamines, such as diphenhydramine, are sometimes used as sleeping pills. They are included in various over-the-counter preparations intended to improve children's sleep patterns.
- Buspirone- $5-HT_{1A}$ receptor agonist, anxiolytic.
- β-Adrenoceptor antagonists (e.g. propranolol)—used particularly where physical symptoms such as sweating, tremor and tachycardia are troublesome.

BENZODIAZEPINES

Mechanism of Action
- Benzodiazepines act selectively on $GABA_A$ receptors, which mediate fast inhibitory synaptic transmission throughout the central nervous system. Benzodiazepines enhance the response to GABA by facilitating the opening of GABA-activated chloride channels. They bind specifically to a regulatory site of the receptor, distinct from the GABA-binding site, and act allosterically to increase the affinity of GABA for the receptor. Benzodiazepines do not affect receptors for other amino acids, such as glycine or glutamate. They are only GABA facilitatory, not GABA mimetic.
- The $GABA_A$ receptor is a ligand-gated ion channel consisting of a pentameric assembly of different subunits, the main ones being α, β and γ, each of which occurs in three or more isoforms. Sensitivity to benzodiazepines requires the presence of both α and β subunits, and mutation of a single amino acid (histidine 101) in the α subunit eliminates benzodiazepine sensitivity.
- $GABA_A$ receptors containing the $α_1$ subunit account for sedative, amnesic and anticonvulsant effects of benzodiazepines, whereas those containing the $α_2$ subunit account for the anxiolytic and muscle relaxant effects.

Effects
- Benzodiazepines have a high therapeutic index. The main effects of benzodiazepines are: reduction of anxiety and aggression, sedation and induction of sleep, reduction of muscle tone and coordination, anticonvulsant effect and anterograde amnesia.
- With the possible exception of alprazolam, benzodiazepines do not have antidepressant effects. Benzodiazepines may paradoxically produce an increase in irritability and aggression in some individuals, probably a manifestation of the benzodiazepine withdrawal syndrome, which occurs with all these drugs but is more acute with drugs whose action wears off rapidly.

- Benzodiazepines are used mainly for treating acute anxiety states, but their use is declining in favor of antidepressants, coupled with behavioral therapies in more severe cases.
- Benzodiazepines decrease the time taken to get to sleep, and increase the total duration of sleep. Both effects tend to decline when benzodiazepines are taken regularly for 1-2 weeks.
- Most hypnotic drugs reduce the proportion of REM sleep, although benzodiazepines affect it less than other hypnotics and zolpidem least of all, which acts on w_1 subtype of receptors. The rebound in REM sleep is seen at the end of a period of administration of benzodiazepines or other hypnotics. The proportion of slow-wave sleep is significantly reduced by benzodiazepines, although growth hormone secretion is unaffected.
- Benzodiazepines reduce muscle tone by a central action that is independent of their sedative effect. Increased muscle tone is a common feature of anxiety states in humans and may contribute to the aches and pains, including headache, which often trouble anxious patients. The relaxant effect of benzodiazepines may therefore be clinically useful.
- All the benzodiazepines are highly effective against chemically induced convulsions caused by pentylenetetrazol, bicuculline and similar drugs but less so against electrically induced convulsions. Benzodiazepines enhance the action of GABA but not glycine, so the selectivity of their anticonvulsant action is explicable. Clonazepam, because of its selective anticonvulsant action, is used to treat epilepsy, as is diazepam, which is given intravenously to control life-threatening seizures in status epilepticus.
- Benzodiazepines obliterate memory of events experienced while under their influence, an effect not seen with other CNS depressants. Minor surgical procedures can thus be performed without leaving unpleasant memories.
- The term *inverse agonist* is applied to drugs that bind to benzodiazepine receptors and exert the opposite effect to that of conventional benzodiazepines, producing signs of increased anxiety and convulsions. Competitive antagonists such as flumazenil bind equally to A and B sites of GABA, and consequently do not disturb the conformational equilibrium but antagonise the effect of both agonists and inverse agonists.

PHARMACOKINETICS

- Benzodiazepines are well absorbed when given orally, usually giving a peak plasma concentration in about 1 hour. Oxazepam and lorazepam are absorbed more slowly. They bind strongly to plasma protein, and their high lipid solubility causes many of them to accumulate gradually in body fat. They are normally given orally but can be given intravenously (e.g. diazepam in status epilepticus, midazolam in anesthesia).
- Benzodiazepines are all metabolised and eventually excreted as glucuronide conjugates in the urine. They are converted to active metabolites such as *N*-desmethyldiazepam (nordazepam), which has a half-life of about 60 hours, and which accounts for the tendency of many benzodiazepines to produce cumulative effects and long hangovers when they are given repeatedly. The short-acting compounds are those that are metabolised directly by conjugation with glucuronide. They undergo redistribution, except midazolam and triazolam.
- Advancing age affects the rate of oxidative reactions more than that of conjugation reactions. Thus, the effect of the long-acting benzodiazepines, which may be used regularly as hypnotics or anxiolytic agents for many years, tends to increase with age.
- CYP 3A4 isoenzyme plays an important role in metabolism of BZD's and hence their action is prolonged by inhibitors of the enzyme.
- The half lives of parent compounds are as follows [in hrs]: Flurazepam [1], Zolpidem [2], midazolam and triazolam [2-4], alprazolam [6-12], lorazepam and oxazepam [8-12], Nitrazepam [16-40], diazepam and chlordiazepoxide [20-40], clonazepam [50].

ADVERSE EFFECTS

Acute Toxicity

Benzodiazepines in acute overdose are considerably less dangerous than other anxiolytic/hypnotic drugs. In overdose, benzodiazepines cause prolonged sleep, without serious depression of respiration or cardiovascular function. The availability of an effective antagonist, flumazenil, means that the effects of an acute overdose can be counteracted, which is not possible for most CNS depressants.

Side Effects during Therapeutic Use

The main side effects of benzodiazepines are drowsiness, confusion, amnesia and impaired coordination. Benzodiazepines enhance the depressant effect of other drugs, including alcohol, in a more than additive way.

Tolerance

- Occurs with all benzodiazepines, as does *dependence*, which is their main drawback. They share these properties with other hypnotics and sedatives. Short-acting benzodiazepines cause more abrupt withdrawal effects. With triazolam, a very short-acting drug and no longer in use, the withdrawal effect occurred within a few hours, even after a single dose, producing early-morning insomnia and daytime anxiety when the drug was used as a hypnotic.

- The physical and psychological withdrawal symptoms make it difficult for patients to give up taking benzodiazepines, but *addiction* is not a major problem.
- The best-known antagonist is flumazenil. Flumazenil can be used to reverse the effect of benzodiazepine overdosage (normally used only if respiration is severely depressed), or to reverse the effect of benzodiazepines such as midazolam used for minor surgical procedures.

BUSPIRONE

- Buspirone is a partial agonist at $5-HT_{1A}$ receptors and is used to treat various anxiety disorders. It also binds to dopamine receptors, but it is likely that its 5-HT-related actions are important in relation to anxiety suppression.
- $5-HT_{1A}$ receptors are inhibitory autoreceptors that reduce the release of 5-HT and other mediators. They also inhibit the activity of noradrenergic locus coeruleus neurons and thus interfere with arousal reactions. Buspirone is ineffective in controlling panic attacks or severe anxiety states.
- Buspirone has side effects quite different from those of benzodiazepines. It does not cause sedation or motor incoordination and do not have withdrawal effects. Its main side effects are nausea, dizziness, headache and restlessness, which generally seem to be less troublesome than the side effects of benzodiazepines.

BARBITURATES

- All Barbiturates have depressant activity on the CNS, producing effects similar to those of inhalation anesthetics.
- Pentobarbital and similar typical barbiturates with durations of action of 6–12 hours are still very occasionally used as sleeping pills and anxiolytic drugs, but they are less safe than benzodiazepines.
- Barbiturates share with benzodiazepines the ability to enhance the action of GABA, but they bind to a different site on the $GABA_A$ receptor/chloride channel, and their action is less specific. Barbiturates act at the GABA: BZD receptor Cl⁻ channel complex. It is both GABA mimetic and GABA facilitatory. As well as being dangerous in overdose, barbiturates induce a high degree of tolerance and dependence.
- Highly lipid soluble thiopentone undergoes redistribution. Others are excreted unchanged in urine.
- They also strongly induce the synthesis of hepatic cytochrome P450 and conjugating enzymes, and thus increase the rate of metabolic degradation of many other drugs, giving rise to a number of potentially troublesome drug interactions. Because of enzyme induction, barbiturates are also dangerous to patients suffering from the metabolic disease porphyria.
- They cause death from respiratory and cardiovascular depression if given in large doses, which is one of the main reasons that they are now little used as anxiolytic and hypnotic agents.
- Acute barbiturate poisoning is treated by gastric lavage, forced alkaline dieresis and hemodialysis.

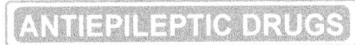

NEURAL MECHANISMS AND ANIMAL MODELS OF EPILEPSY

- The *kindling model* may approximate the human condition more closely than directly evoked seizure models. Low-intensity electrical stimulation of certain regions of the limbic system, such as the amygdala, with implanted electrodes repeated daily for several days shows seizure response. Once produced, the kindled state persists indefinitely which is prevented by NMDA receptor antagonists.
- The *kainate model* entails a single injection of the glutamate receptor agonist kainic acid into the amygdaloid nucleus of a rat. After transient intense stimulation, spontaneous seizures begin to occur 2–4 weeks later, and then continue indefinitely.
- Pentylenetetrazol (PTZ) is involved in absence seizures.
- Neurons from which the epileptic discharge originates display an unusual type of electrical behavior termed the *paroxysmal depolarising shift* (*PDS*), during which the membrane potential suddenly decreases and remains depolarised for up to a few seconds before returning to normal. A burst of action potentials often accompanies this depolarization. This event probably results from the abnormally exaggerated and prolonged action of an excitatory transmitter.
- *Neurotrophins*, particularly brain-derived neurotrophic factor (BDNF), may play a role in epileptogenesis. BDNF, which acts on a membrane receptor tyrosine kinase, enhances membrane excitability and also stimulates synapse formation.

CLASSIFICATION

Based on the type of seizures
- *Tonic-clonic* (grand mal) seizures:
  - Carbamazepine, phenytoin, valproate
  - Newer agents include vigabatrin, lamotrigine, felbamate, gabapentin.
- *Partial (focal) seizures*: Carbamazepine, valproate; Clonazepam or phenytoin.
- *Absence seizures* (petit mal): Ethosuximide or valproate
- *Myoclonic seizures*: Diazepam intravenously or rectally.

Based on Drugs of Choice

Type	First line drugs	Second line
Tonic-clonic	Carbamazepine, valproate, phenytoin	Lamotrigine, oxcarbazepine
Myoclonic	Valproate	Topiramate, levetiracetam, zonisamide
Partial	Carbamazepine, phenytoin	Valproate, lamotrigine, oxcarbazepine, levetiracetam
Absence Antiepileptics of choice	Valproate	Ethosuximide, lamotrigine

BASED ON THE ESTABLISHED AND NEWER DRUGS

ESTABLISHED DRUGS WITH THEIR SALIENT FEATURES

- **Phenytoin**
  - Acts mainly by use-dependent block of sodium channels
  - Effective in many forms of epilepsy, but not absence seizures
  - Metabolism shows saturation kinetics, therefore plasma concentration can vary widely; monitoring is therefore needed
  - Drug interactions are common main unwanted effects are confusion, gum hyperplasia, skin rashes, anemia, teratogenesis
  - Widely used in treatment of epilepsy; also used as antiarrhythmic agent.
- **Carbamazepine**
  - Derivative of tricyclic antidepressants
  - Similar profile to that of Phenytoin but with fewer unwanted effects
  - Effective in most forms of epilepsy (except absence seizures); particularly effective in psychomotor epilepsy; also useful in trigeminal neuralgia
  - Strong inducing agent, therefore many drug interactions
  - Low incidence of unwanted effects, principally sedation, ataxia, mental disturbances, water retention.
- **Valproate**
  - Chemically unrelated to other antiepileptic drugs
  - Mechanism of action is multiple; weak inhibition of GABA transaminase, some effect on sodium channels, attenuation of T type Ca^2 channels.
  - Relatively few unwanted effects: baldness, teratogenicity, liver damage (rare, but serious).
- **Ethosuximide**
  - The main drug used to treat absence seizures; may exacerbate other forms
  - Acts by blocking T-type calcium channels
  - Relatively few unwanted effects, mainly nausea and anorexia.
- **Secondary drugs include**
  - Phenobarbital: Highly sedative
  - Various benzodiazepines (e.g. Clonazepam); Diazepam used in treating status epilepticus.

Newer Drugs

Newer agents that are becoming widely used because of their improved side effect profile include vigabatrin, lamotrigine, felbamate, gabapentin, pregabalin, tiagabine, tiopiramate and Zonisamide.

MECHANISM OF ACTION OF ANTIEPILEPTIC DRUGS

Three main mechanisms appear to be important in the action of antiepileptic drugs:
- Enhancement of GABA action (facilitation of Cl^- channel opening)
- Inhibition of sodium channel function (prolongation of channel inactivation)
- Inhibition of T type calcium channel function.

Enhancement of GABA Action

Several antiepileptic drugs (e.g. Phenobarbital and benzodiazepines) enhance the activation of $GABA_A$ receptors, thus facilitating the GABA-mediated opening of chloride channels. Vigabatrin acts by inhibiting the enzyme GABA transaminase, which is responsible for inactivating GABA, and tiagabine inhibits GABA uptake; both thereby enhance the action of GABA as an inhibitory transmitter. Gabapentin was designed as an agonist at $GABA_A$ receptors and has high affinity for a particular subunit ($\alpha_2\delta$) of voltage-gated calcium channels.

Inhibition of Sodium Channel Function

Several of the most important antiepileptic drugs (e.g. Phenytoin, Carbamazepine, valproate, Lamotrigine) affect membrane excitability by an action on voltage-dependent sodium channels, which carry the inward membrane current necessary for the generation of an action potential. Their blocking action shows the property of use-dependence i.e., they block preferentially the excitation of cells that are firing repetitively, and the higher the frequency of firing, the greater the block produced. This characteristic arises from the ability of blocking drugs to discriminate between sodium channels in their resting, open and inactivated states.

Inhibition of Calcium Channels

Several antiepileptic drugs have minor effects on calcium channels, but only ethosuximide specifically blocks the T- type calcium channel, activation of which plays a role in the rhythmic discharge associated with absence seizures. Gabapentin acts on L-type calcium channels by binding to the $\alpha_2\delta$ subunit.

PHENYTOIN

- Phenytoin is the most important member of the hydantoin group of compounds. Despite its many side effects and unpredictable pharmacokinetic behavior, phenytoin is widely used. It is effective against various forms of partial and generalised seizures, although not against absence seizures, which may even get worse.
- It is well absorbed when given orally, and about 80–90% of the plasma content is bound to albumin. Other drugs, such as salicylates, phenylbutazone and valproate, inhibit this binding competitively. This increases the free phenytoin concentration but also increases hepatic clearance of phenytoin. Phenytoin is metabolised by the hepatic mixed function oxidase system and excreted mainly as glucuronide. It causes enzyme induction, and thus increases the rate of metabolism of other drugs (e.g. oral anticoagulants). The metabolism of phenytoin itself can be either enhanced or competitively inhibited by various other drugs that share the same hepatic enzymes.
- The metabolism of phenytoin shows the characteristic of saturation, which means that over the therapeutic plasma concentration range the rate of inactivation does not increase in proportion to the plasma concentration. The plasma half-life (approximately 20 hours) increases as the dose is increased.
- The steady-state mean plasma concentration, achieved when a patient is given a constant daily dose, varies disproportionately with the dose. A radioimmunoassay for phenytoin in plasma is available, and its use has helped considerably in achieving an optimal therapeutic effect.
- Therapeutic range of phenytoin– 10–20 mcg/mL. Side effects of phenytoin begin to appear at plasma concentrations exceeding 100 imol/l and may be severe above about 150 imol/l. The milder side effects (phenytoin level between 20–40 mcg/mL) include vertigo, ataxia, headache and nystagmus, but not sedation. Lethargy and confusion, coma and seizures occur when level exceeds 40 mcg/mL. Hyperplasia of the gums often develops gradually, as does hirsutism and coarsening of the features, which probably result from increased androgen secretion. Megaloblastic anemia, associated with a disorder of

folate metabolism, sometimes occurs, and can be corrected by giving folic acid. Hypersensitivity reactions, mainly rashes, are quite common. Phenytoin has also been implicated as a cause of the increased incidence of fetal malformations in children born to epileptic mothers, particularly the occurrence of cleft palate called the fetal hydantoin syndrome, associated with the formation of an epoxide metabolite.

CARBAMAZEPINE

- Carbamazepine is well absorbed. Its plasma half-life is about 30 hours when it is given as a single dose, but it is a strong inducing agent, and the plasma half-life shortens to about 15 hours when it is given repeatedly.
- Carbamazepine produces a variety of unwanted effects ranging from drowsiness, dizziness and ataxia to more severe mental and motor disturbances. It can also cause water retention and a variety of gastrointestinal and cardiovascular side effects. Severe bone marrow depression, causing neutropenia, and other severe forms of hypersensitivity reaction can occur.
- Carbamazepine is a powerful inducer of hepatic microsomal enzymes, and thus accelerates the metabolism of many other drugs, such as phenytoin, oral contraceptives, warfarin and corticosteroids. Ozcarbazepine, is a prodrug that is metabolized to a compound closely resembling carbamazepine, with similar actions but less tendency to induce drug-metabolizing enzymes.

VALPROATE

- Valproate is effective in many kinds of epilepsy, being particularly useful in certain types of infantile epilepsy, where its low toxicity and lack of sedative action are important, and in adolescents in whom grand mal and petit mal coexist, because valproate is effective against both. Valproate is also used in psychiatric conditions such as bipolar depressive illness.
- Valproate causes a significant increase in the GABA content of the brain and is a weak inhibitor of two enzyme systems that inactivate GABA, namely GABA transaminase and succinic semialdehyde dehydrogenase. It also inhibits sodium channels, but less so than phenytoin.
- Valproate is well absorbed orally and excreted, mainly as the glucuronide, in the urine, the plasma half-life being about 15 hours.
- The most serious side effect is hepatotoxicity. Valproate is teratogenic, causing spina bifida and other neural tube defects.

ETHOSUXIMIDE

- Ethosuximide, which belongs to the succinimide class is active against PTZ-induced convulsions in animals and against absence seizures in humans, with little or no effect on other types of epilepsy. It is superior to trimethadione, the first drug found to be effective in absence seizures, which had major side effects.
- The mechanism of action of ethosuximide is inhibition of T-type calcium channels, which may play a role in generating the 3 per second firing rhythm in thalamic relay neurons that is characteristic of absence seizures.
- Ethosuximide is well absorbed and metabolised and excreted, with a plasma half-life of about 50 hours. Its main side effects are nausea and anorexia, sometimes lethargy and dizziness.

PHENOBARBITAL

- Phenobarbital closely resembles phenytoin; it affects the duration and intensity of artificially induced seizures, rather than the seizure threshold, and is ineffective in treating absence seizures. The clinical uses of phenobarbital are the same as those of phenytoin, although phenytoin is preferred because of the absence of sedation.
- Phenobarbital is well absorbed, and about 50% of the drug in the blood is bound to plasma albumin. It is eliminated slowly from the plasma (half-life, 50–140 hours). About 25% is excreted unchanged in the urine. its ionisation and hence renal elimination are increased if the urine is made alkaline. Phenobarbital is a powerful inducer of liver P450 enzymes, and it lowers the plasma concentration of several other drugs (e.g. steroids, oral contraceptive, warfarin, tricyclic antidepressants).
- The main adverse effect of phenobarbital is sedation, which often occurs at plasma concentrations within the therapeutic range for seizure control. Other unwanted effects are megaloblastic anemia, mild hypersensitivity reactions and osteomalacia. It must not be given to patients with porphyria. In overdose, phenobarbital produces coma and respiratory and circulatory failure.

BENZODIAZEPINES

Diazepam, given intravenously or rectally, is used to treat *status epilepticus*. Clonazepam and the related compound clobazam are relatively selective as antiepileptic drugs. Sedation is the main side effect of these compounds, withdrawal syndrome occurs, which results in an exacerbation of seizures if the drug is stopped abruptly.

NEWER ANTIEPILEPTIC DRUGS

Vigabatrin

Vigabatrin is a vinyl-substituted analogue of GABA, an inhibitor of the GABA-metabolizing enzyme GABA transaminase. Vigabatrin increases the content of GABA in the cerebrospinal fluid. Although its plasma half-life is short, it produces a long-lasting effect because the enzyme is blocked irreversibly, and the drug can be given orally once daily. The main drawback of vigabatrin is the occurrence of depression, and occasionally psychotic disturbances.

Lamotrigine

- Lamotrigine resembles phenytoin and carbamazepine in its pharmacological effects, acting on sodium channels and inhibiting the release of excitatory amino acids. It has a broader therapeutic profile than the earlier drugs, with significant efficacy against absence seizures and unrelated psychiatric disorders.
- Its main side effects are nausea, dizziness and ataxia, and hypersensitivity reactions (mainly mild rashes, but occasionally more severe). Its plasma half-life is about 24 hours and it is taken orally.

Gabapentin

- Gabapentin, a simple analogue of GABA is an effective anticonvulsant. Its main site of action is on T-type calcium channel function, by binding to a particular channel subunit, and it inhibits the release of various neurotransmitters and modulators. The side effects of gabapentin (mainly sedation and ataxia) are less severe than with many antiepileptic drugs. Its plasma half-life is about 6 hours, requiring dosing two to three times daily.
- It is also used as an analgesic to treat neuropathic pain. A derivative, Pregabalin, is more potent than gabapentin. These drugs are excreted unchanged in the urine, and so must be used with care in patients whose renal function is impaired.

Tiagabine

Tiagabine, an analogue of GABA that is able to penetrate the blood-brain barrier and acts by inhibiting the reuptake of GABA by neurons and glia by depressing transporter GAT-1. It enhances the extracellular GABA concentration and also potentiates and prolongs GABA-mediated synaptic responses in the brain. It has a short plasma half-life, and its main side effects are drowsiness and confusion.

Topiramate

Topiramate acts by blocking sodium channels, enhancing the action of GABA, blocking AMPA receptors and weakly inhibiting carbonic anhydrase. Currently, it is recommended for use as add-on therapy in refractory cases of epilepsy.

Levetiracetam

Levetiracetam, an analogue of piracetam, has little or no effect on known targets (ion channels and GABA-related mechanisms), and its mechanism of action is unknown.

Zonisamide

Zonisamide is a sulfonamide compound which acts by blocking sodium channels. It is free of major unwanted effects, although it causes drowsiness, and of serious interaction with other drugs. It tends to suppress appetite and cause weight loss, has a long plasma half-life of 60–80 hours, and is partly excreted unchanged and partly converted to a glucuronide metabolite.

Felbamate

- Felbamate is an analogue of an anxiolytic drug, meprobamate. It has only a weak effect on sodium channels and little effect on GABA, but causes some block of the NMDA receptor channel. Its acute side effects are mild, mainly nausea, irritability and insomnia, but it occasionally causes severe reactions resulting in aplastic anemia or hepatitis.
- Its use is limited to a form of intractable epilepsy in children (Lennox-Gastaut syndrome) that is unresponsive to other drugs.

Summary of Primary Established Antiepileptics

Drugs	Uses	Half-life	Neurologic effects	Systemic effects
Phenytoin (diphenyl-hydantoin)	Tonic-clonic (grand mal) Focal-onset	24 hours (wide variation, dose-dependent)	Dizziness Diplopia Ataxia Incoordination Confusion	Gum hyperplasia Lymphadenopathy Hirsutism Osteomalacia Facial coarsening Skin rash
Carbamazepine	Tonic-clonic Focal-onset	10–17 hours	Ataxia Dizziness Diplopia Vertigo	Aplastic anemia Leukopenia Gastrointestinal irritation Hepatotoxicity Hyponatremia
Valproic acid	Tonic-clonic Absence Atypical absence Myoclonic Focal-onset	15 hours	Ataxia Sedation Tremor	Hepatotoxicity Thrombocytopenia Gastrointestinal irritation Weight gain Transient alopecia Hyperammonemia
Ethosuximide	Absence (petit mal)	60 hours, adult 30 hours, child	Ataxia Lethargy Headache	Gastrointestinal irritation, Skin rash Bone marrow suppression
Phenobarbital	Tonic-clonic Focal-onset	90 hours (70 hours in children)	Sedation Ataxia Confusion Dizziness Decreased libido Depression	Skin rash

ANTI-PARKINSON'S DRUGS

Parkinson's disease results in an imbalance between dopamine and acetylcholine levels in the nigrostriatal tract. Thus, effective therapy results from lowering acetylcholine levels or activity to correlate with reduced dopamine levels or increasing dopaminergic activity to correlate with normal acetylcholine levels.

Dopamine itself cannot be used for treatment because dopamine is ionized at physiologic pH, and does not effectively cross the blood-brain barrier. In addition, systemic administration of dopamine has effects on major organs (e.g. heart and kidney), resulting in a high degree of adverse effects.

CLASSIFICATION

- Levodopa (dopamine precursor), given with an inhibitor of peripheral dopa decarboxylase (e.g. Carbidopa) to minimise side effects;
- Catechol-o-methyltransferase inhibitor (e.g. entacapone, tolcapone)
- Bromocriptine (dopamine agonist)
- Selegiline (monoamine oxidase B inhibitor)
- Amantadine (which may enhance dopamine release)
- Benztropine, trihexyphenidyl (benzhexol), Procyclidine, Biperiden, and promethazine (muscarinic receptor antagonist used for Parkinsonism caused by antipsychotic drugs).

LEVODOPA

- Levodopa is the first-line treatment for PD and is combined with a peripheral dopa decarboxylase inhibitor, either carbidopa or benserazide, which reduces the dose needed by about 10-fold and diminishes the peripheral side effects.

- It is well absorbed from the small intestine, a process that relies on active transport, although much of it is inactivated by MAO in the wall of the intestine. Bioavailability is affected by gastric emptying and amino acids in food. The plasma half-life is short (about 2 hours). Conversion to dopamine in the periphery is largely prevented by the decarboxylase inhibitor.
- Decarboxylation occurs rapidly within the brain, because the decarboxylase inhibitors do not penetrate the blood-brain barrier. Levodopa can act even when no dopaminergic nerve terminals are present. On the other hand, the therapeutic effectiveness of Levodopa decreases as the disease advances, so part of its action may rely on the presence of functional dopaminergic neurons.
- Most of the patients show initial improvement with Levodopa, particularly of rigidity and hypokinesia, and few are restored virtually to normal motor function. As time progresses, the effectiveness of Levodopa gradually declines. It is likely that the loss of effectiveness of Levodopa mainly reflects the natural progression of the disease, but receptor down regulation and other compensatory mechanisms may also contribute.

Adverse Effects

- Involuntary writhing movements (dyskinesia), which do not appear initially but develop in the majority of patients within 2 years of starting Involuntary writhing movements (dyskinesia), which do not appear initially but develop in the majority of patients within 2 years of starting Levodopa therapy. These movements usually affect the face and limbs, and can become very severe. They occur at the time of the peak therapeutic effect, and the margin between the beneficial and the dyskinetic effect becomes progressively narrower
- Rapid fluctuations in clinical state, where hypokinesia and rigidity may suddenly worsen for anything from a few minutes to a few hours, and then improve again. This is called 'on-off effect'. As with the dyskinesias, the problem seems to reflect the fluctuating plasma concentration of Levodopa, and it is suggested that as the disease advances, the ability of neurons to store dopamine is lost, so the therapeutic benefit of Levodopa depends increasingly on the continuous formation of extraneuronal dopamine, which requires a continuous supply of Levodopa.
- Nausea, alteration in taste sensation and anorexia—*Domperidone,* a dopamine antagonist that works in the chemoreceptor trigger zone (where the blood-brain barrier is leaky) but does not gain access to the basal ganglia, may be useful in preventing this effect.
- *Hypotension:* Postural hypotension is a problem in a few patients.
- Psychological effects. Levodopa, by increasing dopamine activity in the brain, can produce a schizophrenia-like syndrome with delusions and hallucinations.
- Pyridoxine abolishes the therapeutic effect of levodopa.

SELEGILINE

- Selegiline (L-deprenyl) is a MAO inhibitor that is selective for MAO-B, which predominates in dopamine-containing regions of the CNS. It therefore lacks the unwanted peripheral effects of non-selective MAO inhibitors used to treat depression and, in contrast to them, does not provoke the 'cheese reaction' or interact so frequently with other drugs.
- Inhibition of MAO-B protects dopamine from intraneuronal degradation and was initially used as an adjunct to Levodopa. Selegiline might be neuroprotective rather than merely enhancing the action of Levodopa.
- It is contraindicated in epileptic patients.

Dopamine Receptor Agonists

- Bromocriptine, derived from the ergot alkaloids, is a potent agonist at dopamine (D_2) receptors in the CNS. Its duration of action is longer (plasma half-life 6-8 hours) than that of Levodopa, so that it does not need to be given so frequently.
- The main side effects of bromocriptine are nausea and vomiting, and peritoneal fibrosis, as seen with other ergot derivatives.
- Newer dopamine receptor agonists include lisuride, pergolide, ropinirole, Cabergoline and pramipexole. They are longer acting than Levodopa and need to be given only once or twice daily, with fewer tendencies to cause dyskinesias and on-off effects.
- Pramipexole may have antioxidant effects, as well as a protective effect on mitochondria. Piribedil is used as a cerebroactive drug.

Catechol-*o*-methyl Transferase (COMT) Inhibitors

- Combination of Levodopa plus dopa decarboxylase inhibitor with tolcapone and entacapone, inhibitors of Catechol-*o*-methyl transferase (COMT) to inhibit its degradation, is used in patients troubled by 'end of dose' motor fluctuations. But worsening of levodopa adverse effects with yellowish discoloration of urine occurs.

Amantadine

- Amantadine was introduced as an antiviral drug and discovered by accident to be beneficial in PD. Many possible mechanisms for its action have been suggested based on neurochemical evidence of increased dopamine release, inhibition of amine uptake, or a direct action on dopamine receptors.
- Amantadine is less effective than Levodopa or bromocriptine, and its action declines with time. Its side effects are considerably less severe, although qualitatively similar to those of Levodopa, though ankle swelling and Livedo reticularis are particularly common.

Central Anticholinergics

- Muscarinic acetylcholine receptors exert an inhibitory effect on dopaminergic nerve terminals, suppression of which compensates for a lack of dopamine.
- Commonly used drugs are trihexiphenidyl (benzhexol), Procyclidine, Biperiden, and promethazine.
- The side effects of muscarinic antagonists—dry mouth, constipation, impaired vision, urinary retention.
- Used to treat parkinsonian symptoms in patients receiving antipsychotic drugs (which are dopamine antagonists and thus nullify the effect of L-dopa).

ANTIPSYCHOTIC AGENTS

The terms antipsychotic and neuroleptic are used interchangeably to denote a group of drugs that have been used mainly for treating schizophrenia but are also effective in some other psychoses and agitated states.

NEUROLEPTIC DRUGS

Also called antischizophrenic drugs, antipsychotic drugs, or major tranquilizers) are used primarily to treat schizophrenia but are also effective in other psychotic states, such as manic states and delirium.

Pharmacologically, they are characterized as dopamine receptor antagonists, although many of them also act on other targets, particularly 5-hydroxytryptamine (5-HT) receptors, which may contribute to their clinical efficacy.

CLASSIFICATION OF ANTIPSYCHOTIC DRUGS

- First-generation ('typical') antipsychotics(e.g. chlorpromazine, haloperidol, fluphenazine, flupenthixol)
- Second-generation ('atypical') antipsychotics (e.g. clozapine, risperidone, sertindole, quetiapine, amisulpride, aripiprazole, zotepine).

Distinction between typical and atypical groups **is based on**

- Receptor profile
- Incidence of extrapyramidal side effects (less in atypical group)
- Efficacy against negative symptoms.

GENERAL PROPERTIES

Pharmacological investigation showed that phenothiazines, the first drugs used for the purpose block many different mediators, including *histamine, catecholamines, acetylcholine* and *5-HT*, and this multiplicity of actions led to the trade name Largactil for chlorpromazine. Antagonism of *dopamine* is the main determinant of antipsychotic action.

MECHANISM OF ACTION—DOPAMINE THEORY OF SCHIZOPHRENIA

- There are five subtypes, which fall into two functional classes: the D_1 type, comprising D_1 and D_5, and the D_2 type, comprising D_2, D_3 and D_4.
- Antipsychotic drugs owe their therapeutic effects mainly to blockade of D_2-receptors. The first-generation compounds show some preference for D_2 over D_1-receptors, whereas some of the newer agents (e.g. sulpiride, amisulpride, remoxipride) are highly selective for D_2-receptors. Clozapine is relatively non-selective between D_1– and D_2–, but has high affinity for D_4.

- Effects on the mesolimbic/mesocortical dopamine pathways are believed to correlate with antipsychotic effects, whereas effects on the nigrostriatal pathways are responsible for the unwanted motor effects produced by antipsychotic drugs. Haloperidol, a first-generation drug with marked unwanted motor effects, acts on both sets of dopamine neurons, whereas clozapine and other drugs that have much less tendency to cause adverse motor effects affect mainly the ventral tegmental neurons.
- Antipsychotic drugs, like many neuroactive compounds, take several weeks to take effect, even though their receptor-blocking action is immediate.
- Antipsychotic drugs show varying patterns of selectivity in their receptor-blocking effects, some having high affinity for $5-HT_2$ and/or D_4-receptors.

Comparing Major Antipsychotics and their Effects

Drug/Effects	Extrapyramidal	Sedative	Hypotensive	Antiemetic
Chlorpromazine	++	+++	+++	++
Haloperidol	+++	+	+	+++
Pimozide	+++	++	+	+
Clozapine	+/-	++	+++	-
Olanzapine	+	+	++	-

Adverse Effects

Extrapyramidal Motor Disturbances and Tardive Dyskinesia

- Antipsychotic drugs produce two main kinds of motor disturbance in humans: *acute dystonias* and *tardive dyskinesias*, collectively termed *extrapyramidal side effects*. These all result directly or indirectly from D_2-receptor blockade. Extrapyramidal side effects constitute one of the main disadvantages of first-generation antipsychotic drugs.
- *Acute dystonias* are involuntary movements (restlessness, muscle spasms, protruding tongue, fixed upward gaze, torticollis, i.e. involuntary spasm of neck muscles resulting in turning of the head, etc.), often accompanied by symptoms of Parkinson's disease. They occur commonly in the first few weeks, often declining with time, and are reversible on stopping drug treatment. The timing is consistent with block of the dopaminergic nigrostriatal pathway, and the relative selectivity of atypical antipsychotic drugs for the mesolimbic/mesocortical pathway could account for the diminished risk of acute dystonias with these drugs.
- *Tardive dyskinesia* develops after months or years (hence 'tardive') in patients treated with first-generation antipsychotic drugs. An often irreversible condition gets worse when antipsychotic therapy is stopped and is resistant to treatment. The syndrome consists of involuntary movements, often of the face and tongue, but also of the trunk and limbs, which can be severely disabling. It is associated with a gradual increase in the number of D_2-receptors in the striatum, which is less marked during treatment with the atypical than with the first generation of antipsychotic drugs.
- Incidence of acute dystonias and tardive dyskinesia is less with atypical antipsychotics, and particularly low with clozapine, aripiprazole and zotepine. This may reflect relatively strong muscarinic receptor block with these drugs, or a degree of selectivity for the mesolimbic, as opposed to the nigrostriatal, dopamine pathways.

Endocrine Effects

Dopamine, released in the median eminence by neurons of the tuberohypophyseal pathway, acts physiologically to inhibit prolactin secretion via D_2-receptors. Blocking D_2-receptors by antipsychotic drugs can therefore increase the plasma prolactin concentration, resulting in breast swelling, pain and lactation, which can occur in men as well as in women.

Other Effects

- Obstructive jaundice sometimes occurs with phenothiazines.
- Some Other side effects (dry mouth, blurred vision, hypotension, etc.) are due to block of other receptors, particularly α-adrenoceptors and muscarinic acetylcholine receptors.
- Some antipsychotic drugs cause agranulocytosis as a rare and serious idiosyncratic reaction. With clozapine, leucopenia is common and requires routine monitoring.
- Clozapine can cause *agranocytosis* and *wet pillow syndrome*. Olanzapine causes hyperprolactinemia.

Adverse Effects of Antipsychotics

Adverse effects	Features	Duration
Acute dystonias	Muscle spasms; tongue, face, neck, back; terrifying; rarely fatal from asphyxia	1–5 days
Parkinsonism	Bradykinesia, rigidity, variable tremor, mask facies, shuffling gait	1–4 weeks
Malignant syndrome	Catatonia, stupor, fever, unstable pulse, blood pressure and respirations, elevated serum creatine kinase and myoglobin	Days to weeks
Akathisia	Motor "inner" restlessness with anxiety and agitation	Can start immediately
Tardive dyskinesias	Oral-facial dyskinesia, choreoathetosis, variable dystonia	Months to years; gets worse when drug is stopped

Pharmacokinetics

- Chlorpromazine, in common with many other phenothiazines, is erratically absorbed after oral administration. The relationship between the plasma concentration and the clinical effect of antipsychotic drugs is highly variable.
- The plasma half-life of most antipsychotic drugs is 15–30 hours, clearance depending entirely on hepatic transformation by a combination of oxidative and conjugative reactions.
- Most antipsychotic drugs can be given orally or by intramuscular injection once or twice a day. Slow-release (depot) preparations of many are available, in which the active drug is esterified with heptanoic or decanoic acid and dissolved in oil.

ANTIDEPRESSANTS

Majority of antidepressants are Inhibitors of monoamine uptake.

Classification

- Non-selective (noradrenaline/serotonin) uptake inhibitors include tricyclic antidepressants (TCAs) (e.g. imipramine, amitriptyline) and more recent antidepressants such as venlafaxine and duloxetine.
- Selective serotonin reuptake inhibitors (SSRIs) (e.g. fluoxetine, fluvoxamine, paroxetine and sertraline).
- Selective noradrenaline uptake inhibitors (e.g. maprotiline, reboxetine).
- Monoamine oxidase (MAO) inhibitors (MAOIs):
    - Irreversible, non-competitive inhibitors (e.g. phenelzine, tranylcypromine), which are non-selective with respect to the MAO-A and -B subtypes.
    - Reversible, MAO-A-selective inhibitors (e.g. moclobemide).
- Atypical antidepressants: Trazodone, Mianserin, Mirtazapine, Tianeptine, Bupropion.
- The herbal preparation St John's wort, with the active ingredient hyperforin.

TRICYCLIC ANTIDEPRESSANT DRUGS

- Tricyclic antidepressants are closely related in structure to the phenothiazines.
- All the compounds are tertiary amines, with two methyl groups attached to the basic nitrogen atom. They are quite rapidly demethylated in vivo to the corresponding secondary amines (desipramine, nortriptyline, etc.), which are themselves active. Other tricyclic derivatives with slightly modified bridge structures include doxepin.
- The main immediate effect of TCAs is to block the uptake of amines by nerve terminals, by competition for the binding site of the amine transporter. Most TCAs inhibit noradrenaline and 5-HT uptake by brain synaptosomes to a similar degree but have much less effect on dopamine uptake. In addition to their effects on amine uptake, most TCAs affect one or more types of neurotransmitter receptor, including muscarinic acetylcholine receptors, histamine receptors and 5-HT receptors. The antimuscarinic effects of TCAs do not contribute to their antidepressant effects but are responsible for various troublesome side effects.
- TCAs cause sedation, confusion and motor incoordination which occurs in the first few days of treatment, but tend to wear off in 1-2 weeks as the antidepressant effect develops. Atropine-like effects include dry mouth, blurred vision, constipation and urinary retention which are strong with amitriptyline and much weaker with desipramine. Postural hypotension and sedation occurs with TCAs. Tricyclic antidepressants, particularly in overdose, may cause ventricular dysrhythmias associated with

prolongation of the QT interval. The initial effect of TCA overdosage is to cause excitement and delirium, which may be accompanied by convulsions and is followed by coma and respiratory depression. Atropine-like effects are pronounced, including flushing, dry mouth and skin, mydriasis, and inhibition of gut and bladder. Cardiac arrhythmias are common, and sudden death may occur from ventricular fibrillation.

- Tricyclic antidepressants rely on hepatic microsomal metabolism for elimination, and this may be inhibited by competing drugs (e.g. antipsychotic drugs and some steroids). Tricyclic antidepressants potentiate the effects of *alcohol* and anesthetic agents.
- Tricyclic antidepressants are all rapidly absorbed when given orally and bind strongly to plasma albumin, most being 90-95% bound at therapeutic plasma concentrations. They also bind to extravascular tissues and have low rates of elimination. hemodialysis is ineffective as a means of increasing drug elimination. Tricyclic antidepressants are metabolised in the liver by two main routes, N-*demethylation*, whereby tertiary amines are converted to secondary amines and *ring hydroxylation*. The overall half-times for elimination of TCAs are generally long, ranging from 10 to 20 hours for imipramine and desipramine to about 80 hours for protriptyline.

SELECTIVE SEROTONIN UPTAKE INHIBITORS (SSRIS)

- *Selective serotonin reuptake inhibitors (SSRIs)* include fluoxetine, fluvoxamine, paroxetine, citalopram and sertraline. They are the most commonly prescribed group of antidepressants. They show selectivity with respect to 5-HT over noradrenaline uptake and are less likely than TCAs to cause anticholinergic side effects and are less dangerous in overdose. They do not cause 'cheese reactions'. They are also drugs of choice to treat *obsessive compulsive disorder*.
- The SSRIs are well absorbed, and most have plasma half-lives of 15–24 hours (fluoxetine being a longer acting drug with half life of 24–96 hours).
- Common side effects are nausea, anorexia, insomnia, loss of libido and failure of orgasm. In combination with MAOIs, SSRIs can cause a 'serotonin syndrome' characterized by *tremor*, *hyperthermia* and *cardiovascular collapse*.
- 5-HT uptake inhibitors are used in a variety of psychiatric disorders, as well as in depression, including anxiety disorders, panic attacks, impulse disorders and obsessive compulsive disorder.

MONOAMINE OXIDASE INHIBITORS

- Monoamine oxidase inhibitors (MAOIs) are largely superseded by tricyclic and other types of antidepressants, whose clinical efficacies were considered better and whose side effects are generally less than those of MAOIs. The main examples are phenelzine, tranylcypromine and iproniazid.
- Monoamine oxidase is found in nearly all tissues, and exists in two similar molecular forms coded by separate genes. MAO-A has a substrate preference for 5-HT and is the main target for the antidepressant MAOIs. MAO-B has a substrate preference for phenylethylamine, and both enzymes act on noradrenaline and dopamine. Type B is selectively inhibited by selegiline, which is used in the treatment of Parkinsonism. Most antidepressant MAOIs act on both forms of MAO, but antidepressant activity, as well as the main side effects of MAOIs, is associated with MAO-A inhibition. MAO is located intracellularly and is mostly associated with mitochondria.
- Within nerve terminals, MAO regulates the free intraneuronal concentration of noradrenaline or 5-HT, and hence the releasable stores of these transmitters. It is not involved in the inactivation of released transmitter. MAO is important in the inactivation of endogenous and ingested amines that would otherwise produce unwanted effects. An example is *tyramine*, an ingested amine that is a substrate for both MAO-A and MAO-B, and is important in producing some clinically important adverse interactions of MAOIs with foods and other drugs.
- Monoamine oxidase inhibitors cause a rapid and sustained increase in the 5-HT, noradrenaline and dopamine content of the brain, 5-HT being affected most and dopamine least. Similar changes occur in peripheral tissues such as heart, liver and intestine, and increases in the plasma concentrations of these amines are also detectable. In contrast to the effect of TCAs, MAOIs do not increase the response of peripheral organs, such as the heart and blood vessels, to sympathetic nerve stimulation. The main effect of MAOIs is to increase the cytoplasmic concentration of monoamines in nerve terminals, without greatly affecting the vesicular stores that form the pool that is releasable by nerve stimulation.
- Many of the unwanted effects of MAOIs result directly from MAO inhibition, but some are produced by other mechanisms. Hypotension is a common side effect. Excessive central stimulation may cause tremors, excitement, insomnia and, in overdose, convulsions. Increased appetite, leading to weight gain can occur. Atropine-like side effects (dry mouth, blurred vision, urinary retention, etc.) are common with MAOIs, although they are less of a problem than with TCAs.

- Interaction with other drugs and foods is the most serious problem with MAOIs and is the main factor that caused their clinical use to decline. The *cheese reaction* is a direct consequence of MAO inhibition and occurs when normally innocuous amines (mainly tyramine) produced during fermentation are ingested. MAO inhibition allows tyramine to be absorbed, and also enhances its sympathomimetic effect, as discussed above. The result is acute hypertension, giving rise to a severe throbbing headache and occasionally even to intracranial hemorrhage.

Atypical Antidepressant Drugs

- Heterogeneous group including trazodone, mirtazapine and bupropion.
- They have no common mechanism of action. They act mainly as non-selective antagonists at presynaptic receptors, possibly enhancing amine release.
- Mianserin blocks presynaptic alpha 2 receptors. Tianeptine increases 5-HT uptake. Venlafaxine is an SNRI (Serotonin and Noradrenaline Reuptake inhibitor). Mirtazapine is labeled as NaSSA (Noradrenaline and selective serotonin antidepressant). Bupropion is used as a sustained release formulation in aid to smoking cessation.
- Delay in therapeutic response is similar to that with tricyclic antidepressants and monoamine oxidase inhibitors, though Mirtazapine may act more rapidly.
- Unwanted effects and acute toxicity vary but are generally less than with tricyclic antidepressants. Trazodone causes priapism.

Major Antidepressants and their Effects

Drug/Effects	Sedative	Antimuscarinic	Hypotension	Arrhythmogenicity	Seizure precipitation
Amitriptyline	+++	+++	+++	+++	++
Amoxapine	+	+	++	++	++
Fluoxetine	+/-	-	-	-	-
Trazodone	+++	-	+	-	-
Bupropion	+	-	-	-	+++
Mirtazapine	+++	-	+/-	-	-
Venlafaxine	-	-	-	+	-

MOOD-STABILIZING DRUGS

These drugs are used to control the mood swings characteristic of manic-depressive (bipolar) illness. Lithium is most commonly used, but antiepileptic drugs such as carbamazepine, valproate and gabapentin, which have fewer side effects than lithium, have also proved efficacious. Mood-stabilizing drugs prevent the swings of mood and thus reduce both the depressive and the manic phases of the illness.

LITHIUM

- Lithium is clinically effective at a plasma concentration of 0.5-1 mmol/L, and above 1.5 mmol/L it produces a variety of toxic effects, so the therapeutic window is narrow. Lithium is a monovalent cation that can mimic the role of Na^+ in excitable tissues, being able to permeate the voltage-gated Na^+ channels that are responsible for action potential generation, leading to a partial loss of intracellular K^+, and depolarization of the cell.
- Inhibition of inositol monophosphatase, which blocks the phosphatidyl inositol (PI) pathway at the point where inositol phosphate is hydrolysed to free inositol, results in depletion of PI. This prevents agonist-stimulated inositol trisphosphate formation through various PI-linked receptors, and therefore blocks many receptor-mediated effects. Lithium also inhibits hormone-induced cAMP production and blocks other cellular responses.
- Lithium is given orally and is excreted by the kidney. Lithium accumulates slowly over 2 weeks or more before a steady state is reached. The narrow therapeutic window (approximately 0.5–1.5 mmol/L) means that monitoring of the plasma concentration is essential.
- The main toxic effects that may occur during treatment are nausea, vomiting and diarrhea, tremor, and renal effects like polyuria (with resulting thirst) resulting from inhibition of the action of antidiuretic hormone, hypothyroidism and weight gain. acute toxic effects include cerebellar effects, nephrogenic diabetes insipidus.

Clinical Use of Mood-stabilizing Drugs

- Lithium is the main drug used in prophylaxis and treatment of *mania*, and in the prophylaxis of *bipolar* or *unipolar disorder* (manic depression or recurrent depression).
- Carbamazepine and valproic acid are used, respectively, for the prophylaxis and treatment of manic episodes in patients with bipolar disorder unresponsive to lithium. Lamotrigine is also an useful alternative.
- Valproic acid is used in rapid cyclers.

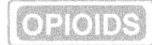

CLASSIFICATION

- Opioid drugs include:
  - Phenanthrene derivatives structurally related to morphine.
  - Synthetic compounds with a variety of dissimilar structures but similar pharmacological effects.
- Morphine-like agonists include diamorphine and codeine
- Partial agonists (e.g. nalorphine and levallorphan) or antagonists (e.g. naloxone, naltrexone).
- Synthetic analogues are pethidine, fentanyl, methadone, pentazocine and the thebaine derivatives (e.g. buprenorphine).

OPIOID ANALGESIC DRUGS

- The term *opioid* applies to any substance, whether endogenous or synthetic, that produces morphine-like effects that are blocked by antagonists such as naloxone. Opium contains many alkaloids related to morphine. In addition to morphine-like compounds, opium also contains papaverine, a smooth muscle relaxant.
- Morphine is a phenanthrene derivative. Pethidine (known as meperidine in the US) was the first fully synthetic morphine-like drug. Its pharmacological actions are very similar to morphine. Fentanyl and sufentanil are more potent and shorter-acting derivatives that are used intravenously, or for chronic pain via patches applied to the skin, to treat severe pain or as an adjunct to anesthesia. Methadone is longer acting than morphine but otherwise very similar to it. Pentazocine and cyclazocine are drugs which differ from morphine in their receptor-binding profile and so have somewhat different actions and side effects. Buprenorphine resembles morphine but is a partial agonist; therefore, although very potent, its maximal effect is less than that of morphine, and it antagonises the effect of other opiates.

Opioid Receptors

- Three types of opioid receptor, termed μ, δ and κ (all of them typical G-protein-coupled receptors) and mediate the main pharmacological effects of opiates. The major pharmacological effects of morphine, including analgesia, are mediated by the μ-receptor.
- μ-Receptors are thought to be responsible for most of the analgesic effects of opioids, and for some major unwanted effects (e.g. respiratory depression, euphoria, sedation and dependence). Most of the analgesic opioids are ì-receptor agonists.
- δ-Receptors are probably more important in the periphery but may also contribute to analgesia.
- κ-Receptors contribute to analgesia at the spinal level and may elicit sedation and dysphoria, but produce relatively few unwanted effects and do not contribute to dependence.
- α-Receptors are not true opioid receptors but are the site of action of certain psychotomimetic drugs, with which some opioids interact.

OPIOID CATEGORIES

- *Pure agonists*—This group includes most of the typical morphine-like drugs. They all have high affinity for ì receptors and generally lower affinity for ä and ê sites.
- *Partial agonists and mixed agonist-antagonists*—These drugs, typified by nalorphine and pentazocine, combine a degree of agonist and antagonist activity on different receptors. Pentazocine and cyclazocine, are antagonists at ì-receptors but partial agonists on ä and ê-receptors.

- *Antagonists*—These drugs produce very little effect when given on their own but block the effects of opiates. The most important examples are naloxone and naltrexone.

MECHANISM OF ACTION OF OPIATES

- All opioid receptors are linked through G-proteins to inhibition of adenylate cyclase. They also facilitate opening of potassium channels (causing hyperpolarization) and inhibit opening of calcium channels (inhibiting transmitter release). These membrane effects are not linked to the decrease in cAMP formation. The overall effect is therefore inhibitory at the cellular level, increasing activity in some neuronal pathways by suppressing the firing of inhibitory interneurons.
- At the spinal level, morphine inhibits transmission of nociceptive impulses through the dorsal horn and suppresses nociceptive spinal reflexes. It can inhibit release of substance P from primary afferent terminals in the dorsal horn neurons. Opiates inhibit the discharge of nociceptive afferent terminals in the periphery, particularly under conditions of inflammation, in which the expression of opioid receptors by sensory neurons is increased.

MORPHINE

- The most important effects of morphine are on the CNS and the gastrointestinal tract, although numerous effects of lesser significance on many other systems have been described.
- Morphine is effective in most kinds of acute and chronic pain. Morphine also reduces the affective component of pain which reflects its supraspinal action, possibly at the level of the limbic system.

Effects

- Morphine causes a sense of contentment and well-being. If morphine or diamorphine (heroin) is given intravenously, the result is a sudden 'rush'. Euphoria appears to be mediated through μ receptors, and to be balanced by the dysphoria associated with κ-receptor activation.
- Respiratory depression, resulting in increased arterial pCO_2, occurs with a normal analgesic dose of morphine or related compounds. Analgesia and respiratory depression are both mediated by μ-receptors. Respiratory depression by opiates is not accompanied by depression of the medullary centers controlling cardiovascular function. respiratory depression is the most troublesome unwanted effect of these drugs and the commonest cause of death in acute opiate poisoning.
- Nausea and vomiting occur due to the effect on area postrema (chemoreceptor trigger zone), a region of the medulla where chemical stimuli of many kinds may initiate vomiting.
- Pupillary constriction is caused by μ and κ receptor-mediated stimulation of the oculomotor nucleus. Pinpoint pupils are an important diagnostic feature in opiate poisoning, because most other causes of coma and respiratory depression produce pupillary dilatation.
- Morphine increases tone and reduces motility in many parts of the gastrointestinal system, resulting in constipation. Pressure in the biliary tract increases because of contraction of the gallbladder and constriction of the biliary sphincter. Opiates should hence be avoided in patients suffering from biliary colic. The rise in intrabiliary pressure can cause a transient increase in the concentration of amylase and lipase in the plasma.
- Morphine releases histamine from mast cells causing local effects, such as urticaria and itching at the site of the injection, or systemic effects, namely bronchoconstriction and hypotension. Morphine should not be given in asthmatic patients.
- *Tolerance* to opiates (i.e. an increase in the dose needed to produce a given pharmacological effect) develops within a few days. *Physical dependence* refers to a state in which withdrawal of the drug causes adverse physiological effects. These phenomena occur to some degree whenever opiates are administered for more than a few days.
- Acute overdosage with morphine results in coma and respiratory depression, with characteristically constricted pupils. It is treated by giving naloxone intravenously.

Pharmacokinetics

- The plasma half-life of most morphine analogues is 3–6 hours. Hepatic metabolism is the main mode of inactivation, usually by conjugation with glucuronide. Morphine glucuronides are excreted in the urine, so the dose needs to be reduced in cases of renal failure. Morphine congeners should not be used in the neonatal period, nor during childbirth.
- Morphine produces very effective analgesia when administered intrathecally, and is often used in this way by anesthetists.

OTHER OPIATE ANALGESICS

Diamorphine (Heroin)
- Heroin is the diacetyl derivative of morphine. It is rapidly deacetylated to morphine, and its effects are indistinguishable following oral administration.
- Because of its greater lipid solubility, it crosses the blood-brain barrier more rapidly than morphine and gives a greater rush when injected intravenously. It is less emetic than morphine and is better soluble, which allows smaller volumes to be given orally, subcutaneously or intrathecally. It exerts the same respiratory depressant effect as morphine, and if given intravenously is more likely to cause dependence.

Codeine
- It is more reliably absorbed by mouth than morphine, but has only 10% or less of the analgesic potency of morphine. It causes little or no euphoria and is rarely addictive. Codeine produces the same degree of respiratory depression as morphine.
- Codeine has marked antitussive activity and is often used in cough mixtures.

Pethidine (Meperidine)
- Pethidine is very similar to morphine in its pharmacological effects, except that it tends to cause restlessness rather than sedation, and it has an additional antimuscarinic action that may cause dry mouth and blurring of vision as side effects.
- It produces a very similar euphoric effect and is equally liable to cause dependence. Its duration of action is similar to that of morphine. Pethidine is partly N-demethylated in the liver to norpethidine, which has a hallucinogenic and convulsant effect.
- Pethidine is preferred to morphine for analgesia during labor, because it does not reduce the force of uterine contraction.

Fentanyl
- Fentanyl and sufentanil are highly potent phenylpiperidine derivatives, with actions similar to those of morphine but with a more rapid onset and shorter duration of action, particularly sufentanil. Other drugs related are alfentanyl and remifentanyl.
- Their main use is in anaesthesia, and they may be given intrathecally.

Methadone
- It is also pharmacologically similar to morphine, but the duration of action is considerably longer (plasma half-life > 24 hours).
- Methadone is widely used as a means of treating morphine and heroin addiction. In the presence of methadone, an injection of morphine does not cause the normal euphoria, and makes it possible to wean addicts from morphine by giving regular oral doses of methadone.

Pentazocine (Fortwin)
Pentazocine is a mixed agonist-antagonist with analgesic Properties similar to those of morphine. However, it causes marked dysphoria, with nightmares and hallucinations, rather than euphoria.

Buprenorphine
- It is a partial agonist on ì receptors, less liable to cause dysphoria than pentazocine but more liable to cause respiratory depression. It has a long duration of action.
- It has a Half-life about 12 h, slow onset and is inactive orally because of first-pass metabolism.
- It is one of the drugs used in opioid detoxification and is useful in chronic pain with patient-controlled injection systems.

Tramadol
A metabolite of the antidepressant trazodone, it is widely used as an analgesic for postoperative pain. It is a weak agonist at μ-opioid receptors, and also a weak inhibitor of noradrenaline reuptake. It is effective as an analgesic, is given orally or by intramuscular or intravenous injection for moderate to severe pain.

OPIOID ANTAGONISTS

- Nalorphine is closely related in structure to. In low doses, it is a competitive antagonist and blocks most actions of morphine. Higher doses are analgesic and mimic the effects of morphine which reflect an antagonist action on μ-receptors, coupled with a partial agonist action on δ and κ-receptors, the latter causing dysphoria. Nalorphine can itself produce physical dependence, and can also precipitate a withdrawal syndrome.

- Naloxone was the first pure opioid antagonist, with affinity for all three opioid receptors. It blocks the actions of endogenous opioid peptides as well as those of morphine-like drugs. naloxone produces a rapid reversal of the effects of morphine and other opiates, including partial agonists such as pentazocine and nalorphine. The main clinical uses of naloxone are to treat respiratory depression caused by opiate overdosage, and occasionally to reverse the effect of opiate analgesics, used during labor. It can be used to detect opiate addiction.
- Naltrexone is very similar to naloxone but with the advantage of a much longer duration of action (half-life about 10 hours).
- It is used in addicts who have been detoxified, to prevent relapse.

Clinical Uses of Analgesic Drugs

- Analgesics are used to treat and prevent pain, for example:
  - Pre- and postoperatively
  - Common painful conditions including headache, dysmenorrhea, labour, trauma, burns
  - Many medical and surgical emergencies (e.g. myocardial infarction and renal colic)
  - Terminal disease (especially metastatic cancer).
- Severe acute pain is treated with strong opioids (e.g. morphine, fentanyl) given by injection. Mild inflammatory pain (e.g. sprains, mild arthralgia) is treated with NSAIDs or paracetamol supplemented by weak opioids (e.g. codeine). Severe pain (e.g. cancer pain) is treated with strong opioid given orally, intrathecally, epidurally or by subcutaneous injection. Patient-controlled infusion systems are useful postoperatively.
- Strong opioids (e.g. morphine) are used for severe pain, particularly of visceral origin.

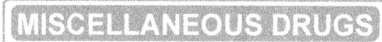

ANALEPTICS

- Convulsants and respiratory stimulants called as *analeptics*. There remains a very limited clinical use for respiratory stimulants in treating acute ventilatory failure, doxapram being most commonly used, because it carries less risk of causing convulsions than earlier compounds.
- Drugs in this group are strychnine, picrotoxin and pentylenetetrazol (PTZ).
- Strychnine is an alkaloid, is a powerful convulsant and acts throughout the CNS but particularly on the spinal cord, causing violent extensor spasms that are triggered by minor sensory stimuli, the head being thrown back and the face fixed. These effects result from blocking receptors for glycine, which is the main inhibitory transmitter acting on motor neurons. In small doses, strychnine causes a measurable improvement in visual and auditory acuity.
- Bicuculline, also a plant alkaloid, resembles strychnine in its effects but acts by blocking receptors for GABA rather than glycine. Its action is confined to $GABA_A$ receptors, which control Cl^- permeability, and it does not affect $GABA_B$ receptors. Its main effects are on the brain rather than the spinal cord.
- Picrotoxin also blocks the action of GABA on chloride channels, although not competitively. Picrotoxin, like bicuculline, causes convulsions and has no clinical uses.
- Pentylenetetrazol acts similarly. Inhibition of PTZ-induced convulsions by antiepileptic drugs correlates quite well with their effectiveness against absence seizures.
- Doxapram is similar to the above drugs but has a bigger margin of safety between respiratory stimulation and convulsions. It is rapidly eliminated, and it is occasionally used as an intravenous infusion in patients with acute respiratory failure.

CNS STIMULANTS

Amphetamines

- Amphetamine and its active dextro isomer dextroamphetamine, together with methamphetamine and methylphenidate are included in the group. All these drugs act by releasing monoamines from nerve terminals in the brain. They are substrates for the neuronal uptake transporters for noradrenaline (norepinephrine), serotonin and dopamine, and cause release of these mediators. With prolonged use, they are neurotoxic, causing degeneration of amine-containing nerve terminals and eventually cell death.
- The main central effects of amphetamine-like drugs are: locomotor stimulation, euphoria and excitement, stereotyped behavior and anorexia.

- Tricyclic antidepressants and monoamine oxidase inhibitors potentiate the effects of amphetamine, presumably by blocking amine reuptake or metabolism. However, reserpine does not block the behavioural effects of amphetamine.
- Amphetamine-like drugs cause marked anorexia, but with continued administration this effect wears off in a few days and food intake returns to normal. The effect is most marked with fenfluramine and its d isomer dexfenfluramine, which preferentially affect 5-hydroxytryptamine (5-HT) release.
- Amphetamine is readily absorbed from the gastrointestinal tract and freely penetrates the blood-brain barrier. Amphetamine is mainly excreted unchanged in the urine. The plasma half-life of amphetamine varies from about 5 hours to 20–30 hours, depending on urine flow and urinary pH.
- The main use of amphetamines is in the treatment of *attention deficit-hyperactivity disorder* (*ADHD*), particularly in children, methylphenidate being the drug most commonly used, at doses lower than those causing euphoria and other side effects.
- The limited clinical usefulness of amphetamine is due to its many unwanted effects, including hypertension, insomnia, anorexia, tremors, risk of exacerbating schizophrenia, and risk of dependence. The drug can induce a condition resembling heatstroke, associated with muscle damage and renal failure, and also causes inappropriate secretion of antidiuretic hormone, leading to thirst, over-hydration and hyponatraemia ('water intoxication').

Melatonin

- Chemically, N-acetyl-5-methoxy tryptamine, is secreted at night by the pineal gland.
- Plays a role in the sleep-wake cycle and the circadian rhythm.
- Reduces jet-lag symptoms and can be used in shift workers and in degenerative diseases.

PSYCHOTOMIMETIC DRUGS

- Psychotomimetic drugs (also referred to as *psychedelic* or *hallucinogenic* drugs) affect thought, perception and mood, without causing marked psychomotor stimulation or depression. Thoughts and perceptions tend to become distorted and dreamlike, rather than being merely sharpened or dulled, and the change in mood is likewise more complex than a simple shift in the direction of euphoria or depression.
- Psychedelic drugs do not cause dependence or addiction, even though their psychological effects overlap those of highly addictive major psychostimulants such as cocaine and amphetamines.
- Drugs that act on 5-HT transporters or receptors include lysergic acid diethylamide (LSD), psilocybin and mescaline, which are agonists at 5-HT_2 receptors, and MDMA (ecstasy), which acts mainly by inhibiting 5-HT uptake. An antagonist at NMDA-type glutamate receptors is phencyclidine.
- LSD is an extremely potent psychotomimetic drug capable of producing strong effects in humans. It is a chemical derivative of lysergic acid, which occurs in the cereal fungus ergot. Mescaline is chemically related to amphetamine and acts as an inhibitor of monoamine transport, in addition to its agonist action on 5HT_2 receptors. Psilocybin is obtained from a fungus and has very similar properties to LSD.
- The main effects of these drugs are on mental function, most notably an alteration of perception in such a way that sights and sounds appear distorted and fantastic. Hallucinations visual, auditory, tactile or olfactory also occur, and sensory modalities may become confused, so that sounds are perceived as visions. Thought processes tend to become illogical and disconnected. LSD might produce a syndrome that is extremely disturbing to the subject 'bad trip', in which the hallucinatory experience takes on a menacing quality and may be accompanied by paranoid delusions. 'Flashbacks' of the hallucinatory experience can occur even after weeks or months.
- LSD and other psychotomimetic drugs, can lead to more persistent mental disorder. LSD may occasionally initiate long-lasting schizophrenia.
- MDMA is an amphetamine derivative with complex effects on monoamine function. It inhibits monoamine transporters, principally the 5-HT transporter, and also releases 5-HT, the net effect being a large increase in free 5-HT in certain brain regions, followed by depletion. MDMA is widely used as a 'party drug' because of the euphoria, loss of inhibitions and energy surge that it induces.
- Phencyclidine, originally intended as an intravenous anesthetic agent was found to produce a period of disorientation and hallucinations following recovery of consciousness. Ketamine is a close analogue of phencyclidine. Its main pharmacological effect is to block the NMDA receptor channel but it is also an antagonist at ó-receptors, which are activated by various opioids of the benzomorphan type.

Drugs against Alzeimer's Disease

Cholinesterase Inhibitors

- Tacrine was the first drug approved for treating AD. It is short acting, reversible, affects both AChE and BuChE. Tacrine has to be given four times daily and produces cholinergic side effects such as nausea and abdominal cramps, as well as hepatotoxicity in some patients, so its use has been reduced.
- Donepezil, rivastigmine and galantamine—These drugs are slowly reversible, affect both AChE and BuChE. Galantamine also enhances nicotinic acetylcholine receptor activation by allosteric mechanism. These cholinesterase inhibitors may act to reduce the formation or neurotoxicity of Aâ, and therefore retard the progression of AD as well as producing symptomatic benefit.
- Memantine, an NMDA receptor antagonist acts by inhibiting glutamate-induced excitotoxicity. It has only mild side effects, and produces a significant improvement in cognitive function in moderate-to-severe AD.

RECENT DRUGS ON CNS

- **GA**
  Dexmeditomidine—Pre– anesthetic medication selective alpha 2a agonist
- **SEDATIVE HYPNOTICS**
  Zaleplon—Decreases sleep latency
- **ANTIEPILEPTICS**
  Felbamate – NMDA receptor blocker
  Ganoxolone – Neurosteroid
  Zonisamide – Carbonic anhydrase inhibitor
- **ANTI-PARKINSON'S**
  Cabergoline – Long acting dopamine agonist
- **ANTI-PSYCHOTICS**
  Aripiprazole – Dopamine serotonin stabilizer
  Ziprasidone/Quetiapine – Atypical antipsychotics
- **ANTI-DEPRESSANTS**
  Atomoxetine – NA reuptake inhibitor in ADHD, drug of choice
  Gepirone/Ispapirone – used in chronic anxiety similar to buspirone
  Milnacipran – NA/Serotonin reuptake inhibitor
- **OPIOIDS**
  Alvimopan – mu antagonist in postoperative paralytic ileus
  Fedotozine – ka opioid antagonist in IBS
- **CNS STIMULANTS**
  Acetyl Carnitine – Alzeimer's disease
  Glatiramer acetate – Myelin basic protein in multiple sclerosis
  Pemoline – ADHD
  Riluzole – NMDA antagonist in ALS
  Modafinil/Armodafinil – Narcolepsy

Multiple Choice Questions

1. Which of the following antiepileptic drug use requires ophthalmological consultation?
   a. Carbamazepine
   b. Topiramate
   c. Valproate
   d. Lamotrigine

2. Which of the following is a gender specific side caused by valproate?
   a. PCOs
   b. Tremor
   c. Alopecia
   d. Weight gain

3. Which drug can cause progressive visual field constriction?
   a. Phenobarbitone
   b. Vigabatrin
   c. Ethosuximide
   d. Valproate

4. When to start folic acid in a patient on antiepileptics?
   a. Any woman who can potentially be pregnant
   b. Three months before planning pregnancy
   c. At confirmation of pregnancy
   d. After pregnancy

5. Prolonged use of which of the following anticonvulsants can produce weight loss?
   a. Gabapentin
   b. Oxcarbazepine
   c. Topiramate
   d. Valproic acid

6. Which statement is true about carbamazepine?
   a. Used in trigeminal neuralgia
   b. Carbamazepine is an enzyme inhibitor
   c. Can cause megaloblastic anemia
   d. It is the drug of choice for status epilepticus

7. Which among the following is the mechanism of action of carbamazepine?
   a. Prolongation of inactivated state of Na⁺ channels
   b. Facilitates GABA
   c. Inhibition of Ca^{2+}
   d. NMDA receptor blockade

8. A patient of juvenile myoclonic epilepsy on valproate comes to you at 5 months of pregnancy with level II scan normal what will you advice?
   a. Change the drug
   b. The drug in same dose
   c. Decrease the dose of drug
   d. Increase the dose of drug

9. Antiepileptic drug not associated with enzyme induction or inhibition property is:
   a. Phenytoin
   b. Valproate
   c. Carbamazepine
   d. Ethosuximide

10. Most serious side effect of valproate is:
    a. Fulminant hepatitis
    b. Spina bifida
    c. Weight gain
    d. Thrombocytopenia

11. Oxcarbazepine true is all *except*:
    a. Metabolises itself
    b. Less chances of hyponatremia than carbazepine
    c. It is less enzyme inducer than carbazepine
    d. Less chances of hepatotoxicity than carbazepine

12. All of the following are adverse effects of sodium valproate *except*:
    a. Weight gain
    b. Alopecia
    c. Liver damage
    d. Osteomalacia

13. Which antiepileptic drug does not act via inhibition of sodium channels?
    a. Vigabatrin
    b. Carbamazepine
    c. Lamotrigine
    d. Phenytoin

14. The drug used in absence seizures and having a narrow spectrum of antiepileptic activity is:
    a. Lamotrigine
    b. Ethosuximide
    c. Sodium valproate
    d. Primidone

Answers

| 1. d | 2. a | 3. b | 4. b | 5. c | 6. a | 7. a |
| 8. b | 9. d | 10. a | 11. b | 12. d | 13. a | 14. b |

15. Antiepileptic drug implicated in causing toxic epidermal necrolysis is:
    a. Felbamate
    b. Gabapentin
    c. Lamotrigine
    d. Vigabatrin

16. Not true about fosphenytoin is:
    a. Used for GTCS
    b. Prodrug of phenytoin
    c. Lipid soluble
    d. Highly protein bound

17. Regarding phenytoin all of the following are correct *except:*
    a. It acts on voltage sensitive neuronal na channels
    b. Used by slow IV injection in status epilepticus
    c. Kinetics change from 1st order to zero order over therapeutic range
    d. It inhibits microsomal enzymes

18. Drug of choice for myoclonic seizures:
    a. Vigabatrin
    b. Phenytoin
    c. Valproate
    d. Carbamazepine

19. Doc for prophylaxis of febrile seizures:
    a. Rectal diazepam
    b. Valproate
    c. Phenytoin
    d. Carbamazepine

20. Felbamate was discontinued due to:
    a. Aplastic anemia
    b. Renal impairment
    c. Gastrointestinal disorder
    d. Seizures

21. Doc for seizures in tuberous sclerosis:
    a. Vigabatrin
    b. Topiramate
    c. lamotrigine
    d. Leveitiracetam

22. The drug of choice for a patient presenting with h/o lennoxgastaut syndrome:
    a. Vigabatrin
    b. Topiramate
    c. Lamotrigine
    d. Leveitiracetam

23. Which of the following benzodiazepine can be used as a muscle relaxant?
    a. Diazepam
    b. Nitrazepam
    c. Clonazepam
    d. Flurazepam

24. Inverse agonist is:
    a. Buspirone
    b. B carboline
    c. Flumazenil
    d. Zolpidem

25. Drug contraindicated in acute intermittent porphyria:
    a. Thiopentone
    b. Ketamine
    c. Propofol
    d. Etomidate

26. True statement regarding methadone are all *except:*
    a. It is a long-acting u-receptor agonist
    b. It is rapidly absorbed from the gastrointestinal tract and is detected in plasma 30 minutes after oral administration
    c. The primary use of methadone is relief of chronic pain
    d. The onset of an algesia is 30-60 minutes after parenteral administration and 1-2 hours after oral administration

27. Which is the mechanism of action of buprenorphine:
    a. Partial agonist at µ and antagonist at κ
    b. Partial agonist at κ and antagonist at µ and δ
    c. Partial agonist at µ and κ and antagonist at δ
    d. Partial agonist at µ and κ and δ

28. Tolerance develops to all of the following action of opioids *except:*
    a. Miosis
    b. Analgesia
    c. Euphoria
    d. Nausea and vomiting

29. Which of the following is least narcotic opioid?
    a. Morphine
    b. Codeine
    c. Heroin
    d. Papaverine

30. Drug of choice for controlling severe pain in cancer patients is:
    a. Morphine
    b. Diclofenac
    c. Ibuprofen
    d. Codeine

31. Actions of opiates include all *except:*
    a. Constipation
    b. Vomiting
    c. Analgesia
    d. Mydriasis

32. Endogenous opioid peptide includes:
    a. Encephalin
    b. Endorphins
    c. Dynorphins
    d. All of the above

33. Morphine is contraindicated in all *except:*
    a. Hepatic insufficiency
    b. Bronchial asthma
    c. Head injury
    d. Preanesthetic medication

34. Dextromethorphan should not be given with which drug?
    a. SSRIs
    b. MAO inhibitors
    c. Atropine
    d. Paracetamol

35. Half-life of lithium is:
    a. 8 hours
    b. 16 hours
    c. 24 hours
    d. 36 hours

Answers

15. c	16. c	17. d	18. c	19. a	20. a	21. a
22. c	23. a	24. b	25. a	26. d	27. a	28. a
29. d	30. a	31. d	32. d	33. d	34. b	35. c

36. Tolcapone is:
    a. Hepatotoxic
    b. Nephrotoxic
    c. Ototoxic
    d. Neurotoxic

37. Peripheral vasospasm is observed with which of the following anti-parkinsonian drugs?
    a. Ropinirole
    b. Levodopa
    c. Bromocriptine
    d. Entacapone

38. Which of the following statement regarding selegeline is false?
    a. May be used in on-off phenomenon
    b. Does not cause cheese reaction
    c. It is used in parkinsonism
    d. It is a MAO-A inhibitor

39. Which drug is used in amyotropic lateral sclerosis:
    a. Riluzole
    b. Glatiramer
    c. Tacrine
    d. Olanzapine

40. Patient on treatment on carbidopa + levidopa for 10 years now has weaning off effect. What should be added to restore action:
    a. Tolcapone
    b. Amantadine
    c. Rasagiline
    d. Benzhexol

41. Natalizumab is used in treatment of:
    a. Multiple sclerosis
    b. Breast carcinoma
    c. Psoriasis
    d. B cell lymphoma

42. Drug of choice for relapsing remitting multiple sclerosis is:
    a. Alpha IFN
    b. B IFN
    c. Gamma IFN
    d. Natalizumab

43. Which of the following drug is used as transcranial patch for Parkinson's disease:
    a. Levodopa
    b. Rotigotine
    c. Selegiline
    d. Carbidopa

44. False statement about selegilline is:
    a. It is a MAO-A inhibitor
    b. Does not cause cheese reaction
    c. May be used in "on-off" phenomenon
    d. It is used in parkinsonism

45. Anti-parkinsonism drug that is a selective comt inhibitor:
    a. Entacapone
    b. Ropinirole
    c. Pergolide
    d. Pramipexole

46. All are side effects of ropinirole *except:*
    a. Sedation
    b. Nausea
    c. Retroperitonea
    d. Hallucination

47. Antiparkinson drug known to cause cardiac valvular fibrosis is:
    a. Bromocriptine
    b. Ropinirole
    c. Pramiprexole
    d. Pergolide and cabergolin

48. All are ergot derivatives used in parkinsonism *except:*
    a. Bromocriptine
    b. Pergolide
    c. Trihexyphenidyl
    d. Cabergoline

49. Which is hepatotoxic:
    a. Entacapone
    b. Ropinirole
    c. Tolcapone
    d. Trihexyphenidy

50. Cb1 antagonist use in smoking cessation is:
    a. Naloxone
    b. Rimonabant
    c. Varenicline
    d. Bupropion

51. Varenicline acts by:
    a. Partial nicotine receptor agonist
    b. Nicotine receptor antagonist
    c. Both agonist and antagonist at nicotine receptor
    d. None of the above

52. A 34-year-old male presents to the outpatient department with a complaint of pain in the right sided jawpain. Each episode of pain is lasting for around 30 seconds. The present complaint was present for the past one month but the increased in the number of episodes per day brought her to the clinic. Those episodes are increasing especially when she walks out in the cold. The mechanism of action of drug of choice in this patient is?
    a. Prevention of Na influx
    b. Increase the time of Cl⁻ channel opening
    c. Increase the frequency of C-channel opening
    d. Decrease in the Ca^{+2} influx

53. Which drug does not cause chorea as a side effect?
    a. Phenytoin
    b. OCPs
    c. Carbamazepine
    d. Clozapine

54. The anti-epileptic drug safe in lactation is:
    a. Valproic acid
    b. Carbamazepine
    c. Phenytoirn
    d. Ethosuximide

Answers

36. a	37. c	38. d	39. a	40. a	41. a	42. b
43. b	44. a	45. a	46. c	47. d	48. c	49. c
50. b	51. a	52. a	53. d	54. a		

55. Following antiepileptics have least interactions other drugs:
    a. Phenytoin
    b. Gabapentin
    c. Valproate
    d. Carbamazepine

56. All of the following are used in nicotine de-addiction *except*:
    a. Bupropion
    b. Clonidine
    c. Nicotine gum
    d. Buspirone

57. Carbamazepine increase medical, neurological and psychiatric symptoms, when used in:
    a. Erthropoietic porphyria
    b. Epilepsy
    c. Bipolar disorder
    d. Trigeminal neuralgia

58. Serum lithium level is increased by all the following drugs *except*:
    a. Aspirin
    b. Chlorthiazide
    c. Tetracycline
    d. Verapamil

59. Which one of the following is not correct regarding the half-life of antiepileptic drugs?
    a. Valproic acid—15h
    b. Carbamazepine—10–17h
    c. Lamotrigine—50–68h
    d. Levetiracetam—6–8h

60. Which one of the following is not correct regarding the side effects of antiepileptics?
    a. Carbamazepine—hypersomnia
    b. Topiramate—renal stones
    c. Lamotrigine—Stevens-Johnson syndrome
    d. Valproic acid—thrombocytopenia

61. All of the following are correct match for drug side effects:
    a. Ziprasidone—cardiac arrhythmias
    b. Risperidone—rise in prolactin levels
    c. Clozapine—hypersalivation
    d. Olanzapine—weight loss

62. Steven-Johnson's syndrome is caused by:
    a. Sodium-valporate
    b. Lamotrigine
    c. Phenobarbitone
    d. Gabapentine

63. Weight gain is not a side effect by using the following drug:
    a. Sodium valproate
    b. Olanzapine
    c. Topiramate
    d. Lithium carbonate

64. Find out the incorrect match:
    a. Fatty liver—tetracycline
    b. Hepatitis—halothane
    c. Granuloma—chlorpromazine
    d. Cholestasis—erythromycin

65. Which one of the following is a benzodizapine antagonist?
    a. Flumazenil
    b. Methadone
    c. Atropine
    d. Naloxone

66. A novel nicotinic agonist approved recently for use in smoking cessation is:
    a. Rimonabant
    b. Varenicline
    c. Nefopam
    d. Pimozide

67. The drug of choice in patients with generalized epilepsy syndromes having mixed seizure type is:
    a. Phenytoin
    b. Oxcarbazepine
    c. Lamotrigine
    d. Valproic acid

68. The shortest acting benzodiazepine:
    a. Midazolam
    b. Lorazepam
    c. Alprozolam
    d. Clonazepam

69. Pimozide belongs to:
    a. Thioxanthines
    b. Phenothiazines
    c. Buprenorhine group
    d. Diphenyl group

70. Picrotoxin is used in case of barbiturate poisoning until:
    a. Respiration normalizes
    b. Pulse returns to normal
    c. Blood pressure normalizes
    d. Pupillary reflex normalizes

Answers

55. b	56. d	57. a	58. d	59. c	60. a	61. d
62. b	63. c	64. c	65. a	66. b	67. d	68. a
69. d	70. d					

CHAPTER 5

Neuro-ophthalmology

COMPONENTS

Retina
- Extends from ora serrata to optic nerve
- Divided into four quadrants by the macula
  - Vertical meridian: Separates superior and inferior retina
  - Horizontal meridian: Separates nasal and temporal retina

Retina Layers

a. Retinal pigment epithelium
   - Deepest layer of retina
   - Forms outer blood-retinal barrier and supports photoreceptors physiologically
b. Photoreceptor layer
   - First neural elements in the retina to react to light
   - Rod and cone cells contain light-sensitive pigment rhodopsin
   - Photoreceptors hyperpolarize (membrane potential becomes more negative) in presence of light
   - Rod cells are sensitive to low levels of light
     - Minimal role in color vision (except blue spectrum)
     - Rods are concentrated in peripheral retina
     - No rods within the macula
   - Cone cells respond to color red, green, and blue
     - Cones are densely concentrated in the macula
   - Macula lutea – 5.5 mm diameter; area rich in cones – situated 2 disk diameters temporal to the optic disk
   - Central 1.5 mm of macula – fovea;
   - foveola – 0.35 mm diameter small central depression in the fovea; vision is most acute at foveola – only cones are found here – each cone directly relays to a ganglion cell
c. Outer nuclear layer: Contains cell bodies of photoreceptors
d. Outer plexiform layer: Contains synapses between photoreceptors and bipolar and horizontal cells
e. Inner nuclear layer
   - Amacrine cells are horizontally oriented, dopaminergic cells that modulate and convey photoreceptor information to ganglion cells
   - Bipolar cells convey photoreceptor information to ganglion cells
   - Horizontal cells provide antagonistic surround signals to bipolar cells
f. Inner plexiform layer: Contains synapses between bipolar and amacrine cells and ganglion cells
g. Ganglion cell layer
   - Most superficial retinal layer
   - They are divided into M and P cells
   - **M** and **P** cell axons project to superior colliculus or lateral geniculate nucleus
   - **M** cells lack color information, but have high contrast sensitivity, fast temporal resolution, low spatial resolution. P cells have color opponency, low contrast sensitivity, and high spatial resolution.

- **M** cell axons project to Magnocellular neurons in layers 1 and 2 of lateral geniculate nucleus, while **P** cell axons project to parvocellular neurons in layers 3, 4, 5, and 6 of lateral geniculate nucleus and these neurons project to layer IVC alpha neurons in cortical area 17.
- Ganglion cell axons traveling to the optic nerve from the retinal nerve fiber layer

Retinal Nerve Fiber Layer

- **Papillomacular bundle:** Nerve fibers extending from macula to optic nerve
- Temporal nerve fibers arch around papillomacular bundle to reach optic disk
- Optic nerve creates a physiologic blind spot on visual field testing (temporal)
- **Scotomas ("blind spots"):** Areas of poor or absent vision within the visual field
- *Monocular scotoma and noncongruous visual field abnormalities (especially monocular) occur from optic nerve and retinal lesions based on arrangement of retinal nerve fiber layer.*

Defects

- Specific scotoma and visual field abnormalities may occur from optic nerve and retinal lesions based on arrangement of retinal nerve fiber layer
  - *Arcuate scotoma or defects:* Arch-shaped, characteristic of nerve fiber bundle defects (e.g. glaucoma)
  - *Central scotoma (macular type of defect):* a blind spot in the visual field represented by the macula (e.g., macular degeneration)
  - *Centrocecal scotoma (optic nerve type of defect):* Affects the visual field in region of the macula and papillomacular bundle
  - *Paracentral scotoma:* Affects retina and visual field just outside the macula
  - *Ring scotoma:* From combined superior and inferior retina and arcuate scotoma
  - Ring scotoma with a horizontal step: typically indicates retinal or nerve fiber layer lesion as opposed to ring scotoma with a vertical step, which may indicate lesion in occipital lobe near calcarine fissure
  - Enlargement of blind spot (e.g., optic disk swelling)
  - *Altitudinal defects:* Blind spots with a horizontal step; typically appear as an abrupt, monocular loss of superior or inferior visual field
  - *Sector scotoma or defects:* Typically caused by retinal lesion (e.g. retinal detachment).

Optic Nerve

- Segments
  - Intraocular segment (optic nerve head)
  - Intraorbital segment
  - Intracanalicular (optic canal) segment
  - Intracranial segment
- Topographic arrangement
  - Macular fibers (papillomacular bundle) are located peripherally (temporal aspect of the optic nerve) in the portion of optic nerve closest to the globe
  - Macular fibers become more centrally located in more distal portion of optic nerve closest to the chiasma.
  - Peripheral retinal fibers travel peripherally.

Defects

- Central field defects are caused by lesions that affect optic nerve, macula, or papillomacular bundle
  1. Unilateral central scotomas, for example, optic neuritis.
  2. Bilateral central or centrocecal defects, for example, suggestive of bilateral optic neuropathies (hereditary, compressive, nutritional, inflammatory) or bilateral occipital lesions.
- Unilateral temporal defects
  - Lesion of nasal retina, optic nerve, or nasal optic nerve fibers at anterior optic chiasm (e.g. junctional scotoma of Traquair)
  - Monocular temporal crescent: retinal disease or lesion of anterior occipital lobe
- *Altitudinal defects:* characteristic of disease of the central retinal artery, with macular sparing (cilioretinal arteries) or posterior ciliary artery (anterior ischemic optic neuropathy).

Optic Chiasma

- Nasal retinal nerve fibers: Cross to contralateral optic tract at level of the optic chiasm (constitute about half of optic nerve fibers)
- Inferior nasal fibers of one optic nerve cross ventrally into contralateral optic nerve proximally and are known as Wilbrand's knee
- Temporal retinal nerve fibers remain ipsilateral in optic chiasma and optic tracts

- *An isolated monocular temporal field defect affecting the contralateral optic nerve or Wilbrand's knee is called a junctional scotoma of Traquair*
- As this is a place where nasal fibers of the retina cross each other and move contralaterally, in case of resection at this region, the binasal retinal fibers are lost which will result in bitemporal hemianopia.

Lesions

- Bitemporal field defects, almost never complete bitemporal field defects and exact field defect depends on localization of the compressive lesion.
- Anterior chiasm
  1. Compressive lesion anterior to optic chiasm generally causes bitemporal field defects involving the upper quadrants and evolves to more extensive bitemporal field defects.
  2. Junctional syndrome of Traquair—Monocular superior temporal field defect in eye contralateral to the lesion
  3. Junctional syndrome—Ipsilateral central scotoma with contralateral superior temporal defect due to compression of Wilbrand's knee and ipsilateral optic nerve.
  4. Bilateral superior temporal field defects due to early anterior compression of both inferonasal crossing fibers.
- *Body of the chiasm syndrome:* Typically bitemporal visual field defects
- Posterior chiasm syndrome
  1. Compressive lesion posterior to optic chiasm generally causes bitemporal field defects involving lower quadrants and evolve to more extensive bitemporal field defects
  2. Bilateral temporal scotomas (involving central vision, peripheral fields spared)
  3. Bitemporal field defects primarily affecting inferotemporal fields due to early compressive lesions.

Optic Tract

Visual field defect related to lesion involving optic tract

- Complete (macular-splitting) homonymous hemianopia
- Wallerian degeneration and dying-back axonal loss causing ganglion cell fiber atrophy of contralateral nasal macula and nasal retina and ipsilateral temporal retina
- *Contralateral relative afferent pupillary defect:* Optic tract lesion on one side may cause the contralateral eye to have a relative afferent pupillary defect and a temporal visual field defect.

Lateral Geniculate Nucleus (LGB)

- It has six layers
- Superior retinal fibers lie superomedial in the nucleus
- Inferior retinal fibers lie lateral in the nucleus.

Defects

- Anterior choroidal artery occlusion causes a quadruple sectoranopia: homonymous defect affecting superior and inferior quadrants, with sparing of the horizontal sectors
- Posterior lateral choroidal artery occlusion causes a horizontal homonymous sector defect: a homonymous defect of horizontal sectors (wedge- or triangle-shaped).

Optic Radiations

- Optic radiations exit the lateral geniculate nucleus in three bundles, which course around the lateral ventricle through white matter to reach calcarine cortex (cortical area 17).
- Three optic radiation bundles
  - *Upper bundle*
    - Originates from medial part of lateral geniculate nucleus
    - Represents superior retina
    - Passes deep in parietal white matter and ends in superior lip of the calcarine fissure
  - *Central bundle*
    - Originates from medial part of lateral geniculate nucleus
    - Represents macular region
    - Traverses posterior temporal and occipital white matter and ends on both lips of posterior part of the calcarine fissure
  - *Lower bundle*
    - Originates from lateral part of lateral geniculate nucleus
    - Represents inferior retina
    - Courses anteriorly from LGB and then turns around temporal horn of lateral ventricle (Meyer's loop) to end on inferior lip of the calcarine fissure.

Defects
- Superior homonymous quadrantic ("pie in the sky") defects may result from lesion of Meyer's loop.
- Inferior homonymous quadrantic ("pie on the floor") defects result from lesion of optic radiations that pass through parietal lobe to occipital lobe superior to the calcarine fissure.

Visual Cortex
- Striate cortex, or primary visual cortex, is Brodmann's area 17: located along superior and inferior banks of calcarine fissure
- Homonymous quadrantic defects can occur from unilateral occipital lobe lesions; the visual field defects typically have a sharp horizontal edge.
- Medial occipital lesions cause congruous homonymous hemianopias, typically with macular sparing and are usually due to infarcts in territory of the posterior cerebral artery.
- Macular sparing is due to dual arterial supply (both posterior and middle cerebral arteries supplying the occipital pole responsible for macular vision) and also a larger cortical representation of the macular region.

Defects
- Striate cortex lesion localization
  - Anterior lesion: causes a temporal crescent or half moon syndrome in contralateral eye to cause a unilateral visual field defect
  - Intermediate lesion: affects from 10 to 60 degrees in contralateral hemifield
  - Posterior lesion: affects macular vision (central 10 degrees in contralateral visual field)
- Cortical blindness: complete blindness or keyhole vision that may result from bilateral occipital lobe disease
- Anton's syndrome: cortical blindness with denial of neurologic impairment
- A wide variety of diseases affect the optic nerve. Clinical features particularly suggestive of optic nerve disease are an afferent pupillary defect, poor color vision, and optic disk changes. Axons can be dysfunctional long before they become atrophic.

Etiologic Classification
One and Half Syndrome
Lesion affecting same side MLF and horizontal gaze center
- *Symptoms:* Horizontal movement of eyes to either side is limited; however abduction of the eye on the opposite side is possible.
- *Causes:* Multiple sclerosis, infarction, hemorrhage, tumor
- *Treatment:* Treat the cause.

Visual Fields Accompanying Damage to Visual Pathways
- Optic nerve—unilateral amaurosis
- Lateral optic chiasm—incongruous, incomplete, contralateral, homonymous hemianopia
- Central optic chiasm—bitemporal hemianopia
- Optic tract – incongruous incomplete homonymous hemianopia
- Temporal (Meyer's) loop of optic radiation – congruous partial or complete (contralateral) homonymous superior quadrantanopia
- Parietal (superior) loop of optic radiation – congruous partial or complete homonymous inferior quadrantanopia
- Complete arieto-occipital interruption of the optic radiation: Complete congruous homonymous hemianopia with psychophysical shift of the foveal point, sparing central vision – macular sparing
- Incomplete damage to the visual cortex: congruous homonymous scotoma encroaching acutely on central vision.

INFLAMMATORY (OPTIC NEURITIS)
- Demyelinating—Idiopathic, Multiple sclerosis, Neuromyelitis optica (Devic's disease)
- Immune-mediated—Postviral optic neuritis (measles, mumps, chickenpox, influenza, infectious mononucleosis), Postimmunization optic neuritis, Acute disseminated encephalomyelitis, Guillain-Barré syndrome, Systemic lupus erythematosus
- Direct infections—Herpes zoster, syphillis, tuberculosis, cryptococcosis, cytomegalovirus
- Granulomatous optic neuropathy—Sarcoidosis
- Contiguous inflammatory disease—Intraocular inflammation, Orbital disease, Sinus disease, including mucormycosis,

Vascular (Ischemic Optic Neuropathy)
- Nonarteritic anterior ischemic optic neuropathy (AION)—Giant cell arteritis (arteritic anterior ischemic optic neuropathy), Systemic vasculitis: systemic lupus erythematosus, anti-phospholipid antibody syndrome, polyarteritis nodosa, Churg-Strauss vasculitis, Sjögren's syndrome, Takayasu's disease.

- Migraine
- **Inherited coagulation defects:** Protein C deficiency, protein S deficiency, antithrombin III deficiency, activated protein C resistance (factor V Leiden mutation), Diabetic papillopathy.

Raised Intracranial Pressure (Papilledema)
- **Intracranial mass:** Cerebral tumor, abscess, subdural hematoma, Arteriovenous malformation, Subarachnoid hemorrhage
- Meningitis or encephalitis—Acquired hydrocephalus, Pseudotumor cerebri, Cerebral venous sinus occlusion.

Optic Nerve Compression
- **Intracranial disease:** Meningioma, pituitary adenoma, craniopharyngioma, supraclinoid internal carotid aneurysm, meningeal carcinomatosis, basal meningitis
- **Orbital disease:** Dysthyroid eye disease, idiopathic orbital inflammatory disease, orbital neoplasm, orbital abscess, Optic nerve sheath meningioma.

Nutritional and Toxic
- **Vitamin deficiencies:** Vitamin B_{12} deficiency, vitamin B_1 (thiamin) deficiency, folate deficiency Tobacco-alcohol amblyopia
- **Heavy metals:** Lead, thalium, arsenic.
- **Drugs:** Ethambutol, isoniazid, quinine, chloramphenicol, amiodarone, halogenated hydroxyquinolines.
- **Chemicals:** Methanol, ethylene glycol.

Trauma
- Direct optic nerve injury
- Indirect optic nerve injury
- Optic nerve avulsion.

Hereditary Optic Atrophy
- Leber's hereditary optic neuropathy (mitochondrial inheritance), Autosomal hereditary optic atrophy, Autosomal dominant (juvenile) optic atrophy, Autosomal recessive (infantile) optic atrophy
- Wolfram's syndrome (DIDMOAD: diabetes insipidus, diabetes mellitus, optic atrophy, deafness).
- Inherited neurodegenerative diseases: Hereditary spinocerebellar ataxia (Friedreich's ataxia), Hereditary motor and sensory neuropathy (Charcot-Marie-Tooth disease), Lysosomal storage disorders.
- *Neoplastic infiltration*: By Glioma, leukemia, lymphoma, meningeal carcinomatosis, astrocytic hamartoma, melanocytoma, hemangioma.

OPTIC ATROPHY

- It is a nonspecific response to optic nerve damage from any cause. Since the optic nerve consists of retinal ganglion cell axons, optic atrophy may be the consequence of primary retinal disease, such as retinitis pigmentosa or central retinal artery occlusion.
- Excavation of the optic nerve head (optic disk cupping) is generally a sign of glaucomatous optic neuropathy, but it may occur with any cause of optic atrophy. Segmental pallor and attenuated retinal blood vessels are often the consequence of anterior ischemic optic neuropathy. Hereditary optic neuropathies usually produce bilateral temporal segmental disk pallor with preferential loss of papillomacular axons.
- Peripapillary exudates occur with optic disk swelling, due to papillitis, ischemic optic neuropathy, or papilledema. The term "neuroretinitis" for the combination of optic disk swelling and retinal exudates, including a macular star. Other helpful signs of prior disk edema are peripapillary gliosis and atrophy, chorioretinal folds, and internal limiting membrane wrinkling.

OPTIC NEURITIS

- Inflammatory optic neuropathy (optic neuritis) may be due to a variety of causes, but the most common is demyelinative disease, including multiple sclerosis.
- Retrobulbar neuritis is an optic neuritis that occurs behind the optic disk that the disk remains normal during the acute episode.
- Papillitis is disk swelling caused by inflammation at the nerve head (intraocular optic nerve).Loss of vision is the cardinal symptom of optic neuritis and is particularly useful in differentiating papillitis from papilledema, with which it may be confused on ophthalmoscopic examination.
- In optic neuritis there is a red green color desaturation while in macular disorders there is blue-yellow desaturation
- Marcus gunn pupil or RAPD is present

- IV methyl prednisolone is preferred to oral steroids which is avoided.
  - **Purtscher retinopathy** is a hemorrhagic and vaso-occlusive, which, in 1912, was first described as a syndrome of sudden blindness associated with severe head trauma.
  - These patients had findings of multiple white retinal patches and retinal hemorrhages that were associated with severe vision loss.
  - Since its original description, Purtscher retinopathy has been associated with traumatic injury, primarily blunt thoracic trauma and head trauma, and numerous nontraumatic diseases.
  - Characteristic fundus findings of Purtscher retinopathy. Multiple cotton-wool spots surround the optic nerve after blunt thoracic trauma.
  - Purtscher-like retinopathy is seen in diverse conditions, including acute pancreatitis; fat embolization; amniotic fluid embolization.
  - Preeclampsia; hemolysis, elevated liver enzymes, and low platelets (HELLP) syndrome; and vasculitic diseases
  - Pathophysiology involves complex pathophysiology, with several contributing factors, including complement-mediated aggregates, fat, air, fibrin clots and platelet clumps. The diseases leads to the formation of cotton wool spots in the retina, a finding observed in several other diseases, and atrophy of the optic nerve.
  - Associated diseases
  - Severe head, chest, or long bone trauma; Acute pancreatitis: Amniotic fluid embolism; Chronic renal failure: Dermatomyositis; Fat embolism syndrome; Scleroderma; Systemic lupus erythematosus (SLE): Thrombotic thrombocytopenic purpura (TTP).
  - Treatment with triamcinolone.

TOXIC OPTIC NEUROPATHY

- This can result in acute visual loss with bilateral optic disk swelling and central or cecocentral scotomas
- Such cases have been reported to result from exposure to ethambutol, methyl alcohol (moonshine), ethylene glycol (antifreeze) or carbon monoxide.
- In toxic optic neuropathy, visual loss also can develop gradually and produce optic atrophy without a phase of acute optic disk edema. Many agents have been implicated as a cause of toxic optic neuropathy, but the evidence supporting the association for many is weak.
  - The following is a partial list of potential offending drugs or toxins: disulfiram, ethchlorvynol, chloramphenicol, amiodarone, monoclonal anti-CD3 antibody, ciprofloxacin, digitalis, streptomycin, lead, arsenic, thallium, d-penicillamine, isoniazid, emetine, and sulfonamides
- Deficiency states induced by starvation, malabsorption, or alcoholism can lead to insidious visual loss. Thiamine, vitamin B12 and folate levels should be checked in any patient with unexplained bilateral central scotomas and optic pallor.

Demyelinative Optic Neuritis

- Optic neuritis affects both eyes simultaneously and produces papillitis more commonly in children than in adults with multiple sclerosis.
- Visual loss is generally subacute, developing over 2–7 days. Color vision and contrast sensitivity are correspondingly impaired. A central scotoma is most commonly found. It is usually circular, varying widely in size and density. The pupillary light response is sluggish, and if the optic nerves are asymmetrically involved, a relative afferent pupillary defect will be present.
- Uhthoff's phenomenon is seen in demyelinating disease in which there is an impairment of vision with increasing body temperature
- Papillitis shows hyperemia of the optic disk and distention of large veins being early signs on ophthalmoscopic examination. There may be slight edema of the nerve head.
- Papillitis needs to be differentiated from papilledema (optic disk swelling due to raised intracranial pressure). In papilledema, which usually causes bilateral optic disk changes, there is often greater elevation of the optic nerve head, normal corrected visual acuity, normal pupillary response to light, and an intact visual field except for an enlarged blind spot. Diagnosis may depend on results of MRI and lumbar puncture, as well as subsequent clinical course.
- During an acute episode of optic neuritis, MRI shows gadolinium enhancement, increased signal, and sometimes swelling of the affected nerve. The visual evoked response (VER) from the affected eye may show reduced amplitude or increased latency during the acute episode of optic neuritis.
- Steroid therapy either intravenously (methylprednisolone, 1 g/d for 3 days with or without a subsequent tapering course of oral prednisolone), orally (methylprednisolone, 500 mg/d to 2 g/d for 3–5 days with or without subsequent oral prednisolone, or prednisolone, 1 mg/kg/d tapered over 10–21 days), or by retrobulbar injection accelerates recovery of vision but does not influence the ultimate visual outcome.

- Without treatment, vision characteristically begins to improve 2–3 weeks after onset and sometimes recovers within a few days. A poor visual outcome is also associated with longer lesions in the optic nerve, especially if there is involvement of the nerve within the optic canal.

In patients with a first episode of optic neuritis and abnormal brain MRI at presentation, interferon β-1a reduces the risk of clinically definite multiple sclerosis and of progression of cerebral white matter lesions.

Multiple Sclerosis

- Multiple sclerosis is typically a chronic relapsing and remitting demyelinating disorder of the central nervous system.
- Optic neuritis may be the first manifestation. There may be recurrent episodes, usually bilateral.
- Diplopia is a common early symptom, due most frequently to internuclear ophthalmoplegia. Diagnosis of multiple sclerosis is based on clinical evidence of white matter disease of the central nervous system disseminated in time and space (Schumacher criteria), subsequently supported by MRI and cerebrospinal fluid abnormalities (Poser criteria).
- Relapses and remissions are characteristic, permanent disability tending to increase with each relapse. Elevation of body temperature may exacerbate disability (Uhthoff's phenomenon), particularly visual impairment.

Steroid treatment, usually oral or intravenous methylprednisolone, is useful in hastening recovery from acute relapses but does not influence the final disability or the frequency of subsequent relapses. Interferon and glatiramer acetate (copolymer 1) reduce the rate and severity of relapses and slow the progression of brain MRI abnormalities.

Neuromyelitis Optica (Devic's Disease)

Diagnostic Criteria

- Required: optic neuritis—acute attacks; may be bilateral or unilateral
- Acute transverse myelitis—can be severe and transverse (rare in MS);
- Supportive (2 of 3 criteria require);
- Longitudinally extensive cord lesion extending over 3 or more vertebral segments
- Brain magnetic resonance imaging normal or not meeting for MS
- Aqua porin 4 seropositivity
- Aquaporin 4 is a protein encoded by the AQP4 gene, which is expressed in the basolateral cell membrane of principal collecting duct cells in kidney and thus provide a pathway for water to escape the cells
- AQP4 is expressed in astrocytes and is upregulated by direct insult to CNS and aquaporin 4 has been proposed as the primary autoimmune target in NMO.
- Histopathologically, these lesions reveal thickening of blood vessel walls, demyelination, deposition of antibody and compliment, a characteristic loss of astrocytes and aquaporin 4 staining not seen in MS.

Treatment is with systemic steroids for the acute episodes followed by long-term immunosuppression according to disease activity. A serum autoantibody, NMO-IgG, has been reported to be specific for neuromyelitis optica.

Anterior Ischemic Optic Neuropathy

Anterior ischemic optik neuropathy is characterized by pallid disk swelling associated with acute loss of vision. The disorder is due to infarction of the retrolaminar optik nerve (the region just posterior to the lamina cribrosa) from occlusion or decreased perfusion of the short posterior ciliary arteries.

Nonarteritic Anterior Ischemic Optic Neuropathy

- It occurs generally in the sixth or seventh decade and is associated with arteriosclerosis, diabetes, hypertension, and hyperlipidemia. Low optic cup to disk ratio is present. Optic nerve head drusen and increased intraocular pressure are predisposing factors. Low-dose aspirin therapy may reduce the risk of involvement of the fellow eye.

Giant Cell Arteritis

- This causes severe visual loss with the risk of complete blindness if treatment is delayed. It occurs in elderly people and is associated with painful and tender temporal arteries, jaw claudication, general malaise, and muscular aches and pains (polymyalgia rheumatica).
- The diagnosis is usually based on an anterior ischemic optic neuropathy and high erythrocyte sedimentation rate (ESR) and C-reactive protein (CRP) in an elderly patient, with or without associated local or systemic features, but the ESR and CRP may be normal.
- Other ocular manifestations of giant cell arteritis are central retinal artery occlusion, cilioretinal artery occlusion, retinal cotton-wool spots, ophthalmic artery occlusion, and diffuse ocular ischemia.
- Treatment with high-dose systemic steroids should be started. Temporal artery biopsy should be performed within 1 week after starting treatment.

Papilledema

- Papilledema is by definition optic disk swelling due to raised intracranial pressure, of which the most common causes are cerebral tumors, abscesses, subdural hematoma, arteriovenous malformations, subarachnoid hemorrhage, hydrocephalus, meningitis, and encephalitis.
- Idiopathic intracranial hypertension is characterized by raised intracranial pressure, no neurologic or neuroimaging abnormality except for anything attributable to the raised intracranial pressure, such as sixth cranial nerve palsy, and normal cerebrospinal fluid constituents. It is a diagnosis of exclusion, commonly seen in young fat females and a number of other causes of the syndrome of pseudotumor cerebri must be excluded, such as cerebral venous sinus occlusion, steroid, OCP's, Amiodarone, tetracycline or vitamin A (retinoid) therapy, uremia, and respiratory failure.
- For papilledema to occur, the subarachnoid space around the optic nerve must be patent and connect the retrolaminar optic nerve through the bony optic canal to the intracranial subarachnoid space, thus allowing increased intracranial pressure to be transmitted to the retrolaminar optic nerve. Slow and fast axonal transport is blocked and axonal distention is seen at the superior and inferior poles of the optic disk, occurs as the first sign of papilledema. Hyperemia of the disk with dilated surface capillaries, blurring of the peripapillary disk margin, and loss of spontaneous venous pulsations are the signs of mild papilledema. Circumferential peripapillary retinal folds (Paton's lines) also develop.
- In acute papilledema, there are hemorrhages and cotton-wool spots on and around the optic disk, indicating vascular and axonal decompensation with the attendant risk of acute optic nerve damage and visual field defects.
- In chronic papilledema, which is likely to be the consequence of prolonged, moderately raised intracranial pressure, a process of compensation appears to limit the optic disk changes such that there are few if any hemorrhages or cotton-wool spots. Vintage papilledema is characterized by the presence of drusen-like deposits within the swollen optic nerve head.
- Papilledema is often asymmetric. **Foster Kennedy's syndrome** is papilledema on one side with optic atrophy due to optic nerve compression on the other, commonly due to skull-base meningiomas. However, it can be mimicked (pseudo-Foster Kennedy syndrome) by ischemic optic neuropathy when optic disk swelling due to a new episode of ischemic optic neuropathy is associated with optic atrophy in the fellow eye due to a previous episode.
- The treatment of papilledema must be directed to the underlying cause. Oral acetazolamide 250 mg one to four times daily or diuretics such as furosemide are usually effective in reducing optic disk swelling. Cerebrospinal fluid shunting or optic nerve sheath fenestration may be undertaken if there is severe or progressive loss of vision or if medical therapy is not tolerated.

Abnormality	Cause	Visual loss	Pupils
Papilledema	Increased intracranial pressure	None or transient blurring; constriction of visual fields and enlargement of blind spot	Normal
Anterior ischemic optic neuropathy	Infarction of disk and intraorbital optic nerve due to atherosclerosis or temporal arteritis	Acute visual loss, monocular	Afferent pupillary defect
Optic neuritis ("papillitis")	Inflammatory changes in disk and intraorbital part of optic nerve— usually due to MS	Rapidly progressive visual loss; usually monocular	Afferent pupillary defect

Tobacco-Alcohol Amblyopia

- Usually it occurs in individuals with poor dietary habits, with heavy alcohol consumption and heavy smoking often being associated.
- There is bilateral loss of central vision, but it can be asymmetric. Central visual fields reveal scotomas that nearly always include both fixation and the blind spot (centrocecal scotoma).
- Adequate diet plus thiamine, folic acid, and vitamin B12 supplements are nearly always effective if presentation is not delayed. Withdrawal of tobacco and alcohol is advisable to hasten the cure.

Optic Nerve Trauma

- Direct optic nerve injury occurs in penetrating orbital trauma, including local anesthetic injections for ocular surgery, and in fractures involving the optic canal.
- Visual loss occurs due to indirect optic nerve trauma, which refers to optic nerve damage secondary to distant skull injury. The site of injury is usually the forehead, often without skull fracture, and the probable mechanism of optic nerve injury is transmission of shock waves through the orbital walls to the orbital apex.

- Optic nerve avulsion usually results from an abrupt rotational injury to the globe, such as from being poked in the eye with a finger.
- Surgery may be indicated to relieve orbital, subperiosteal, or optic nerve sheath hemorrhage or to treat orbital fractures. There is no effective treatment for optic nerve avulsion.

Leber's Hereditary Optic Neuropathy

- Leber's hereditary optic neuropathy is a rare disease characterized by sequential subacute optic neuropathy usually in adolescent males. The underlying genetic abnormality is a point mutation in mitochondrial DNA (mtDNA). mtDNA is exclusively derived from the mother, and thus, in accordance with the general pattern of mitochondrial (maternal) inheritance, the mutation is transmitted through the female line.
- Blurred vision and a central scotoma usually appears first in one eye and later within days, weeks, or months in the other eye. Typical visual field defects are centrocaecal which eventually become absolute. During the acute episode, there may be swelling of the optic disk and peripapillary retina with dilated telangiectatic small blood vessels on their surface
- It causes uniocular, sudden painless, progressive and permanent visual loss. The papillary light reactions frequently remain fairly brisk despite severe visual loss.
- Both optic nerves eventually become atrophic. Total loss of vision or recurrences of visual loss usually do not occur.
- Diagnosis is by identification of one of the three mtDNA point mutations.
- No treatment is known to be effective.

Optic atrophy also occurs in other mitochondrial disorders, either as a manifestation of primary optic neuropathy—e.g., myoclonic epilepsy and ragged red fibers (MERRF) and mitochondrial myopathy, lactic acidosis, and stroke-like episodes (MELAS) or secondary to retinal degeneration in Kearns-Sayre syndrome.

HEREDITARY OPTIC ATROPHY

- Autosomal dominant (juvenile) optic atrophy generally has an insidious onset in childhood, with slow progression of visual loss throughout life. There is characteristically a centrocecal scotoma with impaired color vision. Temporal optic disk pallor is usually present, although often mild, and mild disk cupping is occasionally seen. Diagnosis is by identification of other affected family members. The genetic defect has been mapped to the long arm of chromosome 3.
- Autosomal recessive (infantile) optic atrophy manifests as severe visual loss, present at birth or within 2 years and accompanied by nystagmus. It can be associated with progressive hearing loss, spastic quadriplegia, and dementia, although an inborn error of metabolism must first be considered. Wolfram's syndrome consists of juvenile diabetes insipidus, diabetes mellitus, optic atrophy, and deafness (DIDMOAD).

Optic Nerve Anomalies

- Optic nerve hypoplasia, dysplasia, and coloboma have all been associated with basal encephaloceles and with varying intracranial anomalies, including agenesis of the corpus callosum (de Morsier's syndrome) and pituitary-hypothalamic dysfunction (especially growth hormone deficiency).
- Tilted disks may be seen with hypertelorism or the craniofacial dysostoses (Crouzon's disease, Apert's disease). Megalopapilla may be mistaken for optic atrophy due to the prominence of the lamina cribrosa.
- Remnants of the embryonic hyaloid system range from tissue fragments on the optic disk (Bergmeister's papilla) to strands extending to the posterior lens capsule.

Neoplastic Optic Nerve Infiltration

- In leukemia (usually acute leukemia), non-Hodgkin's lymphoma, and disseminated carcinoma, optic nerve infiltration with marked visual loss and optic disk swelling may develop.
- Gliomas of the anterior visual pathway, more commonly arising in the optic nerve but sometimes arising in the optic chiasm, are rare, usually indolent disorders of children, particularly associated with neurofibromatosis 1. Visual field defects reveal an optic nerve or chiasmal syndrome. Neuroimaging may reveal optic nerve expansion or a mass in the region of the chiasm and hypothalamus.
- Treatment depends on the location of the tumor and its clinical course. Irradiation can be given during a tumor growth spurt, and optic nerve resection is sometimes done when an optic nerve tumor aggressively starts to extend intracranially toward the chiasm.

The size of the normal pupil varies at different ages, from person to person, and with different emotional states, levels of alertness, degrees of accommodation, and ambient room light. The normal pupillary diameter is about 3–4 mm, smaller in infancy, and tending to be larger in childhood and again progressively smaller with advancing age. Evaluation of pupillary responses is important in localizing lesions involving the optic pathways.

Light Reflex Pathway

- The pupillary response to light is a pure reflex with an entirely subcortical pathway. The afferent pupillary fibers are included within the optic nerve and visual pathways until they exit the optic tract just prior to the lateral geniculate nucleus. Fibred decussate in the chiasm and enter the midbrain through the brachium of the superior colliculus and synapse in the pretectal nucleus.
- Each pretectal nucleus decussates neurons dorsal to the cerebral aqueduct to the ipsilateral and contralateral Edinger-Westphal nucleus via the posterior commissure and the periaqueductal gray matter. A synapse then occurs in the Edinger-Westphal nucleus of the oculomotor nerve.
- The efferent pathway is via the third nerve to the ciliary ganglion in the lateral orbit. The postganglionic fibers go via the short ciliary nerves to innervate the sphincter muscle of the iris.

Near Response

- When the eyes look at a near object, three responses occur—accommodation, convergence, and constriction of the pupil, bringing a sharp image into focus on corresponding retinal points. The final common pathway is mediated through the oculomotor nerve with a synapse in the ciliary ganglion.
- The afferent pathway enters the midbrain ventral to the Edinger-Westphal nucleus and sends fibers to both sides of the cortex. Bilateral overaction of the near response is accommodative spasm.

Afferent Pupillary Defect

- If an optic nerve lesion is present, the pupillary light response (both the direct response in the stimulated eye and the consensual response in the fellow eye) is less intense when the involved eye is stimulated than when the normal eye is stimulated. This phenomenon is called a relative afferent pupillary defect (RAPD) and it is a characteristic sign of lesion of optic nerve. Swinging flash light test is used in its detection.
- Absolute afferent pupillary defect is the term applied when there is no pupillary response to light stimulation of a completely blind (amaurotic) eye. Light shone into the normal eye would still induce a consensual response in the blind eye.

Argyll Robertson Pupil (ARP)

- They are usually bilateral, are typically small (less than 3 mm in diameter), commonly irregular and eccentric, do not respond to light stimulation but do respond to a near stimulus, and dilate poorly with mydriatics as a consequence of concomitant iris atrophy. They are seen in central nervous system syphilis. (Remember ARP = Accommodation reflex present)

Tonic Pupil

- Tonic pupil is characterized by light-near dissociation, delayed dilation after a near stimulus (tonic near response), segmental iris constriction, and constriction in response to a weak (0.1%) solution of pilocarpine due to denervation hypersensitivity (confirmatory test).
- It results from post viral illness that causes damage to the ciliary ganglion (ganglionitis) or the short ciliary nerves which leads to parasympathetic nerve fibers damage. In the acute stage, the pupil is dilated and accommodation is impaired.
- Tonic pupil is usually an isolated benign entity, presenting in young women. It may be associated with loss of deep tendon reflexes (Adie's syndrome).

Horner's Syndrome

- Horner's syndrome is caused by a lesion of the sympathetic pathway either
    1. In its central portion, which extends from the posterior hypothalamus through the brainstem to the upper spinal cord (C8–T2);
    2. In its preganglionic portion, which exits the spinal cord and synapses in the superior cervical (stellate) ganglion;
    3. In its postganglionic portion, from the superior cervical ganglion via the carotid plexus and the ophthalmic division of the trigeminal nerve, by which it enters the orbit.
- Melanocyte maturation in the iris of a neonate depends on sympathetic innervation; thus, less pigmented Heterochromia irides occur if a congenital sympathetic lesion is present. Paresis of Müller's muscle produces ptosis. Unilateral miosis, ptosis, and absence of sweating on the ipsilateral face and neck make up the complete syndrome.

- Central Horner's syndrome may be due to brainstem infarction, particularly lateral medullary infarction (Wallenberg's syndrome), syringomyelia, or cervical cord tumor. Preganglionic Horner's syndrome may be due to cervical rib, cervical vertebral fractures, bronchogenic carcinoma (Pancoast's syndrome) and brachial plexus injuries. Postganglionic Horner's syndrome may be due to carotid artery dissection, skull base tumors, or cluster headache.
- The neural control of eye movements is ultimately controlled by alterations in activity in the nuclei and nerve fibers of the oculomotor, trochlear, and abducens nerves, referred to as the nuclear and infranuclear pathways. Coordination of eye movements requires connections between these ocular motor nuclei, the internuclear pathways. The supranuclear pathways are responsible for generation of the commands necessary for the execution of the appropriate movement, whether it be voluntary or involuntary.
- Disorders of the supranuclear pathways characteristically produce a dissociation of effect upon the various types of eye movements. Destructive lesions cause transient deviation to the same side, and the eyes cannot be turned quickly and voluntarily (saccadic movement) to the opposite side. This is called frontal gaze palsy, and recovery occurs when the opposite frontal eye field substitutes.

Disease of the internuclear pathways results in a disruption of the conjugacy of eye movements. In infranuclear disease, the pattern of eye movement disturbance is similar to a lesion involving one or more cranial nerves or their nuclei.

Brainstem

- Lesions of the posterior commissure of the midbrain cause impairment of conjugate upgaze. Lesions dorsal and medial to the red nuclei produce a downgaze paresis.
- **Dorsal midbrain syndrome** (Parinaud's syndrome) is characterized by loss of voluntary upward gaze, convergence-retraction nystagmus, pupillary light-near dissociation, and eyelid retraction (Collier's sign). There may also be accommodative paresis or spasm, loss of voluntary downward gaze, or loss of convergence. Conjugate horizontal ocular movements are usually not affected. The syndrome results from tectal or pretectal lesions affecting the periaqueductal area.
- Lesions of the paramedian pontine reticular formation produce an ipsilateral horizontal gaze palsy affecting saccadic and pursuit movements. Vestibular slow-phase movements are preserved owing to the direct pathway from the vestibular nuclei to the abducens and oculomotor nuclei.

Internuclear Ophthalmoplegia

- The medial longitudinal fasciculus is an important fiber tract extending from the rostral midbrain to the spinal cord. It contains many pathways connecting nuclei within the brainstem, particularly those concerned with extraocular movements. The most common manifestation of damage to the medial longitudinal fasciculus is an internuclear ophthalmoplegia, in which conjugate horizontal eye movements are disrupted owing to failure of coordination between the abducens nerve nucleus in the pons and the oculomotor nerve nucleus in the midbrain.
- The lesion in the brainstem is ipsilateral to the eye with the adduction failure and contralateral to the direction of horizontal gaze that is abnormal. In the most severe form, there is complete loss of adduction on horizontal gaze, producing constant diplopia on lateral gaze with nystagmus in the abducting eye on attempted horizontal gaze.
- In bilateral internuclear ophthalmoplegia, there may also be an upbeating nystagmus on upgaze due to failure of control of gaze holding in the upward direction, and the eyes may be divergent; known as the wall-eyed bilateral internuclear ophthalmoplegia (WEBINO) syndrome.
- Internuclear ophthalmoplegia may be due to multiple sclerosis (particularly in young adults), brainstem infarction (particularly in older patients), tumors, arteriovenous malformations, Wernicke's encephalopathy, and encephalitis. Bilateral internuclear ophthalmoplegia is most commonly due to multiple sclerosis.

Ocular Motor Nerve Palsies

Oculomotor Palsy

- Lesions of the third nerve nucleus typically affect the ipsilateral medial and inferior rectus and inferior oblique muscles, both levator muscles, and both superior rectus muscles. There will be bilateral ptosis and bilateral limitation of elevation as well as limitation of adduction and depression ipsilaterally.
- From the fascicle of the nerve in the midbrain to its eventual termination in the orbit, third nerve palsy produces purely ipsilateral dysfunction. The eye may only be moved laterally. There can be a dilated fixed pupil, absent accommodation, and ptosis of the upper lid, often severe enough to cover the pupil. Concomitant Horner's syndrome (sympathetic paresis) resulting in a relatively small unreactive pupil may be present.
- Ischemia, intracranial aneurysm, head trauma, and intracranial tumors are the most common causes of third nerve palsy in adults. Aneurysm usually arises from the junction of the internal carotid and posterior communicating arteries. Intracranial tumor may cause oculomotor palsy by direct damage to the nerve or due to mass effect. Pupillary dilation, initially unilateral and then bilateral, is an important sign of herniation of the medial temporal lobe through the tentorial hiatus (tentorial herniation) due to a rapidly expanding supratentorial mass. Bilateral peripheral third nerve palsies can occur secondary to other interpeduncular lesions, such as basilar artery aneurysm.

Etiology is Classified Anatomically Based on the Location

- Nuclear—Vascular (stroke), Demyelination (multiple sclerosis), Tumors
- Fasiculus—Weber's syndrome, Benedikt's syndrome, Nothnagel's syndrome
    1. In *Nothnagel's syndrome*, injury to the superior cerebellar peduncle causes ipsilateral oculomotor palsy and contralateral cerebellar ataxia.
    2. In *Benedikt's syndrome*, injury to the red nucleus results in ipsilateral oculomotor palsy and contralateral tremor, chorea, and athetosis.
    3. *Claude's syndrome* incorporates features of both the aforementioned syndromes, by injury to both the red nucleus and the superior cerebellar peduncle.
    4. In *Weber's syndrome*, injury to the cerebral peduncle causes ipsilateral oculomotor palsy with contralateral hemiparesis. Basilar aneurysm (between posterior communicating and internal carotid arteries), Raised intracranial pressure (uncal herniation)
- Intracavernous—cavernous sinus syndrome
- Intraorbital—Vascular (DM), Trauma.

THIRD CN PALSY FEATURES

	Medical 3rd CN palsy	Surgical 3rd CN palsy
Features	• Age > 60 • Vascular risk factors (DM, HPT, smoking) • Pupil sparing (80%) • Pupil continues to be spared after 1 week • Complete 3rd CN palsy • Isolated 3rd CN palsy • No aberrant regeneration • Recovery within 3 months	• Young • No vascular risk factors • Pupil involved (90%) • Progression of pupil involvement • Incomplete 3rd CN palsy • Multiple CN palsies • Aberrant regeneration • No recovery
Etiology	• DM • Giant cell arteritis (GCA) • Ophthalmic migraine • Inflammatory • Tolosa-Hunt syndrome • Miller Fisher syndrome	• Cerebral aneurysm • Raised intracranial pressure (from uncal herniation) • Tumor
Evaluation	• History of DM and HPT • Check BP (HPT) • Headache (GCA, ophthalmic migraine) • Painful 3rd CN palsy (DM, migraine, Tolosa-Hunt) • Ataxia, areflexia (Miller Fisher)	• Check fundus for papilledema uncal herniation) • Examine neurologically • History of head injury • History of headache, nausea and vomitting (raised intracranial pressure) • History of HPT (aneurysm)
Investigations	• CBC, ESR • Fasting blood sugar level • VDRL, FfA • Autoimmune markers	• CT scan (CNS bleed, meningioma, stroke, trauma)

Cyclic oculomotor palsy can complicate congenital third nerve palsy with a unilateral third nerve palsy showing cyclic spasms every 10–30 seconds. During these intervals, ptosis improves and accommodation increases. This phenomenon continues unchanged throughout life but decreases with sleep and increases with greater arousal. It is probably a periodic discharge by damaged neurons of the oculomotor nucleus that summate subthreshold stimuli until a discharge occurs.

- *Marcus gunn phenomenon (jaw winking syndrome)*
    - This congenital condition consists of elevation of a ptotic eyelid upon movement of the jaw. Acquired cases occur after damage to the oculomotor nerve with subsequent innervation of the lid (levator palpebrae superioris) by a branch of the fifth cranial nerve.

Trochlear Palsy
- It may present in childhood with an abnormal head posture or in childhood or adult life with eyestrain or diplopia due to reduced ability to overcome the vertical ocular deviation (decompensation). The nerve is vulnerable to injury at the site of exit from the dorsal aspect of the brainstem. Both nerves may be damaged by severe trauma as they decussate in the anterior medullary velum, resulting in bilateral superior oblique palsies.
- Superior oblique palsy results in upward deviation (hypertropia) of the eye, which increases when the patient looks down and to the opposite side. In addition in acquired palsy, there is excyclotropia; therefore, one of the diplopic images will be tilted with respect to the other. Tilting the head toward the involved side increases the vertical ocular deviation. Tilting the head away from the side of the involved eye may relieve the diplopia, and patients frequently adopt such a head tilt.

Abducens Nerve Palsy
- This is the most common single extraocular muscle palsy. Abduction of the eye is reduced or absent; esotropia is present in the primary position and increases with distance fixation and upon gaze to the affected side. Ischemia secondary to arteriosclerosis, diabetes, migraine, and hypertension is a common cause.
- Abducens palsy is a false localizing sign in increased intracranial pressure.
- Mobius' syndrome (congenital facial diplegia) can be associated with a sixth nerve or conjugate gaze palsy. Pseudo-sixth nerve palsies can occur in Duane's syndrome, spasm of the near response, thyroid eye disease, myasthenia, or long-standing strabismus and in medial rectus entrapment by an ethmoid fracture.
- Duane's syndrome is a stationary, nearly always unilateral condition consisting of deficient horizontal ocular motility characterized by complete or partial deficiency of abduction.
- Gradenigo's syndrome is characterized by pain in the face (from irritation of the trigeminal nerve) and abducens palsy. The syndrome is produced by petrositis and occurs as a complication of otitis media with mastoiditis or petrous bone tumors.

5th Cranial Nerve Palsy
- Nasociliary branch of the ophthalmic branch (V1) of the 5th cranial nerve, i.e. trigeminal nerve mediates the corneal reflex by acting as the afferent and sensing the stimulus on the cornea, lid or conjunctiva. Damage to this cranial nerve branch results in absent corneal reflex when the affected eye is stimulated.
- Temporal and zygomatic branches of the facial nerve act as the efferent of this reflex by initiating the motor response with the center (nucleus) as the pons of the brainstem.
- This reflex is absent in infants under 9 months of age and is diminished or abolished by use of contact lens while testing.
- The corneal reflex/blink reflex is an involuntary blinking of the eyelids caused by stimulation of the cornea (touching/foreign body)
- The reflex should elicit both direct and consensual response (stimulation of one cornea elicits closing of both eyelids) and is usually rapid (0.1 seconds).
- Purpose of this reflex is to protect eyes from foreign bodies or even bright light (optical reflex – slower; mediated by visual cortex which resides in the occipital part of the brain).

Multiple Cranial Nerve Palsies
Syndromes Affecting Cranial Nerves III, IV, and VI
Superior Orbital Fissure Syndrome
- All the ocular motor nerves pass through the superior orbital fissure and can be involved by trauma or by tumor encroaching on the fissure.

Orbital Apex Syndrome
- This syndrome is similar to the superior orbital fissure syndrome with the addition of optic nerve signs and usually greater proptosis. It may be caused by tumor, inflammation, or trauma.

Sudden Complete Ophthalmoplegia
- Complete ophthalmoplegia of sudden onset can be due to extensive brainstem vascular disease, Wernicke's encephalopathy, Fisher's syndrome, bulbar poliomyelitis, pituitary apoplexy, basilar aneurysm, meningitis, diphtheria, botulism, or myasthenic crisis.

Myasthenia Gravis
- Myasthenia gravis is characterized by abnormal fatigability of striated muscles after repetitive contraction that improves after rest and often is first manifested by weakness of the extraocular muscles. Unilateral fatiguing ptosis is a frequent first sign, with subsequent bilateral involvement of extraocular muscles, so that diplopia is often an early symptom. The weakness shows diurnal variations and often worsens as the day progresses but can be improved by a nap.

- The differential diagnosis includes chronic progressive external ophthalmoplegia, oculopharyngeal muscular dystrophy, myotonic dystrophy, ocular motor cranial nerve palsies, brainstem lesions, epidemic encephalitis, bulbar and pseudobulbar palsy, postdiphtheritic paralysis, botulism, and multiple sclerosis.

Chronic Progressive External Ophthalmoplegia

- This disease is characterized by a slowly progressive inability to move the eyes and severe early ptosis yet normal pupillary responses. It may begin at any age and progresses over a period of 5–15 years to complete external ophthalmoplegia.
- It is a form of mitochondrial myopathy and may be associated with other manifestations of mitochondrial disease, such as pigmentary degeneration of the retina, deafness, cerebellar-vestibular abnormalities, seizures, cardiac conduction defects, and peripheral sensorimotor neuropathy.
- Onset before 15 years of age of chronic progressive external ophthalmoplegia, heart block, and pigmentary retinopathy constitutes the Kearns-Sayre syndrome.

Vascular Diseases

CRVO

- **Causes:**
  - Uncontrolled hypertension
  - Uncontrolled diabetic mellitus
  - Hypercholesterolemia
  - Atherosclerosis
  - Collagen vascular diseases
  - Hyperviscosity diseases
  - Dysproteinemia
  - Leukemia
  - glaucoma
- **Clinical features:**
  - Usually occurs in females in the 6th–7th decade
  - Presents with floaters and decreased vision; Characterised by sudden painless loss of vision
- **Signs:**
  - Optic disk edema, macular edema, cotton wool spots, hard exudates, dilated vessels in all quadrants
  - The retinal is full of flame shaped hemorrhages (splashed tomato/tomato ketchup retina)
  - Glaucoma associated with CRVO is called hundred day glaucoma since it takes 90–100 days for the developmet of glaucoma after CRVO due to neovascularization.

Pathogenesis

CRVO–occlusion just posterior to lamina cribosa – hypoxia – secretion of VEGF – neovascularization – Glaucoma in 3 months/90 days–neovascular glaucoma in CRVO.

Treatment

- Treat underlying medical causes
- Anti–VEGF agents, steroids, intravitreal medications for macular edema.

RETINAL DETACHMENT

- CSR causes exudative retinal detachment; Shifting fluid is a hallmark of exudative RD
- Photopsia is absent; RD is without any breaks
- Rhegmatogenous RD: Holes/breaks in the retina lead to the detachment of Retinal pigment, Epithelium and Neurosensory layer.

Diagnosis

1. **Ophthalmoscopy:** RD best examined by indirect ophthalmoscopy with sclera indentation. Freshly detached retina gives gray reflex and is raised anteriorly.
   Shaffer sign (tobacco dusting): posterior vitreous detachment with pigment in the anterior vitreous

2. Perimetry
3. Goldmann three mirror fundus lens and indirect slit lamp biomicroscopy
4. Electroretinography
5. B scan USG

TELANGIECTASIA

- Refers to the abnormal dilated conjunctival capillary formation
- May present as only an asymptomatic red spot on eye
- Depending on the etiology patient may also have epistaxis or GI bleeding
- Some may present with subconjunctival hemorrhage
- Evaluation includes a complete ophthalmic history with detailed examination of the conjunctiva, cornea and lens
- CT scan and medical consultation is necessary to rule out other systemic diseases
- *DD:* Fabry's disease, Osler-Weber-Rendu syndrome, Sturge-Weber syndrome. Usually no treatment is recommended.

Vascular Insufficiency and Occlusion of the Internal Carotid Artery

- Transient episodes of visual loss (amaurosis fugax) most often result from retinal emboli, usually from carotid disease but possibly from cardiac valvular disease or cardiac arrhythmia.
- They also occur in thrombotic disorders such as hyperviscosity states or antiphospholipid syndrome and from other causes of impaired ocular or cerebral perfusion such as giant cell arteritis, migraine, vertebrobasilar ischemia (see below), severe hypotension, or shock.
- The visual loss from retinal emboli is characteristically described as a curtain descending across the vision of one eye, with complete loss of vision for 2–10 minutes, and then completes recovery.
- There may be associated transient ischemic attacks (TIAs) or completed strokes of the ipsilateral cerebral hemisphere. In other causes of amaurosis fugax, there may be constriction of the visual field from the periphery to the center, "graying" rather than complete loss of vision, and involvement of both eyes simultaneously.
- Fleeting episodes of visual loss that last a few seconds (transient visual obscurations) may occur in papilledema, affecting one or both eyes together or monocularly with orbital tumors.
- Cholesterol, platelet-fibrin, and calcific are the three main types of retinal emboli. Cholesterol emboli (Hollenhorst plaques) may be visible with the ophthalmoscope as small, glistening, yellow-red crystals situated at bifurcations of the retinal arteries.

Occlusion of the Middle Cerebral Artery

This may produce severe contralateral hemiplegia, hemianesthesia, and homonymous hemianopia. The lower quadrants of the visual fields (upper radiations) are most apt to be involved. Aphasia may be present if the dominant hemisphere is involved.

Vascular Insufficiency of the Vertebrobasilar Arterial System

- Brief episodes of transient bilateral blurring of vision commonly precede a basilar artery stroke. The blurring is described as a graying of vision just as if the house lights were being dimmed at a theater. Episodes last less than 5 minutes (often only a few seconds) and may be associated with other transient symptoms of vertebrobasilar insufficiency.
- Antiplatelet drugs can decrease the frequency and severity of vertebrobasilar symptoms.

Occlusion of the Basilar Artery

Complete or extensive thrombosis of the basilar artery nearly always causes death. With partial occlusion or basilar "insufficiency" due to arteriosclerosis, a wide variety of brainstem and cerebellar signs may be present. These include nystagmus, supranuclear oculomotor signs, and involvement of cranial nerves III, IV, VI, and VII.

Occlusion of the Posterior Cerebral Artery

Occlusion of the cortical branches (most common) cause homonymous hemianopia, usually superior quadrantic (the artery supplies primarily the inferior visual cortex).

Nystagmus

This is a rhythmical oscillation of the eyes, occurring physiologically from vestibular and optokinetic stimulation or pathologically in a wide variety of diseases. Abnormalities of the eyes or optic nerves, present at birth or acquired in childhood, can produce a complex, searching nystagmus with irregular pendular (sinusoidal) and jerk features. This nystagmus is commonly referred to as *congenital sensory nystagmus.*

Jerk Nystagmus

This is characterized by a slow drift off the target, followed by a fast corrective saccade. The nystagmus is named after the quick phase. Jerk nystagmus can be downbeat, upbeat, horizontal (left or right), and torsional. The pattern of nystagmus may vary with gaze position.

Gaze-Evoked Nystagmus

This is the most common form of jerk nystagmus. When the eyes are held eccentrically in the orbits, they have a natural tendency to drift back to primary position. The subject compensates by making a corrective saccade to maintain the deviated eye position. Many normal patients have mild gaze-evoked nystagmus. Exaggerated gaze-evoked nystagmus can be induced by muscle paresis; myasthenia gravis; demyelinating disease; and cerebellopontine angle, brainstem, and cerebellar lesions.

Vestibular Nystagmus

Vestibular nystagmus results from dysfunction of the labyrinth (Meniere's disease), vestibular nerve, or vestibular nucleus in the brainstem. Peripheral vestibular nystagmus often occurs in discrete attacks, with symptoms of nausea and vertigo. There may be associated tinnitus and hearing loss. Sudden shifts in head position may provoke or exacerbate symptoms.

Downbeat Nystagmus

- *Downbeat nystagmus* occurs from lesions near the craniocervical junction (Chiari malformation, basilar invagination). It has also been reported in brainstem or cerebellar stroke, lithium or anticonvulsant intoxication, alcoholism, and multiple sclerosis. *Upbeat nystagmus* is associated with damage to the pontine tegmentum, from stroke, demyelination, or tumor.
- The phakomatoses are a group of diseases characterized by multiple hamartomas occurring in various organ systems and at variable times.

Neurofibromatosis

- Neurofibromatosis is a generalized hereditary disease characterized by multiple tumors of the skin, central nervous system, peripheral nerves, and nerve sheaths. Other developmental anomalies, particularly of the bones, may be associated. There are two distinct dominant conditions, both due to inactivating mutations of tumor suppressor genes.
- Neurofibromatosis 1 is associated with tumors primarily of astrocytes and neurons, whereas neurofibromatosis 2 is associated with tumors of the meninges and Schwann cells. The manifestations may be present at birth but often become apparent during pregnancy, during puberty, and at menopause.
- **Neurofibromatosis 1** (Recklinghausen's disease) is characterized by multiple café au lait spots (six or more greater than 1.5 cm in diameter), peripheral neurofibromas, which are usually nodular but may be diffuse (plexiform) and usually cutaneous but may involve deep structures, axillary freckling, and Lisch nodules (iris hamartomas). Its gene lies on chromosome 17.
- Neurofibromas may need to be removed to relieve spinal nerve root compression. They may undergo sarcomatous degeneration.
- A defining feature of **neurofibromatosis 2** is bilateral vestibular schwannomas, but unilateral vestibular schwannoma, other intracranial or spinal schwannoma, multiple intracranial or intraspinal meningiomas, or gliomas may occur. Café au lait spots and peripheral neurofibromas may be present. Its gene lies on chromosome 22.
- In neurofibromatosis 1, there may be neurofibromas of the lids, either cutaneous nodular or subcutaneous plexiform (rubbery "bag of worms"). Corneal nerves are often prominent. There may be congenital glaucoma. Anterior visual pathway glioma is particularly associated with neurofibromatosis 1.
- About 75% of patients with neurofibromatosis 2 have early posterior subcapsular lens opacities. Epiretinal membranes, combined pigment epithelial and retinal hamartomas, optic disk gliomas, and optic nerve sheath meningiomas occur with increased frequency in neurofibromatosis 2.

Von Hippel-Lindau Disease

- Von Hippel-Lindau disease is due to a mutation on chromosome 3. Inheritance is autosomal dominant with high penetrance.
- The most common manifestation is retinal capillary hemangioma. Other manifestations are cerebellar hemangioblastoma; cysts of the kidneys, pancreas, and epididymis; pheochromocytoma; and renal cell carcinoma.
- Retinal capillary hemangioma usually develops in the peripheral retina and initially manifests as dilation and tortuosity of retinal vessels, followed by development of an angiomatous lesion with hemorrhages and exudates.
- Retinal capillary hemangiomas may be treated with laser photocoagulation, cryotherapy, or plaque radiotherapy. First-degree relatives of patients with von Hippel-Lindau disease also need to undergo regular screening. Genetic testing increasingly allows identification of individuals specifically at risk.

Sturge-Weber Syndrome

- This nonfamilial disease with unknown inheritance is recognizable at birth by a characteristic nevus flammeus (port wine stain, or venous angioma) on one side of the face. There is corresponding angiomatous involvement (leptomeningeal angiodysplasia) of the meninges and brain, which causes seizures, mental retardation, and cerebral atrophy.
- There is no effective treatment for Sturge-Weber syndrome. The glaucoma is difficult to control. Choroidal hemangioma may require treatment with laser photocoagulation or radiotherapy.

Wyburn-Mason Syndrome

- Wyburn-Mason syndrome is a rare disorder of multiple arteriovenous malformations, variably involving the retina, other portions of the anterior visual pathway, the midbrain, the maxilla, and the mandible, all on the same side of the head.
- Headaches and seizures are the common presenting symptoms. Large, tortuous, dilated vessels covering extensive areas of the retina are an important diagnostic clue and can cause cystic retinal degeneration with decreased vision. Optic atrophy without retinal lesions can also occur.

Ataxia-telangiectasia

- Ataxia-telangiectasia is an autosomal recessive disorder characterized by skin and conjunctival telangiectases, cerebellar ataxia, and recurrent sinopulmonary infections.
- The recurrent infections relate to thymic deficiencies, corresponding T cell abnormalities and low levels of immunoglobulins.

Tuberous Sclerosis (Bourneville's Disease)

- Tuberous sclerosis is characterized by the triad of adenoma sebaceum, epilepsy, and mental retardation. Adenoma sebaceum (angiofibromas) are flesh-colored papules are 1–2 mm in diameter and have a butterfly distribution on the nose and malar area; they can also occur in the subungual and periungual areas.
- Ashleaf-shaped hypopigmented ovals can be present on the skin even of neonates and are best seen under Wood's light examination.
- Retinal hamartomas appear as oval or circular white areas in the peripheral fundus and, like optic nerve hamartomas, characteristically have a mulberry-like appearance. Subependymal nodules in the periventricular areas of the brain can calcify and appear as candle wax gutterings or drippings on radiologic studies. Seizures occur in most patients, often starting within the first year of life.
- The disease is inherited sporadically or as an autosomal dominant disorder with low penetrance. The prognosis for life relates to the degree of central nervous system involvement. In severe cases, death can occur in the second or third decade; if there is minimal central nervous system involvement, life expectancy should be normal.

Cerebromacular Degeneration

- The genetically determined (autosomal recessive) lysosomal storage disorders may affect the neural elements of the retina. The clinical forms are classified by the age at onset and the enzyme deficiency. The pathologic changes are present prenatally.
- Clinical manifestations occur as a critical level of intraneuronal lipid deposition is reached, resulting in a progressive disease, including dementia, visual disturbance, and neuromotor deterioration.
- The striking ocular finding of a cherry-red spot in the macula is seen in a number of lysosomal storage disorders, e.g., gangliosidosis (Tay-Sachs disease, Sandhoff disease, and generalized GM_1), Niemann-Pick type A (sphingomyelin lipidosis), neuraminidase deficiency (sialidosis and Goldberg syndrome), and Farber disease.

MAJOR PHAKOMATOSES AND THEIR FEATURES

Syndrome	Inheritance	Genetics	Cutaneous findings	Neurologic findings
Neurofibromatosis 1	Autosomal *dominant*	*NF1* gene (17q11)	Café au lait spots	Neurofibroma Lisch nodules Optic glioma
Neurofibromatosis 2	Autosomal *dominant*	*NF2* gene (22q12)	Cutaneous and subcutaneous schwannomas	Bilateral vestibular schwannoma, Meningioma, ependymoma, Subcapsular cataracts
Tuberous sclerosis complex	Autosomal *dominant*	*TSC1* gene (9q34) *TSC2* gene (16p13)	Ash-leaf spot, Shagreen patches, Adenoma sebaceum	Vogt's triad: seizures, mental retardation, adenoma sebaceum subependymal giant cell astrocytoma (SEGA)
Sturge-Weber syndrome	Sporadic	—	Port wine stain	Leptomeningeal angiomatosis, Skull X-ray or CT may show tram-track sign
von Hippel-Lindau disease	Autosomal *dominant*	*VHL* gene (3p)	Retinal hemangioblastoma	Cerebellar Hemangioblastoma
Incontinentia pigmenti	X-linked *dominant*	NEMO/IKKā gene	"Marble cake" hyper-pigmentation, Diffuse hypopigmented retina	Mental retardation and seizures

EALES DISEASE: PERIPHLEBITIS RETINAE

- It consists of the classical triad of spontaneous and recurrent hemorrhage in young males. The vitreous will be filled with blood.
- The symptoms consist of floaters and sudden painless loss of vision, though flashes are characteristically absent
- *Treatment:* ATT followed by steroids.

STARGARDT'S DISEASE

- Most common macular dystrophy – 80% show silent choroid in early stage
- Inheritance:
  - Autosomal recessive trait;
  - Typical form STGD1 – caused by mutations involving ABCA4 gene – maps to the short arm of chromosome 1 (1p22.1)
  - Accumulation of lipofuscin throughout RPE leads to the characteristic hallmark of the disease – an accumulation of discrete "pisciform" flecks at the level of RPE.

FUNDOSCOPY

Examination of the optic fundus usually involves assessing the following parameters:
- Shape of the disk
- Color of the disk—coloboma
- Size of the optic cup—normal cup:disk ratio – less than 0.7. greater ratios indicate nerve fiber loss as seen in glaucoma
- Vascular architecture—trifurcation seen in optic nerve head drusen
- Evidence of papilledema—absence of pulsation; worsening is indicated by optic disk being raised with exudates and hemorrhages
- Changes in surrounding retina such as hard and soft exudates, microaneurysms, hemorrhages, new vessel formation, pigmentary changes (bone spicules–retinitis pigmentosa, salt and pepper in mitochondrial diseases; Macular changes – cherry red spot.

OCULAR SARCOIDOSIS

- Uveitis secondary to sarcoidosis: candle wax drippings and punched out lesions
- Anterior uveitis: 22–70%; granulomatous and chronic
- Conjunctival involvement is seen
- Sarcoid granuloma—solitary yellow millet seed nodules; iris nodules–12.5%
- Hypercalcemia leads to corneal band keratopathy in a few
- Posterior segment: vitritis, intermediate uveitis, panuveitis, posterior uveitis, choroid nodules, exudative retinal detachment
- Complications: posterior synechiae, cataract and glaucoma; more in patients with chronic posterior uveitis and panuveitis.

VISUAL FIELD DEFECTS

- **Causes:** Tumor compressing optic nerves or chiasma leading to axonal damage.
- Visual field defects vary in severity and symmetry based on size and location of tumor.
- **Chiasmal field defects:** Lesions at the level of optic chiasma such as pituitary adenomas (compress chiasma from below) typically produce bitemporal hemianopia.
- **Junctional field defects:** Commonly seen in meningioma, aneurysm, inflammation and as the presenting sign of pituitary adenomas.
- **Junctional scotoma:** Central scotoma in one eye with temporal visual field loss in the other eye.
- **Monocular visual field defects:** Asymmetric tumors may preferentially involve one side of the chiasm or an optic nerve and most commonly presents as a supertemporal quadrantanopia.
- Sudden monocular visual loss can be due to pituitary adenoma (missed) pituitary apoplexy. When not found associated with RAPD or optic atrophy, suspicion of functional vision loss is raised. This is confirmed by the persistence of temporal hemianopia on binocular visual field testing.

- **Lesions of optic tract:** Characterized by incongruous homonymous hemianopia associated with contralateral hemianopic papillary reaction–Wernickes reaction.
- **Causes:** Syphilitic meningitis, tuberculosis and tumors of optic thalamus, aneurysm of superior cerebellar or posterior cerebral arteries
- These lesions lead to partial descending optic atrophy.

ORBITAL TUMORS

Mostly benign in both childhood and adult age groups.
- **MC benign orbital tumors:**
  - **In children:** Dermoids, capillary and cavernous hemangioma
  - **In adults:** Hemangioma, lymphangioma, A-V malformations
  - **Less common orbital tumors:** Schwannomas, lipoma, mucocele
- **Orbital malignancies:**
  - **In children:** Rhabdomyosarcoma (MC), Burkitt's lymphoma, granulocytic sarcoma;
  - **Metastatic orbital tumors:** Neuroblastoma, Ewing sarcoma, Wilms tumor, Leukemia
  - **In adults:** Lymphoma (MC), hemangiopericytoma, chondrosarcoma, malignant neurofibroma
  - **Lymphoma:** Initially confined to orbit without systemic manifestations
  - **Metastatic orbital tumors:** Mainly arise from breast and prostate
  - **Direct invasion:** Squamous and basal cell carcinomas – from surrounding skin and sinuses.

RETINOBLASTOMA

- **Congenital**—more common in infants and very young children
- Due to deletions or mutation of QL4 band of chromosome 13
- *Symptoms:* Leucocoria/amaurotic cat eye – yellow reflex from pupil
- Cauliflower like growth from the retina extending into the vitreous – chiefly consists of small round cells with large nuclei
- 75% tumors have calcification– pathognomonic–can be detected by X-ray. However CT more sensitive to delineate tumor
- *Treatment:*
  - Small tumors – brachytherapy with 60Co or 125I; cryotherapy for anterior lesions, photocoagulation for posterior lesions
  - Large tumors – enucleation, external beam radiation therapy – radiation only to affected areas of posterior segment; avoids damage to lens and surrounding retina
  - Prognosis – fatal if left untreated; fair if extraocular extension is avoided

CATARACT

Chronic, slowly progressive painless loss of vision; loss of vision is usually bilateral, asymmetrical and develops over weeks to years.

Causes
- Age
- Genetics—Down syndrome, Turner syndrome, Edward syndrome, Patau syndrome, cri-du-chat syndrome, neurofibromatosis type 2, Alport syndrome, Conradis syndrome, Lowe syndrome
- Skin diseases—Eczema, atopic dermatitis, pemphigus, basal cell nevus
- Radiation—UV light, glassblowers, lasers
- Medications—Steroids, antipsychotics, miotics
- Infections—Cysticercosis, leprosy, toxoplasmosis, varicella, onchocerciasis
- Postoperative—Vitrectomy, cataract surgery
- Trauma—Blunt trauma, electrical injuries
- Smoking and alcohol
- Congenital—Congenital syphilis, CMV, rubella
- Metabolic and nutritional diseases—Fabrys disease, galactosemia, homocystinuria, hyperparathyroidism, hypothyroidism, hypocalcemia, Wilson's disease, mucopolysaccharidoses.

Types of Cataract

- Sunflower cataract—Wilson's disease
- Oil drop cataract—Galactosemia
- Christmas tree opacity—Dystrophia myotonica
- Snow flake/snow storm cataract—Diabetes mellitus
- Shield like anterior subcapsular cataract—atopic dermatitis (syndermatotic)
- Stellate posterior subcapsular cataract—Myotonic dystrophy
- Rosette shaped cataract—Traumatic cataract (vossius ring – imprinting of iris pigment on the anterior lens capsule)
- Polychromatic lustre—Complicated cataract
- Morgagnian cataract—hypermature senile cataract
- Glass blowers cataract—infrared radiation.

Glaucoma

Open Angle

- Progressive peripheral visual field loss followed by central field loss
- Associated with elevated intraocular pressure – due to increased aqueous production and decreased outflow
- Optic disk – cupping – associated with loss of ganglion cell axons.

Angle Closure

- Narrowing or closure of anterior chamber angle
- Normal anterior chamber angle provides drainage for the aqueous humor and this upon being blocked or narrowed leads to increased IOP and damage to optic nerve due to inadequate drainage.
- Acute angle closure glaucoma can occur in certain anatomically predisposed individuals; can present as painful red eye and must be treated within 24 hours to prevent permanent blindness.

Symptoms

- Severe eye pain and headache accompanied by nausea or vomiting
- Blurred vision/appearance of rainbow colored circles around bright lights
- Sudden loss of vision.

Vitreous Hemorrhage

Causes

- Diabetic retinopathy (MC-adults) hemorrhage due to proliferation of new and abnormal blood vessels in the retina which are weak and more prone to breakage
- Trauma (more common in the young)
- Retinal detachment – break in the retina leads to fluid leakage behind the retina leading to detachment; this is turn causes retinal blood vessels to leak into the vessels
- Posterior vitreous detachment
- Age related macular degeneration
- Macroaneurysm
- Retinal neovascularization due to CRVO
- Proliferative sickle cell retinopathy.

Symptoms

- Blurred vision; photopsia
- Small hemorrhage – sudden development of floaters
- Extensive hemorrhage – sudden painless loss of vision
- *Fate:* organization or complete absorption

Complications

- Vitreous liquefaction
- Degeneration
- Khaki cell glaucoma
- Retinitis proliferans

Treatment
- Conservative
- Treat the cause
- Vitrectomy

Major Causes of Blindness
- Cataract
- Glaucoma
- Uncorrected refractive errors

Causes of Sudden Loss of Vision
- Central retinal artery occlusion
- Retinal detachment
- Central retinal vein occlusion
- Retrobulbar neuritis

Causes of Transient Loss of Vision
- Carotid artery disease
- Migraine
- Papilloedema
- Severe hypertension

Diabetic Retinopathy
- Important cause of avoidable blindness in India
- No early warning signs
- *Early symptoms:* Blurred vision—difficulty in carrying out daily activities;
- Earliest manifestation—microaneurysms
- *Diagnosis:* by visual acuity test
- Pupillary dilation
- Ophthalmoscopy
- Cotton wool spots/soft exudates are commonly found in diabetics
- Neovascularization forms the hallmark of the disease.

Pterygium
- Elevated, superficial, external ocular mass which forms over the perilimbal conjunctive and extends onto the corneal surface
- Usually follows a pingecula
- They can be small and quiescent to large aggressive fibrovascular lesions which erode and distort the corneal surface and obscure the optical center of the cornea.

Treatment
- Simple excision
- Sliding flaps of conjunctiva
- External beta radiation therapy
- Topical chemotherapeutic agents–mitomycin C.

Multiple Choice Questions

1. Swinging test is positive in:
   a. Retrobulbar neuritis
   b. Open angle glaucoma
   c. Immature senile cataract
   d. Vitreous hemorrhage

2. Which of the following is false about central serous retinopathy?
   a. More common in anxious males
   b. Sudden painless loss of vision
   c. Smoke stack appearance on FA
   d. Treatment should be started as early as possible

3. The most common cause of loss of vision in diabetic retinopathy is:
   a. Vitreous hemorrhage
   b. Tractional retinal detachment
   c. CSME
   d. Neovascularization

4. All of the following are true about retinal detachment except:
   a. Floaters are present
   b. Flashes of light due to pulling of vitreous
   c. Curtain falling in front of eye
   d. Gradual painless loss of vision

5. All of the following are true about Eale's disease except:
   a. Spontaneous vitreous hemorrhage
   b. Recurrent vitreous hemorrhage
   c. Flashes are present
   d. Floaters are present

6. Resection at optic chiasma will lead to:
   a. Homonymous hemianopia
   b. Binasal hemianopia
   c. Bitemporal hemianopia
   d. Bitemporal quadrant pain

7. All are true about pseudotumor cerebri except:
   a. Papilloedema present
   b. CT/MRI normal
   d. Vit a deficiency
   c. ICT increased

8. "Silent choroid" on FFA is feature of:
   a. Best's disease
   b. Age related macular degeneration
   c. Stargardt's disease
   d. Cystoid macular edema

9. Leber's optic neuropathy has the following features except:
   a. LT commonly affects healthy males
   b. It causes uniocular, sudden painless, progressive and permanent visual loss
   c. Pupillary reflexes are affected early in the disease
   d. Typical visual field defects are centrocaecal which eventually become absolute

10. Uhthoff's sign is seen in:
    a. Diabetic retinopathy
    b. Demyelinating optic neuritis
    c. Craniopharyngioma
    d. Diabetes insipidus

11. Which of the following diagnostic studies is indicated in evaluation of age-related maculardegeneration (AMD) to detect the presence of choroidal neovascularization (CNV)?
    a. Fluorescein angiography
    b. Magnetic resonance imaging
    c. Corneal topography
    d. Computerized axial tomography

12. Hallmark of diabetic retinopathy:
    a. Microaneurysms
    b. Soft exudates
    c. Neovascularization
    d. Cotton wool spots

13. "Pie in the floor" field defects are seen in:
    a. Optic tract lesions
    b. Lateral geniculate lesions
    c. Temporal lobe lesions
    d. Parietal lobe lesions

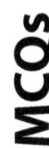

Answers

| 1. a | 2. d | 3. c | 4. d | 5. c | 6. c | 7. d |
| 8. c | 9. c | 10. b | 11. a | 12. c | 13. d | |

14. Hundred-day glaucoma is associated with:
    a. Neovascular glaucoma
    b. CRAO
    c. CRVO
    d. Steroid related glaucoma

15. The following are incorrect *except*:
    a. Wernicke's hemianopic pupillary response: occurs in optic tract field defect
    b. Gerstmanns syndrome: lesion in the non-dominant parietal lobe
    c. Marcus Gunn's pupil: diagnostic of optic neuritis
    d. Foster-Kennedy syndrome: lesion in the optic tract

16. The best treatment for MX of CRAO:
    a. Ocular massage
    b. Paracentesis
    c. Carbogen inhalation
    d. IV TPA

17. The best treatment for wet ARMD:
    a. Antioxidants
    b. Photodynamic phototherapy
    c. B carotene
    d. Anti VEGF

18. The causes of rhegmatogenous retinal detachment are all *except*:
    a. Myopia
    b. Aphakia
    d. CSR
    c. Trauma

19. Adie's pupil:
    a. Young females
    b. Accommodation reflex present
    c. Mydriatic test is performed
    d. Light reflex absent

20. All are true about Horner's syndrome *except*:
    a. Enophthalmos
    b. Miosis
    a. Anhydrosis
    d. Ptosis

21. Popcorn simulating lesion between normal and avascular retina is which stage of ROP?
    a. ROP 1
    b. ROP 2
    c. ROP 3
    d. ROP 4

22. A 25-year-old lady presents with sudden, severe bilateral loss of vision more so on right side with no perception of light. Rest of the examination including pupillary reflex, fundus and optokinetic nystagmus are normal. She was able to touch tips of her finger with right eye closed but not with left eye closed. Most likely diagnosis:
    a. Optic neuritis
    b. Anterior ischemic optic neuropathy
    c. CMV retinitis
    d. Functional visual loss

23. Which retinal layer accounts for the petalloid cystic appearance of cystoid macular edema (CME)?
    a. Nerve fiber layer
    b. Inner plexiform layer
    c. Outer plexiform layer
    d. Outer nuclear layer

24. Differentiating classic and occult neovascular membranes is possible using:
    a. Amsler grid
    b. Fundus fluorescein angiography
    c. Optical coherence tomography
    d. B-scan ultrasound

25. Which of the following is not a typical feature of nonarteritic anterior ischemic optic neuropathy (NAION):
    a. Complete visual recovery over time
    b. Swollen optic nerve (rarely retrobulbar) with ipsilateral relative afferent pupil defect
    c. Usually painless, acute, unilateral loss of vision
    d. Older patient

26. Palinopsia occurs in all *except*:
    a. Use of hallucinogens
    b. Parietal lobe lesion
    c. Occipital lobe lesion
    d. Frontal lobe lesion

27. Retinal detachment is best demonstrated by:
    a. Presence of shaffer's sign
    b. Gray reflex on distant direct retinoscopy
    c. Scleral indentation on indirect ophthalmoscopy
    d. Absent reflex on retinoscopy

Answers

| 14. c | 15. a | 16. b | 17. d | 18. d | 19. c | 20. a |
| 21. b | 22. d | 23. c | 24. b | 25. a | 26. d | 27. c |

Neuroanesthesia

EFFECTS OF ANESTHESIA ON CNS PHYSIOLOGY

Specific anesthetic regimen is a combination of drugs that favorably affects cerebral hemodynamics, cerebral metabolism, and intracranial pressure (ICP) to provide good operating conditions and to enhance the probability of a quality outcome.

INTRAVENOUS DRUGS AND THEIR EFFECTS

Drug	CBF/CMRO$_2$	Autoregulation and CO$_2$ reactivity	CSF dynamics	ICP	Spinal cord metabolism
Barbiturates	Decreases in a parallel fashion-up to the point of isoelectricity on the electroencephalogram (EEG)	Does not appear to abolish cerebral autoregulation or CO$_2$ reactivity	No change in the rate of CSF formation	Decreases	Significant reduction seen
Etomidate	Reduces CBF and CMRO$_2$	Reactivity to CO$_2$ is maintained	Low-dose - no change; High-dose - decrease	Reduces ICP	–
Propofol	Dose-related reductions in both	Preserved	No change	Reduces ICP	Decreases local spinal cord metabolism
Fentanyl	Low doses of narcotics have little effect whereas higher doses progressively decrease both CBF and CMRO$_2$	Maintained	Decreases rate of CSF formation; increases resistance to CSF reabsorption at high doses	Produce either no change or a no change or a slight decrease in ICP	–
Ketamine	Increase in CBF and CMRO$_2$	Maintained	Increases resistance to CSF reabsorption and causes no change in rate of formation	Increase in PaCO$_2$ and ICP	–
Benzo-diazepines	Small decreases in CBF and CMRO$_2$ in both small and large doses.	Maintained	No change in rate of formation at low doses and a decrease at high doses	No change or a slight reduction	–

INHALATIONAL DRUGS AND THEIR EFFECTS

Drug	CBF/CMRO$_2$	Autoregulation and CO$_2$ reactivity	CSF dynamics	ICP	Spinal cord metabolism
Nitrous oxide	Cause large increases in CBF	Preserved	No change	Can increase ICP in patients who have mass lesions	Increases the spinal cord's utilization of glucose
Isoflurane	Increases CBF; most potent depressant of CMRO$_2$	Cerebral autoregulation is impaired; CO$_2$ reactivity is maintained	Low dose –no change; high dose-decreases	Increase	Isoflurane produces an increase in SCBF and an attenuation of autoregulation

Contd...

Contd...

Drug	CBF/CMRO$_2$	Autoregulation and CO$_2$ reactivity	CSF dynamics	ICP	Spinal cord metabolism
Desflurane	Similar to those of isoflurane	Similar to those of isoflurane	Normocapnia—no change; hypocapnia and increased CSF pressure—increases rate of formation	Increase in ICP	–
Sevoflurane	Similar to those of isoflurane	Cerebral autoregulation and CO$_2$ reactivity are preserved	Decreases rate of CSF formation; increases resistance to CSF reabsorption	Minimal change in ICP in patients with mass lesions	–

Muscle Relaxants

Nondepolarizing Muscle Relaxants

- *Short-acting drugs*—When large doses are given rapidly, some histamine release can occur with the potential for an increase in CBF and ICP.
- *Intermediate-acting drugs*—causes histamine release when given in large bolus doses, does not alter ICP or CSF dynamics
- *Long acting drugs*—decrease in cerebral input from paralyzed muscle spindles is seen with increase CBF and ICP.

Depolarizing Muscle Relaxants

Succinylcholine can cause an increase in CBF that is associated with an increase in ICP. This is secondary to increases in muscle spindle activity, which increase cerebral afferent input.

ANESTHETIC MANAGEMENT OF HEAD TRAUMA

Head trauma is Characterized by:

- Systemic effects of head trauma
    - Cardiovascular responses to head trauma include hypertension, tachycardia, and increased cardiac output and those suffering from multiple systemic injuries with substantial blood loss, however, may develop hypotension and a decrease in cardiac output.
    - Respiratory responses to head trauma include apnea and abnormal respiratory patterns
    - Temperature regulation may be disturbed, and hyperthermia, if it occurs, can provoke further brain damage
- Changes in cerebral circulation and metabolism
    - Cerebral blood flow (CBF) and cerebral metabolic rate for oxygen consumption (CMRO$_2$) decrease in the core area of injury and in the penumbra, an area of hypoperfused tissue that surrounds the damaged tissue. The combination of hypotension and impaired autoregulation exacerbates cerebral ischemia
- Acute brain swelling and cerebral edema
    - Acute brain swelling is provoked by a decrease in vasomotor tone and a marked increase in the volume of the cerebral vascular bed.
    - Cerebral edema following head trauma is often a mixture of vasogenic and cytotoxic types caused by blood-brain barrier disruption and ischemia, respectively
- Excitotoxicity
    - Excessive release of glutamate from neurons and glia, increasing the concentration of glutamate in the cerebrospinal fluid (CSF), an increase in intracellular calcium ion, which triggers a number of events that lead to the damage.
- Inflammatory cytokines and mediators
    - Cytokines increase in response to cerebral ischemia. Interleukin-6 (IL-6) and tumor necrosis factor alpha are known to be released.

Emergency Management

- Initial assessment of the patient's condition
    - Neurologic assessment—GCS is a simple and universally accepted method for assessing consciousness and neurologic status in patients with head injuries. GCS score of <8 characterizes severe head injury. Pupillary responses (size, light reflex) and symmetry of motor function in the extremities can be quickly assessed.
    - Assessment of injuries to other organs - patients often suffer from injuries to multiple organ systems. Particular attention should be paid to determine whether there is evidence of intrathoracic or intraperitoneal (intrapelvic) hemorrhage. Treatment of hemorrhagic shock takes precedence over neurosurgical procedures.

- Establishment of airway and ventilation:
  - Tracheal intubation—first step in emergency therapy is to secure an open airway and ensure adequate ventilation. If facial fractures and soft tissue edema prevent direct visualization of the larynx, either fiberoptic intubation or intubation with an illuminated stylet may be attempted. In the presence of either severe facial injuries or laryngeal trauma a cricothyrotomy may be required.
  - Mechanical ventilation—As soon as the trachea has been intubated, a nondepolarizing muscle relaxant is administered and mechanical ventilation to a partial arterial pressure of carbon dioxide ($PaCO_2$) of approximately 35 mm Hg is instituted. Aggressive hyperventilation ($PaCO_2$ of < 30 mm Hg) should be avoided unless transtentorial herniation is suspected.
- Cardiovascular stabilization:
  - Fluid resuscitation—fluid resuscitation should be guided not only by blood pressure but also by urinary output and central venous pressure (CVP). Isotonic and hypertonic crystalloid solutions and colloid solutions may be given to maintain adequate intravascular volume. Hydroxyethyl starch (HES) and human plasma products can be administered to maintain intravascular volume for longer periods. Glucose-containing solutions are avoided because hyperglycemia is associated with worsened neurologic outcomes.
  - Blood and blood products—Patients who have a low hematocrit may require a transfusion to optimize oxygen delivery; the hematocrit ideally is maintained above 30%
  - Inotropics and vasopressors—If the blood pressure and cardiac output cannot be restored through fluid resuscitation, the administration of intravenous inotropic and vasopressor drugs may be necessary to maintain cerebral perfusion pressure (CPP), the difference between the mean arterial pressure (MAP) and the ICP, above 60 mm Hg.
- Management of elevated ICP:
  - When evidence of transtentorial herniation in patients with severe head injuries exists, hyperventilation to a $PaCO_2$ of 30 mm Hg should be instituted. Mannitol, 1 g/kg i.v infused over 10 minutes, is administered. A head-up tilt of 10° to 30° facilitates cerebral venous and CSF drainage and lowers ICP.
  - Barbiturates are known to exert cerebral protective and ICP-lowering effects. However Corticosteroids, have no place in the treatment of head injury despite their proven efficacy in spinal cord injury.

Anesthetic Management

- ***Induction of anesthesia***—The patient who comes to the operating room without endotracheal intubation is treated with immediate oxygenation and securing of the airway. Patients often have a full stomach, decreased intravascular volume, and a potential cervical spine injury. Direct arterial pressure monitoring by an indwelling arterial catheter inserted before the induction of anesthesia is recommended.
- ***Rapid sequence induction***—Although this procedure can produce an elevation in blood pressure and ICP, it is desirable. During administration of 100% oxygen, an induction dose of thiopental, 3 to 4 mg/kg, or propofol, 1 to 2 mg/kg, and succinylcholine, 1.5 mg/kg, is administered and the trachea is intubated.
- ***Intravenous induction***—When the patient is stable and does not have a full stomach, anesthesia can be induced by titrating the dose of either thiopental or propofol to minimize circulatory instability. An intubating dose of a nondepolarizing muscle relaxant is given with or without priming to facilitate intubation within a short period of time. Fentanyl, 1 to 4 mcg/ kg i.v., is administered to blunt the hemodynamic response to laryngoscopy and intubation. A large-bore oral gastric tube is inserted after intubation, and gastric contents are initially aspirated and then passively drained during the operation.
- ***Maintenance of anesthesia***—Maintenance of anesthesia should reduce ICP, maintain adequate oxygen supply to the brain tissue, and protect the brain against ischemic-metabolic insult.
- ***Intravenous anesthetics***—Barbiturates; Thiopental and pentobarbital decrease CBF, cerebral blood volume (CBV), and ICP. Barbiturates can be detrimental in patients with head injuries because of their cardiovascular-depressant effect. As with barbiturates, etomidate reduces CBF, $CMRO_2$, and ICP. Systemic hypotension occurs less frequently than with barbiturates. Propofol might be useful in patients who have intracranial pathology if hypotension is avoided. Emergence from anesthesia is rapid, even after prolonged administration. Diazepam and midazolam may be useful either for sedating patients or inducting anesthesia because these drugs have minimal hemodynamic effects and are less likely to impair cerebral circulation.
- ***Inhalational anesthetics***—A potent metabolic depressant, isoflurane has less effect on CBF and ICP than halothane has. Because isoflurane depresses cerebral metabolism, it may have a cerebral protective effect when the ischemic insult is not severe. Sevoflurane's effect on cerebral hemodynamics is similar to or milder than that of isoflurane. The disadvantage of sevoflurane is that its biodegraded metabolite may be toxic in high concentrations. Patients who have intracranial hypertension or a decrease in intracranial compliance should, therefore, not receive N_2O.
- Respiratory and circulatory management
- ***Mechanical ventilation***—Mechanical ventilation is adjusted to maintain a $PaCO_2$ of around 35 mm Hg. The fraction of inspired oxygen (FiO_2) is adjusted to maintain a PaO_2 of >100 mm Hg.

- Circulatory management—CPP should be maintained between 60 and 110 mm Hg. When hypotension persists despite adequate oxygenation, ventilation, and fluid replacement, careful elevation of the blood pressure with a continuous infusion of an inotrope or vasopressor may be necessary.
- Intraoperative management of elevated ICP
    - A slight head-up tilt of 10 to 30° is desirable as the patient's posture.
    - Mannitol decreases cerebral volume and reduces ICP. Furosemide may be coadministered in severe cases as well as in the patient who has compromised cardiac function and the potential for heart failure.
    - If an intraventricular catheter is in place, CSF drainage is an effective and reliable technique for reducing ICP.
- **Cerebral protection**
    - A reduction of body temperature to 33°C to 35°C may confer cerebral protection. Protective mechanisms include a reduction in metabolic demand, excitotoxicity, free radical formation, and edema formation.
    - When induction of hypothermia is elected, meticulous care is necessary to avoid adverse side effects such as hypotension, cardiac arrhythmias, coagulopathies, and infections. Rewarming should be carried out slowly.
- **Postoperative management**
    - Patients who had a normal level of consciousness before the operation and who have undergone an uneventful procedure can be awakened and their tracheas extubated in the operating room, assuming that emergence criteria have been satisfactorily met. Smooth emergence with control of systemic blood pressure and avoidance of coughing is necessary to prevent postoperative cerebral edema and hematoma formation
    - Extubation in the operating room is discouraged for patients whose level of consciousness was depressed preoperatively and in whom brain swelling is either marked during operation or expected to occur postoperatively.
    - Patients who are hypothermic during emergence should be mechanically ventilated postoperatively and their tracheas extubated after careful rewarming.

Clinical Criteria for Brain Death in Adults and Children

- Coma
- Absence of motor responses
- Absence of pupillary responses to light and pupils at midposition with respect to dilatation (4-6 mm)
- Absence of corneal reflexes
- Absence of caloric responses
- Absence of gag reflex
- Absence of coughing in response to tracheal suctioning
- Absence of sucking and rooting reflexes
- Absence of respiratory drive at a $PaCO_2$ of 60 mm Hg or 20 mm Hg above normal base-line values[a]
- Interval between two evaluations, according to patient's age:
    - Term to 2 months old, 48 hr
    - >2 months to 1 year old, 24 hr
    - >1 year to <18 years old, 12 hr
    - >18 years old, interval optional
- Confirmatory test:
    - Term to 2 months old, 2 confirmatory tests
    - >2 months to 1 year old, 1 confirmatory test
    - >1 year to <18 years old, optional
    - >18 years old, optional

Relative Indications of Intra-arterial Pressure Monitoring

- Elevated intracranial pressure
- Ischemia or incipient ischemia of neurologic tissue
    - Recent subarachnoid hemorrhage
    - Recent head injury
    - Recent spinal-cord injury
    - Intended or potential temporary vessel occlusion
- Circulatory instability
    - Trauma
    - Spinal-cord injury (spinal shock)
    - Sitting position

- Possible barbiturate coma
- Possibility of induced hypo/ hypertension
- Anticipated/potential major blood loss
  - Aneurysm clipping
  - Arteriovenous malformations
  - Vascular tumors
  - Tumors involving major venous sinuses
  - Craniofacial reconstruction
  - Extensive craniosynostosis procedures
- Anticipated light anesthesia without paralysis
- Brain-stem manipulation/compression/dissection
- Anticipated cranial nerve manipulation (especially CN V)
- Advantageous for postoperative intensive care
  - Hypervolemic therapy
  - Head injury
  - Diabetes insipidus
- Incidental cardiac disease

SPECIFIC PROCEDURES

Supratentorial Tumors

- The relevant preoperative considerations include the patient's ICP status and the location and size of the tumor. Location and size give the anesthesiologist an indication of the surgical position and the potential for blood loss, and occasionally they reveal a risk of venous air embolism (VAE).
- Full VAE precautions, including an atrially placed CVP catheter, are usually reserved only for supratentorial tumors that lie near the posterior half of the sagittal sinus.
- Patients with a significant tumor-related mass effect, especially if there is tumor-related edema, should receive preoperative steroids. Preinduction placement of an arterial line may be appropriate in patients with severe mass effect and little residual compensatory latitude.
- Patients with craniopharyngiomas and pituitary tumors with suprasellar extension may undergo procedures that involve dissection in and around the hypothalamus. Irritation of the hypothalamus can elicit sympathetic responses including hypertension. Diabetes insipidus is the most likely disorder, although the cerebral salt-wasting syndrome can potentially occur.
- Patients who undergo a craniotomy involving a subfrontal approach manifest a disturbance of consciousness in the immediate postoperative period. Retraction/irritation of the inferior surfaces of the frontal lobes can result in a patient who is lethargic and does not awaken cleanly.

Intracranial Hypertension and Brain Bulging

Prevention	Treatment
Preoperative: adequate anxiolysis and analgesia	Cerebrospinal fluid drainage (lumbar catheter or ventricle)
Preinduction: hyperventilate on demand, head-up position, head straight, no jugular vein compression	Osmotic diuretics
Avoid overhydration	Hyperventilation
Osmotic diuretics (mannitol, hypertonic saline); steroids for tumor	Augment depth of anesthesia using intravenous
Loop diuretics (furosemide)	Anesthetics (propofol, thiopental, etomidate)
Optimize hemodynamics: MAP, central venous pressure, pulmonary capillary wedge pressure, heart rate; use beta-blockers, clonidine, or lidocaine if necessary	Muscle relaxation
Ventilation: PaO_2 >100; $PaCO_2$ ~ 35 mm Hg, low intrathoracic pressure	Improve cerebral venous drainage: head up, no positive end-expiratory pressure, reduce inspiratory time
Use of intravenous anesthetics for induction and maintenance	Mild controlled hypertension if cerebral autoregulation intact (MAP ~ 100 mm Hg)

Aneurysms and Arteriovenous Malformations

- The management of the ischemia caused by vasospasm, the period of maximal vasospasm risk being days 4 to 12 after SAH involves volume loading and induced hypertension. Early clipping of the aneurysm eliminates the risk of rebleeding associated with this therapy.

- Some patients develop syndrome of inappropriate antidiuretic hormone (SIADH) after SAH and are appropriately managed with fluid restriction. Cerebral salt wasting is also associated with contracted intravascular volume.
- When neurologic deterioration occurs subsequent to the patient's initial period of stabilization, vasospasm is frequently the cause. In the ICU, the regimens employed to treat vasospasm usually involve some combination of hypervolemia, hemodilution, and hypertension
- Calcium channel blockers are an established part of the management of SAH. Administration of nimodipine has been shown to decrease the incidence of morbidity from cerebral ischemia after SAH.
- Anesthetic Technique involves the provision of intraoperative brain relaxation to facilitate surgical access to the aneurysm, the maintenance of a high-normal MAP in order to prevent critical reduction of CBF in recently insulted and now marginally perfused areas of brain and be prepared to perform precise manipulations of MAP as the surgeon attempts to clip the aneurysm and/or control bleeding from a ruptured aneurysm.
- Elective lumbar CSF drainage to facilitate exposure of the operative site is extremely effective; Drainage should be discontinued promptly after final withdrawal of the retractors after dural opening is made in order to allow CSF to reaccumulate and thereby to reduce the size of the potential pneumocephalus.
- EEG monitoring can be used as a guide to management during the period of flow interruption and/or to guide the administration of CMR-reducing anesthetic agents given prior to occlusion. If the EEG shows significant slowing, the usual practice is to reposition the clip and/or elevate MAP by some combination of phenylephrine and lightening of anesthesia in order to find a way of temporary clipping without a major EEG disturbance.
- For the majority of intracranial AVMs, avoidance of acute hypertension and the capability to manipulate blood pressure accurately in the event of bleeding is practiced. A problem that is specific to AVM is the phenomenon known as perfusion pressure breakthrough or cerebral dysautoregulation. It is characterized by an often sudden engorgement and swelling of the brain, sometimes with a relentless cauliflower-like protrusion from the cranium. It has been attributed to the acute obliteration of the high-volume, low-resistance pathway (the AVM) that, for many years, has been stealing blood from the surrounding tissue. With severe episodes of swelling, combination of hypotension, hypocapnia, hypothermia, and barbiturates is used.
- **Predictors of mortality after subarachnoid hemorrhage**
    - Poor neurologic condition at hospital admission, a function of rate and volume of bleed
    - Depressed level of consciousness after initial bleed
    - Older age
    - Preexisting illness
    - Elevated blood pressure
    - Thick clot in the brain substance or ventricles on initial computed tomographic scan
    - Repeat hemorrhage
    - Basilar aneurysmal location

Posterior Fossa Procedures

- The use of the sitting position to facilitate surgery in the posterior fossa increases the likelihood of cardiovascular effects and complications (quadriplegia, macroglossia), pneumocephalus.
- Irritation of the lower portion of the pons and of the upper medulla and of the extra-axial portion of the fifth cranial nerve can result in a number of cardiovascular perturbations which may include bradycardia and hypotension, tachycardia and hypertension, bradycardia and hypertension, and ventricular dysrhythmias.
- Procedures involving dissection on the floor of the fourth ventricle entail the possibility of injury to cranial nerve nuclei and/or postoperative swelling in that region. Relatively little swelling can result in disorders of consciousness, respiratory drive, and cardiomotor function.
- Various electrophysiologic monitoring techniques may be used which include somatosensory evoked responses, brain-stem auditory evoked responses, and EMG monitoring of the facial nerve.

Transsphenoidal Hypophysectomy

- The important preoperative considerations relate to the patient's endocrine status. In general, as a pituitary lesion expands and compresses the pituitary tissue, the sequence in which hormonal function is lost is as follows: (1) gonadotropins; (2) growth hormone; (3) ACTH; and (4) TSH.
- The procedure is performed with the patient in a supine position, usually with some degree of head-up posture to avoid venous engorgement. During the approach, the mucosal surfaces within the nose are infiltrated with a local anesthetic and epinephrine solution, and the patient should be observed for the occurrence of dysrhythmias, as the surgical approach is via the nasal cavity through an incision made under the upper lip.

- In some instances, hypocapnia is requested to reduce brain volume and thereby to minimize the degree to which the arachnoid bulges into the sella though when there is suprasellar extension of a tumor, a normal or increased CO_2 helps to deliver the lesion into the sella for excision.
- Diabetes insipidus is a potential complication of this procedure. This disorder usually occurs 4 to 12 hours postoperatively and very rarely arises intraoperatively. When the diagnosis of diabetes insipidus is established, an appropriate fluid management regimen is hourly maintenance fluids plus two-thirds of the previous hour's urine output. In general, the patient is losing fluid that is hypo-osmolar and relatively low in sodium. Half-normal saline and 5 percent dextrose in water are commonly used as replacement fluids.

Awake Craniotomy

- Prior to the resection, most patients have undergone either or both a Wada test and videotelemetry.
- The Wada test involves selectively anesthetizing the cerebral hemispheres by injection of sodium amytal into the carotid artery to localize the hemisphere that controls speech and/or to confirm that there is bilateral representation for short-term memory.
- Videotelemetry is performed to permit localization of the seizure focus that is responsible for the clinically problematic events. This usually requires prior placement of either subdural strip electrodes (via bur holes) or a subdural electrode grid (requiring a craniotomy). Occasionally, electrodes are placed deep into parenchyma, usually within the temporal lobe (placed stereotaxically via bur holes), or they are positioned so as to look at the inferior surfaces of the temporal lobe. The latter is commonly accomplished with so-called foramen ovale electrodes. These are placed using a needle similar to an epidural needle. Typically, this procedure is performed as a "MAC," although doses of methohexital or propofol are usually required at the time of stimulation by the needle of the periosteum at the base of the skull.
- ***The objectives of the anesthetic technique are as follows:***
  - To minimize patient discomfort associated with the potentially painful portions of the procedure and with the prolonged restriction of movement.
  - To ensure patient responsiveness and compliance during the phases of the procedure that requires assessment of either speech or motor/sensory responses to cortical stimulation.
  - To select anesthetic techniques that produce minimal inhibition of spontaneous seizure activity.
- Reliable capnography, to provide breath-by-breath confirmation of airway patency and respiratory drive, is an essential component of the technique if deep sedation is intended for any portion of the procedure.
- In general, after the dural opening is complete, cortical surface EEG recording is performed to locate the seizure focus. After localization by EEG, functional testing may be performed by stimulating the cortical surface electrically and observing for motor, sensory, or speech interruption effects. During stimulation, the anesthesiologist should be prepared to treat grand mal convulsions that are not self-limited for which Thiopental in 1 mg/kg increments is appropriate.

Interventional Neuroradiology

- The duration of a procedure, individual patient factors, and, occasionally, the necessity for precise physiologic control may result in requests for monitored anesthesia care or general anesthesia.
- Anesthesiologists may become involved during the resuscitation stage in the event of vascular rupture or of the migration of an intravascular device to an incorrect location. When detachable devices are misplaced and ischemia ensues, fluid loading and pressor administration may be requested to improve collateral CBF while the device is retrieved.
- Vasospasm can be treated by selective intra-arterial instillation of papaverine or more commonly by balloon dilation.
- Hyperventilation may be appropriate in an attempt to divert flow away from normal brain and toward a lesion that is intended to receive the occlusive device or material.

Cerebrospinal Fluid Shunting Procedures

- Invasive monitoring is generally not required. The anesthetic technique should be chosen to avoid further increases in ICP. Moderate hyperventilation ($PaCO_2$, 25-30 mm Hg) is customary.
- Ventriculoperitoneal shunting is usually performed with the patient supine, with the table turned 90° and the patient's head turned toward the anesthesiologist.
- Inhalation inductions using volatile agents are empirically well tolerated even in children with closed fontanelles. However it is better to avoid induction technique in a child who is already stuporous.
- If, in the absence of sevoflurane, halothane were employed for induction, immediately following loss of consciousness, we would generally change to isoflurane and control ventilation manually using the bag and mask.
- For children older than 6 months of age who are not stuporous at the outset, we commonly administer 2 to 3 mcg/kg of fentanyl as this procedure is not entirely pain-free postoperatively and, in addition, that a smoother emergence from anesthesia can be accomplished with a narcotic background.

Carotid endarterectomy (CEA)

Local Anesthesia
- Local Anesthetic techniques like Superficial and deep cervical plexus blocks are the most commonly used regional anesthetic techniques for CEA.
- Intraoperative monitors include the following:
  - Intra-arterial cannula for blood pressure measurement
  - Continuous electrocardiogram (ECG)
  - Pulse oximetry
  - Capnography sampled via nasal prongs for monitoring respiratory rate
- Supplemental oxygen should be provided through a mask or nasal prongs positioned to avoid the site of surgery.
- Carefully titrated sedation using small, repeated, intravenous doses of fentanyl, 10 to 25 mcg, and/or midazolam, 0.5 to 2 mg, should render the patient comfortable and cooperative during the operation. Propofol is a reasonable alternative.

General Anesthesia
- General anesthesia represents the most common anesthetic technique for CEA.
- The key consideration during the induction of anesthesia is the maintenance of stable hemodynamic conditions during intubation, positioning, and draping.
- All of the nondepolarizing neuromuscular-blocking drugs facilitate tracheal intubation. Succinylcholine is a reasonable alternative.
- General anesthesia is usually maintained with a combination of volatile anesthetic (typically isoflurane, desflurane, or sevoflurane) and opioid. Neuromuscular blockade is maintained throughout the procedure.

Neurosurgery in the Pregnant Patient
- Sedative premedication may be appropriate in extremely anxious patients, but the risk of hypoventilation, hypercarbia, and subsequent increases in intracranial pressure (ICP) should be considered and guarded against.
- A rapid-sequence induction designed to prevent aspiration does little to prevent the hemodynamic response to intubation that can be catastrophic for the patient who has an intracranial aneurysm or increased ICP. At the same time, a slow neuroinduction with thiopental, a narcotic, a nondepolarizing muscle relaxant, and mask ventilation does little to decrease the risk of aspiration.
- Cricoid pressure should be maintained from the point at which consciousness is lost until intubation is confirmed by capnography. If cesarean delivery is performed as part of a combined procedure, the physician caring for the newborn should be alerted to the likelihood of neonatal depression and the need to provide ventilatory support.
- In addition to the standard maternal monitors, fetal heart rate (FHR) monitoring can be extremely useful during craniotomy, not because an ominous FHR indicates when cesarean delivery should be performed but because it should lead to a rapid search for potentially reversible causes of decreased uteroplacental perfusion, such as hypotension or hypoxemia.
- Maternal hyperventilation can facilitate surgical exposure by decreasing cerebral blood volume. Controlled hypotension is becoming less common during aneurysm surgery because of the growing use of temporary clip occlusion of proximal vessels.

MANAGEMENT OF NEUROLOGIC CATASTROPHES

Initial Resuscitation
- Secure the airway and hyperventilate with 100% O_2. Determine if problem is hemorrhagic or occlusive.
  - *Hemorrhagic:* Immediate heparin reversal (1 mg protamine for each 100 U heparin given) and low-normal pressure.
  - *Occlusive:* Deliberate hypertension, titrated to neurologic examination, angiography, or physiologic imaging studies (e.g., TCD, CBF).

Further Resuscitation
- Head-up 15° in neutral position. Titrate ventilation to a $PaCO_2$ of 26 to 28 mm Hg. Give 0.5 g/kg mannitol, rapid intravenous infusion.
- Anticonvulsants: phenytoin (give slowly, 50 mg/min) and phenobarbital. Titrate thiopental infusion to electroencephalogram burst suppression.
- Allow body temperature to fall as quickly as possible to 33°C to 34°C. Add dexamethasone 10 mg.

Neurosurgery

Disordered primary neurulation results in defects in the axial skeleton, meninges, and overlying dermal structures. Ex: craniorachischisis totalis, anencephaly, encephalocele, and myelomeningocele.

Disorders of *caudal neural tube formation* result in occult dysraphic states. Ex: lipomyelomeningocele, diastematomyelia, and congenital dermal sinus.

These caudal spinal anomalies may be associated with other abnormalities, such as imperforate anus, malformed genitalia, and renal dysplasias as part of a broader caudal regression syndrome.

MYELOMENINGOCELES

- Represent the most important clinical examples of disordered neurulation; most severe form of dysraphism involving the vertebral column
- Incidence – 1/ 4000 live births; Most common site – lumbosacral region (75%)
- The essential defect is a failure of closure of the caudal neuropore. The resulting lesion by definition involves the spinal cord, a deficient axial skeleton, and an incomplete meningeal and dermal covering. Spinal defects include a lack of fusion of the vertebral arches, laterally displaced pedicles, and a widened spinal canal.
- The cause of myelomeningocele has not been determined precisely, but both environmental and genetic factors have been implicated.
- Associated anomalies of the skull, brain, spine, and spinal cord have been collectively described as the *Chiari II malformation*.
- Several types of Chiari malformations are classified into three types. In each case, abnormal descent of cerebellar tissue into the cervical canal is demonstrated.
  - A Chiari I malformation consists of elongated peg-like cerebellar tonsils below the foramen magnum, while the brain stem is normal in location.
  - In cases where the tonsils, vermis, pons, medulla, and an elongated fourth ventricle are displaced inferiorly into the upper cervical canal, a Chiari II malformation is diagnosed.
  - Chiari III malformations are associated with occipital or high cervical encephaloceles, containing cerebellar tissue, with or without brain stem.
- The cause of this anomaly is unknown, but the failure of neural tube closure with drainage of CSF through the open neural tube into the amniotic fluid has been implicated.
- Major features of this complex include a small posterior fossa with inferior displacement of the medulla, fourth ventricle, and cerebellar vermis through the foramen magnum; formation of a medullary kink within the cervical spinal canal; and various midbrain anomalies such as a beaked tectum and abnormalities of the ventricular system.

Management

- Careful clinical assessment with particular emphasis on motor, sensory, reflex, and sphincter function.
- Open defects should be covered with a saline-moistened nonadherent dressing to prevent injury to and desiccation of the neural placode.
- Surgical goals include elimination of CSF leakage, preservation of neurologic function, and the prevention of infection. The general procedure for closure includes separation of the neural placode from the surrounding epithelial tissue, followed by Identification and mobilization of the dura mater. Reconstruction of the neural placode to prevent retethering when the dura is closed followed by fascial and multilayer skin closure is also advocated.

ENCEPHALOCELES

- Disordered closure of *the cranial neuropore* results in anencephaly, due to failure of cranial neuropore closure.
- Failure of the development of the overlying mesenchymal tissue with local cerebral herniation occurring at approximately 8 to 12 weeks of gestation is implicated as the cause.
- They are frequently associated with other intracranial abnormalities, such as partial or complete agenesis of the corpus callosum, Dandy-Walker malformations, hydrocephalus, or holoprosencephaly.

Management

- Neurosurgical intervention is indicated in most situations with the exception of patients with large defects and associated microcephaly.
- The goals of surgery are to obtain a watertight dural closure, after either the relocation of the encephalocele contents into the cranium or their resection, and an acceptable cosmetic result.

OCCULT SPINAL DYSRAPHISM

- Refers to those embryologic defects that occur due to *disordered retrogressive differentiation*.
- Majority of these disorders occur in the lumbar region and are not infrequently associated with abnormal cutaneous markings such as hemangiomas, focal hirsutism, soft tissue masses, or a sinus tract.
- Persistent urinary tract infections in a child or the new onset of incontinence in a child who was previously toilet trained as well as lower extremity weakness, sensory abnormalities, or radicular pain is also associated with an occult dysraphic disorder.

Lipomyelomeningoceles

- Skin-covered malformations in which a subcutaneous lipoma is connected through a fibroadipose stalk to an intramedullary, intradural lipoma. Occur when the superficial ectoderm separates prematurely from the underlying neural ectoderm, allowing the migration of mesenchymal tissue into the neural tube.
- The goals of treatment include the release of the tethering elements, preservation of neurologic function, debulking of the intramedullary mass, dural reconstruction, and acceptable cosmesis.

Diastematomyelia

- Uncommon dysraphic lesion in which the spinal cord is split longitudinally at one or more continuous levels and separated by a bony, cartilaginous, or fibrous spur.
- Surgical goals include untethering the spinal cord by removing the bony or fibrous median septum and reconstructing the dural sac.

Craniosynostosis

- Refers to the premature closure or fusion of a cranial suture. It can also occur as part of a recognized syndrome or secondary to a systemic disorder.
- Isolated sagittal synostosis is the most common form of craniosynostosis. Closure of the sagittal suture typically results in scaphocephaly, with a long, narrow skull with varying degrees of compensatory frontal and occipital bossing.
- Premature fusion of the metopic suture results in a skull with a characteristic triangular shape, or trigonocephaly, with a prominent midline frontal ridge, recessed orbital rims, and hypotelorism.
- The specific surgical technique will vary depending on the affected suture, most craniofacial surgeons agree that early surgery is preferable for the simple reason that one can capitalize on the period of rapid brain growth to ameliorate any minor postoperative asymmetries in skull shape. The timing of surgery is usually between 3 and 9 months of age.

Hydrocephalus

Condition that results from an imbalance between the production and absorption of CSF, leads to the accumulation of CSF within the intracranial compartment and, ultimately, ventricular enlargement and intracranial hypertension.
- *Communicating hydrocephalus* is present when an obstruction to the flow of CSF occurs outside of the ventricular system, usually at the level of the basal subarachnoid cisterns or at the arachnoid granulations.
- *Noncommunicating hydrocephalus* results from lesions that create an obstruction to CSF flow within the ventricular system which most commonly occurs at the level of the aqueduct of Sylvius but is also seen at the foramina of Monro or at the foramina of Luschka and Magendie in the fourth ventricle.

- Can occur in either congenital or acquired forms.
  - Aqueductal stenosis is a major cause of hydrocephalus in the newborn and is responsible for nearly one third of congenital cases. The Dandy-Walker malformation is another cause of congenital hydrocephalus and is characterized by the absence of the cerebellar vermis, cystic expansion of the fourth ventricle, and hydrocephalus. Intracranial tumors, arachnoid cysts, and other abnormalities such as vein of Galen malformations are other causes.
  - Acquired forms of hydrocephalus usually occur after intraventricular hemorrhage or after an episode of meningitis
- Clinical features of hydrocephalus are related to the development of elevated ICP. In the newborn, excessive head enlargement with an enlarged, tense anterior fontanelle and open cranial sutures are common presentations. Irritability, vomiting, and lethargy may also be present.
- Ultrasonography can easily determine the presence of ventriculomegaly, however CT scanning remains the most commonly used imaging technique for screening or emergent indications and is preferred when a more detailed assessment of intracranial morphology is required.

Management

- The goal of any treatment for hydrocephalus is to prevent or possibly even reverse the neurologic injury that may occur as a result of distortion of the normal intracranial structures or that due to the effects of elevated ICP.
- Diversion of CSF from the cerebral ventricles to the peritoneal cavity via a *ventriculoperitoneal shunt* is preferred. Other less favored sites for diversion include the pleural cavity and the superior vena cava. Lumboperitoneal shunt created either by open surgery or percutaneously is rarely performed.
- A valve is incorporated in the shunt system, whose pressures range from 5-150 mm H_2O.
  - Fixed opening pressure valves. Ex: *Heyer-Schulte, Hakim*
  - Variable opening pressure valves. Ex: *Orbis Sigma, Delta*
  - Programmable valves. Ex: *Medos, Sophy*
- *Endoscopic third ventriculostomy* is another technique where a small fenestration is created in the floor of the anterior third ventricle under endoscopic guidance, thus allowing CSF to directly enter the subarachnoid space.

The term brain attack has been coined to increase the awareness of stroke. A brain attack is considered a sudden onset of neurologic worsening, including a loss of consciousness and focal neurologic deficits, and causes can be classified as either ischemic or hemorrhagic as diagnosed by a computed tomography (CT) scan of the brain.

Ischemic causes for brain attack includes thromboembolism leading to infarction. The term hemorrhage stroke is used whenever a patient presents with a brain attack and a CT scan reveals the cause to be intracranial hemorrhage.

Intracerebral Hemorrhage

Causes

- *Cranial trauma*—Penetrating/nonpenetrating
- Coup and contra coup injury during brain deceleration; intraparenchymal: affects the frontal lobes, anterior temporal lobes, subarachnoid
- Nontraumatic intracerebral hemorrhage:
  - Hypertensive damage to blood vessel walls due to hypertension, eclampsia, drug abuse; affects putamen, pons, globus pallidus and cerebellar hemisphere
  - *Altered hemostasis*—Thrombolysis, anticoagulation, bleeding diathesis
  - Hemorrhagic necrosis due to tumor or infection
  - Venous outflow obstruction as in cerebral venous thrombosis
  - *Rupture of an aneurysm/A-V malformation*—Rupture of microaneurysms–charcot-bouchard aneurysm, Rupture of berry aneurysm; causes hemorrhage in lobar, intraventricular, intraparenchymal and subarachnoid regions
  - *Amyloid angiopathy*—Lobar hemorrhage
  - *Metastatic brain tumor*—Lobar hemorrhage; primaries from lung, thyroid, RCC, melanoma
  - *Drug abuse*—Hemorrhage in lobar and subarachnoid; e.g., cocaine, amphetamine, phenylpropranolamine
- Two main forms of hemorrhage stroke are recognized: subarachnoid hemorrhage and intracerebral hematoma.

SPONTANEOUS SUBARACHNOID HEMORRHAGE

- Defined as blood in the subarachnoid space and basal cisterns of the brain that is not caused by trauma
- The most frequent cause of spontaneous subarachnoid hemorrhage is *rupture of an intracranial aneurysm.*
- It is characterized by a sudden explosive onset of very severe headaches that patients describe as the *worse headaches of their lives*. Other symptoms include nausea and vomiting and loss of consciousness with or without a concomitant seizure.

Cerebral Aneurysms

- Cerebral arterial aneurysms (*berry aneurysms*) account for slightly more than half of all cases of spontaneous subarachnoid hemorrhages. These congenital cerebral aneurysms typically develop at vessel bifurcations and have been postulated to follow congenital deficiencies or degenerative changes in the wall of the vessel. As the aneurysm enlarges, its internal elastic lamina frays and its dome consist primarily of intima and the remaining adventitial connective tissue.
- They are especially common at the junction of the posterior communicating artery and the internal carotid artery, at the junction of the anterior communicating artery and one of the anterior cerebral arteries, or at the first major branches of the middle cerebral artery.
- Rebleeding is the single most important cause of death if the patient survives the initial bleed, with the peak incidence of rebleeding in the first few days after the initial bleed.
- Blood in the subarachnoid space obliterates the arachnoidal villi and other arachnoidal channels that are important in the normal absorption of cerebrospinal fluid. This frequently causes communicating hydrocephalus that can last for days to weeks until the blood has been absorbed.

Hunt-Hess Grading of SAH	
Hunt-Hess grade	Presentation
0	Unruptured aneurysm
1	Awake; symptomatic or mild headache with mild nuchal rigidity
2	Awake; moderate to severe headache; cranial nerve palsy(3rd or 4th), nuchal rigidity
3	Lethargic; mild focal neurological deficit (e.g., Pronator drift)
4	Stuporous; significant neurological deficit (e.g., Hemiplegia)
5	Comatose; posturing

Management of Subarachnoid Hemorrhage

- Subarachnoid hemorrhages are identified as areas of increased density in the subarachnoid spaces along the base of the skull within the sylvian fissure. The location of the subarachnoid hemorrhage may frequently suggest the site of the aneurysm, and in some cases, the aneurysm itself might be visible. MRI and magnetic resonance angiography are excellent screening procedures to detect and categorize unruptured intracranial aneurysms.
- *Management of Vasospasm*
    - Prevention of arterial narrowing
        - Subarachnoid blood removal
        - Prevention of dehydration and hypotension
        - Calcium-channel blockers (nimodipine)
    - Reversal of arterial narrowing
        - Intra-arterial papaverine
        - Transluminal balloon angioplasty
    - Prevention and reversal of ischemic neurologic deficit
        - Hypertension, hypervolemia, and hemodilution
- The final step in the radiologic evaluation of patients who are suspected of having a subarachnoid hemorrhage is a complete four-vessel cerebral angiogram with complete evaluation of the vasculature to both cerebral hemispheres and the posterior fossa.

Surgical Treatment of Aneurysms

- *Craniotomy and clipping*—After a craniotomy is performed, microsurgical techniques with the operative microscope are used to dissect free the aneurysm neck from the feeding vessels without rupturing the aneurysm. Final treatment involves the placement of a surgical aneurysm clip around the neck of the aneurysm, thereby obliterating flow into the aneurysm. The goal at surgery is to obliterate the aneurysm from the normal circulation without compromising any of the adjacent vessels or small perforating branches of these vessels.
- *Endovascular methods*—Guglielmi described a detachable platinum microcoil for use in the treatment of intracranial aneurysms. These coils are soft and can be detached from the stainless steel guide by passing a very small direct current that causes electrolysis at the solder junction. Separation usually occurs within 2 to 10 minutes after satisfactory coil placement.
- *Supportive*—Blood in the subarachnoid space obliterates the arachnoidal villi and can cause acute hydrocephalus, which can lead to neurologic worsening because of the raised ICP for which an immediate intraventricular catheter is placed with CSF drainage.

SPONTANEOUS INTRACEREBRAL HEMORRHAGE

A spontaneous intracerebral hematoma (SICH) is a blood clot in the parenchyma of the brain that arises without immediately preceeding trauma and has a variety of causes, with the most important being hypertension. The most likely cause of an SICH varies with patient's age. In young adults, it is more likely due to AVM, aneurysm, or drug abuse, whereas in elderly persons, hypertension, tumors, and coagulopathies lead the list.

- Hypertensive intracerebral hemorrhage (or hematoma) most frequently occurs in the putamen, thalamus, cerebellum, or pons. These hemorrhages follow bleeding from the small perforating arteries of the brain such as the thalamoperforating, lenticulostriate, or midline perforating basilar artery branches. Although these arteries can usually withstand high pressure when subjected to long-standing hypertension, their walls undergo fibrinoid necrosis, and miliary microaneurysms known as *Charcot-Bouchard aneurysms* appear.
- If the hemorrhage involves the dominant hemisphere, aphasia is usually present. Patients with a thalamic hemorrhage usually manifest a hemisensory loss greater than their motor deficit. Small reactive pupils and downward eye deviation characteristically occur with this lesion.
- Cerebellar hemorrhage characteristically presents with headache, dizziness, nausea, and vomiting. Examination may demonstrate an inability to walk, ataxia, facial weakness, and paresis of conjugate gaze.

CT scan of the brain reveals not only the size and location of the hematoma but also whether there is hydrocephalus, brain shift, and brain stem compression.

Treatment

- The treatment plan should be aimed at preventing and reversing secondary brain damage caused by intracranial hypertension, brain shift, and direct pressure on the surrounding brain parenchyma.
- The role and timing of surgical intervention for a hypertensive intracerebral hemorrhage remain controversial. In elderly moribund patients with a large dominant hemispheric hematoma, surgery is probably not indicated. Likewise, in an alert, awake patient with minimal neurologic deficit with a small hematoma, surgery might not be beneficial.
- Clearly, patients with an initial good neurologic examination who are deteriorating, especially if the clot is on the nondominant side, should undergo immediate surgery.
- The goal of surgery is to remove the hematoma, therefore removing the pressure on the surrounding brain and restoring the ICP to normal; to reverse midline shift and herniation; and by removing the blood clot and blood breakdown products to minimize the secondary molecular events, leading to less edema and ischemia.

Surgical Methods for Removing Intracerebral Hematomas

- *Stereotactic needle aspiration* of the blood clot with fibrinolytic or mechanical assistance.
- More commonly used method is through a craniotomy and open removal of the hematoma
- For supratentorial hematomas, a *suboccipital craniectomy* and surgical evacuation of the hematoma are indicated to reverse brain stem compression and to relieve obstructive hydrocephalus.

ANGIOMATOUS MALFORMATIONS

- *Venous angiomas*—an extensive network of veins separated by normal parenchyma
- *Telangiectasia (capillary angiomas)*—benign lesions of the brain stem
- *Cavernous angiomas*—may manifest clinically as a growing mass, intracerebral hemorrhage, or intractable seizures
- *Arteriovenous malformations*—consist of a feeding artery or arteries, a nidus, and draining veins. The superficial portion of a malformation may cover part of the cerebral surface, but the lesion frequently extends like a cone down to the ventricular surface. AVMs usually present with an intracranial bleed, they tend to bleed earlier in life than aneurysms, with a peak incidence in individuals between 30 and 40 years old.

Management

- *Microsurgical excision*—Gamma knife radiation or linear accelerator radiosurgery is reserved for surgically inaccessible lesions that are usually smaller than 3 cm.
- *Embolization* with glue or thrombogenic particles—Reduce the size and blood flow through the malformation
- *Focused radiation*—Large inoperable AVMs in eloquent cortex can be candidates for focused radiation if embolization can diminish lesion size or divide the larger AVM into smaller sections that can then be individually radiated.

Vein of Galen Malformation

- Direct communication between a cerebral artery and a cerebral vein results from a congenital vascular malformation.
- The vein of Galen abnormality is the most frequent arteriovenous malformation in neonates. The vein of Galen is located under the cerebral hemispheres, is formed by the confluence of two cerebral veins (receives entire deep venous drainage of cerebrum) – joins the inferior sagittal sinus and empties the venous drainage into the straight sinus.
- The vein of Galen aneurysmal malformation is a choroidal type of arteriovenous malformation.
- The congenital malformation develops during weeks 6-11 of fetal development as a persistent embryonic prosencephalic vein of Markowski; thus, VGAM is actually a misnomer. The vein of Markowski actually drains into the vein of Galen.
- Parenchymatous AVMs can be distinguished from true VOG malformations by retrograde filling of the internal cerebral vein in the former
- True VOG malformations are fed from the medial and lateral choroidal, circumferential, mesencephalic, anterior choroidal, pericallosal and meningeal arteries.

Manifestation

- High-output heart failure in the newborn—due to decreased resistance and high blood flow in the lesion
- Cerebral ischemic changes—strokes or steal phenomena—progressive hemiparesis and seizures
- Hemorrhage
- Mass effects—progressive neurological impairment
- Hydrocephalus—obstruction of the cerebrospinal fluid (CSF) outflow
- Marked continuous cranial bruit

Diagnostic Imaging

- Cranial USG (IOC)
- MRI and angiography—Defines lesion better

EXTRADURAL HAEMATOMA

- It occurs usually as a result of squamous temporal bone fractures with laceration of the middle meningeal artery. They can also arise from fractured bone edges or rarely from the dural venous sinuses. The potential space between the dura and bone is developed by the expanding haematoma allowing it to take on the familiar convex configuration due to the adherence of the dura to the inside of the calvarium.
- The degree of trauma might not be severe and there is typically a lucid interval following the trauma. Frequently, patients present in coma and require urgent evacuation via a burr hole prior to formal craniotomy.

SUBDURAL HAEMATOMAS

- They are the most common intracranial mass lesions resulting from head injury. Most result from torn bridging veins draining blood from the cortex to the dura. They can also arise from cortical lacerations or bleeding from the dural venous sinuses. They are usually associated with more severe, high-velocity trauma with a poorer outcome, usually in older patients.
- The blood follows the subdural space over the convexity of the brain and appears as a concave hyperdense lesion. Acute subdural haematomas are more rapidly evolving lesions and early evacuation is mandatory.
- Chronic subdural haematomas—These haematomas are most common in infants and in adults over 60 years of age. They present with progressive neurological deficits more than 2 weeks after the trauma. Often the initial head injury has been completely forgotten and the pathology has been attributed to either dementia or a brain tumour until patients are scanned. The initial haemorrhage may be relatively small or may occur in elderly patients with large ventricles or a dilated subarachnoid space. Membranes deriving from the dura and arachnoid mater encapsulate the haematoma which remains clotted for 2-3 weeks then liquefies. The acute clotted blood initially appears white on a CT scan. As it liquefies it slowly becomes black. These collections can be removed by drilling burr holes and washing them out with warmed saline.

Severe head injury is generally defined as a coma-producing injury where coma is not related to extracranial conditions (e.g., severe intoxication) and is sustained at least beyond the period of acute resuscitation.

Periorbital ecchymosis: Raccoon eyes or panda eyes
- Sign of basal skull fracture: B/L subconjunctival hemorrhage occurs, tears the meninges, causes the venous sinuses to bleed into the arachnoid villi and the cranial sinuses; blood from the skull fracture seeps into the soft tissue around the eyes

- Raccoon eyes may be associated with anterior cranial fossa; may be a sign of disseminated neuroblastoma or of amyloidosis (multiple myeloma)
- Craniotomy that ruptured the meninges
- Cancer
- Battle sign: Ecchymosis behind the ear
- Glove and Stocking anaesthesia
- The well-established Glasgow Coma Scale (GCS) is the most common method for the diagnosis of traumatic coma.

GLASGOW COMA SCORE

Eye opening	Verbal (Nonintubated)	Verbal (Intubated)	Motor activity
4—Spontaneous	5—Oriented and talks	5—Seems able to talk	6—Verbal command
3—Verbal stimuli	4—Disoriented and talks	3—Questionable ability to talk	5—Localizes to pain
2—Painful stimuli	3—Inappropriate words	1—Generally unresponsive	4—Withdraws to pain
1—No response	2—Incomprehensible sounds		3—Decorticate
	1—No response		2—Decerebrate
			1—No response

DIFFUSE AXONAL INJURY

Diffuse axonal injury (DAI) is a type of traumatic brain injury (TBI) that results from a blunt injury to the brain.
- It is an injury to the white matter, can occur in minor as well as severe brain injury and is due to anatomic or functional disruption of axons.
- The CT scan "foot print" of diffuse axonal injury consists of small petechial hemorrhages in the white matter, most frequently seen in the corpus callosum and the dorsal rostral brain stem.
- Extensive diffuse axonal injury in the brain stem can cause coma and is in fact the most likely cause of coma in patients without evidence of mass effect and herniation.

Secondary brain stem injury frequently occurs from mass effect, which is almost always supratentorial; herniation then occurs across the tentorium with secondary brain stem compression. Herniation can cause destruction of the brain stem as the downward movement of the stem exceeds the dislocation of its nutrient arteries, resulting in hemorrhagic infarctions (Duret's *hemorrhages*)

Traumatic brain injury is classified as mild, moderate, and severe based on Glascock Coma Scale (GCS). Traumatic brain injury patients with

GCS score: 13 to 15—mild (majority of traumatic brain injury patients)
GCS score: 9 to 12—moderate traumatic brain injury
GCS score: < 8—severe traumatic brain injury.

Etiology
- The most common etiology—high-speed motor vehicle accident.
- The most common mechanism—an accelerating and decelerating motion or angular strain that leads to shearing forces to the white matter tracts of the brain.
- This leads to microscopic and widespread damage to the axons in the brain at the junction of the gray and white matter.
- Diffuse axonal injury commonly affects white matter tracts involved in the corpus callosum and brainstem
- The primary insults of diffuse axonal injury lead to disconnection or malfunction of neurons interconnection.

Clinical Presentation
- Varies from concussion to coma
- LOC–common; it's the most common cause of post traumatic vegetative state
- Bilateral neurological examination deficits frequently affecting the frontal and temporal white matter, corpus callosum, and brainstem.

The Adams Diffuse Axonal Injury Classification

Grade 1
- A mild diffuse axonal injury with microscopic white matter changes in the cerebral cortex(frontal lobes and periventricular temporal lobes), corpus callosum, and brainstem;
- Inapparent on conventional imaging; may be seen in MRS

Grade 2
- A moderate diffuse axonal injury with gross focal lesions in the corpus callosum (in addition to stage 1 locations)
- Seen in 20% patients;
- Most frequently unilateral
- Seen to affect most commonly posterior body and splenium
- Can be visualized in SWI

Grade 3
- A severe diffuse axonal injury with finding as Grade 2 and additional focal lesions in the brainstem.
- Most commonly seen to involve rostral midbrain, superior cerebellar peduncles, medial lemnisci and corticospinal tracts

Pathology
- Hemorrhagic/non-hemorrhagic white matter tears in bilateral hemispheres
- Axonal portions of neurons—mechanical disruption of cytoskeletons resulting in proteolysis, swelling, and other microscopic and molecular changes to the neuronal structure

Evaluation
- DAI is diagnosed after a TBI with GCS <8 for more than six consecutive hours
- MRI, specifically Diffuse Tensor Imaging (DTI)—imaging modality of choice for diagnosis of DAI (MRI will enhance the detection of axonal injury in grade 3 diffuse axonal injury patients)

Treatment and Prognosis
- Goal of DAI patients' treatment is supportive care and prevention of secondary injuries and facilitating rehabilitation.
- The secondary injuries, which include hypoxia with coexistent hypotension, edema, and intracranial hypertension, can lead to increased mortality. Therefore, prompt care to avoid hypotension, hypoxia, cerebral edema, and elevated intracranial pressure (ICP) is advised.
- DAI carries an extremely poor prognosis.

Management
- The initial management is assessment and treatment of shock and hypoxia, as well as the search for other injuries and an evaluation of the patient's clotting ability with rapid correction if necessary.
- ICP should be maintained below 20 mm Hg, and CPP should be maintained above 70 mm Hg. Hypotension, particularly a mean arterial blood pressure of less than 90 mm Hg, should be prevented or treated, and dehydration should be avoided. ICP elevations of more than 20 mm Hg should be managed by drainage of ventricular fluid.
- If ICP elevations still occur, mannitol or other diuretics are used. Mannitol is given in boluses of 0.25 to 1 g per kg and repeated every 4 to 6 hours.

Operative Management
- Clots or contusions larger than 25 to 30 cm^3 are generally considered to cause significant mass effect capable of causing neurologic deterioration and progressive brain injury. Clots on the lateral surface of the brain are most often removed by creating a large "trauma flap" that extends down to the zygoma to expose the middle fossa and a large portion of the lateral surface of the brain.
- *Decompressive craniotomy*—The decompression should include the dura, and expansion of the dura using a graft is generally recommended; the opening, however, should be large enough so that the brain does not herniate through the created hole and strangulate its blood supply.

Herniations
- Herniation refers to displacement of brain tissue into a compartment that it normally does not occupy.
- The most common herniations are those in which a part of the brain is displaced from the supratentorial to the infratentorial compartment through the tentorial opening; this is referred to as *transtentorial* herniation.

Types

- **SUPRATENTORIAL HERNIATION:**
  - **Central (transtentorial) herniation**
  - **Uncal herniation**
  - **Cingulate herniation**—cingulated gyrus herniates under falx—subfalcine herniation
  - Usually asymptomatic; warning sign of impending transtentorial herniation
- **INFRATENTORIAL HERNIATION:**
  - **Upward cerebellar** – seen in posterior fossa masses; exacerbated by ventriculostomy; cerebellar vermis ascends above tentorium leading to compression of midbrain, occlusion of SCA's—cerebellar infarction; may cause hydrocephalus due to compression of Sylvian aqueduct.
  - **Tonsillar herniation** – cerebellar tonsils cone through foramen magnum, leading to compression of medulla and respiratory arrest – rapidly fatal; occurs with supra or infra tentorial masses or elevated ICP.
- *Uncal transtentorial* herniation refers to impaction of the anterior medial temporal gyrus (the uncus) into the tentorial opening just anterior to and adjacent to the midbrain.
- The uncus compresses the third nerve as it traverses the subarachnoid space, causing enlargement of the ipsilateral pupil (putatively because the fibers subserving parasympathetic pupillary function are located peripherally in the nerve). The coma that follows is due to compression of the midbrain against the opposite tentorial edge by the displaced parahippocampal gyrus.
- Herniation may also compress the anterior and posterior cerebral arteries as they pass over the tentorial reflections, with resultant brain infarction.
- The distortions may also entrap portions of the ventricular system, resulting in hydrocephalus
- **Diagnosis:** CT criteria
- **Impending uncal/hippocampal herniation:** Encroachment on lateral aspect of suprasellar cistern–flattening of normal pentagonal shape

Established Herniation

- Brainstem displacement and flattening
- Compression of contralateral cerebral peduncle
- Midbrain rotation with slight increase of ipsilateral subarachnoid space
- Contralateral hydrocephalus
- Obliteration of parasellar and interpeduncular cisterns (as uncus/hippocampus are forced through hiatus)

Stages

Early 3rd Nerve Stage

- Oculocephalic reflex (dolls eye)—normal or dysconjugate
- Oculovestibular reflex—slow ipsilateral deviation, impaired nystagmus

Late 3rd Nerve Stage

- Midbrain dysfunction occurs almost immediately after the symptoms extend to those beyond focal cerebral lesion (may skip diencephalic stage due to lateral pressure on brain)
- Delay in treatment can result in irreversible damage:
  - Fully dilated pupil
  - Lateral displacement of the midbrain may compress the opposite cerebral peduncle, producing a babinski's sign and hemiparesis contralateral to the original hemiparesis (the kernohan-woltman sign). False localizing sign
  - Sustained hyperventilation
  - Bilateral decerebration

Midbrain Upper Pons Stage

- Contralateral pupil fixes in mid position or full dilation; eventually both fix mid position (5-6 mm)
- Bilateral decerebrate rigidity

Following Midbrain Upper Pons Stage

- Similar to central herniation
- *Central transtentorial* herniation denotes a symmetric downward movement of the thalamic medial structures through the tentorial opening with compression of the upper midbrain.

- Both temporal and central transtentorial herniations have been considered causes of progressive compression of the brainstem, with initial damage to the midbrain, then the pons, and finally the medulla.
- The result is a sequence of neurologic signs that corresponds to each affected level.
- The diencephalon is gradually forced through the tentorial incisura; the pituitary stalk may be sheared leading to diabetes insipidus
- PCA may be trapped along the open edge of the incisura and may occlude producing cortical blindness
- The brainstem may suffer ischemia due to compression and shearing of perforating arteries from basilar artery – hemorrhages within the brainstem (duret hemorrhages)
- Miotic pupils and drowsiness are the heralding signs.
- More chronic than uncal herniation (due to tumour in frontal, parietal or occipital lobes)

Diagnosis
- Compression of perimesencephalic cisterns may be seen in CT/MRI
- Downward displacement of pineal gland in skull X-ray

Stages of Central Herniation

Diencephalic Stage
- Early and reversible
- Small range of pupillary contraction
- Parinauds syndrome: Impaired upgaze due to compression of superior colliculi and diencephalic pretectum
- Later: Decorticate

Midbrain—Upper Pons Stage
- Extreme ischemia of midbrain – poor prognosis
- Sustained tachypnea
- Fixed, moderately dilated pupils in midposition
- Dolls eye impaired
- Decorticate—Bilaterally decerebrate.

Lower Pons—Upper Medullary Stage
- Rapid shallow regular respiration
- Fixed pupils in mid position
- Absent dolls eye
- Flaccid tone

Medullary Stage—Terminal Stage
- Gasping
- Wide dilation of pupils with hypoxia

Other forms of herniation are *transfalcial herniation* (displacement of the cingulate gyrus under the falx and across the midline), and *foraminal herniation* (downward forcing of the cerebellar tonsils into the foramen magnum), which causes compression of the medulla, respiratory arrest, and death.

Decerebrate posturing: indicates brainstem damage below the level of red nucleus (mid collicular lesion). Commonly seen in pontine strokes. Progression from decorticate to decerebrate posturing is indicative of uncal (transtentorial) or tonsillar brain herniation. Activation of gamma motor neurons occurs in decerebrate rigidity.
- Involuntary extension of upper extremities in response to external stimuli
- Head is arched back, arms are extended by the sides and legs are extended; hallmark is extended elbows
- Arms and legs are extended and rotated internally
- Patient is rigid with teeth clenched

STEPWISE APPROACH TO TREATMENT OF ELEVATED ICP
- Insert ICP monitor—ventriculostomy versus parenchymal device
- **General goals**: maintain ICP < 20 mm Hg and CPP 60 mm Hg
- For ICP >20–25 mm Hg for >5 min:
- **Drain CSF via ventriculostomy** (if in place)
- Elevate head of the bed; midline head position

- **Osmotherapy**—Mannitol 25–100 g q4h as needed (maintain serum osmolality < 320 mOsmol) or hypertonic saline (30 mL, 23.4% NaCl bolus)
- **Glucocorticoids**—Dexamethasone 4 mg q6h for vasogenic edema from tumor, abscess (avoid glucocorticoids in head trauma, ischemic and hemorrhagic stroke)
- **Sedation** (e.g., morphine, propofol, or midazolam); add neuromuscular paralysis if necessary (patient will require endotracheal intubation and mechanical ventilation at this point, if not before)
- **Hyperventilation**—To $PaCO_2$ 30–35 mm Hg
- **Pressor therapy**—Phenylephrine, dopamine, or norepinephrine to maintain adequate MAP to ensure CPP 60 mm Hg (maintain euvolemia to minimize deleterious systemic effects of pressors)
- Consider **second-tier therapies** for refractory elevated ICP
  - High-dose barbiturate therapy ("pentobarb coma")
  - Aggressive hyperventilation to $PaCO_2$ <30 mm Hg
  - Hypothermia
  - Hemicraniectomy

Management of Head Trauma has been Explained in Detail Under Neuro-anesthesia

Traumatic injury of the spinal cord can result from vertebral fracture or subluxation, hyperextension of the cervical spine in the presence of a narrow spinal canal, herniation of intervertebral disc material into the canal, and penetrating injuries such as gunshots or stabbings.

- Neurologic involvement ranges from mild and transient to severe and permanent. Spinal fracture and cord injury should be suspected in head-injured patients with or without coma and in those with multiple injuries.
- Clinical findings can include spinal tenderness, extremity weakness, numbness or paresthesia, respiratory compromise, and hypotension. Spinal root involvement produces a radiculopathy characterized by motor and sensory impairment in the corresponding myotome and dermatome. Spinal cord involvement produces a myelopathy of variable manifestations.
- Complete lesions, signifying total loss of function below the level of injury, are often referred to as transections of the cord. Acute transections are characterized by areflexia, flaccidity, anesthesia, and autonomic paralysis below the level of the lesion. Arterial hypotension is invariably present when the transection is above T-5 because of the loss of sympathetic vascular tone.
- Incomplete lesions can result in the Brown-Séquard syndrome, which is manifested by ipsilateral loss of motor function and position-vibratory sensation with contralateral loss of pain and temperature sensation below the level of injury. Anatomically, this presentation is explained by hemisection of the cord.
- *The central cord syndrome* is characterized by bilateral loss of motor function and pain and temperature sensation in the upper extremities, with relative preservation of these functions in the lower extremities. Typically, the distal upper extremities are more severely affected because the most medial portions of the corticospinal and spinothalamic tracts subserve these areas. Motor impairment > sensory; UL>LL; some control over bladder and bowel is present; recover is possible. Causes: hyperextension of neck; spinal stenosis, syringomyelia, tumours.
- *The anterior spinal artery syndrome* involves the bilateral loss of motor function and pain and temperature sensation below the level of the lesion, with sparing of position-vibratory and light touch sensation. This incomplete lesion develops when the anterior spinal artery is occluded. This renders the cord ischemic within the anterior spinal artery distribution, affecting the anterior and lateral columns bilaterally.
- Trauma to the lumbar spine can produce signs and symptoms of *cauda equina compression*. Presentation consists of multiple lumbosacral radiculopathies of variable severity. Lower extremity motor, sensory, and reflex functions can be affected, producing variable degrees of weakness, sensory loss (all modalities in the specific distribution of the roots involved), and diminution or absence of reflexes. Bladder distention from detrusor muscle paralysis, flaccidity of the anal sphincter, and loss of perineal sensation are common in severe injuries.

In addition to the neurologic deficit, acute spinal cord injury is accompanied by many systemic responses. If the spinal cord is damaged above C-3, respiratory efforts cease, accounting for this injury's high mortality rate at the scene of the accident. Although spontaneous ventilatory efforts can be initiated with injuries involving C-4 to C-6, tidal volumes are often insufficient accounting for progressive hypoxia and carbon dioxide retention. Airway obstruction, atelectasis, and pneumonia are common complications. Assisted ventilation may be indicated, especially early after injury.

Management

- The goals of treatment are:
  - To correct spinal alignment
  - To protect undamaged neural tissue
  - To restore function to reversibly damaged neural tissue
  - To achieve permanent spinal stability.

Reduction and immobilization of any fracture or dislocation must receive top priority to meet these objectives.
- Cervical spine malalignment can almost always be reduced by skeletal traction. Traction can be applied with skull tongs or halo apparatus. Both are seated percutaneously through the outer table of the skull while the patient is kept supine and immobilized. The patient is then transferred to a special bed and placed in cervical traction, usually in the neutral position. Once the spinal injury is reduced, traction should be maintained.
- Patients with thoracic and lumbar spine fractures are also treated with immobilization initially. Patients are kept flat in bed without traction, and flexion, extension, lateral bending, and rotational movements are avoided. Typically, fewer systemic complications are associated with these neurologic injuries, but vigilance is required to prevent neurologic deterioration and to provide the best chance for neurologic recovery.
- **Indications for early operation on patients with spinal cord injury include:**
    - The inability to reduce the fracture or dislocation satisfactorily by closed methods
    - Neurologic deterioration in a patient with an initially incomplete cord lesion
    - Severe compression of the spinal cord by an intraspinal mass shown by myelography or MRI
    - A penetrating injury with or without a CSF leak.

CNS Causes of Vomiting
- Meningitis/encephalitis
- Causes of increased intracranial pressure: trauma, stroke, meningitis, vascular headache, malignant hypertension
- Vertigo/motion sickness
- Idiopathic epilepsy
- Increased ICP can also cause projectile vomiting upon waking up from sleep – late feature, accompanies headache

Intracranial Tumors
- *Primary* intracranial tumors—Arise from cells found in the brain, the pituitary gland, or the coverings of the brain
- *Secondary* intracranial tumors—derived from tumors that arise from outside the coverings of the brain. They may represent local extension of regional tumors such as chordoma or glomus tumors, or more commonly, they are blood-borne metastases from primary malignancies outside the brain.

Clinical Presentation
- A generalized increase in ICP—by direct mass effect from tumor bulk or hemorrhage into a tumor, or indirectly through hydrocephalus. A tumor may obstruct the ventricular system at the foramen of Monro, aqueduct of Sylvius, or the fourth ventricle, thus producing noncommunicating hydrocephalus. Alternatively, tumor debris or hemorrhage can obstruct the arachnoid villi, causing the symmetric enlargement of the entire ventricular system (communicating hydrocephalus)
- Vital sign changes include an elevation of the systolic blood pressure, bradycardia, and abnormal ventilatory patterns (Cushing's response)
- Focal compression or irritation of the brain - loss of neurologic function or Irritation of the cerebral cortex by a tumor causing a seizure.

Principles of Surgical Management
- Diagnosis may be accomplished by image-directed stereotactic needle biopsy or from specimens obtained at craniotomy.
- Any tumor causing mass effect or neurologic symptoms in a relatively noneloquent area of the brain should be removed, provided the patient can undergo general anesthesia. Exceptions are made for tumors that are unusually sensitive to radiation or chemotherapy, such as lymphoma or germinoma. All other tumors should undergo stereotactic biopsy.

Surgery Options
- *Bipolar electrocautery* to precisely cauterize tissues and vessels between two points.
- The *ultrasonic aspirator* simultaneously breaks up tough tumors and sucks away the debris. This device allows for internal debulking of large tumors and reduces the amount of brain retraction needed for tumor removal.
- Fusion of stereotactic systems with the operating microscope.

Primary Brain Tumors
- *Intra-axial*—Those that arise from either within the brain parenchyma. Majority are derived from neuroglia and are called gliomas.
    - Astrocytomas

- Oligodendrogliomas
- Ependymomas
- Medulloblastomas
- Primary central nervous system lymphomas
- Germ cell tumors
■ *Extra-axial*—Those that arise outside the parenchyma
- Meningiomas
- Schwannomas
- Pituitary adenomas.

Astrocytomas

- Most common type of glioma and account for 50% of all primary brain tumors
- Four criteria are evaluated by pathologists: degree of cellularity, mitotic figures, endothelial proliferation, and necrosis under WHO classification.
    - Grade 1 astrocytomas are a special category reserved for well-circumscribed tumors with essentially no ability to transform into higher grades.
    - Grade 2 or Low grade astrocytomas contain only one attribute, usually increased cellularity, and have a lower growth rate than higher-grade tumors.
    - Grade 3 or anaplastic astrocytomas have two attributes, usually increased cellularity and either endothelial proliferation or mitotic figures.
    - Grade 4 or glioblastoma multiforme have three or more attributes and characteristically have necrosis. Glioblastoma multiformes are the most aggressive and most common of all gliomas.

Pilocytic Astrocytoma

- The most common Grade 1 astrocytoma, most frequently seen in the cerebellar hemisphere and third ventricular region of children and young adults.
- On MRI, they appear as peripherally enhancing lesions, often with a mural nodule.
- In the cerebrum and cerebellum they are well circumscribed, surgically accessible, and therefore curable by complete resection

CLASSIFICATION AND GRADING OF ASTROCYTIC TUMOURS

Tumor	WHO Classification	St.Anne/Mayo grade based on number of criteria
Pilocytic astrocytoma	I	1
Astrocytoma	I, II	1 [No criteria]
		2 [Nuclear atypia]
Anaplastic astrocytoma	III	3 [Nuclear atypia + Mitosis]
Glioblastoma	IV	4 [Nuclear atypia + Mitosis + Endothelial proliferation and/or necrosis]

Treatment

- High-grade astrocytomas have mass effect and extensive areas of edema and infiltrating tumor cells. The best treatment involves surgical resection followed by fractionated external beam radiation to a dose of 60 Gy (6000 rads).
- Chemotherapy may slightly improve survival in selected patients. Bischloroethyl nitrosourea (BCNU) impregnated absorbable wafers also offer a small survival advantage and may replace intravenous chemotherapy in some patients.

Oligodendrogliomas

- Typically found in the supratentorial (90%), frontal(45%), temporal or parietal lobes (outside frontal lobes – 40%), third or lateral ventricle – 15%
- On CT scans, calcification and hemorrhage are more often seen in oligodendrogliomas than in other primary brain tumors.
- Chemotherapy may be more effective in oligodendroglioma.

Ependymomas

- Most frequently diagnosed in younger patients. The peak incidence is in childhood, where it typically presents as a mass in the fourth ventricle and causes hydrocephalus.
- Ependymomas are glial tumors that arise from ependymal cells or ependymal lining of the cerebral hemispheres and spinal cord-central canal remnants
- More predominantly manifest in children and young adults; they tend to be intracranial in children and spinal in adults
- The World Health Organization (WHO) divides ependymomas into the following types:
  - Subependymoma (WHO Grade I)
  - Myxopapillary ependymoma (WHO Grade I)
  - Ependymoma (with papillary, clear cell, and tanycytic variants; WHO Grade II)
  - *RELA* fusion–positive ependymoma (WHO Grade II or Grade III with change in the *RELA* gene)
  - Anaplastic ependymoma (WHO Grade III)
  - MC type in adults—Myxopapillary ependymoma (arises from filum terminale of the spinal cord – most commonly in the lumbosacral region)
- **Signs and symptoms:** Varies according to the age of the patient and the location of the lesion.
- **Masses in the fourth ventricle:** Progressive lethargy, headache, nausea, and vomiting; multiple cranial-nerve palsies (primarily VI-X), as well as cerebellar dysfunction
- In children who present before closure of cranial sutures, enlarging head circumference secondary to obstructive hydrocephalus
- Changes in personality, mood, and concentration; seizures; focal neurologic deficits reflecting location of the tumour
- **Spinal ependymomas:** Progressive neurologic deficit
- **Infratentorial ependymomas:** Papilledema ataxia; nystagmus
- **Supratentorial ependymomas:** Hemiparesis, sensory loss, visual loss, aphasia, and cognitive impairment; with increased ICP symptoms.

Diagnosis

- CT/MRI: They appear as diffusely enhancing masses; well demarcated from adjacent neural tissue
- MRI findings: Well circumscribed lesion; ventricular or brainstem displacement and hydrocephalus are frequent

Treatment

- Gross total resection (GTR) (maximal possible without causing neurologic deficits) followed by limited field fractionated external beam radiotherapy
- Craniospinal radiation is recommended as ependymomas have the potential to spread through neuraxis by seeding of the CSF

Medulloblastomas

- Most common primary brain tumor in children; very radiosensitive.
- Chromosomal alterations: 1q, 8p, 10q, 16q, 17p deletion; deletion of 1q, 10q (20–40%); SHH, WNT ErB signaling are defective
- Derived from an undifferentiated precursor to both astrocytes and neurons, medulloblastomas are most often found in the cerebellar vermis. Outside the posterior fossa, these tumors are called primitive neuroectodermal tumors.
- Histologically, they are highly cellular with the potential for both astrocytic and neuronal differentiation.

Primary Central Nervous System Lymphomas

- Rising in incidence during the past 20 years, seen in elderly and immunocompromised patients, especially those with end-stage AIDS.
- This tumor is very sensitive to radiation, and surgical resection is not indicated. Suspected patients should undergo a stereotactic biopsy followed by radiation therapy.

Germ Cell Tumors

- Includes germinoma, embryonal carcinoma, choriocarcinoma, and endodermal sinus tumor, these tumors are characteristically found in the pineal or hypothalamic region of children and young adults.

- *Alpha-fetoprotein* is characteristic of endodermal sinus tumors, and *beta-human chorionic gonadotropin* is secreted by choriocarcinoma. The finding of alpha-fetoprotein or human chorionic gonadotropin in CSF is pathognomonic for germ cell tumor and can preclude the need for biopsy.
- Craniotomy is preferred over stereotactic needle biopsy due to the presence of large veins in the pineal region.

Meningiomas
- Arising from arachnoidal cap cells, meningiomas are benign tumors that originate in the dura and displace the brain as they grow
- Do not invade the brain unless they are malignant, but they can invade and erode the skull or cause a hyperostotic reaction
- Most common locations are the parasagittal region, cerebral convexities, subfrontal region, and cerebellopontine angle, are usually found in adults and are more common in women.
- Appear isointense to brain on T1 and T2 MRI sequences but enhance strongly and homogeneously
- Meningiomas in the medial sphenoid wing or petroclival region are entwined with critical blood vessels and cranial nerves
- The Primary treatment is surgery with complete resection though the development of stereotactic radiosurgery using the gamma knife or linear accelerator offers a new tool for the control of residual tumor growth.
- Large (>4 cm) residual or recurrent meningiomas may require treatment with conventional fractionated radiation therapy. Chemotherapy does not play a significant role in the treatment of this tumor

Schwannomas
- Benign tumors arising from Schwann cells that form the myelin sheath around cranial nerves after their emergence from the brain stem, most commonly affected nerve is the vestibulocochlear nerve
- They present with the following symptoms: hearing loss (98%), tinnitus (70%), disequilibrium (67%) and facial numbness, weakness, diplopia
- Although surgery is still the primary treatment, small schwannomas can also be treated with stereotactic radiosurgery

Craniopharyngioma
- Slowly growing tumours of the sellar region
- At the time of diagnosis, patients have neurologic and endocrine signs and symptoms related to disruption of hypothalamo-pituitary function and ICP/increased mass effect
- Originates from the anterior superior margin of the pituitary
- Lined by stratified squamous epithelium
- Cyst contents are cholesterol crystals
- With thick walls
- 5% of CNS tumours and majority of sellar tumours in childhood
- Bimodal distribution; peak incidences from 5–14 years and again from 65 –74 years
- Manifestations:
  - *Endocrine:* Varying degrees of hypopituitarism and precocious puberty; growth spurt typically expected at puberty may be masked by concomitant growth hormone deficiency
  - Hyperphagia and obesity
  - Psychomotor retardation
  - Emotional immaturity
  - Apathy
  - Short term memory deficits
  - Incontinence
- *Diagnosis:*
  - CT–Identifies pathognomonic calcification–radiologic hallmark
  - MRI–preferred secondary to its superiority in detailing anatomy and tumour extent
- *Treatment:*
  - Total surgical removal is the treatment; recurrence–15% despite complete resection
  - Selective debulking along with adjunctive radio therapy

Rathke's Cleft Cyst
- Originates from the pars intermedia of pituitary
- Lined by single layer cuboidal epithelium
- Cyst wall is thin and consists of content which resembles motor oil
- Surgical treatment is partial excision and drainage

EPIDURAL HEMATOMA

Pituitary Adenoma
- *Functional tumors*—Diagnosed on the basis of an endocrinopathy caused by excessive hormone production. These endocrine abnormalities are often clinically evident in microadenomas (<1 cm), which is a tumor too small to cause neurologic deficit.
    - The most common functional tumor is the prolactinoma, which causes amenorrhea and galactorrhea in women.
    - Overproduction of adenocorticotrophic hormone by a pituitary adenoma causes Cushing's disease, which is characterized by centripetal obesity, moon facies, buffalo hump, purple striae, glucose intolerance, and psychiatric disturbance.
    - A growth hormone-secreting adenoma causes acromegaly, which results in growth of the hands, feet, lower jaw, and supraorbital ridge.
    - Tumors that secrete thyroid-stimulating hormone, luteinizing hormone, or follicle-stimulating hormone are rare.
- *Nonfunctional pituitary adenomas*—Typically present with mass effect on adjacent structures, notably the optic chiasm. Because the optic pathways serving the medial half of each retina cross in the chiasm, compression in this area affects both temporal visual fields. The patient experiences a loss of peripheral vision and manifests a bitemporal field cut on formal visual field testing.
- On MRI, the anterior pituitary enhances strongly and rapidly because it lacks a blood-brain barrier. Due to this effect, pituitary microadenomas appear as a nonenhancing area within the pituitary gland. Macroadenomas erode and enlarge the sella turcica in addition to elevating the optic chiasm

Surgical Treatment
- The unique anatomy of the pituitary sella allows tumors in this region to be approached through the nose via a transseptal, transsphenoidal craniotomy
- Residual tumor may be observed for evidence of regrowth, alternatively, radiosurgery may be used to control regrowth.
- Intracranial surgery is used only if there is extensive suprasellar extension.

METASTATIC BRAIN TUMORS
- The brain is a common site for metastases, by virtue of its disproportionately high blood flow.
- The most common primary sites are lung > breast > skin (melanoma) > kidney > gastrointestinal tract.
- Management is dependent on the number of lesions, their size, and the condition of the patient. A large (>4 cm) metastasis causing neurologic compromise should be resected, if surgically accessible, and then followed with whole-brain radiation therapy (WBRT).
- A smaller, single metastasis causing neurologic deficit may be removed or treated with radiosurgery followed by WBRT. Multiple metastases are also usually treated with radiosurgery and WBRT or with WBRT alone.

Intraspinal Tumors

1. Extradural Tumors
- Originate in the vertebral body or, less commonly, the epidural space
- Majority are malignant and represent metastatic tumors, particularly from lung, breast, and prostate
- As these tumors grow, they destroy the vertebrae, causing pathologic fractures and spinal cord compression. The thoracic spine is most commonly involved, and the earliest symptom is usually pain both along the axial spine and around the trunk in a radicular pattern. As the tumor enlarges, progressive spinal cord injury ensues. Myelopathic symptoms such as motor weakness, spasticity, and hyperreflexia are common findings.

Treatment
- Always a combination of surgery and radiation therapy.
- Surgery is required if the biopsy is inadequate or if there is a progressive neurologic deficit. Tumor found in the posterior epidural space or posterior bony elements is best treated by laminectomy

- A transthoracic or a lateral extracavitary approach may be used to perform a vertebrectomy along with stabilization by a bone graft with metal plate internal fixation or a methyl methacrylate construct.
- External beam radiation is indicated if multilevel extradural disease exists or if there is minimal neurologic compromise.

2. Intradural, Extramedullary Tumors
- Found within the dura but outside the substance of the spinal cord
- Mostly benign, arising from the meninges (meningioma) or nerve roots (schwannoma and neurofibroma)
- Primary tumors from outside the brain can also seed the spinal subarachnoid space, resulting in meningeal carcinomatosis.

Treatment
- A laminectomy is usually adequate to gain access to the tumor, although certain tumors may require a lateral or even an anterior approach to facilitate complete removal.
- External beam radiation therapy is the best treatment for these patients.

3. Intramedullary Tumors
- Originate in the substance of the spinal cord, most common tumors are astrocytoma and ependymoma.
- Patients usually experience myelopathy and sensory disturbance below the spinal level of involvement. Tumors at the level of the conus medullaris can cause a cauda equina syndrome, which classically presents with perineal anesthesia, bowel and bladder incontinence, and lower extremity pain and weakness.
- MRI with contrast medium is the preferred imaging study. Contrast enhancement within the spinal cord is suggestive of an intramedullary tumor

Treatment
- Laminectomy followed by tumor resection or biopsy.
- Intraoperative ultrasound is useful for determining the extent of tumor and location of a syrinx. Ultrasonic aspiration and the operating microscope are indispensable in the surgical treatment of intramedullary tumors.

Glioblastoma Multiforme
- Most common form of primary intracranial neuroepithelial tumour
- 25% of intracranial tumours; 50% of CNS origin tumours
- Heterogenous glial cell tumours derived from the malignant degeneration of an astrocytoma or anaplastic astrocytoma
- Found in cerebral hemispheres in fifth decade
- CT/MRI – irregular lesion with hypodense central necrosis
  - Peripheral ring enhancement of the highly cellular tumour tissue
  - Surrounding edema ad mass effect
- *Treatment:*
  - Diagnostic biopsy followed by radiotherapy to slow tumour growth
  - Curative resections are rare

Cerebellopontine Angle Tumours
- Most common neoplasms in the posterior fossa; 5-10% intra cranial tumours
- Most CPA tumours are benign; >85% are vestibular schwannomas (acoustic neuromas), lipomas, vascular malformations, hemangiomas
- MC non acoustic CPA tumours: meningiomas, epidermoids, facial or lower cranial nerve schwannomas <2% CPA tumours – primary malignancies/metastatic lesions

Presenting Symptoms
- Hearing loss
- Tinnitus
- Vertigo
- Headache, facial hypesthesia
- Diplopia (presentation varies based on size and location of tumour)
- Tumours within nerve canaliculi–unilateral sensorineural hearing loss, tinnitus or disequilibrium. Speech discrimination out of proportion to hearing loss
- Tumours extending into CPA–disequilibrium/ataxia
- Tumours with brainstem extension–midfacial and corneal hypesthesia, hydrocephalus.

LUMBAR RADICULOPATHY

- Disk herniations can occur in any direction but most commonly follow a posterolateral direction at the site where the posterior longitudinal ligament is thinnest. Disk material extruded in this location can compress a nerve root, leading to low back pain and radicular symptoms in a specific dermatomal distribution.
- Large, more central disk herniations may compress the cauda equina with resultant cauda equina syndrome, consisting of saddle anesthesia, urinary retention with possible overflow incontinence, and significant motor weakness.
- An initial period of nonsurgical management for at least 4 to 8 weeks is indicated unless the patient presents with cauda equina syndrome, progressive neurologic deficit, recurrent episodes of incapacitating pain, or profound motor weakness. Conservative therapy includes rest, activity modification, physical therapy, weight loss, analgesics, muscle relaxants, oral steroids, and epidural steroid injections.
- The standard treatment of these herniations involves a midline approach centered over the affected interspace followed by a hemilaminectomy to expose the thecal sac and nerve root.
- A minimally invasive procedure through a 1-cm paramedian incision with a muscle-splitting technique can also be used under either microscopic or endoscopic visualization with less postoperative morbidity.

COMMON LUMBAR DISC HERNIATIONS AND THEIR FEATURES

Disk	Incidence	Root	Pain	Muscle involved	Sensory deficits	Reflex lost
L3-L4	Least	L4	Anterior thigh	Quadriceps femoris	Medial malleolus and medial foot	Knee jerk
L4-L5	2nd most common	L5	Posterolateral thigh and leg	Tibialis anterior Extensor hallucis longus	Large toe web and dorsum of foot	None
L5-S1	Most common	S1	Posterolateral thigh and leg down to ankle	Gastrocnemius	Lateral malleolus Lateral foot	Ankle jerk

LUMBAR SPINAL STENOSIS

- Advanced degeneration of the lumbar spine may result in spondylosis with arthrosis and hypertrophy of the facet joint as well as thickening and buckling of the ligamentum flavum. These changes lead to narrowing of the spinal canal with resultant constriction of the thecal sac and development of neurologic deficits.
- Patients classically present with neurogenic claudication: unilateral or bilateral dermatomal discomfort precipitated by standing or walking or prolonged maintenance of the same posture
- Neurogenic claudication is thought to arise from ischemic changes of roots as a result of increased metabolic demands from exercise in the presence of a vascular compromise of the root from the surrounding constriction.
- Surgical decompression is warranted in patients with recurrent and disabling pain that limits their daily activity. Laminotomies or laminectomies of the involved levels with undercutting of the superior articular facet are required to decompress the nerves in the foramina.

CERVICAL RADICULOPATHY

- The most common present upon awakening in the morning without identifiable trauma or stress. The pain usually radiates from the proximal arm distally, together with numbness and paresthesia, in a dermatomal distribution. The pain may be intensified by neck movements. In severe cases, a motor weakness along the same nerve may be noticed.
- On examination, pain with downward pressure on the vertex while tilting the head toward the symptomatic side (*Spurling's sign*) is a mechanical sign of disk herniation.
- MRI is the study of choice for the initial evaluation of a herniated cervical disk. A CT myelogram is indicated for patients who cannot undergo MRI or when anatomic bony details are required. A cervical spine X-ray is always recommended to evaluate the degree of spondylosis in the cervical spine before surgery. Electromyography and nerve conduction studies can be useful when other causes need to be excluded, such as plexopathies or peripheral nerve entrapment.
- Conservative therapy includes a combination of oral steroids, nonsteroidal anti-inflammatory drugs, analgesics, muscle relaxants, intermittent cervical traction, and physical therapy. Surgery is indicated for those who fail to improve and those with progressive neurologic deficit while undergoing the conservative therapy.

- With anterior pathology (paracentral herniation or large uncovertebral osteophyte), an anterior cervical discectomy, nerve root decompression, and fusion are indicated.
- A posterior approach, also called *keyhole foraminotomy,* is indicated in patients with unilateral radiculopathy with soft disk herniation or small lateral osteophyte and in patients with a short thick neck.

STEREOTACTIC NEUROSURGERY

- Uses a coordinate system to provide accurate navigation to a point or region in space. The coordinate system may be a fixed stereotactic frame that is rigidly attached to the skull, or it may be based on a frameless system that uses fiducial markers placed on the scalp that are then correlated with MRI or CT results.
- The most commonly used frame-based systems are the *Leksell Model G* and the *Cosman-Roberts-Wells frames.*
- The most common frame-based stereotactic procedures are biopsies and the implantation of electrodes to make lesions or chronic stimulation of the brain.
- Gamma knife and modified linear accelerator (many different systems) are the most widely used radiosurgery devices. Coordinates of a lesion within the brain are used to determine where to focus the radiation beams. This treatment is used to treat brain tumors that are inoperable or multiple in number as well as AVMs. It is also effective for patients with trigeminal neuralgia.
- The primary risk of radiosurgery is *radionecrosis,* which may occur 6 to 12 months after treatment and is related to the dose delivered and the volume treated.
- The new generation of frameless stereotactic devices allows the neurosurgeon to correlate MRI and CT images with pointing devices that may be a simple probe, a robotic arm, or an actual surgical instrument such as an endoscope or biopsy probe.

EPILEPSY SURGERY

- The most frequent performed is *temporal lobectomy*. Usually, the lateral and inferior cortices are removed after a temporal craniotomy exposes the anterior temporal lobe. The mesiotemporal structures, including the amygdala and hippocampus, are excised. The extent of the resection is guided by the location of the focus and language mapping in the dominant lobe
- Cortical resections can also be made to remove a focus in other parts of the hemisphere. Ex. Frontal cortex. Instead of resection, multiple gyral cortical incisions perpendicular to the axis of the involved gyrus are also made, interrupting the local association fibers but sparing the deeper projecting fibers.
- *Corpus callosum callosotomy* is used to interrupt the spread of severe seizures and mitigate generalization.
- *Hemispherectomy* is an operation usually restricted to children with extensive unilateral epileptiform activity.
- *Vagal nerve stimulators* are a newly approved method to manage intractable seizures

PSYCHOSURGERY

- *Prefrontal leucotomy*—Initially performed surgery for wide range of disorders.
- Latest procedures using stereotactic radiosurgery
  - *Subcaudate tractotomy*—Endogenous depression
  - *Limbic leucotomy*—Obsessional neurosis
  - *Amygdalotomy*—Severe uncontrolled aggression.

NEUROABLATION PROCEDURES FOR PAIN MANAGEMENT

- *Neurectomy:* Transection of a peripheral nerve results in numbness and may temporarily relieve pain.
- *Rhizotomy:* Open ablation of the sensory root can be performed via an intradural or extradural approach or percutaneously using radiofrequency coagulation or phenol injection.
- *Dorsal root entry zone lesion:* Using a specially designed radiofrequency electrode, multiple lesions are made along the dorsal roots that ablate the dorsal horn gray matter, including the second-order neurons. This treatment is most successful for nerve root or brachial plexus avulsion and spinal cord injury.

- *Cordotomy:* Performed percutaneously with radiofrequency lesioning of the spinothalamic tract in the anterior portion of the cervical spinal cord. Bilateral cordotomy is not advised because of the risk of Ondine's curse (loss of involuntary respiratory drive).
- *Myelotomy:* Splitting the spinal cord at and above the level of pain divides the spinothalamic tract as it crosses in the anterior spinal cord.
- *Midbrain tractotomy:* Ablation of the spinothalamic tract in the brain stem with the use of stereotactic guidance, commonly indicated for face and shoulder pain from head and neck cancer.
- *Cingulotomy:* Using stereotactic guidance, bilateral radiofrequency lesions are made in the white matter deep to the cingulate gyrus, resulting in interference to Papez's limbic circuit, most useful when depression is the dominant feature of the pain syndrome.
- *Sympathectomy:* Indicated for the treatment of causalgia, reflex sympathetic dystrophy, or Raynaud's phenomenon.

NEUROAUGMENTATION PROCEDURES FOR PAIN MANAGEMENT

- *Spinal cord stimulation:* Based on the gate control theory, which postulates that nonpainful stimuli carried through large, myelinated nerves that continued in the dorsal columns of the spinal cord could modulate perception of painful stimuli through unmyelinated fibers, indicated for neuropathic pain syndromes, including peripheral nerve injury, reflex sympathetic dystrophy, deafferentation pain, and postherpetic neuralgia.
- *Intrathecal narcotic infusion:* Direct application of narcotics provides a more potent activation of opioid receptors in the substantia gelatinosa of the spinal cord. Usually used for nociceptive cancer pain.

DEEP BRAIN STIMULATION [DBS]

- A *surgical* treatment involving the implantation of a medical device called a brain pacemaker, which sends electrical impulses to specific parts of the brain.
- Consists of three components: the implanted pulse generator (IPG), the lead, and the extension.
- DBS leads are placed in the brain according to the type of symptoms to be addressed. For example, in non-Parkinsonian *essential tremor* the lead is placed in the ventrointermedial nucleus (VIM) of the *thalamus*. For dystonia and symptoms associated with *Parkinson's disease* (rigidity, bradykinesia/akinesia and *tremor*), the lead may be placed in either the globus pallidus or subthalamic nucleus.
- DBS is approved by the FDA for the treatment of Parkinson's disease.

OSLER-WEBER-RENDU SYNDROME

- Rare autosomal dominant disorder causing vascular dysplasia - tendency for bleeding.
- Also known as hereditary hemorrhagic telangiectasia (HHT)
- *Capillary telangiectasia*—Slightly enlarged capillaries with low flow and have intervening neural tissue as opposed to cavernous malformations
- Telangiectases of the skin and mucous membranes, epistaxis, and a positive family history make up the classic triad of Osler-Weber-Rendu disease 90% of patients manifest by age 40 years or later.
- The diagnosis of HHT is made clinically on the basis of the Curaçao criteria
- The four clinical diagnostic criteria are as follows:
  - Epistaxis (MC presentation–can lead to severe anemia) (90%)
  - Telangiectasias (75%)
  - Visceral lesions (can affect lung liver spleen, GI tract, conjunctiva nasopharynx, CNS) (30%)
  - Pulmonary AVMs affect approximately 50% of patients with HHT
  - Pulmonary AVMs may cause enough right-to-left shunting to cause cyanosis, hypoxemia, and secondary polycythemia. Pulmonary AVMs also increase the incidence of infection as a result of septic emboli formation in the pulmonary vasculature.
  - Family history (a first-degree relative with HHT)

ETIOLOGY

- Mutations of *ENG* (encoding endoglin)—chromosome 9, 9q33–34
- Mutations of *ALK1* (encoding ALK-1)—chromosome 12, 12q13

- Mutations of chromosome 5 (5q31.1–32)
- Mutations of *SMAD4/MADH4* (encoding Smad4)
- The first two (HHT types 1 and 2) account for approximately 85% of cases.

PROGNOSIS

- The prognosis is highly dependent on the severity of the disease/the degree of systemic involvement, especially pulmonary, hepatic, and CNS involvement.
- 10% of patients die of complications of HHT.

Investigations
CT—a well demarcated homogenous or mottled high density

Treatment
Surgery—evacuation of hematoma when favorably located, recurrent hemorrhage, medically intractable seizures

DANDY-WALKER MALFORMATION

Dandy-Walker malformation (also known as Dandy-Walker syndrome): having a small cerebellar vermis, large fourth ventricle, and enlarged posterior fossa.

Variants

- Isolated cerebellar vermis hypoplasia (sometimes known as Dandy-Walker variant): having a small cerebellar vermis without other features of Dandy-Walker complex
- Mega-cisterna magna: having an enlarged posterior fossa with a typically developed cerebellum. This may be a normal variant and may not cause any health problems.
- Posterior fossa arachnoid cyst: the development of a cyst on the posterior fossa without any other features of Dandy-Walker complex
- **Key features** of this syndrome are an cystic enlargement of the fourth ventricle and midline cerebellar hypoplasia or complete absence (agenesis) of the cerebellar vermis and corpus callosum (associated anomalies)
- Results due to failure in the development of the roof of the 4th ventricle and a partial or complete congenital failure to develop the cerebellar vermis which blocks the CSF circulation (hydrocephalus – 90%)

Presentation

- Rapid progressive enlargement in head size (increased head circumference); transillumination of skull - positive
- Delayed motor and cognitive milestones (due to structural abnormalities) and long tract signs
- Symptoms of increased intracranial pressure such as irritability, vomiting, and convulsions
- Signs of cerebellar dysfunction such as unsteadiness ataxia and lack of muscle coordination or nystagmus

Treatment
Shunting of cystic cavity (in the presence of hydrocephalus)

NELSON SYNDROME

- Nelson syndrome refers to a spectrum of symptoms and signs arising from an adrenocorticotropin (ACTH)–secreting pituitary macroadenoma after a therapeutic bilateral adrenalectomy.
- The spectrum of clinical features observed relates to
  - The local effects of the tumor on surrounding structures
  - The secondary loss of other pituitary hormones
  - The effects of the high serum concentrations of ACTH on the skin
- The first case was reported by Nelson et al. in 1958.
- Almost all cases of Nelson syndrome follow bilateral adrenalectomy in patients who have Cushing disease due to an ACTH-secreting pituitary adenoma.
- Following bilateral adrenalectomy and normalization of cortisol levels that had suppressed hypothalamic CRH production, an increase in CRH occurs, which then has a trophic effect on the tumor, stimulating its growth.

BALINT'S SYNDROME

- Psychic impairment of visual fixation and alteration in visual attention
- The patient has normal visual acuity and field yet he has inability to reach out for objects using visual guidance.
- Lesions in B/L parieto-occipital region can result in optic ataxia and inability to voluntary direct gaze.

TOLOSA-HUNT SYNDROME

- *Lesion at the orbital apex*—Hence also known as orbital apex syndrome
- Characterized by acute, painful ophthalmolegia, with/without involvement of the optic nerve and ophthalmic division of the trigeminal nerve; prompt response seen to steroid treatment
- Tolosa described a case wherein a amass of granulation tissue around the carotid artery in the cavernous sinus and there was an asymmetrical enlargement of the cavernous sinus

Brain Abscess

- A brain abscess is a focal, suppurative infection within the brain parenchyma, typically surrounded by a vascularized capsule.
- The term *cerebritis* is often employed to describe a nonencapsulated brain abscess.
- Relatively uncommon intracranial infection
- Predisposing conditions include:
  - Otitis media and mastoiditis
  - Paranasal sinusitis
  - Pyogenic infections in the chest or other body sites
  - Penetrating head trauma
  - Neurosurgical procedures
  - Dental infections.
- In immunocompetent individuals the most important pathogens are *Streptococcus* spp., Enterobacteriaceae [*Proteus* spp., *E. Coli* sp., *Klebsiella* spp.], anaerobes (e.g., *Bacteroides* spp.) and staphylococci.
- In immunocompromised hosts with underlying HIV infection, organ transplantation, cancer, or immunosuppressive therapy, most brain abscesses are caused by *Nocardia* spp., *Toxoplasma gondii*, *Aspergillus* spp., *Candida* spp., and *C. Neoformans*.
- Brain abscess in congenital heart disease occur due to hematogenous seeding of blood borne bacteria which bypass the capillary bed due to right to left shunt. They commonly infect parietal and frontal lobes (middle cerebral artery territory)
- In India and the Far East, mycobacterial infection (tuberculoma) remains a major cause of focal CNS mass lesions.

Etiology

A brain abscess may develop
- By direct spread from a contiguous cranial site of infection, such as paranasal sinusitis, otitis media, mastoiditis, or dental infection;
  - Otogenic abscesses occur predominantly in the temporal lobe and cerebellum;
  - Abscesses that develop as a result of direct spread of infection from the frontal, ethmoidal, or sphenoidal sinuses and those that occur due to dental infections are usually located in the frontal lobes.
- Following head trauma or a neurosurgical procedure;
- Hematogenous spread from a remote site of infection: Hematogenous abscesses are:
  - Often multiple
  - Show a predilection for the territory of the middle cerebral artery (i.e., posterior frontal or parietal lobes).
  - Often located at the junction of the gray and white matter and poorly encapsulated.
  - The microbiology is dependent on the primary source of infection.
- In up to 25% of cases, no obvious primary source of infection is apparent (cryptogenic brain abscess).
- **Clinical presentation**: depends on its location, the nature of the primary infection if present, and the level of the ICP;
  - Hemiparesis is the most common localizing sign of a frontal lobe abscess.
  - Dysphasia) or an upper homonymous quadrantanopia - temporal lobe abscess
  - Signs of raised ICP— papilledema, nausea and vomiting, and drowsiness or confusion – cerebellar abscess

- Typically presents as an expanding intracranial mass lesion
- The classic clinical triad of headache (mc symptom >75%; constant dull aching sensation which progressively becomes severe and refractory to treatment), fever, and a focal neurologic deficit (hemiparesis, aphasia, or visual field defects).
- The new onset of focal or generalized seizure activity is a presenting sign in 15–35% of patients.
- **Diagnosis** is made by neuroimaging studies.
  - MRI > CT for demonstrating abscesses in the early (cerebritis) stages and in the posterior fossa.
  - On a contrast-enhanced CT scan, a mature brain abscess appears as a focal area of hypodensity surrounded by ring enhancement with surrounding edema (hypodensity).

Treatment

- Combination of high-dose parenteral antibiotics and neurosurgical drainage. Empirical therapy includes a third- or fourth-generation cephalosporin (e.g., cefotaxime, ceftriaxone, or cefepime) and metronidazole
- Aspiration and drainage of the abscess under stereotactic guidance are beneficial for both diagnosis and therapy.
- Medical therapy alone should be reserved for patients whose abscesses are neurosurgically inaccessible, for patients with small (< 2–3 cm) or nonencapsulated abscesses (cerebritis), and patients whose condition is too tenuous to allow performance of a neurosurgical procedure. All patients should receive a minimum of 6–8 weeks of parenteral antibiotic therapy.
- Prophylactic anticonvulsant therapy [high risk (35%) of focal or generalized seizures] continued for at least 3 months after resolution
- Glucocorticoids (Intravenous dexamethasone therapy—10 mg every 6 h) is usually reserved for patients with substantial periabscess edema and associated mass effect and increased ICP.

Prognosis

- The mortality rate is typically <15%.
- Significant sequelae, including seizures, persisting weakness, aphasia, or mental impairment, occur in 20% of survivors.

Neurological Centres

- *Major causes of TBI*—Vehicle accidents
- *Prevention of accidents*—Reduction in intensity and gravity of TBI
- Damage reduction in accidents:
  - Use of seat belts, child safety seats, presence of roll bars and airbags, motorcycle helmets
- *Education programs:*
  - Change in public policy/safety laws—speed limits, compulsory helmets and seat belts, road engineering practices.

NEUROGENIC SHOCK

Severe CNS damage due to trauma causes sudden loss of background sympathetic stimulation to the blood vessels which can result in vasodilation and sudden decrease in blood pressure (secondary to decrease in peripheral vascular resistance). The sympathetic stimulation usually triggers compensatory mechanisms in other forms of shock, such as increased neurotransmitters such as epinephrine and norepinephrine and helps to keep the blood pressure and heart rate up by causing vasoconstriction and shunting blood from the extremities to the vital organs. In neurogenic shock these compensatory mechanisms are not activated due to loss of sympathetic tone; in end stage shock patient exhibits very low blood pressure, weak and fast pulse, rapid shallow breathing.

Neurogenic shock results from damage to spinal cord above the level of 6th thoracic vertebra.

Occurs in 50% of patients who suffer spinal cord injury within 24 hours and lasts 1-3 weeks

Clinical Presentation

- Instantaneous hypotension–sudden massive vasodilation–warm flushed skin
- Priapism
- Bradycardia
- Diaphragmatic breathing when injury is below C5 vertebra (loss of nervous control over intercostal muscles)
- Respiratory arrest if injury above C3 vertebra (loss of nervous control over diaphragm).

HYPOVOLEMIC SHOCK

MC cause of shock after trauma–hypovolemia (due to hemorrhage)

Severity Classification

- **Class 1 hemorrhage**: Loss of 15% blood volume; manifestation – mild anxiety
- **Class 2 hemorrhage**: Loss of 15 – 30% blood volume; manifestation – tachycardia, tachypnea, anxiety, decreased urinary output
- **Class 3 hemorrhage**: Loss of 30 – 40% blood volume; manifestation – extreme anxiety, combativeness, marked tachycardia, tachypnea and decrease in urine output
- **Class 4 hemorrhage**: Loss of more than 40% blood volume; manifestation – marked hypotension and tachycardia; complete urine output shutoff; can be lethal

CARDIOGENIC SHOCK: CLINICAL PRESENTATION

- Hypotension, tachycardia
- Weak thread pulse
- Cool, pale, moist skin
- Urine output < 30 mL/hr
- Decreased cardiac output

SEPTIC SHOCK

- Hypotension, tachycardia, decreased cardiac output
- Full bounding pulse, tachypnea
- Pink warm flushed skin
- Fever decreased urine output

ANAPHYLACTIC SHOCK

- Hypotension, tachycardia, decreased cardiac output
- Cough, dyspnea
- Pruritis, urticaria
- Restlessness, loss of consciousness

DAMAGE TO MOTOR NERVES may produce the following symptoms:

- Weakness; Muscle atrophy: Twitching, also known as fasciculation; Paralysis

Sensory nerve damage may produce the following symptoms:

- Pain: Sensitivity: Numbness: Tingling or prickling; Burning: Problems with positional awareness
- Distal axonopathies usually present with sensorimotor disturbances that have a symmetrical "stocking and glove" distribution.
- Deep tendon reflexes and autonomic nervous system functions are also lost or diminished in affected areas.

Multiple Choice Questions

1. Most common location of Oligodendroglioma?
   a. Frontal lobes
   b. Hemispheres
   c. Infratentorial and spinal cords
   d. Within third and lateral ventricle

2. Myxopapillary ependymoma most commonly occurs in:
   a. Intratentorial
   b. Supratentorial
   c. Cervical segment
   d. Cauda region

3. The second most common symptom of Vestibular schwannoma:
   a. Headache
   b. Tinnitus
   c. Hearing loss
   d. Dysequilibrium

4. All of the following are true about Rathke's Cleft Cyst *except:*
   a. Thin cyst wall
   b. Contents resemble motor oil
   c. Lined by single layer of cuboidal epithelium
   d. Originates from anterior superior margin of pituitary

5. Difference between a dermoid and an epidermoid tumor are all *except:*
   a. Epidermoid is more common in occurrence than dermoid
   b. Epidermoid located more towards the midline
   c. Dermoid is associated with congenital anomalies up to 50% cases
   d. Dermoid may be associated with repeated Bouts of bacteria meningitis

6. All of these patients can be observed at home *except:*
   a. Head CT done and its normal
   b. Initial GCS E3M6V4
   c. Patient having amnesia of for the event
   d. Patient stays nearby the Hospital ER

7. Normal ICP for term infants:
   a. 0.5 to 1.5 mm of HgC. 3.5 to 7 mm of Hg
   b. 1.5 to 6 mm of Hg
   c. 3.5 to 7 mm of Hg
   d. 6.5 to 8 mm of Hg

8. All of the following are true regarding posterior fossa EDH *except:*
   a. More common in first 2 decades of life
   b. Presence of cerebellar signs are common
   c. Source of bleeding is usually not found
   d. Overall mortality is 26%

9. All of the following are true regarding EDH *except:*
   a. EDH measuring 10 cc with GCS E1M3VT should undergo immediate surgery
   b. EDH measuring 25 cc with 4 mm midline shift can be managed medically
   c. Temporal EDH measuring 10 cc with pupillary asymmetry can be managed medically
   d. EDH with thickness of 10 mm and midline shift of 1 cm should be managed with surgery

10. All of the following are true regarding acute SDH *except:*
    a. Patients operated within 4 hours have 30% mortality
    b. ICP need to be monitored in all patients with GCS less than 9 with a diagnosis of acute SDH
    c. If there is no newly developed pupillary asymmetry. Acute SDH can be managed medically despite a drop of GCS by 2 points

11. All of the following about Osler-Weber-Rendu syndrome are true *except:*
    a. May be associated with AVMs
    b. Rare Autosomal recessive genetic disorder
    c. There are slightly enlarged capillaries with low flow
    d. 95% of patients have recurrent epistaxis

12. Difficulty in walking but not needing assistance and unable to work full time is classified as:
    a. Nurick Grade- 1
    b. Nurick Grade- 2
    c. Nurick Grade- 3
    d. Nurick Grade- 4

13. All are true regarding vein of Galen malformation *except:*
    a. Congenital malformation, usually develops 3 months embryo stage
    b. New born presents with heart failure and cranial bruit
    c. Straight sinus is always very well developed
    d. Untreated VOGM presenting at neonatal Period has 100% mortality

14. Characteristic of early subacute haemorrhage in MRI:
    a. T1-Hyper, T2- Hypo
    b. T1-Hypo, T2-Hyper
    c. T1-Hypo, T2 Hypo
    d. T1-Iso, T2-Hyper

15. Most common cause of spontaneous ICH in young adults:
    a. Ruptured aneurysm
    b. Arterial hypertension
    c. Intracerebral SOL
    d. Ruptured AVM

Answers

1. a	2. d	3. b	4. d	5. b	6. b	7. b
8. b	9. c	10. c	11. b	12. c	13. d	14. a
15. d						

16. All of the following are true regarding SRS dosage *except:*
    a. Non-secretory pituitary adenoma: 16-18 Gy
    b. Meningioma 14 Gy
    c. Secretory pituitary adenoma: 25 Gy
    d. Vestibular schwannoma: 14-16 Gy

17. Witzelsucht syndrome is seen in:
    a. Frontal lobe tumours
    b. Parietal lobe tumours
    c. Temporal lobe tumours
    d. Interventricular tumours

18. Which of the following brain tumour is noted for its radiosensitivity?
    a. Astrocytoma
    b. Ependymoma
    c. Meningioma
    d. Medulloblastoma

19. Which of the following is often the site of origin of Jacksonian epilepsy?
    a. Orbitofrontal area
    b. Frontal lobe
    c. Prerolandic gyrus
    d. Postrolandic gyrus

20. In ICH, LP can be negative for first:
    a. 8–10 hrs
    b. 12–16 hrs
    c. 16–24 hrs
    d. 24–48 hrs

21. You are a surgeon posted at CHC. A patient of head injury comes to you with rapidly deteriorating sensorium and progressive dilatation and fixation of pupil. Neurosurgeon and CT scan is not available. You decide to make a burr hole to emergently relieve the intracranial pressure. Which of the following sites will you choose?
    a. In the temporal region contralateral to the side of papillary Dilatation
    b. In the midline if both pupils are equal or it is not known which side dilated first
    c. In the tHe left temporal region if no localizing sign is found
    d. Refer to higher centre if both pupils are equal or it is not known which side dilated first

22. Triple H therapy for subarachnoid hemorrhage consists of all *except:*
    a. Hypertension
    b. Hypervolaemia
    c. Hemodilution
    d. Hypothermia

23. An adult hypertensive male presented with sudden onset severe headache and vomiting. On examination, there is marked neck rigidity and no neurological deficit was found. The symptoms are most likely due to:
    a. Intracranial parenchymal hemorrhage
    b. Ischemic stroke
    c. Meningitis
    d. Subarachnoid haemorrhage

24. Brain abscess in cyanotic heart disease is commonly located in:
    a. Cerebellar hemisphere
    b. Thalamus
    c. Temporal lobe
    d. Parietal lobe

25. A young female patient with long history of sinusitis presented with frequent fever along with personality changes and headache of recent origin. The fundus examination revealed papilledema. The most likely diagnosis is:
    a. Frontal lobe abscess
    b. Meningitis
    c. Encephalitis
    d. Frontal bone osteomyelitis

26. A newborn with meningomyelocele has been posted for surgery. The defect should be immediately covered with:
    a. Normal saline gauze
    b. Povidone iodine gauze
    c. Tincture benzoin gauze
    d. Methylene blue gauze

27. In causalgia, the nerve most commonly affected are:
    a. Radial and ulnar
    b. Median and sciatic
    c. Radial and peroneal
    d. Ilioinguinal and sural

28. A newborn present with congestive heart failure. On examination has bulging anterior fontanelle with a bruit on auscultation. Trans-fontanellar USG shows a hypoechoic midline mass with dilated lateral ventricles. Most likely diagnosis:
    a. Medulloblastoma
    b. Encephalocele
    c. Vein of Galen malformation
    d. Arachnoid cyst

29. Cells from the neural crest are involved in all *except:*
    a. Hirschsprung's disease
    b. Neuroblastoma
    c. Primitive neuroectodermal tumour
    d. Wilms' tumour

30. Commonest site of meningocele is:
    a. Lumbosacral
    b. Occipital
    c. Frontal
    d. Thoracic

31. Transtentorial uncal herniation causes all *except:*
    a. Ipsilateral dilated pupils
    b. Ipsilateral hemiplegia
    c. Cheyne stokes respiration
    d. Decorticate rigidity

32. A patient presents with unilateral painful ophthalmoplegia. Imaging revealed an enlargement of cavernous sinus on the affected side. The likely diagnosis is:
    a. Gradenigo syndrome
    b. Cavernous sinus thrombosis
    c. Tolosa-Hunt syndrome
    d. Orbital pseudotumor

Answers

16. d	17. a	18. d	19. c	20. a	21. c	22. d
23. d	24. d	25. a	26. a	27. b	28. c	29. d
30. a	31. d	32. c				

33. All of the following statements about Diffuse Axonal Injury (DAI) are true *except:*
    a. Caused by shearing force
    b. Predominant white matter hemorrhages, in basal ganglion and corpus callosum
    c. Increased intracranial tension is seen in all cases
    d. Most common at junction of grey and white matter

34. The nerve of Kuntz is an important landmark in:
    a. Lumbar sympathectomy
    b. Cervicodorsal sympathectomy
    c. Obturator neurectomy
    d. Splanchnicectomy

35. Enlargement of pituitary tumour after adrenalectomy is called as:
    a. Nelson syndrome
    b. Steel-Richardson syndrome
    c. Hamman-Rich syndrome
    d. Job's syndrome

36. Highly vascular tumor of brain and spinal cord in adults:
    a. Metastasis
    b. Pilocytic astrocytoma
    c. Hemangioblastoma
    d. Cavernous malformation

37. A 55-year-old female presents with grade I. Ependymoma extending from C7-T1 with no neural defect. Surgery is done next management is:
    a. Post-op chemotherapy
    b. Post-op chemoradiation
    c. Imaging, regular follow up, chemotherapy if required
    d. Imaging, regular follow up, radiotherapy if required

38. All of the following lower intracranial pressure *except:*
    a. Mannitol
    b. Furosemide
    c. Corticosteroids
    d. Hyperventilation

39. Not true regarding Dandy-Walker cyst:
    a. Cerebellar vermis hypoplasia
    b. Hydrocephalus
    c. Arachnoid cyst
    d. Posterior fossa cyst

40. In Balint's syndrome there is:
    a. Oculomotor apraxia
    b. Optic ataxia
    c. Results from b/l dorsal parietal lesions
    d. All of the above

41. About Prolactin levels after seizures:
    a. Repetitive seizures are associated with progressively smaller serum prolactin level elevation
    b. No rise following absence seizures
    c. Greater than two fold serum prolactin level elevation consistently follow seizures that produce intense widespread high frequency mesial temporal lobe discharges
    d. All of the above

42. Which of the following antiepileptic drug level increases during pregnancy:
    a. Carbamazepine
    b. Phenobarbitol
    c. Phenytoin
    d. Valproic acid

43. Which of the following AED leads to withdrawal seizures even Status and has to be withdrawn over 3-6 months?
    a. Phenytoin
    b. Clonazepam
    c. Phenobarbitone
    d. Valproic acid

44. All of the following are true following head injury *except:*
    a. Decreased glutamine intracellularly
    b. Decreased adenosin
    c. Increased intracellular Ca^{2+}
    d. Increased extracellular K^+

45. A patient is having diffuse axonal injury, histologically there are axonal swelling (retraction ball) in cerebral white matter, corpus callosum, dorsolateral quadrant upper brainstem and superior cerebellar peduncle and a focal lesion in the corpus callosum. He is having:
    a. Grade I DAI
    b. Grade II DAI
    c. Grade III DAI
    d. None of the above

46. Chromosomal alteration associated with Medulloblastoma is:
    a. 17 q
    b. 6 q
    c. 16 q
    d. 1 p

47. About olfaction and gustation:
    a. There are four types of primary taste
    b. Alphas Gustducin is related to salty and sour taste
    c. Conscious perception of smell take place in Pyriform cortex
    d. Entorhinal cortex (area 28) is the association olfactory cortex

48. Normal position of optic chiasma is:
    a. Sulcus chiasmaticus
    b. Diaphgram sellae
    c. Dorsum sellae
    d. Posterior to dorsum sellae

49. According to Collins law, the risk of recurrence of tumor for a patient presented at an age of 2 years with Medulloblastoma is within:
    a. 32 months
    b. 33 months
    c. 34 months
    d. 35 months

50. Brain tumor responsible for highest risk of DVT and pulmonary embolism include:
    a. Meningioma
    b. Malignant glioma
    c. Metastasis
    d. Medulloblastoma

Answers

33. c	34. b	35. a	36. c	37. d	38. b	39. c
40. d	41. d	42. d	43. b	44. b	45. b	46. c
47. d	48. c	49. b	50. a			

Neuroradiology

Neuroradiologic examinations of the brain consisted primarily of plain films of the skull, cerebral arteriography, pneumoencephalography, and conventional nuclear medicine studies until in 1974, Computed tomography (CT) revolutionized the radiologic workup of central nervous system abnormalities allowing normal and abnormal structures could be directly visualized with minimal risk to the patient.

Recent technologic advances in radiology include the development of new pulse sequences such as MR angiography (MRA), MR spectroscopy (MRS), diffusion-weighted (DW) and perfusion-weighted (PW) MR imaging, and functional MR imaging (fMRI).

Recent advances in nuclear medicine functional imaging techniques, including single photon emission computed tomography (SPECT) and positron emission tomography (PET).

TECHNIQUES IN NEURORADIOLOGY

- Anatomic modalities—Provide information mostly of a structural nature, include plain films of the skull, computed tomography, magnetic resonance imaging, cerebral arteriography, and ultrasonography
- Functional modalities—include SPECT and PET imaging, CTP, DW and PW MR imaging, fMRI, and MRS are primarily functional modalities, which give information about brain perfusion or metabolism
- Both—Cerebral arteriography and ultrasonography of the carotid bifurcation provide both anatomic and functional information.

PLAIN RADIOGRAPHS

- Obtained by placing a patient's head between an X-ray source and a recording device. Bones of the skull can block a large number of X-rays and, therefore, cast a white "shadow" on the X-ray film. Soft tissues such as scalp or brain cast little, if any, shadow on the film.
- Multiple routine views of the skull, including frontal, lateral, and axial projections, may be needed to adequately assess the calvarium and to accurately localize a lesion.
- Skull radiograph primarily gives information about the bones of the skull, but no direct information about the intracranial contents.
- They have been largely replaced today by more sensitive techniques such as CT or MR imaging.

Different Views and Structures Best seen

- Caldwell view (occipito-frontal)—Supraorbital fissure; frontal sinus
- Water's view (occipito-mental)—Maxillary and sphenoid sinuses
- Basal view (submentovertical)—Sphenoid, posterior ethmoid sinuses; zygoma.
- Lateral skull view—Sella turcica

COMPUTED TOMOGRAPHY

Plain Studies

- Consist of computer-generated cross-sectional images obtained from a rotating X-ray beam and detector system.
- The resultant images, unlike plain films, exquisitely depict and differentiate between soft tissues, thus allowing direct visualization of intracranial contents and abnormalities associated with neurologic diseases. The contrast or brightness ("window" or "level," respectively) of these images can be adjusted to highlight particular tissues

- A head CT consists of images adjusted to emphasize soft-tissue detail (soft-tissue windows) as well as images adjusted to visualize bony detail (bone windows)
- **Appearances**
  - Cortical bone appears white (has a high attenuation value or Hounsfield unit), whereas air within the paranasal sinuses appears black (has a low attenuation value)
  - Cerebral white matter has a slightly lower Hounsfield number than does cerebral gray matter and consequently appears slightly darker than gray matter on a head CT scan
  - Intracranial pathologic conditions can be either dark (low attenuation) or bright (high attenuation), depending on the particular abnormality. For example, acute intracranial hemorrhage is typically very bright, whereas an acute cerebral infarction demonstrates low attenuation when compared to the surrounding normal brain because of the presence of edema.
- Axial images are most commonly obtained, but coronal images can be obtained with hyperextension of the patient's neck.

Contrast Studies

- CT examinations performed after intravenous administration of an iodinated contrast agent, "light up" or enhance normal blood vessels and dural sinuses, as well as intracranial structures that lack a blood–brain barrier (BBB), such as the pituitary gland, choroid plexus, or pineal gland.
- Pathologic conditions that interrupt the BBB also demonstrate enhancement after contrast material administration
- Volumetric images of intravenously injected contrast as it passes through the arterial circulation, or CT Angiogram, are routinely performed. High spatial resolution 3-D CTA images of the cervical and intracranial vasculature have been implemented into recently developed acute stroke protocol examinations. CTA accurately identifies the location and extent of large vessel occlusions, which may predict response to reperfusion therapies.
- CTA can additionally be supplemented by a more detailed, quantitative evaluation of the cerebral microvascular hemodynamics (CTP) during the early phase of bolus passage.
- CTA is also used in the screening evaluation of blunt cerebrovascular injury, including closed head injuries, seat belt abrasion (or other soft tissue injury) of the anterior neck, basilar skull fracture extending through the carotid canal, and cervical vertebral body fracture. It is an accurate technique for detecting internal carotid artery (ICA) dissections and for assessing stenoses.
- Data acquisition during the venous phase following intravenous contrast administration (CT venography) can be used to identify dural sinuses and cerebral veins, evaluate for dural venous sinus thrombosis, and distinguish partial sinus obstruction from venous occlusion in the setting of adjacent brain masses.

Advantages

- It is inexpensive, widely available, can be used in patients with MR-incompatible hardware, and allows a relatively quick assessment of intracranial contents in the setting of a neurological deficit.
- Patients are reasonably accessible for monitoring during the examination

Disadvantages

- Patients are exposed to ionizing radiation and iodine-based contrast agents
- Imaging artifacts can interfere with accurate interpretation. Ex: Streak artifacts from metallic objects like fillings, braces, surgical clips.
- Images can be severely degraded by patient motion

MAGNETIC RESONANCE IMAGING

- MRI consists of computer-reconstructed cross-sectional images. Unlike CT scans or plain radiographs, the information collected is not X-ray beam attenuation. The MR image is a visual display of nuclear magnetic resonance data collected principally from nuclei within body tissues—especially hydrogen nuclei within water and fat molecules.
- Sequences that emphasize T_1 decay are commonly referred to as T_1-weighted, images; sequences that accentuate T_2 relaxation properties are called T_2-weighted images. T_2-weighted images are usually easy to identify because fluid (e.g., cerebrospinal, globe vitreous) is very bright; fluid on a T_1-weighted scan is usually dark. Fat is bright on T_1-weighted scans, but darker on T_2-weighted images.

- The most commonly used agent for MR imaging is gadopentetate-dimeglumine or Gd-DTPA [Gadolinium], which is very well tolerated and extremely safe. Its major use in the central nervous system (CNS) is to improve lesion detectability by "lighting up" pathologic conditions that either lack a BBB or have a disrupted BBB.

Applications

- MR Angiogram has proven to be a useful tool for evaluation of the cervical or intracranial carotid vasculature. These methods permit distinction between blood flow and adjacent soft tissue, with or without administration of intravenous contrast. MRA serves as one of the first-line studies for evaluation of arterial occlusive disease and for screening of intracranial aneurysms.
- Perfusion MR imaging measures cerebral blood flow (CBF) at the capillary level of an organ or tissue region. Perfusion-weighted MR imaging has applications in the evaluation of cerebral ischemia and reperfusion, brain tumors, epilepsy, and blood flow deficits in Alzheimer's disease.
- Functional MR imaging is an important brain mapping technique that uses fast imaging techniques to depict regional cortical blood flow changes in space and time during performance of a particular task. The utilization of this technique to localize brain activity is based on measurable increases in cerebral blood flow (and blood volume) with increased neural activity, referred to as *neurovascular coupling*. fMRI techniques are considered an indirect approach to imaging brain function and provide excellent spatial resolution and can be precisely matched with anatomic structures. Changes in blood oxygenation and perfusion can also be imaged. fMRI is applied in presurgical mapping. Ex: in a patient with complex partial seizures, prior to undergoing temporal lobectomy.
- MR spectroscopy provides qualitative and quantitative information about brain metabolism and tissue composition. This functional analysis is based on detecting variations in the precession frequencies of spinning protons in a magnetic field. MRS complements the conventional MR imaging study and is commonly applied in the pre- and post-treatment evaluation of brain tumors, with MRS playing an important role in assessing for residual or recurrent tumor following surgical resection.

Advantages

- Soft-tissue contrast resolution is superior to that of CT, and lesions that may be subtle or invisible on CT are frequently obvious on MR imaging.
- MRI also allows acquisition of multiplanar views in the sagittal, axial, coronal, and oblique projections that may be impossible to obtain with CT
- MRI gives information about blood flow without the need for a contrast agent, and bony streak artifacts that obscure lesions of the brain stem and cerebellum on CT scans are not present on MR images.
- It does not expose the patient to ionizing radiation.

Intensities in Different Modalities			
Tissue	*CT*	*MRI T1 Signal*	*MRI T2 Signal*
Brain	Gray	Gray	Gray
Air	Black	Black	Black
CSF	Black	Black	White
Fat	Black	White	Black
Bone	Very white	Black	Black
Blood	White	White	Black
Inflammation	Contrast enhancing	Gray, gadolinium enhancing	White
Tumor	Gray or white and contrast enhancing	Gray or white and gadolinium enhancing	White

CEREBRAL ARTERIOGRAPHY

- Involves the injection of water-soluble contrast material into a carotid or vertebral artery. Contrast material is injected into the desired vessel via a small catheter, which has been introduced into the body through the femoral or brachial artery
- It is the gold standard for assessing vascular stenosis and atherosclerosis or vasculitis, and it is indispensable in identifying and evaluating cerebral aneurysms and certain intracranial vascular malformations or fistulae. It is useful in assessing carotid or vertebral artery integrity after trauma to the neck, especially in the setting of acute neurologic deficit.

Disadvantages

- Cerebral arteriograms are expensive (two to three times as much as MR examinations).
- The major risk of the procedure is stroke, which occurs either from an embolic event (e.g., inadvertent injection of air, thrombus formation on catheter tip, atherosclerotic plaque dislodged by catheter manipulation) or from catheter-related local vessel trauma.

ULTRASONOGRAPHY

- Major applications of ultrasonography in CNS disease include gray-scale imaging and Doppler evaluation of carotid artery patency and flow in the setting of atherosclerosis, assessment of vasospasm in the setting of subarachnoid hemorrhage using transcranial Doppler, screening evaluation of intracranial abnormalities in the newborn and young infant
- Also used intraoperatively to demonstrate the spinal cord and surrounding structures during spine surgery and to define tumor and cyst margins during craniotomies.
- Transcranial Doppler is a recently developed tool in the evaluation of cerebrovascular disorders. It uses low-frequency sound waves to adequately penetrate the skull, and produces spectral waveforms of the major intracranial vessels for evaluation of flow velocity, direction, amplitude, and pulsatility. Present clinical applications include diagnosis of cerebral vasospasm, evaluation of stroke and transient ischemic attack, detection of intracranial emboli, serial monitoring of vasculitis in children with sickle cell disease, and assessment of intracranial pressure and cerebral blood flow changes in patients with head injury or mass lesions.

SINGLE PHOTON EMISSION COMPUTED TOMOGRAPHY (SPECT)

- SPECT uses a rotating gamma camera to reconstruct cross-sectional images of the distribution of a radioactive pharmaceutical that has been administered to a patient (usually intravenously). For brain imaging, radioactive iodine (^{123}I) or technetium (^{99m}Tc) is combined with a compound that rapidly crosses the BBB and localizes within brain tissue (HMPAO) in proportion to regional blood flow.
- The rotating gamma camera detects gamma rays emitted by the radiopharmaceutical and produces cross-sectional images of the brain that are really a map of brain perfusion
- It gives indirect information about brain metabolism, because perfusion is usually highest to parts of the brain with high metabolic activity and lowest to areas with low metabolic demand

Disadvantages

- SPECT studies are moderately expensive and they provide limited anatomic information.
- SPECT also exposes patients to ionizing radiation.

POSITRON EMISSION TOMOGRAPHY (PET)

- PET scans consist of computer-generated cross-sectional images of the distribution and local concentration of a radiopharmaceutical similar to SPECT imaging. The main difference is that PET studies use radiopharmaceuticals labeled with a cyclotron-produced positron emitter.
- The most widely used radiotracer is ^{18}F-deoxyglucose. PET scanning with this agent gives a measurement of brain glucose metabolism. Other agents are useful in assessing regional cerebral blood flow and neuroreceptor function.
- Areas of high metabolic activity (i.e., cerebral cortex, deep gray nuclei) demonstrate greater radiopharmaceutical uptake than do areas of low metabolic activity, such as white matter or cerebrospinal fluid, the bones of the skull and scalp soft tissues being invisible.

Advantages

It is extremely versatile, providing *in vivo* information about brain perfusion, glucose metabolism, receptor density, and, ultimately, brain function

Disadvantages

- PET scans are very expensive, due to the high cost of operating the PET facility, which requires an on-site cyclotron for radiotracer production.
- Patients undergoing PET examinations are exposed to ionizing radiation.
- Anatomic resolution is not as good as with CT or MR imaging.

CLINICAL APPLICATIONS IN NEURORADIOLOGY

DIAGNOSTIC FEATURES AND SPECIFIC SIGNS

Tumors

- **Craniopharyngioma:**
  - On CT and X-ray—Suprasellar calcification with cystic lesion; On MRI–Mixed cystic and solid suprasellar mass.
  - Signs of Raised ICT seen.
- **Ependymoma:** On CT—Isodense to slightly hypodense with calcification; mild to moderate in homogenous enhancement
- **Meningioma:**
  - On Plain X-ray—ball like amorphous calcification in the parasagittal site; bony hyperostosis with increased meningeal vascular markings
  - Hyperdense on non-contrast CT; with calcification
  - Subarachnoid space widened on the side of lesion as seen in myelography
  - Isointense with the cord on both T1 and T2 weighed images; Homogenous enhancement on contrast; *Dural tail sign.* MRI with contrast is the investigation of choice.
- **Common neoplasms showing calcification**
  - Craniopharyngioma
  - Meningioma
  - Ependymoma
  - Choroid plexus papilloma
  - Pinealoma
  - Chordoma
  - Medulloblastoma

Choroid plexus and Pineal gland are the most common physiological causes of intracranial calcification in a skull X-ray.

HYDROCEPHALUS

Investigation of choice in infants is Ultrasonography. In older patients CT and MRI are preferred. NPH seen in elderly is best diagnosed by MRI.

CT scan findings in non-communicating hydrocephalus may include sulci effacement, transependymal spread of CSF, and dilation of all the ventricles proximal to the level of blockage. The entire ventricular system, including the 4th ventricle, is dilated in communicating hydrocephalus.

- **Signs of Raised ICT**
  - In children—Suture diastasis is the hallmark Increased convolutional markings or copper beating of the skull vault; sellar erosion.
  - In adults—Thinning or erosion of the dorsal sellae is the hallmark, starting as slight porosis of anterior cortex of dorsum and floor of sella; pineal displacement.

	Cerebrovascular Accidents	
	CT	*MRI*
Diffuse axonal injury	Multiple small petechial haemorrhages <2 cm diameter in the cerebral hemisphere	Multiple small face of decreased signal intensity of T!WI with increased signal on T2WI
Cerebral contusion	Early—Patchy ill-defined low density lesion mixed with small hyperdense foci of petechial haemorrhages Late—Delayed hemorrhage with increased mass effect; enhances with contrast	On T2WI–decreased intensity surrounded by hyperdense edema
Subdural hemorrhage	Crescentic extra-axial hematomas crossing the suture lines	
Multiple infarcts	Cortical and subcortical infarcts with large ventricles and cortical sulci; white matter lucencies.	

DISORDERS OF THE CNS

Disorders of the White Matter

- **Dysmyelinating**
  - *Adrenoleukodystrophy*—X-linked recessive trait, Involvement of the parieto-occipital regions and thin serrated or curvilinear rim of contrast enhancement. Posterior central white matter show low attenuation on CT, low signal on T1WI and high signal on T2WI MRI
  - *Pelizaeus-Merzbacher disease*—X-linked recessive, Severe hypomyelination on T2WI compared to T1
  - *Alexanders disease*—Presentation in the first year with developmental delay, macrocephaly, spasticity and seizures, large cystic components in the frontal and temporal regions; contrast enhancement along the ventricular ependyma, periventricular area and caudate nucleus.
  - *Krabbe's disease*—galactosylceramide β-galactosidase deficiency, AR, presentation in the first 6 months of life with death in early childhood. Symmetrical abnormalities in the posterior white matter of the optic radiations, centrum semiovale, thalami and caudate nuclei are seen. Increased density in the thalamus and basal ganglia; hypodensity of the white matter. Hypointense in T2WI with cavitatory changes adjacent to the frontal horns.
  - *Metachromatic leukodystrophy*—Due to arylsulphatase-A deficiency, AR, usually presents at 2-3 years, is rapidly progressive. Diffuse symmetrical abnormalities with sparing of the subcortical arcuate fibres and cerebellar lesions may be present. Hypodense in deep and peripheral supratentorial white matter in CT; Low density in T2WI

- **Demyelinating**
  - Multiple sclerosis—MRI is the investigation of choice showing either 4 lesions involving the white matter or 3 lesions in the periventricular region. Typical lesions are hyperintense ovoid lesions on T2WI. Lesions of the corpus callosum are best seen in FLAIR.
  - Schilders disease—Lesions extending through the corpus callosum into both parieto-occipital regions
  - Central pontine myelinosis—Low density of the pontine white matter on CT; increase in density in T1WI and T2WI MRI.

- **Others**
  - Canavan's disease—AR, manifests in the first few months of life; progressive increase in head size, hypotonia, seizures, progressing to spasticity and death by 2 years of age. Bilaterally symmetrical changes are seen, most severe in the subcortical white matter and globus pallidus with relative sparing of the brainstem and internal capsule.

Disorders of Neuronal Migration

- Agyria-pachygyria—Poorly formed gyri and sulci, the former being more severe.
  - *Type I lissencephaly*—Small brain with few gyri; smooth, thickened four-layer cortex resembling that of a 13-week fetus with diminished white matter and shallow vertical sylvian fissures ('figure-of-eight' appearance on axial images). Agenesis of the corpus callosum is seen.
  - *Type II lissencephaly (Walker-Warburg syndrome)*—Smooth cortex, cerebellar hypoplasia and vermian aplasia and hydrocephalus due to cisternal obstruction by abnormal meninges or aqueduct stenosis.
- *Polymicrogyria*—The neurons reach the cortex but are distributed abnormally. Macroscopically the surface of the brain appears as multiple small bumps. The cortex is isointense to grey matter. Polymicrogyrias may be present in the vicinity of a porencephalic cyst, be associated with heterotopic grey matter or agenesis of the corpus callosum.
- *Schizencephaly*—clefts which extend through the full thickness of the cerebral mantle from ventricle to subarachnoid space. The cleft is lined by heterotopic grey matter and microgyrias.
- *Heterotopic grey matter*—collections of neurons in a subependymal location, i.e. at the site of the germinal matrix or arrested within the white matter on their way to the cortex. Isointense to normal grey matter.
- *Cortical dysplasia*—Focal disorganization of the cerebral cortex. A single enlarged gyrus resembling focal pachygyria may be seen.

HIGH SIGNAL ON T1W MRI

Normal
- *Posterior lobe of pituitary*—The pituitary gland is uniformly high signal up to 6 months.
- *Moving structures*—Flow-related 'enhancement'.
- Ossification of the falx.
- Calcification within the basal ganglia.
- Rathke's cleft cyst.
- Fat.

Pathological
- *Haemorrhage*—Methaemoglobin in 'subacute' hematomas causes markedly increased T1W signal.
- Thrombus
- *Fat*—lipoma of the corpus callosum, perimesencephalic and chiasmatic cisterns.
- Proteinaceous fluid – e.g., craniopharyngioma, colloid cyst.
- Melanin—melanoma, neurocutaneous melanosis.
- Heavy metals – e.g., manganese in total parenteral nutrition and Wilson's disease.

SIGNAL VOID ON T2W MRI

Normal
- Normal arterial and venous flow
- Densely packed bone
- Dural calcification
- Air
- CSF flow.

Pathological
- Aneurysms
- Arteriovenous malformations
- Acute/Chronic haemorrhage

Amyotrophic Lateral Sclerosis
Axial T2WI through the lateral ventricle reveals abnormal high signal intensity within the corticospinal tracts.

Leigh's Disease
- Bilateral symmetrical signal change within brainstem, deep cerebellar gray matter, subthalamic ganglia; hyperintense on T2WI.
- Panda face—Midbrain changes with involvement of substantia nigra and tegmentum

Basal Ganglia Calcification
- Endocrinal—Hypoparathyroidism and pseudohypoparathyroidism; secondary hyperparathyroidism
- Toxic—Hypoxia
- Infection—TORCH; HIV
- Metabolic–Fahr's disease
- Vascular malformation—Mineralizing microangiopathy
- Chemotherapy/Radiotherapy
- Tumors.

Conditions Causing Ring Enhancement on Contrast CT
- Toxoplasmosis
- Tuberculoma
- Cysticercosis
- Craniopharyngioma.

CONGENITAL SYNDROMES ASSOCIATED WITH ENLARGED VENTRICLES

- Achondroplasia.
- X-linked hydrocephalus syndrome.
- Soto's syndrome—Cerebral gigantism, Advanced skeletal maturity.
- Acrocephalosyndactyly—Types Apert and Pfeiffer.
- Crouzon's syndrome
- Fetal alcohol syndrome
- Lissencephaly
- Osteopetrosis.

SOLITARY INTRACEREBRAL MASS

- Glioblastoma multiforme
- Metastasis
- Arterial infarct
- Abscess
- Demyelination
- Haematoma
- Encephalitis
- Aneurysm.

Stroke

- Ischemic—On CT scans, this entity may have a normal appearance for the first 12 hours. The first manifestations of an infarct are subtle and include a white clot in one of the vessels, loss of normal gray-white differentiation, and sulcal flattening *(effacement)*. Thereafter, the appearance often progresses to a wedge-shaped dark area, extending to the edge of the brain, involving both the gray and white matter.
- Hemorrhagic—On CT scan, this entity appears as an abnormal area of bright blood within the brain tissue.

Space Occupying Lesions

- Subfalcine herniation—On the film, when the septum pellucidum is bowed to one side because of mass effect.
- Uncal herniation—On CT scan, the star *(suprasellar cistern)* may be deformed. In addition, the brainstem is pushed away by the mass
- Tonsilar herniation—This entity is difficult to visualize on CT scan. It occurs when the cerebellar tonsils slip through the foramen magnum out of the skull.

INTERVENTIONAL NEURORADIOLOGY

Many different procedures are performed for the evaluation and treatment of intracranial and extracranial disease. These include principally attempts to obliterate aneurysms or to devascularize tumors and AVMs using balloons, coils, or glue. Stenting of extracranial carotid disease is occasionally performed. Vasospasm can be treated by selective intra-arterial instillation of papaverine or more commonly by balloon dilation.

Multiple Choice Questions

1. Presence of calcification on an intracranial lesion is best made out by:
   a. CT
   b. MRI
   c. Ultrasound
   d. Contrast study

2. Radiological findings in Meningioma are all *except:*
   a. Calcification
   b. Vascular markings
   c. Osteosclerosis
   d. None of the above

3. Hydrocephalus in children, first seen on X-ray:
   a. Large head
   b. Sutural diastasis
   c. Thinned out vault
   d. Post clinoid erosion

4. Most serious complication of myelogram is:
   a. Allergy
   b. Headache
   c. Arachnoiditis
   d. Transient neurological deficit

5. Extradural haematoma CT scan finding is:
   a. Hypodense biconvex lesion
   b. Hyperdense biconvex lesion
   c. Low attenuated biconvex lesion
   d. Concavo convex hyperdense lesion

6. First investigation of choice for spinal cord tumor:
   a. CT scan
   b. MRI
   c. Plain X-ray
   d. Myelography

7. For Traumatic paraplegia investigation of choice is:
   a. MRI
   b. USG
   c. X-ray
   d. CT scan

8. In case of subarachnoid haemorrhage investigation of choice is:
   a. MRI
   b. CT scan
   c. Carotid angiogram
   d. MRI angio with MRI imaging

9. Calcification in basal ganglia is seen in:
   a. Hypopituitarism
   b. Hypothyroidism
   c. Hypoparathyroidism
   d. Hypoaldosteronism

10. Which of the following is best test for screening a case of proximal internal carotid artery stenosis:
    a. CT angiogram.
    b. Digital subtraction angiography
    c. Magnetic resonance angiography
    d. Colour Doppler ultrasonography

11. Investigation of choice for Multiple sclerosis is:
    a. MRI
    b. EEG
    c. X-ray
    d. CT scan

12. On CT scan, all are seen as hypodense area *except:*
    a. Glioblastoma
    b. Cerebral infarct
    c. Cerebral edema
    d. Cerebral haemorrhage

13. Bracket calcification in skull X-ray is seen in:
    a. Meningioma
    b. Sturge-Weber syndrome
    c. Tuberous sclerosis
    d. Corpus callosum lipoma

14. All of the following calcify, *except:*
    a. Oligodendroglioma
    b. Medulloblastoma
    c. Meningioma
    d. Ependymoma

Answers

| 1. a | 2. d | 3. b | 4. c | 5. b | 6. b | 7. a |
| 8. b | 9. c | 10. d | 11. a | 12. d | 13. d | 14. None > b |

15. Which of the following is the best choice to evaluate radiologically a posterior fossa tumour?
    a. MRI
    b. CT scan
    c. Angiography
    d. Myelography

16. Which view is used to visualize the foramina of the skull?
    a. AP view
    b. Lateral view
    c. Towne's view
    d. Base of skull view

17. Best view for evaluating sella turcica is:
    a. Lateral X-ray skull
    b. AP X-ray skull
    c. Towne's view
    d. Open mouth

18. Which of the following is wrong regarding "J Shaped sella"?
    a. Normal variant in 30% of cases
    b. Seen in optic glioma
    c. Mucopolysaccharidoses
    d. Low grade hydrocephalus

19. X-rays skull characteristically shows "hair on end" appearance in one of the following disease:
    a. Still's disease
    b. Scurvy
    c. Thalassemia major
    d. Cirrhosis of liver

20. Punched out lesions in skull X-ray is seen in:
    a. Multiple myeloma
    b. Sickle cell anemia
    c. Thalassemia
    d. Acute leukaemia

21. Punched out translucencies in the skull does not occur in one of the conditions given below:
    a. Multiple myeloma
    b. Metastatic deposits
    c. Leukaemia
    d. Fluorosis

22. Craniopharyngioma arises from:
    a. Rathke's pouch
    b. First branchial arch
    c. Tuber cinereum
    d. Pituitary

23. Optic foramen enlargement on X-ray skull is suggestive of:
    a. Meningioma
    b. Retinoblastoma
    c. Optic nerve glioma
    d. Carotico-cavernous fistula

24. 'Bare Orbit' appearance of skull is seen in:
    a. Multiple myeloma
    b. Meningioma
    c. Neurofibromatosis
    d. Craniopharyngioma

25. Geographic lytic lesion in vault of skull with bevelled edges:
    a. Multiple myeloma
    b. Eosinophilic granuloma
    c. Hyperparathyroidism
    d. Paget's disease

26. In Haemolytic anaemia, patient's skull bones show characteristic feature of:
    a. Erosion of cortex
    b. Thickening of outer table of skull
    c. Narrow diploic space
    d. Widened diploic space

27. On X-ray skull "Intracranial calcification", which may be due to:
    a. Cysticercosis
    b. Pineal calcification
    c. Dural calcification
    d. All of the above

28. Which of the normal calcifications may be considered abnormal and suggestive of Pseudohypoparathyroidism:
    a. Choroid plexuses
    b. Basal ganglia
    c. Pineal gland
    d. Petroclinoid ligament

29. Procedure of choice in diagnosing empty sella syndrome is:
    a. Pneumoencephalography
    b. Caldwell X-ray view
    c. CT scan
    d. MRI

30. Commonest calcified brain tumour is:
    a. Craniopharyngioma
    b. Meningioma
    c. Tuberculoma
    d. Medulloblastoma

31. Alzheimer's disease is associated with:
    a. Atrophy of frontal and temporal poles of brain
    b. Atrophy of parietal and temporal lobes of brain
    c. Transient episodes of hemiplegia
    d. Hemianesthesia

32. Which of the normal calcifications may be considered abnormal and suggestive of Pseudohypoparathyroidism?
    a. Choroid plexuses
    b. Basal ganglia
    c. Pineal gland
    d. Petroclinoid ligament

Answers

15. a	16. d	17. a	18. a	19. c	20. a	21. d
22. a	23. c	24. c	25. b	26. d	27. d	28. b
29. d	30. a	31. b	32. b			

33. On usual CT scale of densities (– to +), brain tissue measures:
    a. –10 to +10
    b. 0 to 20
    c. +10 to 30
    d. +20 to +45
    e. +50 to +100

34. CT scan of a 60-year-old male who had a fall presenting with confusion is most likely to reveal:
    a. Cerebral atrophy
    b. Glioma
    c. Normal pressure hydrocephalus
    d. Subdural haematoma

35. CT scan will reveal all *except*:
    a. Cerebral tumours
    b. Cerebral hemorrhages
    c. Cerebral atrophy
    d. Grey and a white matter differentiation

36. Procedure of choice in diagnosing empty sella syndrome:
    a. Pneumoencephalography
    b. Caldwell X-ray view
    c. CT scan
    d. MRI

37. 5th ventricle is:
    a. Cavum vergae
    b. Cavum septipellucidi
    c. Cavum veli interpositi
    d. Colloid cyst

38. The crescent sign on a brain scan commonly indicates a subdural haematoma. It may also be seen in:
    a. Dural metastases
    b. Pachymeningitis
    c. Both
    d. Neither

39. After acoustic neuroma, the second commonest cerebellopontine angle tumor is:
    a. Trigeminal neuroma
    b. Epidermoid tumor
    c. Glioma
    d. Medulloblastoma

40. Most common cause of suprasellar enlargement with calcification in children is:
    a. Meningioma
    b. Suprasellar tuberculid
    c. Craniopharyngioma
    d. Astrocytoma

41. A 4-year-old child may have physiologic intracranial calcification of:
    a. Pineal gland
    b. Habenular commissure
    c. Choroid plexus
    d. Petroclinoid ligament

42. The metastatic lesions may be present as subarachnoid haemorrhage:
    a. Seminoma
    b. Lymphoma
    c. Malignant melanoma
    d. Ovarian cystadenoma

43. The commonest cause of intracerebral calcified shadow found in skull X-ray is:
    a. Astrocytoma
    b. Glioma
    c. Pituitary adenoma
    d. Oligodendroglioma

44. Presence of calcification in an intracranial lesion is best made out by:
    a. Contrast study
    b. Ultrasound
    c. CT scan
    d. MRI

45. Best investigation for spontaneous subarachnoid haemorrhage is:
    a. CT scan
    b. Angiography
    c. Pneumoencephalogram
    d. Ultrasound

46. Investigation done in cerebral and cerebellar abscess is:
    a. MRI
    b. CT
    c. L.P.
    d. Angiography

47. Commonest cause of intracranial calcification in a childs:
    a. Craniopharyngioma
    b. Medulloblastoma
    c. Meningioma
    d. Ependymoma

48. Subdural haemorrhage is common because of rupture of:
    a. Middle cerebral artery
    b. Anterior cerebral artery
    c. Posterior cerebral artery
    d. Dural sinuses

49. Which investigation is not done in a brain abscess?
    a. L.P.
    b. CT scan
    c. Blood culture
    d. X-ray chest

50. Diagnostic procedure of choice in brain tumour is:
    a. X-ray skull
    b. Computerized axial tomography scan
    c. Radionuclide study
    d. MRI

Answers

33. d	34. d	35. d	36. d	37. b	38. c	39. b
40. c	41. c	42. c	43. d	44. c	45. a	46. a
47. a	48. d	49. a	50. d			

51. **The most common cerebello-pontine angle tumour is:**
    a. Acoustic neuroma
    b. Cholesteatoma
    c. Meningioma
    d. All of the above

52. **Calcification is most frequently seen in:**
    a. Astrocytoma
    b. Ependymoma
    c. Medulloblastoma
    d. Oligodendroglioma

53. **Intracranial calcification is characteristic of:**
    a. Sturge-Weber syndrome
    b. Steven-Johnson syndrome
    c. Papillou-Letre syndrome
    d. Hallermann-Streiff syndrome

54. **Pneumocephalus is seen in:**
    a. Laceration of brain
    b. Occipital bone fracture
    c. Frontal bone fracture
    d. Gun-shot injuries

55. **Most useful investigation in head injury is:**
    a. X-ray lateral view
    b. Angiogram
    c. Ventriculography
    d. CT scan

56. **Fresh blood in CT scan appears as:**
    a. Hyperdense
    b. Isodense
    c. Hypodense
    d. Any of the above

57. **Ideal modality to diagnose hydrocephalus in a one month baby is:**
    a. Plain X-ray
    b. Ultrasound
    c. CT scan
    d. MRI

58. **Which is the most sensitive investigation for detecting secondary bony deposits at base of skull?**
    a. MRI
    b. CT scan
    c. Radionuclide scan
    d. X-ray skull

59. **An X-ray of the skull of an eight year old child presenting with growth failure, progressive visual loss and papilloedema showed suprasellar calcification. The most likely diagnosis is:**
    a. Craniopharyngioma
    b. Toxoplasmosis
    c. Cytomegalovirus disease
    d. Sturge-Weber syndrome

Answers

51. a	52. d	53. a	54. c	55. d	56. a	57. b
58. a	59. a					

Psychiatry

PERSONALITY DISORDERS

- Common and chronic disorders occurring in 10–20% of the general population and over 50% of patients with psychiatric illnesses
- Personality disorder symptoms are **ego-syntonic** (acceptable to the ego) and **alloplastic** (adapt by trying to alter the environment than themselves) hence patients mostly deny their problems, refuse psychiatric help, often seem disinterested in treatment and are impervious to recovery.

Defined by DSM-5 as

- An enduring pattern of behavior and inner experiences that deviates significantly from the individuals cultural standard
- Is rigidly pervasive
- Has an onset in adolescence or early childhood
- Is stable through time
- Leads to unhappiness and impairment
- Manifests in at least two of the following four areas:
  - Cognition
  - Affectivity
  - Interpersonal function
  - Impulse control

Subtypes **classified** in DSM-5

Cluster A

Disorders with odd/aloof features
- Schizotypal
- Schizoid
- Paranoid

Cluster B

Disorders with dramatic, impulsive, erratic features
- Narcissistic
- Borderline
- Antisocial
- Histrionic

Cluster C

Disorders sharing anxious and fearful features
- Obsessive-compulsive
- Dependent
- Avoidant.

ETIOLOGY

- **Genetic factors:**
  - Cluster A disorders are more common in the biological relatives of patients with schizophrenia and more relatives with schizotypal personality disorder occur in the family histories of persons with schizophrenia
  - Cluster B disorders:
    - Antisocial personality disorder is associated with alcohol use disorders.
    - Depression is more common in the family backgrounds of patients with borderline personality disorder
    - Persons with borderline personality disorder often have a mood disorder
    - A strong association is found between histrionic personality disorder and somatization disorder
  - Cluster C:
    - Patients with avoidant personality disorder often have high anxiety levels
    - Patients with obsessive-compulsive disorders show signs associated with depression such as shortened REM latency and abnormal dexamethasone suppression test results.
- **Biological factors:**
  - High levels of testosterone, 17-estradiol and estrone are seen in persons who exhibit impulsive traits
  - Low platelet MAO levels is found to be associated with increased sociability; also sometimes with schizotypal personalities
  - Smooth pursuit eye movements are saccadic in introverted people with low self-esteem, who tend to withdraw, and those who have schizotypal personality disorders
  - Levels of 5-hydroxyindoleaceticacid (5-HIAA), a metabolite of serotonin, is found to be low in persons who attempt suicide and in patients who are impulsive and aggressive.

Table 9.1: Personality disorders

Sl. no	Type	Epidemiology	Characteristics (DSM-5 criteria)	Treatment: Psychotherapy	Treatment: Pharmacology
1.	Paranoid personality disorder	• 2–4% of general population • More commonly diagnosed in men • Relatives of patients with schizophrenia show higher level of incidence • Specific familial relationship with delusional disorder persecutory type	• A pervasive distrust and suspiciousness of others interpreting all their motives as malevolent; beginning in early adulthood • Persistently bears grudges, perceives attacks on their character and is quick to react • Preoccupied with unjustified doubts on the loyalty of friends and the fidelity of spouse, reluctant to confide in others because of unwarranted fear that the information will be used against them • Refuse responsibility for their own feelings and assign responsibility to others • Hostile, irritable, angry, humorless and serious	• Treatment of choice • Individual psychotherapy requires professional style and not excessive warmth or overzealous use of interpretation which increases patients mistrust significantly • They do not do well in group therapy and cannot handle the over intrusiveness of behavior therapy	• Useful in dealing with anxiety and agitation • Diazepam can be used as an anti-anxiety drug • Haloperidol may be used in small doses for brief periods to manage severe agitation or quasi-delusional thinking • Antipsychotic drug pimozide is said to reduce paranoid ideation
2.	Schizoid personality disorder	• May affect 5% of general population • 2:1 male:female ratio • Gravitate towards solitary jobs requiring little contact with others and prefer night jobs	• Detachment from social relationships and a restricted range of emotions in interpersonal settings beginning in early adulthood • Neither desires nor enjoys close relationships including being part of family • Has little interest in sexual pleasures, lacks close friends and appears indifferent to praise or criticism of others • Shows emotional coldness, detachment or flattened affectivity • Quiet, distant, aloof, seclusive, unsociable	• Patients tend towards introspection • Become devoted, if distant, patients • In group therapy, they should be protected against aggressive attack by group members for their proclivity to remain silent	• Serotonergic agents may make patients less sensitive to rejection • Benzodiazepines may help to diminish interpersonal anxiety

Contd...

Contd...

Sl. no	Type	Epidemiology	Characteristics (DSM-5 criteria)	Treatment: Psychotherapy	Treatment: Pharmacology
3.	Schizotypal personality disorder	• Occurs in 3% of general population • May be slightly more in males • Frequently diagnosed in females with fragile x syndrome • Increased prevalence was found in families of schizophrenic patients	• Social and interpersonal deficits acute discomfort and reduced capacity for close relationships and eccentricities of behavior such as • Ideas of reference • Odd beliefs and magical thinking (belief in clairvoyance, sixth sense, telepathy, bizarre fantasies) • Unusual perceptions including bodily illusions • Odd thinking or speech • Suspiciousness or paranoid ideation • Inappropriate or constricted affect • Behavior or appearance that is odd • Lack of close friends or relatives	• Patients have peculiar patterns of thinking and some are involved in cults, strange religious practices and the occult. Therapists must deal with them sensitively and must not ridicule or be judgmental of such activities	• Antipsychotic medication is used to deal; with ideas of reference, illusions and other symptoms; can be used in conjunction with psychotherapy • Antidepressants are useful when a depressive component of the personality is present

4.	Antisocial personality disorder	• 12 months prevalence rates are 0.2–3% in general population
		• Increased prevalence found in:
		  – Poor urban areas
		  – Mobile residents
		  – Prison inmates
		  – Males with alcohol disorder
		  – More common in males especially those who hail from large families
		  – Onset is before the age of 15 years
		  – Familial pattern is present; 5 times more common in first degree relatives of the men with the disorder
			• Disregard for and violation of rights of others
			• Failure to conform to social norms with respect to lawful behavior; repeatedly performing acts that are ground for arrest
			• Deceitfulness, repeated lying, conning others for personal pleasure or profit
			• Impulsivity, failure to plan ahead, reckless disregard for safety of self or others
			• Irritability and aggressiveness (physical fights or assaults)
			• Consistent irresponsibility, repeated failure to sustain consistent work behavior or honor financial obligations
			• Lack of remorse; being indifferent to or rationalizing having hurt, mistreated or stolen from another
				• Patients become amenable to treatment if immobilized; when amongst peers, their lack of motivation for change disappears
				• Firm limits are essential before the start of therapy
					• Used to deal with incapacitating symptoms such as anxiety, rage and depression but must be judiciously used as most of them are substance abusers
					• Methylphenidate may be useful if they show evidence of ADHD
					• Antiepileptic drugs can be used to control impulsive behavior
					• Beta adrenergic receptor antagonists have been used to reduce aggression

5.	Borderline personality disorder	• 1-2% of the general population • Twice as common in women • Increased prevalence of major depressive disorder and substance abuse in 1st degree relatives of patients with this disorder	• Unstable, intense interpersonal relationships alternating between extremes of idealizing and devaluation • Identity disturbance • Self-destructive impulsivity in spending, sex, substance use, reckless driving or binge eating • Recurrent suicidal or self-mutilating behavior • Affective instability with chronic feelings of emptiness • Inappropriate anger difficult to control	• Difficult for patient and therapist alike • Dialectical behavior therapy is useful especially for patients with parasuicidal behavior • Mentalization behavior therapy • Transference focused psychotherapy	• Antipsychotics have been used to control anger, hostility and brief psychotic episodes • Antidepressants to improve depressed mood in patients • MAOI have successfully modulated impulsivity • Benzodiazepines especially alprazolam helps to allay anxiety and depression • Anticonvulsants and SSRIs have shown to improve global functioning in patients

Contd...

Contd...

Sl. no	Type	Epidemiology	Characteristics (DSM-5 criteria)	Treatment: Psychotherapy	Treatment: Pharmacology
6.	Histrionic personality disorder	• 1–3% of general population • 10–15% of inpatient and outpatient population in mental health institutions • More common in women • Increased association found with somatization disorder and alcohol use disorders	• Interaction with others characterized by inappropriate sexually seductive/provocative behaviors • Self-dramatization, theatrical, exaggerated expression of emotions using physical appearance to draw attention to self • Is suggestible and is uncomfortable in situations where he/she is not the center of attention • Rapidly shifting and shallow expression of emotions	• Psychoanalytic oriented psychotherapy, whether individual or group, is the treatment of choice as the individual often unaware of his/her own feelings	Adjunctive when symptoms are targeted such as • Antidepressants for depression and somatic complaints • Antipsychotics for derealization and illusions • Anti-anxiety agents for anxiety
7.	Narcissistic personality disorder	• 1–6% in community samples • Offspring of parents with the disorders have a higher risk for developing the disorder	• Preoccupied with fantasies of unlimited success, power, brilliance, beauty or ideal love • Believes he/she is special/unique and requires excessive admiration • Has sense of entitlement and is interpersonally exploitative • Lacks empathy and shows arrogant, haughty behavior attitudes • Grandiose sense of self importance and believes others are envious of him/her	• Treatment is difficult • Group therapy may be effective for patients to learn to share with others and under ideal circumstances develop an empathetic response to others	• Lithium can be used for patients with mood swings • Antidepressants can be used as patients with this disorder tolerate rejection poorly and are susceptible to depression
8.	Avoidant personality disorder	• Occurs in about 2–3% of general population	• A pervasive pattern of inadequacy and hypersensitivity to negative evaluation beginning by early adulthood • Exhibits restraint in intimate relationships for fear of being shamed • Preoccupied with being criticized in social situations • Is inhibited in new interpersonal situations and views self as inadequate, socially in adept and inferior to others • Reluctant to take personal risks or engage in new activities because they may prove embarrassing • Avoids occupational activities that involve significant personal contact because of fear of criticism, disapproval or rejection	• Group therapy may help patients understand how their sensitivity to rejection affects themselves and others • Assertiveness training may teach patients to express their needs openly and to enlarge their self-esteem	• Beta adrenergic receptor antagonists to manage autonomic system hyperactivity when patients approach feared stimulus • Serotonergic agents may help rejection sensitivity
9.	Dependent personality disorder	• 0.6% of general population • 2.5% of all personality disorders fall under this category • More common in women and persons with chronic physical illness in childhood	• Excessive need to be taken care of that leads to submissive and clinging behavior and fear of separation beginning by early adulthood • Difficulty in making everyday decisions without excessive amount of advice/reassurance from others • Difficulty in expressing disagreement with others for fear of loss of support • Feels uncomfortable when left alone and goes to excessive lengths to obtain nurturance from others • Urgently seeks another relationship as source of care when a close relationship	• Treatment is often successful • Insight oriented therapy helps patients to become more independent, assertive and self-reliant • Behavioral therapy, assertiveness training, family therapy and group therapy have all been used with successful outcomes	• Imipramine helps patients who experience panic attacks/high levels of separation anxiety • Benzodiazepines and serotonergic agents have also been useful to allay specific symptoms of anxiety and depression

Contd...

Contd...

Sl. no	Type	Epidemiology	Characteristics (DSM-5 criteria)	Treatment: Psychotherapy	Treatment: Pharmacology
10.	Obsessive-compulsive personality disorder	• 2–8% in general population • More common in men • Most often diagnosed in oldest siblings • More common in 1st degree relatives of persons with the disorder than general population • Patients with backgrounds of harsh discipline	Preoccupation with orderliness, perfectionism, mental and interpersonal control, details, rules, lists, order, organization or schedules • Excessive devotion to work and productivity with exclusion of leisure activities and friendships showing perfectionism that interferes with work completion • Reluctant to delegate work or to discard worn out objects even without sentimental value • Shows rigidity, stubbornness and lives like a miser, treating money as something to be hoarded	• Patients are often aware of their suffering and they seek treatment • Treatment however is long, complex and counter transference problems are common • Group therapy and behavior therapy offer advantages in that interrupting patients in the midst of their maladaptive interactions and preventing completion of their habitual behavior raises their anxiety and leaves them susceptible to learning new coping strategies	• Clonazepam has reduced symptoms in severe obsessive compulsive disorder • Clomipramine for obsessive compulsive signs and symptoms break through • Nefazodone

AMNESTIC DISORDERS

The amnestic disorders are coded in DSM-5 as 'Major or Minor Neurocognitive Disorder Due to Another Medical Condition'. They form a broad category that results from a variety of diseases and conditions that have amnesia as the major complaint. Three major different etiologies exist:

1. Amnestic disorder caused by a general medical condition (e.g. Head trauma)
2. Substance-induced persisting amnestic disorder (chronic alcohol consumption or carbon monoxide poisoning)
3. Amnestic disorder not otherwise specified.

Affected Anatomy

1. Diencephalic structures: dorsomedial and midline nuclei of the thalamus
2. Midtemporal lobe structures: hippocampus, amygdala and the mammillary bodies

Though amnesia mostly results from bilateral damage to these structures, some may result from unilateral damage especially with the left hemisphere being more critical than the right.

MAJOR CAUSES OF AMNESTIC DISORDERS

- Thiamine deficiency (Korsakoff syndrome)
- Hypoglycemia
- Primary brain conditions
  - Seizures
  - Head trauma (closed and penetrating)
  - Cerebral tumors (especially thalamic and temporal)
  - Cerebrovascular diseases (especially thalamic and temporal lobe)
  - Surgical procedures on the brain
  - Encephalitis due to herpes simplex
  - Hypoxia (including nonfatal hanging attempts and carbon monoxide poisoning)
  - Transient global amnesia
  - Electroconvulsive therapy
  - Multiple sclerosis

- Substance-related causes
  - Alcohol use disorders
  - Neurotoxins
  - Benzodiazepines (and other sedative-hypnotics)
  - Many over the counter preparations.

DIAGNOSIS AND CLINICAL FEATURES (DSM-5 CRITERIA)

- The recognition of amnestic disorders occurs when
  - Impairment in the ability to learn new information (anterograde amnesia) or
  - The inability to recall previously learned information (retrograde amnesia) as a result of which
  - There is a significant impairment in social or occupational functioning and
  - Which is caused by a general medical condition
- Short term and recent memory are usually impaired; Remote memory and immediate memory is intact
- The onset of symptoms can be abrupt as in trauma, cerebrovascular events and neurochemical assaults or gradual as in nutritional deficiency and cerebral tumors
- Orientation is seldom lost;
- Patients characteristically lack good insight.

DIFFERENTIAL DIAGNOSES

Alcoholic Blackouts

Persons with severe alcohol abuse characteristically wake up in the morning with a conscious awareness of being unable to remember a period the night before during which they were intoxicated.

Korsakoff Syndrome

Causes

- Thiamine deficiency–due to poor nutritional habits of chronic alcohol abusers
- Starvation
- Gastric carcinoma
- Hemodialysis
- Hyperemesis gravidarum
- Prolonged IV hyperalimentation
- Gastric placation

Clinical Features

- Change in personality–lack of initiative, diminished spontaneity and interest; similar to frontal lobe lesions as they exhibit executive function deficits involving planning, attention, set shifting
- Onset- gradual
- Affects recent memory > remote memory
- Confabulation, apathy, passivity are prominent symptoms
- Most commonly associated with **Wernicke's encephalopathy**–associated syndrome of confusion, ataxia and ophthalmoplegia. Although delirium clears up in a month, the amnestic syndrome either accompanies or follows untreated Wernicke's encephalopathy in 85% of cases.

Treatment

- With treatment patients may remain amnestic upto 3 months following which there is gradual improvement in the ensuing year. Approximately 1/3rd recover completely and 1/3rd of patients have no improvement in their symptoms.
- Administration of thiamine may prevent the development of additional amnestic symptoms but treatment seldom reverses severe amnestic symptoms when present.

TRANSIENT GLOBAL AMNESIA

- Characterized by the abrupt loss of the ability to recall recent events or to remember new information, mild confusion, lack of insight and clear sensorium
- Episodes last from 6–24 hours
- **Pathophysiology**: SPECT has shown to involve ischemia to the temporal lobe, parietotemporal regions and the diencephalic brain regions especially in the left hemisphere
- Patients universally show complete improvement with 20% having recurrence and 7% having epilepsy.

COURSE AND PROGNOSIS

- Static course–show little improvement but also no progression of the disease
- With the exception of transient global amnesia which shows a complete recovery over hours to days and those associated with head trauma which improves steadily.

TREATMENT

Treat the cause with supportive prompts about date, time, place.

DELIRIUM

- Characterized by acute decline in level of consciousness and cognition with particular impairment to attention
- Classically has
  - Sudden onset
  - A brief and fluctuating course
  - Rapid improvement when the causative factor is identified and eliminated.

EPIDEMIOLOGY AND ETIOLOGY

- Increased prevalence in:
  - Elderly
  - ICU patients (70–80%)
  - Patients treated for hip fracture (50%)
  - Open heart surgery patients (30%)
  - End of life care patients (83%)
  - Severe burns patients (21%)
  - HIV patients (30–40%)
  - Terminally ill patients (80%)
- The major neurotransmitter involved is **acetylcholine**
- The major neuroanatomical area is **reticular formation**–principle area regulating attention and arousal
- The major pathway implicated is **dorsal tegmental pathway, the tectum and thalamus**
- Delirium associated with alcohol withdrawal is associated with locus coeruleus and noradrenergic neurons.

DSM-5 DIAGNOSIS AND CLINICAL FEATURES

A. A disturbance in attention (i.e. reduced ability to direct, focus, sustain and shift attention) and awareness (reduced orientation to the environment)
B. The disturbance develops over a short period of time (usually hours to a few days) and tends to fluctuate in severity over the course of the day
C. An additional disturbance in cognition (e.g. Memory deficit, disorientation, language, visuospatial ability or perception)
D. The above disturbances are not explained by a pre-existing, established or evolving neurocognitive disorder or reduced level of consciousness such as coma
E. There is evidence from history or physical examination that the disturbance is a direct consequence of another medical condition, due to the direct effect of substance intoxication or toxin exposure.

DELIRIUM VS DEMENTIA

Table 9.2: Dementia vs Delirium

Feature	Dementia	Delirium
Onset	Slow	Rapid
Duration	Months to years	Days to weeks
Attention	Preserved	Fluctuates
Memory	Impaired remote memory	Impaired recent and immediate memory
Speech	Word finding difficulty	Incoherent (slow or rapid)
Sleep–Wake Cycle	Fragmented sleep	Frequent disruptions (e.g. Day night reversals)
Thoughts	Impoverished	Disorganized
Awareness	Unchanged	Reduced
Alertness	Usually normal	Hypervigilant or reduced vigilance

COURSE AND PROGNOSIS

- Symptoms of delirium persist as long as the causative factors are present. After identification and removal of the factors, symptoms recede over a 3 to 7 day period.
- The older the patient and the longer the patient has been delirious, the longer it takes to resolve.

TREATMENT

- Treat the underlying cause
- Physiostigmine—if the cause is anticholinergic toxicity
- Physical support, family support, familiarity orientation.

Pharmacology

Required for two major symptoms of delirium:
- Psychosis: Haloperidol, dexmedetomedine
- Insomnia: Short acting benzodiazepines.

PANIC DISORDER

An acute intense attack of anxiety accompanied by feelings of impending doom is known as panic disorder. The anxiety is characterized by discrete periods of intense fear that can vary from several attacks a day to a few attacks a year.

EPIDEMIOLOGY

- Lifetime prevalence–1-4%
- 6 months prevalence–0.5-1%
- 2–3 times more common in women, more in those with recent history of divorce or separation
- 4–8 fold higher risk in 1st degree relatives of patients with the disorder
- Common age of presentation–25 years.

COMORBIDITY

- 91% have one other psychiatric disorder.
- 1/3rd diagnosed with major depressive disorder before onset and 2/3rd experience panic disorder after diagnosis of major depressive disorder.

ETIOLOGY

- Abnormal regulation of brain noradrenergic system with studies implicating both peripheral and central nervous system dysregulation-ANS in panic disorder patients exhibit increased sympathetic tone, to adapt slowly to repeated stimuli and to respond excessively to moderate stimuli
- Serotonergic dysfunction caused by post-synaptic serotonin hypersensitivity
- Attenuation of local inhibitory GABAergic transmission in the basolateral amygdala, midbrain and hypothalamus
- Foci on:
  - The brainstem
  - The limbic system–responsible for the anticipatory anxiety
  - The prefrontal cortex–generation of phobic avoidance.
- Panicogens–panic producing substances induce panic attacks in patients with panic disorder, e.g. Respiratory panicogens—Carbon monoxide, sodium lactate and bicarbonate neurochemical substances–yohimbine, flumazenil, cholecystokinin, caffeine.

PANIC ATTACK (DSM-5 CRITERIA)

- It is a sudden period of abrupt surge of intense fear or apprehension, reaches a peak within minutes, that may last from minutes to hours with any of these symptoms:
  - Palpitations, pounding heart or accelerated heart rate
  - Sweating
  - Trembling or shaking
  - Sensation of shortness of breath or smothering
  - Feelings of choking
  - Chest pain or discomfort
  - Nausea or abdominal distress
  - Feeling dizzy, unsteady, light headed or faint
  - Chills or heat sensation
  - Derealization or depersonalization
  - Fear of losing control or going crazy
  - Fear of dying
- Seen in:
  - Panic disorder
  - Specific phobia
  - Social phobia
  - PTSD
- They can occur at any time not associated with any identifiable social stimulus or they can also occur in phobias, cued to a recognizable stimulus–**situationally predisposed panic attacks**.

DIAGNOSIS AND CLINICAL FEATURES (DSM-5 CRITERIA)

A. Recurrent unexpected panic attacks
B. At least one of the attacks has been followed by 1 month of:
  1. Persistent concern or worry about panic attacks or their consequences
  2. Significant maladaptive changes in behavior related to the attacks
C. The disturbance not attributable to the physiological effects of any substance or medical condition
D. The disturbance is not better explained by any other mental disorder.

COURSE AND PROGNOSIS

- Chronic disorder with a variable course
- 30–40% patients become symptom free at long term follow-up
- 50% have mild symptoms that do not affect their life significantly
- 10–20% have significant symptoms.

TREATMENT

Pharmacotherapy: Required for 8–12 months
- Selective Serotonin Reuptake Inhibitors: Paroxetine, escitalopram, sertraline.
  Since their onset of action is slow, to abort panic attack immediately patient can be started with alprazolam and SSRI at the same time and after SSRI take action in a few weeks slowly taper the alprazolam
- Benzodiazepines: Alprazolam, lorazepam, clonazepam.
  Most rapid onset of action against panic attacks but have increased risk of abuse, dependence and tolerance and withdrawal effects.
  Tricyclic Antidepressants: Clomipramine, imipramine.
  These have more side effects than SSRI and require higher dose for effective treatment.
  Psychotherapy: Cognitive behavior therapy.

GENERALIZED ANXIETY DISORDER

Etiology

- **Biological factors**: Treatment efficacies of benzodiazepines and buspirone focused research efforts on GABA neurotransmitter system and the 5HT neurotransmitter system
- The brain areas hypothesized to be involved are:
  - Occipital lobe–Increased benzodiazepine receptors
  - Basal ganglia
  - Limbic system
  - Frontal cortex
- **Brain imaging studies:** PET study showed decreased basal metabolic rate in basal ganglia/white matter
- **EEG studies:** Patterns in GAD was found to be different from the sleep EEG pattern in depression by the following:
  - Increased sleep discontinuity
  - Reduced REM
  - Reduced stage 1 sleep
  - Reduced delta wave sleep
- **Psychosocial factors:**
  1. **CBT school of thought:**
     - The patient responds to incorrectly and inaccurately perceived dangers
     - The inaccuracy is generated
       - From selective attention to negative detail
       - Distortions in the information processing
       - And by an overly negative view of the persons ability to cope.
  2. **Psychoanalytic school of thought:** Anxiety is a symptom of unresolved conflict.

EPIDEMIOLOGY

- 2:1 ratio in female:Male
- Lifetime prevalence–5%
- 1 year prevalence–3–8%
- Onset in late adolescence/early adulthood
- 50–90% comorbidities present such as:
  - Panic attacks
  - Dysthymia
  - Social phobia/specific phobia
  - Depression
  - Substance related disorder

DIAGNOSIS AND CLINICAL FEATURES (DSM-5 CRITERIA)

A. It is characterized by the pattern of frequent, persistent worry and anxiety about a number of events, that is out of proportion of the impact of the event, for at least 6 months.
B. The individual finds it difficult to control the worry.
C. The worry/ anxiety is associated with at least 3 of the following 6 symptoms (for the past 6 months)
   - Restlessness or feeling keyed up or on the edge
   - Being easily fatigued
   - Difficulty concentrating or mind going blank
   - Irritability
   - Muscle tension
   - Sleep disturbance (difficulty falling or staying asleep, restless or unsatisfied sleep).
D. The anxiety/worry or physical symptoms cause significant distress or impairment in social, occupational or other areas of functioning.
E. The disturbance is not attributable to the physiological effects of a substance or another medical condition.
F. The disturbance is not better explained by any other medical/mental disorder.

COURSE AND PROGNOSIS

Chronic and life long.

TREATMENT PHARMACOTHERAPY

Sometimes seen as 6-12 months treatment course, mostly patients need to take drugs life long 25% relapse in the first year after discontinuation of the therapy and 60–80% relapse in the course of the next year.

- Benzodiazepines:
  - Longer-acting agents, such as diazepam, chlordiazepoxide, flurazepam, and clonazepam, tend to accumulate active metabolites, with resultant sedation, impairment of cognition, and poor psychomotor performance.
  - Shorter-acting compounds, such as alprazolam and oxazepam, can produce daytime anxiety, early morning insomnia, and, with discontinuation, rebound anxiety and insomnia.
- Buspirone-nonbenzodiazepine anxiolytic agent, nonsedating, does not produce tolerance or dependence
- Venlafaxin, SSRI
- Anticonvulsants with GABAergic properties–gabapentin, oxcarbazepine, pregabalin, divalproex.

AUTISM SPECTRUM DISORDER

Differences in DSM-5 from ICD-10 and DSM-IV-TR

- The classification system used in ICD-10 is not congruent with the revisions made in DSM-5 for autistic disorders.
- ICD-10 still includes separate designations for:
  - Autistic disorder
  - Rett syndrome
  - Childhood disintegrative disorder
  - Asperger's disorder
  - Pervasive developmental disorder not otherwise specified
- However according to DSM-5, each is subsumed under the rubric of autism spectrum disorder and should not be diagnosed
- Autistic disorder was initially characterized by impairments in three domains:
  - Social communication
  - Restricted and repetitive behaviors
  - Aberrant language development and usage
- But in the recently developed DSM-5, the core diagnostic impairments are collapsed into two domains:
  - Social communication
  - Restricted and repetitive behavior

- Aberrant language development and usage is no longer considered a core feature as it is not a defining feature but an associated feature in some individuals with autism spectrum disorder and the less extensive form of autism spectrum disorder, Asperger's disorder, did not include language impairment as a diagnostic criterion.
- Autism spectrum disorder is typically evident in the second year of life

EPIDEMIOLOGY

- Diagnosed 4 times more frequently in male children.
- Girls diagnosed with autism spectrum disorder exhibit increased prevalence of intellectual disability.
- Though it occurs in the early developmental period, as it is not diagnosed until much later, it is seen more commonly at a much older age in young children.

ETIOLOGY/PATHOGENESIS

Psychosocial Theories

No significant differences in child rearing skills of parents of autistic children.

Comorbid CNS Disorders

- 4–32% have associated grand mal seizures.
- 20–25% have ventricular enlargement revealed by CT scans
- 10–83% have EEG disorders—specifically failed cerebral lateralization is revealed in EEG patterns.

Prenatal Factors

- Associated with risk factors for hypoxia
- Advanced maternal/ paternal age at birth
- Maternal gestational bleeding
- 1st born baby.

Perinatal Factors

- Umbilical cord complications
- Birth trauma
- Fetal distress
- Small for gestational age, low birth weight
- Poor 5 minutes apgar score
- ABO/Rh incompatibility, hyperbilirubinemia

BIOMARKERS

- Elevated platelet serotonin levels (5HT)—was the first found biomarker for autistic spectrum disorder
- mTOR—mammalian target of rapamycin linked synaptic plasticity mechanism appeared to be disrupted

DIAGNOSIS AND CLINICAL FEATURES (DSM-5 CRITERIA)

A. Persistent deficits in social communication and social interaction across multiple contexts such as:
- Deficits in social-emotional reciprocity:
  - Abnormal social approach
  - Failure or normal back and forth conversation
  - Reduced sharing of interests
  - Emotions or affect
  - Failure to initiate or respond to social interactions
- Deficits in non-verbal communicative disorders used for social interaction:
  - Poorly integrated verbal and non-verbal communication
  - Abnormalities in eye contact and body language
  - Deficits in understanding and use of gestures
  - Total lack of facial expressions and nonverbal communication
- Deficits in developing, maintaining and understanding relationships:
  - Difficulties adjusting behavior to suit various social contexts

- Difficulties in sharing imaginative play
- In making friends
- Absence of interest in peers

Severity is based on social communication and restricted, repetitive patterns of behavior.

B. Restricted, repetitive patterns of behavior, interests or activities as manifested by at least two of the following (either by history or currently):
  1. Stereotyped or repetitive motor movements, use of objects or speech
  2. Insistence on sameness, inflexible adherence to routines or ritualized patterns of verbal or non-verbal behavior
  3. Highly restricted, fixated interests that are abnormal in intensity or focus
  4. Hyper-or hypo-reactivity to sensory input or unusual interest in sensory aspects of the environment
C. Symptoms must be present in early developmental period (though may not become fully manifest until social demands exceed limited capacities.
D. Symptoms cause clinically significant impairment in social, occupational or other important areas of current functioning.
E. These disturbances are not better explained by intellectual disability or global developmental delay.

Specifications must be made whether Autism Spectrum Disorder is accompanied by intellectual impairment, language impairment, associated with a known medical, genetic condition or environmental factor, neurodevelopmental disorder, mental or behavioral disorder or with catatonia.

ASSOCIATED BEHAVIORAL SYMPTOMS

1. **Disturbances in language development and usage:**
   - Language deviance as much as language delay is a characteristic of more severe subtypes of Autism Spectrum Disorder
   - The patients have difficulty putting meaningful sentences together and even when they learn to converse fluently, it lacks typical prosody or inflection
   - Difficulties in articulation are common and use peculiar voices and rhythm.
   - 50% never develop useful speech
2. **Intellectual disability:**
   - 30% children with ASD have mild to moderate intellectual disability
   - 45–50% children with ASD are severely to profoundly intellectually disabled
3. **Instability of mood/affect:** Sudden mood changes with bursts or laughing or crying without obvious reason are common in children with ASD associated with aggression, irritability, temper tantrums without an obvious trigger and self-injurious behaviors such as head banging, skin picking, biting oneself which are often difficult to control.
4. **Response to sensory stimuli:**
   - Children with ASD over respond to some stimuli and under respond to other sensory stimuli.
   - Some children have a heightened pain threshold/altered response to pain.
   - Some children with ASD perseverate on a sensory experience.
5. **Hyperactivity/Inattention:**
   - Both are common in children with ASD.
   - Short attention span, poor ability to focus on a task may also interfere with daily functioning.
6. **Precocious skills:** Some children with ASD have 'splinter skills' of great proficiency, well beyond the capacity of their normal peers, such as:
   - Hyperlexia–an early ability to read well (even though they cannot understand what they read)
   - Memorizing and reciting
   - Musical abilities (singing or playing tunes or recognizing musical pieces)
   - Prodigious rote memories
   - Calculating abilities
   1. **Insomnia:**
      - 44–83% of children with ASD have insomnia
      - Pharmacological treatment: melatonin
      - Behavioral treatment:
        - Modification of parental behavior at bed times
        - Providing routines that remove reinforcers for remaining awake
   2. Increased incidence of upper respiratory infections, gastrointestinal problems and febrile seizures.

ASSESSMENT TOOLS

Autism Diagnostic Observation Schedule–Generic (ADOS-G).

COURSE AND PROGNOSIS

- Lifelong; heterogenous disorder with highly variable severity and prognosis
- Best prognosis for those with IQ >70 with average adaptive skills, who develop communicative language by ages 5 to 7 years.

TREATMENT

Psychosocial Interventions

These help children with ASD to develop skills in social conventions, increase social acceptable and prosocial behavior with peers and to decrease odd behavioral symptoms.
- UCLA/Lovaas-based model
- Early start denver method (ESDM)
- Parent training approaches
- Social skills training
- Behavioral interventions and cognitive behavioral therapy for repetitive behaviors and associated symptoms
- Neuro-feedback and management of insomnia as interventions for comorbid symptoms.

PHARMACOLOGICAL INTERVENTIONS

- Second generation antipsychotics such as risperidone and aripiprazole to control symptoms of irritability
- Methylphenidate for symptoms of hyperactivity, impulsivity and inattention
- Mood stabilizers such as valproate, second generation antipsychotics and SSRIs for repetitive and stereotypic behavior
- Quetiapine, clozapine, ziprasidone and lithium to treat behavioral impairment.

Table 9.3: Pervasive developmental disorders

Features	Autism	Asperger	Rett
Social disturbance	Severe	Moderate-severe	Variable
Language/communication impairment	Marked	Good verbal ability, poor communication	Very marked
Restricted interests	Marked, mannerisms, trouble with change, occasionally savant ability	Usually highly circumscribed interests (interfering with normal functioning)	Significant psychomotor retardation
Motor issues	Often preserved early but poor later when imitation is required	Often clumsy, with fine and gross motor difficulties	Significant loss of motor abilities, handwashing sterotypies
Onset	Always before age 3 years, often before age 1 year	Problems often recognized in preschool	Before age 5 years (typically onset with loss of skills)

ATTENTION DEFICIT HYPERACTIVE DISORDER

Epidemiology

- Occurrence of ADHD:
  - 7–8% in pre pubertal school children
  - 5% of youth including children and adolescents
  - 2.5% in adults
- More prevalent in boys than girls, with a ratio of 2:1 ranging up to 9:1
- Prevalence increased by 2–8 times in 1st degree relatives of children with ADHD
- Siblings of children with ADHD are at a higher risk for learning disorders and academic difficulty
- Parents of children with ADHD show an increased incidence of substance abuse disorder
- Most common presentation age is 3 years.

ETIOLOGY

Genetic Factors

- Etiology of ADHD is largely genetic with a heritability of approximately 75%
- Studies have shown the association **of dopamine transporter gene (DAT1)** and **dopamine 4 receptor seven-repeat allele gene (DRD4)** and ADHD.

Neurochemical Factors
- Brain regions involved are:
  - Prefrontal cortex–has a role in attention and regulation of impulse control
  - Locus ceruleus–consists of noradrenergic neurons which play an important role in attention
- Dysfunction in both adrenergic and dopaminergic systems is seen in ADHD with dopamine being the major focus of investigations.

Neurophysiological Factors
Increased theta activity in the frontal regions and beta-activity has been found in the EEG studies conducted in ADHD children and it was found that these youth showed increased mood lability and temper tantrums.

Neuroanatomical Aspects
- MRI, PET AND SPECT studies that children with ADHD show evidence of decreased volume and activity in:
  - Prefrontal regions
  - Anterior cingulated
  - Globus pallidus
  - Caudate
  - Thalamus
  - Cerebellum
- Another theory postulate that the frontal lobes of children with ADHD do not adequately inhibit lower brain structures, an effect leading to disinhibition.

Development Factors
Higher rates of ADHD occurred in children:
- Born prematurely
- Born to mothers who had maternal infection during their pregnancy
- Who had perinatal insult to brain during early infancy caused by infection, inflammation and trauma
- Born in September, due to prenatal exposure to winter infections in the first trimester.

DIAGNOSIS AND CLINICAL FEATURES (DSM-5 CRITERIA)

A. A persistent pattern of inattention and/or hyperactivity–impulsivity that interferes with functioning or development as characterized by:
  1. **Inattention: Six or more symptoms of inattention for children up to age 16, or five or more for adolescents 17 and older and adults; symptoms of inattention have been present for at least 6 months, and they are inappropriate for developmental level:**
     a. Often fails to give close attention to details or makes careless mistakes in schoolwork, at work, or with other activities.
     b. Often has trouble holding attention on tasks or play activities.
     c. Often does not seem to listen when spoken to directly.
     d. Often does not follow through on instructions and fails to finish schoolwork, chores, or duties in the workplace (e.g. loses focus, side-tracked).
     e. Often has trouble organizing tasks and activities.
     f. Often avoids, dislikes, or is reluctant to do tasks that require mental effort over a long period of time (such as schoolwork or homework).
     g. Often loses things necessary for tasks and activities (e.g. school materials, pencils, books, tools, wallets, keys, paperwork, eyeglasses, mobile telephones).
     h. Is often easily distracted
     i. Is often forgetful in daily activities.
  2. **Hyperactivity and Impulsivity: Six or more symptoms of hyperactivity-impulsivity for children up to age 16, or five or more for adolescents 17 and older and adults; symptoms of hyperactivity-impulsivity have been present for at least 6 months to an extent that is disruptive and inappropriate for the person's developmental level**
     a. Often fidgets with or taps hands or feet, or squirms in seat.
     b. Often leaves seat in situations when remaining seated is expected.
     c. Often runs about or climbs in situations where it is not appropriate (adolescents or adults may be limited to feeling restless).
     d. Often unable to play or take part in leisure activities quietly.
     e. Is often "on the go" acting as if "driven by a motor".

f. Often talks excessively.
g. Often blurts out an answer before a question has been completed.
h. Often has trouble waiting his/her turn.
i. Often interrupts or intrudes on others (e.g. butts into conversations or games)
B. Several inattentive or hyperactive-impulsive symptoms were present before age 12 years.
C. Several symptoms are present in two or more setting, (e.g. at home, school or work; with friends or relatives; in other activities).
D. There is clear evidence that the symptoms interfere with, or reduce the quality of, social, school, or work functioning.
E. The symptoms do not happen only during the course of schizophrenia or another psychotic disorder. The symptoms are not better explained by another mental disorder (e.g. Mood disorder, Anxiety disorder, Dissociative disorder, or a Personality disorder).

Based on the types of symptoms, three kinds (presentations) of ADHD can occur:
- **Combined presentation**: If enough symptoms of both criteria inattention and hyperactivity-impulsivity were present for the past 6 months
- **Predominantly inattentive presentation**: If enough symptoms of inattention, but not hyperactivity-impulsivity, were present for the past six months
- **Predominantly hyperactive-impulsive presentation**: If enough symptoms of hyperactivity-impulsivity but not inattention were present for the past six months.

Because symptoms can change over time, the presentation may change over time as well.

COURSE AND PROGNOSIS

- Course is variable
- 60–85% cases persist into adolescence. Those who persist with the disorder are at higher risk for developing conduct disorder and children with both ADHD and conduct disorder are at a risk for developing substance use disorder
- 60% cases persist into adulthood. Those who persist with the disorder may show diminished hyperactivity but remain impulsive and accident prone
- 40% cases may remit at puberty, around 12–20 years of age
- Overactivity is the first symptom to remit and distractibility is the last.

TREATMENT

Pharmacotherapy: 1st line treatment
- **Stimulants:**
  - Methylphenidate
  - Amphetamine, dextroamphetamine
- **Nonstimulants:**
  - Alpha agonists–Clonidine/guanfacine
  - Norepinephrine reuptake inhibitor–atomoxetine

PSYCHOSOCIAL INTERVENTIONS

- Psychoeducation
- Academic organization skills remediation
- Parent training
- Behavioral modification in the classroom and at home
- Cognitive behavioral therapy
- Social skills training.

UTAH CRITERIA FOR ADULT ADHD

I. Retrospective childhood ADHD diagnosis
   a. Narrow criterion: Met DSM criteria in childhood by parent interview
   b. Broad criterion: Both 1 and 2 are met as reported by patient
      1. Childhood hyperactivity
      2. Childhood attention deficits

II. Adult characteristics: Five additional symptoms, including on going difficulties with inattentiveness and hyperactivity and at least three other symptoms
   a. Inattentiveness
   b. Hyperactivity
   c. Mood lability
   d. Irritability and hot temper
   e. Impaired stress tolerance
   f. Disorganization
   g. Impulsivity
III. Exclusions: Not diagnosed in presence of severe depression, psychosis or severe personality disorder.

NARCOLEPSY

- A condition characterized by excessive sleepiness that represents the intrusion of REM sleep in the waking state.
- 0.02–0.16% adults show familial tendency
- Sleep attacks represent episodes of irresistible sleepiness for about 10–20 min occurring at inappropriate times following which patient feels refreshed at least briefly
- It is an abnormality of sleep mechanism, specifically REM inhibiting mechanism–dysfunction of REM sleep generator gating mechanism
- Patients may experience depression, social isolation, difficulty with academics and employment and fear of driving contributing to a sense of loss.

Classic form–Tetrad of Symptoms
- Excessive day time sleepiness
- Cataplexy
- Sleep paralysis
- Hypnagogic hallucinations

DIAGNOSIS AND CLINICAL FEATURES (DSM-5 CRITERIA)

A. Recurrent periods of an irrepressible need to sleep, lapsing into sleep, or napping occurring within the same day. These must have been occurring at least three times per week over the past 3 months.
B. The presence of at least one of the following:
   1. Episodes of cataplexy, defined as either (a) or (b), occurring at least a few times per month:
      a. In individuals with long-standing disease, brief (seconds to minutes) episodes of sudden bilateral loss of muscle tone with maintained consciousness that are precipitated by laughter or joking.
      b. In children or in individuals within 6 months of onset, spontaneous grimaces or jaw-opening episodes with tongue thrusting or a global hypotonia, without any obvious emotional triggers
   2. Hypocretin deficiency, as measured using cerebrospinal fluid (CSF) hypocretin-1 immunoreactivity values (less than or equal to one-third of values obtained in healthy subjects tested using the same assay, or less than or equal to 110 pg/mL). (Low CSF levels of hypocretin-1 must not be observed in the context of acute brain injury, inflammation, or infection).
   3. Nocturnal sleep polysomnography showing rapid eye movement (REM) sleep latency less than or equal to 15 minutes, or a multiple sleep latency test showing a mean sleep latency less than or equal to 8 minutes and two or more sleep-onset REM periods.

Narcolepsy Subtypes–Diagnostic Criteria DSM-5 Narcolepsy without cataplexy but with hypocretin deficiency:
- Criterion B requirements of low CSF hypocretin-1 levels and positive polysomnography/multiple sleep latency test are met
- But no cataplexy is present (Criterion B1 not met).

Narcolepsy with cataplexy but without hypocretin deficiency:
- In this rare subtype (less than 5% of narcolepsy cases), Criterion B requirements of cataplexy and positive polysomnography/multiple sleep latency test are met
- But CSF hypocretin-1 levels are normal (Criterion B_2 not met).

Autosomal dominant cerebellar ataxia, deafness, and narcolepsy:
This subtype is caused by exon 21 DNA (cytosine-5)- methyltransferase-1 mutations characterized by:
- Late-onset (age 30-40 years) narcolepsy (with low or intermediate CSF hypocretin-1 levels)

- Deafness
- Cerebellar ataxia
- Eventually dementia.

Autosomal dominant narcolepsy, obesity, and type 2 diabetes:
Narcolepsy, obesity, and type 2 diabetes and low CSF hypocretin-1 levels have been described in rare cases and are associated with a mutation in the myelin oligodendrocyte glycoprotein gene.

Narcolepsy secondary to another medical condition:
This subtype is for narcolepsy that develops secondary to medical conditions that cause infectious (e.g. Whipple's disease, sarcoidosis), traumatic, or tumoral destruction of hypocretin neurons.

TREATMENT

- **Modafinil:** An alpha adrenergic receptor agonist, approved by FDA to reduce number of sleep attacks and improve psychomotor performance
- TCAs and SSRIs to reduce cataplexy
- Scheduled naps
- Lifestyle adjustment
- Psychological counseling
- Drug holidays to reduce tolerance
- Careful monitoring of drug refills
- General health
- Cardiac status

PHOBIA

Phobia—Excessive fear of a specific object, circumstance or situation.
Specific phobia—A strong persisting fear of an object or situation causing intense anxiety to the point of panic, when exposed to the feared object.

EPIDEMIOLOGY

- Lifetime prevalence of specific phobia 10%
- 14–16% prevalence in women was twice that of the prevalence in men (5–7%)
- Specific phobia most common mental disorder among women and the second most common among men after substance related disorder
- Peak age of onset of natural environment phobia and the blood-injection-injury type is in the range of 5 to 9 years
- Peak age of onset for the situational type (except fear of heights) is in the mid 20s similar to the age of onset of agoraphobia
- Prevalence of comorbidities with phobias is found to be as high as (50–80%) with anxiety, mood and substance related disorders being the most common.

ETIOLOGY

General Principles of Phobias

Behavioral Factors

Watson's hypothesis: Pavlovian Stimulus-Response model of the conditioned reflex:
- Anxiety is aroused by a naturally frightening stimulus that occurs in contiguity with a second inherently neutral stimulus. As a result of the contiguity, especially on being paired on several successive occasions, the originally neutral stimulus becomes capable of arousing anxiety itself. Thus, the neutral stimulus becomes a conditioned stimulus for anxiety production
- In classical stimulus-response theory, the conditioned stimulus gradually loses its potency to arouse a response if not reinforced by a periodic repetition of the unconditioned stimulus, but in phobias, this attenuation of response does not occur; the symptoms last for years without reinforcement.
- Operant conditioning theory explains this phenomenon by this model: Anxiety is a drive that motivates an organism to do what it can to obviate a painful affect. In course of its random behavior, the organism learns that certain actions enable it to

avoid the anxiety provoking stimulus. These avoidance patterns remain stable for long periods as a result of reinforcement they receive from their capacity to diminish anxiety. This model is accept-able to phobias. Such avoidance behavior becomes fixed as a stable symptom because of its effectiveness in protecting the person from phobic anxiety.
- Learning theory is particularly relevant to phobias.

Psychodynamic themes in phobia:
- Principle defense mechanisms include displacement, projection and avoidance
- Environmental stressors including humiliation and criticism interact with a genetic-constitutional diathesis
- A characteristic pattern of internal object relations is externalized in social situations in social phobias
- Shame and embarrassment are the principle affect states
- Self-exposure to the feared situation is the basic principle of all treatment

Counter-phobic attitude:
Phobic anxiety can be hidden inside attitudes that represent a denial, that either the dreaded object is dangerous or that the person is afraid. Instead of being a passive victim, they reverse the situation and actively attempt to confront and master whatever is feared

Genetic factors:
Blood-injection-injury type has a high familial tendency.

Common types of phobias:
- Acrophobia: Fear of heights
- Agoraphobia: Fear of open spaces
- Ailurophobia: Fear of cats
- Hydrophobia: Fear of water
- Claustrophobia: Fear of closed spaces
- Cynophobia: Fear of dogs
- Mysophobia: Fear of dirt and germs
- Pyrophobia: Fear of fire
- Xenophobia: Fear of strangers
- Zoophobia: Fear of animals

DIAGNOSIS AND CLINICAL FEATURES (DSM-5 CRITERIA)

a. Marked fear or anxiety about a specific object or situation
b. The phobic object or situation almost always provokes immediate fear or anxiety
c. The phobic object or situation is actively avoided or endured with intense fear or anxiety
d. The fear or anxiety is out of proportion to the actual danger posed by the specific object or situation and to the socio cultural context
e. The fear or anxiety or avoidance is persistent, typically lasting for 6 months or more
f. The fear, anxiety or avoidance causes clinically significant distress or impairment in social, occupational or other important areas of functioning
g. The disturbance is not better explained by the symptoms of other mental disorder.

COURSE AND PROGNOSIS

The severity is believed to remain constant in contrast with the waxing and waning course seen in other anxiety disorders.

TREATMENT

- Behavior therapy:
  - Systemic desensitization
  - Imaginal flooding
  - Flooding
- Insight oriented psychotherapy
- Virtual therapy
- Hypnosis
- Supportive treatment
- Family therapy
- Pharmacotherapy: Beta adrenergic receptor antagonists for performance anxiety.

SOCIAL ANXIETY DISORDER (SOCIAL PHOBIA)

- Fear of social situations, including situations that involve scrutiny or contact with strangers
- It is fear of embarrassment to oneself, that may occur in the situation, not of the situation itself
- Lifetime prevalence: 3–13%; epidemiological studies show females are more affected than males
- Peak age of onset is in the teens
- Anxiety disorders, mood disorders, substance related disorders and bulimia nervosa are the common comorbidities
- Studies showed that the children affected had a trait characterized by a consistent pattern of behavioral inhibition, common in children whose parents had panic disorder and were less caring, more rejecting and more overprotecting of their children than were other parents
- Noradrenergic and dopaminergic dysfunction seen in patients with social phobia
- 1st degree relatives of patients with social phobia were three times more likely to be affected
- Chronic course with disruption in school or academic achievement and interference with job performance and social development
- SSRIs, benzodiazepines, buspirone and venlafaxine are the effective drugs of choice for social anxiety disorder
- Combination of behavioral and cognitive methods including cognitive retraining, desensitization are the psychotherapy methods of treatment for social phobia.

AGORAPHOBIA

- Fear or anxiety regarding places from which escape might be difficult. It can be the most disabling of the phobias
- Although agoraphobia coexists with panic disorder DSM-5 classifies it as a separate condition
- 0.4% prevalence in elderly (>65 years); Lifetime prevalence: 2–6%
- DSM-5 criteria stipulates fear or anxiety about at least one situation from two or more of the five situation groups, persisting for at least 6 months
    - Using public transportation
    - In an open space
    - In an enclosed space
    - In a crowd or standing in a line
    - Alone outside of home
- Patients rigidly avoid situations in which it will be difficult to obtain help
- Patients insist that they be accompanied each time they leave the house
- Agoraphobia caused by panic disorder improves with time when the panic disorder is treated; Agoraphobia not accompanying panic disorder is incapacitating and chronic
- Benzodiazepines, SSRIs and TCAs form the pharmacotherapy treatment.
- Supportive psychotherapy, insight oriented psychotherapy, behavior and cognitive therapy, virtual therapy are the commonly used psychotherapy treatment options.

POSTTRAUMATIC STRESS DISORDER

Epidemiology

- Lifetime incidence–9–15%
- Lifetime prevalence of
    - General population– 8%
    - Males–4%
    - Females–10%
- More likely to occur in those who are single, divorced, widowed, socially withdrawn or of low socio economic level
- The most important risk factors are the severity, duration and proximity of a person's exposure to the actual trauma
- 2/3rd of the patients with PTSD have comorbidities such as depressive disorders, substance related disorders, anxiety disorders and bipolar disorders.

ETIOLOGY

Stressor

- It is the prime causative factor though it alone does not suffice to cause the disorder
- The stressors subjective meaning to a person is also important

- The response to the traumatic event must involve intense fear or horror and it depends on the individuals preexisting biological and psychosocial factors and events that happened before and after the trauma.

Predisposing Vulnerability Factors
- Presence of childhood trauma
- Borderline, paranoid, dependant or antisocial personality disorder traits
- Inadequate family or peer support system
- Being female
- Genetic vulnerability to psychiatric illness
- Recent stressful life changes
- Perception of an external locus of control (natural cause) rather than an internal one (human cause)
- Recent excessive alcohol intake.

Psychodynamic themes in PTSD
- The subjective meaning of a stressor may determine its traumatogenicity
- Traumatic events can resonate with childhood trauma
- Inability to regulate affect may result from trauma
- Somatization and alexithymia may be the after effects of trauma
- Common defenses used include denial, minimization, splitting, projective disavowal, dissociation, and guilt (as a defense against underlying helplessness)
- Mode of object relatedness involves projection and introjections of the following roles: omnipotent rescuer, abuser, victim.

Biological Factors
- Opioid system hyperregulation characterized by low plasma beta endorphin levels in patients with PTSD
- Hyperregulation of HPA axis characterized by low plasma and urinary free cortisol concentrations in patients with PTSD
- Altered functioning of noradrenergic system in PTSD characterized by increased 24 hour urine epinephrine concentrations and increased urine catecholamine concentrations with downregulation of platelet alpha-2 and lymphocyte beta-adrenergic receptors.

DIAGNOSIS AND CLINICAL FEATURES (DSM-5 CRITERIA)

a. Exposure to actual or threatened death, serious injury, or sexual violence in one (or more) of the following ways:
   1. Directly experiencing the traumatic event(s).
   2. Witnessing, in person, the event(s) as it occurred to others.
   3. Learning that the traumatic event(s) occurred to a close family member or close friend. In cases of actual or threatened death of family member or friend, the event(s) must have been violent or accidental.
   4. Experiencing repeated or extreme exposure to aversive details of the traumatic event(s) (e.g. first responders collecting human remains; police officers repeatedly exposed to details of child abuse).
b. Presence of one (or more) of the following intrusion symptoms associated with the traumatic event(s), beginning after the traumatic event(s) occurred:
   1. Recurrent, involuntary, and intrusive distressing memories of the traumatic event(s).
   2. Recurrent distressing dreams in which the content and/or effect of the dream are related to the traumatic event(s).
   3. Dissociative reactions (e.g., flashbacks) in which the individual feels or acts as if the traumatic event(s) were recurring.
   4. Intense or prolonged psychological distress at exposure to internal or external cues that symbolize or resemble an aspect of the traumatic event(s).
   5. Marked psychological reactions to internal or external cues that symbolize or resemble an aspect of the traumatic event(s).
c. Persistent avoidance of stimuli associated with the traumatic event(s), beginning after the traumatic event(s) occurred, as evidenced by one or both of the following:
   1. Avoidance of or efforts to avoid distressing memories, thoughts, or feelings about or closely associated with the traumatic event(s).
   2. Avoidance of or efforts to avoid external reminders (people, places, conversations, activities, objects, situations) that arouse distressing memories, thoughts, or feelings about or closely associated with the traumatic event(s).
d. Negative altercations in cognitions and mood associated with the traumatic event(s), beginning or worsening after the traumatic event(s) occurred, as evidenced by two (or more) of the following:
   1. Inability to remember an important aspect of the traumatic event(s) (typically due to dissociative amnesia)
   2. Persistent and exaggerated negative beliefs or expectations about oneself, others, or the world
   3. Persistent, distorted cognitions about the cause or consequences of the traumatic event(s) that lead the individual to blame himself/herself or others.
   4. Persistent negative emotion state (e.g., fear, horror, anger, guilt, or shame).

5. Markedly diminished interest or participation in significant activities.
6. Feelings of detachment or estrangement from others.
7. Persistent inability to experience positive emotions (e.g., inability to experience happiness, satisfaction, or loving feelings).
- e. Marked alterations in arousal and reactivity associated with the traumatic event(s), beginning or worsening after the traumatic event(s) occurred, as evidence by two (or more) of the following:
    1. Irritable behavior and angry outbursts (with little or no provocation) typically expressed as verbal or physical aggression toward people or objects.
    2. Reckless or self-destructive behavior.
    3. Hypervigilance.
    4. Exaggerated startle response.
    5. Problems with concentration.
    6. Sleep disturbance (e.g. difficulty falling or staying asleep or restless sleep).
- f. Duration of the disturbance (Criteria B, C, D, and E) is more than 1 month.
- g. The disturbance causes clinically significant distress or impairment in social, occupational, or other important areas of functioning.
- h. The disturbance is not attributable to the physiological effects of a substance (e.g. medication, alcohol) or another medical condition.

COURSE AND PROGNOSIS

- Left untreated:
  - 30% recover completely
  - 40% continue to have mild symptoms
  - 20% continue to have moderate symptoms
  - 10% remain unchanged
- After 1 year, 50% patients will recover
- Good prognosis is predicted by rapid onset of symptoms, short duration of symptoms, good premorbid functioning, strong social supports, absence of other psychiatric, medical or substance related disorders
- PTSD comorbid with other diseases is chronic and hard to treat.

TREATMENT

Pharmacotherapy
- SSRI: sertraline, paroxetine
- TCA: imipramine, amitriptyline
- MAOI: phenelzine, trazodone
- Anticonvulsants: carbamazepine, valproate

Psychotherapy
- Behavior therapy
- Cognitive therapy
- Hypnosis
- Eye movement desensitization and reprocessing
- Group therapy
- Family therapy

OBSESSIVE-COMPULSIVE DISORDER

Epidemiology
- Lifetime prevalence in general population: 2–3%
- 4th most common psychiatric disorder after phobias, substance abuse and major depressive disorder
- Mean age of onset about 20 years. Males have an earlier onset at 19 years than women who have it around 22 years
- Lifetime prevalence for major depressive disorder in patients with OCD is about 67%, for social phobia is 25%, tourettes disorder is 5–7%. Other common comorbidities are alcohol use disorder, generalized anxiety disorder, specific phobia, panic disorder, eating disorders and personality disorders.

Etiology

- Dysfunction in serotonergic and noradrenergic neurotransmitter systems
- Group A beta-hemolytic streptococcal infection can lead to development of 10–30% of Sydenham chorea with OCD symptoms
- **Brain imaging studies** have shown increased metabolism and blood flow in the:
  - Frontal lobes
  - Basal ganglia–especially the caudate (CT and MRI studies have shown bilaterally smaller caudate)
  - Cingulum of patients with OCD
- **Genetics:** Relatives of probands with OCD consistently have a threefold to fivefold higher chance of having OCD
- Sleep EEG studies showed decreased REM latency similar to depressive disorders.

Behavioral Factors

Obsessions are conditioned stimuli. A relatively neutral stimulus becomes associated with fear or anxiety through a process of respondent conditioning by being paired with noxious or anxiety provoking events. Thus previously neutral objects or thoughts become conditioned stimuli capable of producing anxiety.

When a person discovers that a certain action reduces anxiety attached to an obsessional thought, he/she develops active avoidance strategies in the form of compulsions or ritualistic behaviors to control the anxiety. Gradually because of their efficacy in reducing the anxiety, the avoidance strategies become fixed as learned patterns of compulsive behavior.

Psychosocial Factors

One of the striking features of patients with OCD is the degree to which they are preoccupied with aggression or cleanliness, indicating the psychogenesis of OCD may lie in the disturbances in the growth and development related to the anal-sadistic phase of development.

- **Ambivalence:** Patients with OCD often consciously experience both love and hate towards an object. This conflict of opposing emotions is often evident in a patients doing and undoing patterns of behavior and in paralyzing doubt in the face of choices
- **Magical thinking:** Persons believe that merely by thinking about an event in the external world they can cause the event to occur without immediate physical actions. This causes them to have a fear of having an aggressive thought.

DIAGNOSIS AND CLINICAL FEATURES (DSM-5 CRITERIA)

A. Presence of obsessions, compulsions or both:
   Obsessions are defined by 1 and 2.
   1. Recurrent and persistent thoughts, urges or images that are experienced, at some time during the disturbance, as intrusive and unwanted (ego-dystonic), and that in most individuals cause marked anxiety or distress
   2. The individual attempts to ignore such thoughts, urges or images or to neutralize them with other thought or action (i.e. by performing a compulsion).

   Compulsions are defined by:
   - Repetitive behaviors (e.g. handwashing, checking, ordering) or mental acts (e.g. praying, counting, repeating words silently) that the individual feels driven to perform in response to an obsession or according to rules that must be applied rigidly
   - The behaviors or mental acts are aimed at preventing or reducing anxiety or distress or preventing some dreaded event or situation; however, these behaviors or mental acts are not connected in a realistic way with what they are designed to neutralize or prevent, or are clearly excessive.

B. The obsessions and compulsions are time consuming or cause clinically significant distress or impairment in social, occupational or other areas of functioning.

C. The obsessive-compulsive symptoms are not attributable to the physiological effects of a substance or any other medical condition.

D. The disturbance is not better explained by symptoms of any other mental disorder.

COURSE AND PROGNOSIS

- The onset of symptoms for about 50–70% of patients is sudden, after a stressful event
- 1/3rd of the patients have major depressive disorder and suicide is a risk for all patients with OCD
- Good prognosis is indicated by:
  - Good social and occupational adjustment
  - The presence of precipitating event
  - Episodic nature of symptoms

- Bad prognosis is indicated by:
  - Yielding to compulsions
  - Childhood onset
  - Bizarre compulsions
  - Need for hospitalization
  - Comorbid major depressive disorder
  - Delusional beliefs
  - Presence of overvalued ideas
  - Presence of personality disorder especially schizotypal personality.

TREATMENT

Pharmacotherapy: Initial effects are seen after 4–6 weeks, although 8–16 weeks are required to obtain maximal therapeutic benefit.
- SSRIs-best clinical outcomes when combined with behavioral therapy
- Clomipramine–most selective drug; first approved by the FDA for treatment of OCD.

BEHAVIORAL THERAPY

- Exposure response prevention
- Desensitization
- Thought stopping
- Flooding
- Implosion therapy
- Aversive conditioning

MOOD DISORDERS

Major Depressive Disorder:

- A major depressive disorder occurs without a history of manic, mixed or hypomanic episode and must last at least two weeks
- Typically to fit the diagnosis the patient must experience at least four of the following symptoms:
  - Changes in appetite or weight
  - Changes in sleep or activity
  - Lack of energy
  - Feelings of guilt
  - Problems thinking and making decisions
  - Recurring thoughts of death or suicide.

EPIDEMIOLOGY

- Life time prevalence: 5–17% (higher than any psychiatric disorder)
- More prevalent by at least two times in women
- Mean age of onset–40 years
- More common in persons who are divorced or separated (without close interpersonal relationships)
- More common in rural areas than urban areas
- Substance abuse disorder, panic disorder, OCD, eating disorders are the common comorbidities.

ETIOLOGY

- **Biological factors:**
  - Norepinephrine and serotonin are the two neurotransmitters most implicated in the pathophysiology of mood disorders
  - Serotonin is the biogenic amine neurotransmitter most commonly associated with depression
  - Depletion of serotonin may precipitate depression and patients with suicidal impulses have been shown to have low CSF concentrations of serotonin metabolites and low concentrations of serotonin uptake sites on platelets
  - Dopamine levels are decreased in depression

- Reduction of GABA have been observed in plasma, CSF and brain GABA levels in depression and cholinergic agonists have shown to induce changes in HPA axis activity and sleep that mimic those associated with severe depression
- Elevated HPA activity is a hallmark of mammalian stress responses and one of the clearest links between depression and the biology of chronic stress.
- **Immunological disturbance:** Depressive disorders are associated with severe immunological abnormalities including decreased lymphocyte proliferation in response to mitogens and other forms of impaired cellular immunity.
- **Alterations of sleep neurophysiology:**
  - Depression is associated with a premature loss of deep (slow wave) sleep and an increase in nocturnal arousal
  - The combination of reduced REM latency, increased REM density and decreased sleep maintenance identifies around 40% of depressive outpatients and 80% of depressed in patients. Patients manifesting with abnormal sleep profiles are found to be less responsive to psychotherapy and have a greater risk of relapse or recurrence and may benefit from pharmacotherapy
- **Structural and functional brain imaging:**
  - The most consistent abnormalities observed in depressive disorders is increased frequency of abnormal hyperintensities in subcortical regions such as periventricular regions, the basal ganglia, and the thalamus.
  - PET findings in depression show decreased anterior brain metabolism more pronounced on the left side
  - Other studies have shown more specific reductions of reduced cerebral blood flow or metabolism or both in dopaminergically innervated tracts of the mesocortical and mesolimbic systems in depression
  - In addition to global reduction of anterior cerebral metabolism, increased glucose metabolism has been observed in several limbic regions especially in patients with severe recurrent depression and a family history of mood disorder.
- **Genetic disorders**
  - A twofold increase in unipolar disorder is seen in the biological relatives of bipolar probands
  - Gene mapping studies of unipolar depression have found very strong linkage to the locus for c-AMP response element binding protein (CREB1) on chromosome 2.
- **Psychosocial factors:**
  - A long standing clinical observation is that stressful life events (unemployment, loss of spouse) often precede the first episode, rather than the subsequent episodes. A theory explained this observation by proposing that the stress accompanying the first episode results in long lasting changes in the brains biology such as loss of neurons and excessive reduction in synaptic contacts, altering the various neurotransmitter and intraneural signaling systems. As a result, a person has a high risk of undergoing subsequent episodes of mood disorder without an external stressor.
  - Persons with histrionic, OCD and borderline personalities have a greater risk for depression.
- **Psychodynamic theory of depression:**
  1. Disturbances in the oral phase (1st 10–18 months of life) predispose to subsequent vulnerability to depression
  2. Depression can be linked to real or imagined object loss
  3. Introjections of the departed objects is a defense mechanism invoked to deal with the distress connected with the objects loss
  4. Since the lost object is viewed with a mixture of love and hate, feelings of anger are directed inward at the self
- **Cognitive theory of depression:**
  - Aaron Beck postulated a cognitive triad of depression that consists of:
    - Views about the self—a negative self-percept
    - About the environment—a tendency to experience the world as hostile and demanding
    - About the future—the expectation of suffering and failure.

DIAGNOSIS AND CLINICAL FEATURES (DSM-5 CRITERIA)

a. Five (or more) of the following symptoms have been present during the same 2-week period and represent a change fromt previous functioning; at least one of the symptoms is either (1) depressed mood or (2) loss of interest or pleasure.
   Note: Do not include symptoms that are clearly due to a general medical condition.
   1. Depressed mood most of the day, nearly every day, as indicated by either subjective report (e.g. feels sad or empty) or observation made by others (e.g. appears tearful).
      Note: In children and adolescents, can be irritable mood
   2. Markedly diminished interest or pleasure in all, or almost all, activities most of the day, nearly every day (as indicated by either subjective account or observation made by others)
   3. Significant weight loss when not dieting or weight gain (e.g. a change of more than 5% of body weight in a month), or decrease or increase in appetite nearly every day.
      Note: In children, consider failure to make expected weight gains.
   4. Insomnia or hypersomnia nearly every day

5. Psychomotor agitation or retardation nearly every day (observable by others, not merely subjective feelings of restlessness or being slowed down)
6. Fatigue or loss of energy nearly every day
7. Feelings of worthlessness or excessive or inappropriate guilt (which may be delusional) nearly every day (not merely self-reproach or guilt about being sick)
8. Diminished ability to think or concentrate, or indecisiveness, nearly every day (either by subjective account or as observed by others)
9. Recurrent thoughts of death (not just fear of dying), recurrent suicidal ideation without a specific plan, or a suicide attempt or a specific plan for committing suicide.

b. The symptoms cause clinically significant distress or impairment in social, occupational or other important areas of functioning
c. The symptoms are not due to the direct physiological effects of a substance (e.g. a drug of abuse, a medication) or a general medical condition (e.g. hypothyroidism).
d. The symptoms are not better explained by schizoaffective disorder, schizophrenia, schizophreniform disorder, delusional disorder, or other specified and unspecified schizophrenia spectrum and other psychotic disorders.
e. There has never been a manic or hypomanic episode.

DEPRESSION WITH PSYCHOTIC FEATURES

- This reflects severe disease and is a poor prognostic factor
- The psychotic symptoms are classified into mood congruent and mood incongruent
- Factors associated with poor prognosis for patients with mood disorders:
  - Long duration of episodes
  - Temporal dissociation between the mood disorder and the psychotic symptoms
  - Poor premorbid history of social adjustment
- These patients require antipsychotic medication along with antidepressants and may require ECT to obtain clinical improvement.

DEPRESSION WITH MELANCHOLIC FEATURES

- Also known as endogenous depression–depression that arises in the absence of external life stressors or precipitants
- Used to describe the dark mood of depression–characterized by severe anhedonia, early morning awakening, weight loss, profound feelings of guilt
- It is associated with changes in the autonomic nervous system and in endocrine functions

DEPRESSION WITH ATYPICAL FEATURES

- Patients have specific predictable characteristics: Overeating and oversleeping
- These symptoms are also known as 'reversed vegetative symptoms' or 'hysteroid dysphoria'
- Patients with atypical features are found to have
  - A younger age of onset
  - More severe psychomotor slowing
  - More frequent coexisting diagnoses of panic disorder, substance abuse or dependence and somatization disorder

DEPRESSION WITH CATATONIA FEATURES

- The presence of catatonic features in patients with mood disorders may have prognostic and treatment significance
- The hallmark symptoms of catatonia:
  - Stuporousness
  - Blunted affect
  - Extreme withdrawal
  - Negativism
  - Marked psychomotor retardation
- Can be seen in both catatonic and noncatatonic schizophrenia, major depressive disorder and medical and neurological disorders.

COURSE AND PROGNOSIS

- An untreated depressive episode lasts 6–13 months
- Most treated cases last 3 months. The withdrawal of antidepressants before 3 months has elapsed almost always results in the return of the symptoms
- As the course of the disorder progresses, patients tend to have more frequent episodes that last longer

TREATMENT

Psychotherapy

- Hospitalization–indications:
  - Risk of suicide or homicide
  - Patients grossly reduced ability to get food and shelter
  - Need for diagnostic procedures
  - History of rapidly progressing symptoms
  - Rupture of a patients usual support system
- Psychosocial therapy:
  - Cognitive therapy
  - Behavior therapy
  - Interpersonal therapy
- Psychoanalytically oriented therapy
- Family therapy
- Vagal nerve stimulation
- Transcranial magnetic stimulation
- Phototherapy

PHARMACOTHERAPY

- 5HT reuptake inhibitors: Fluoxetine, paroxetine, escitalopram, sertraline
- NE reuptake inhibitors: Desipramine, protriptyline, nortriptyline, maprotiline
- NE and 5HT reuptake inhibitors: Venlafaxine, duloxetine
- Dopamine reuptake inhibitor: Bupropion

Depressive Pseudodementia

The geriatric equivalent of semistupor in younger persons with depressive disorder, depressive pseudodementia, is distinguished from primary degenerative dementia by its

- Acute onset without prior cognitive disturbance
- A personal or family history of past affective episodes
- Marked psychomotor retardation with reduced social interaction
- Self-reproach
- Diurnal cognitive dysfunction (worse in the morning)
- Subjective memory dysfunction in excess of objective findings
- Circumscribed memory deficits that can be reversed with proper coaching and a tendency to improve with sleep deprivation.

The main clinical message here is not to miss treatable and/or potentially reversible depressive and bipolar states in elderly patients with dementiform manifestations or early and even mid-stage dementia.

Normal Bereavement

Bereaved persons exhibit many depressive symptoms during the first 1 to 2 years after their loss, 5 percent of bereaved persons progress to a depressive disorder

- Grieving persons and their relatives perceive bereavement as a normal reaction, whereas those with depressive disorder often view themselves as sick and may actually believe they are losing their minds.
- Unlike the melancholic person, the grieving person reacts to the environment and tends to show a range of positive effects.
- Marked psychomotor retardation is not observed in normal grief.

- Although bereaved persons often feel guilty about not having done certain things that they believe might have saved the life of the deceased loved one (guilt of omission), they typically do not experience guilt of commission.
- Delusions of worthlessness or sin and psychotic experiences in general point toward mood disorder.
- Active suicidal ideation is rare in grief but common in major depressive disorder.
- "Mummification" (i.e. keeping the belongings of the deceased person exactly as they were before his or her death) indicates serious psychopathology.
- Severe anniversary reactions should alert the clinician to the possibility of psychopathology.

In another form of bereavement depression, the patient simply pines away, unable to live without the departed person, usually a spouse.

Their immune function is often depressed, and their cardiovascular status is precarious. Death can ensue within a few months of that of a spouse, especially among elderly men. It would be clinically unwise to withhold antidepressants from many persons experiencing an intensely mournful form of grief.

Cross-sectional profiles of clinical anxiety and depression:

Anxiety	Depression
Hypervigilance	Psychomotor retardation
Severe tension and panic	Severe sadness
Perceived danger	Perceived loss
Phobic avoidance	Loss of interest-anhedonia
Doubt and uncertainty	Hopelessness-suicidal
Insecurity	Self-deprecation
Performance anxiety	Loss of libido Early-morning awakening Weight loss

Postpsychotic Depressive Disorder of Schizophrenia

A postpsychotic depression can occur during the residual phase of schizophrenia. It is characterized by the persistence of negative symptoms or positive symptoms that are in an attenuated form (e.g. odd beliefs, unusual perceptual experiences).

The depression is characterized by loss of interest or pleasure and sad or depressed mood.

Most typically, the Major Depressive Episode follows immediately after remission of the active phase of the psychotic episode. Sometimes it may follow after a short or extended interval during which there are no psychotic symptoms.

In all postpsychotic depressions, one must first exclude a missed bipolar diagnosis. Negative symptoms due to classic antipsychotics—especially depot phenothiazines and those due to the residuum of schizophrenia once positive symptoms are brought under control—should be distinguished from the depressive episodes that complicate the course of schizophrenia in young, intelligent patients.

This phenomenon is so common (at least 30% of patients with schizophrenia) that it can be considered as part of the natural course of schizophrenia rather than a separate nosological entity.

BIPOLAR DISORDER

- **Bipolar I disorder** is defined as having a clinical course of one or more manic episodes and sometimes major depressive episodes.
- **A mixed episode** is a period of at least 1 week in which both a manic episode and a major depressive episode occur almost daily
- A variant of bipolar characterized by episodes of major depression and hypomania rather than mania is known as **bipolar II disorder**
- A **manic episode** is a distinct period of an abnormally and persistently elevated, expansive or irritable mood lasting for at least 1 week or less if a patient must be hospitalized
- A **hypomanic episode** lasts at least for 4 days and is similar to a manic episode except that it is not sufficiently severe enough to cause impairment in social or occupational functioning and no psychotic features are seen
- Both mania and hypomania are associated with
  - Inflated self-esteem
  - A decreased need for sleep
  - Distractibility
  - Great physical and mental activity
  - Overinvolvement in pleasurable behavior.

Psychiatry

EPIDEMIOLOGY AND ETIOLOGY

- The annual incidence of bipolar illness is less than 1 percent
- In contrast to major depressive disorder, bipolar I disorder has an equal prevalence among men and women.
- Manic episodes are more common in men; depressive episodes are more common in women.
- When manic episodes occur in women, they are more likely than men to present a mixed picture (e.g. mania and depression).
- Women also have a higher rate of being rapid cyclers, defined as having four or more manic episodes in a 1-year period.
- The age of onset for bipolar I disorder ranges from childhood (as early as age 5 or 6) to 50 years or even older in rare cases, with a mean age of 30.
- Bipolar I disorder is more common in divorced and single persons than among married persons, but this difference may reflect the early onset and the resulting marital discord characteristic of the disorder.
- A higher than average incidence of bipolar I disorder is found among the upper socioeconomic groups.
- The most frequent comorbid disorders are alcohol abuse or dependence, panic disorder, obsessive compulsive disorder (OCD), and social anxiety disorder.
- Three-fold increase in rate of bipolar disorder in biological relatives of bipolar probands.
- DNA MARKERS: Chromosomes 18q and 22q are the two regions with strongest evidence for linkage to bipolar disorder
- Psychodynamic factors in mania:
  - Defense against underlying depression—defensive reaction to depression, using manic defenses such as omnipotence, in which person develops delusion of grandeur
  - The manic state may also result from a tyrannical super ego, which produces intolerable self-criticism which is then replaced by euphoric self-satisfaction.

CLINICAL FEATURES PREDICTIVE OF BIPOLAR DISORDER

- Early age at onset
- Psychotic depression before 25 years of age
- Postpartum depression, especially one with psychotic features
- Rapid onset and offset of depressive episodes of short duration (<3 months)
- Recurrent depression (more than five episodes)
- Depression with marked psychomotor retardation
- Atypical features (reverse vegetative signs)
- Seasonality
- Bipolar family history
- High-density, three-generation pedigrees
- Trait mood lability (cyclothymia)
- Hyperthymic temperament
- Hypomania associated with antidepressants
- Repeated (at least three times) loss of efficacy of antidepressants after initial response
- Depressive mixed state (with psychomotor excitement, irritable hostility, racing thoughts, and sexual arousal *during* major depression).

DIAGNOSTIC CRITERIA FOR BIPOLAR 1 DISORDER (DSM-5 CRITERIA)

For a diagnosis of bipolar 1 disorder, it is necessary to meet the following criteria for a manic episode. The manic episode may have been preceded by and may be followed by hypomanic or major depressive disorder.

Manic Episode

a. A distinct period of abnormally and persistently elevated, expansive, or irritable mood, and abnormally and persistently increased goal-directed activity or energy, lasting at least 1 week and present most of the day, nearly every day (or any duration if hospitalization is necessary).
b. During the period of mood disturbance and increased energy or activity, three (or more) of the following symptoms have persisted (four if the mood is only irritable) and have been present to a significant degree and represent a noticeable change from usual behavior:
   1. Inflated self-esteem or grandiosity
   2. Decreased need for sleep (e.g. feels rested after only 3 hours of sleep)
   3. More talkative than usual or pressure to keep talking

4. Flight of ideas or subjective experience that thoughts are racing
5. Distractibility (i.e. attention too easily drawn to unimportant or irrelevant external stimuli)
6. Increase in goal-directed activity (either socially, at work or school, or sexually) or psychomotor agitation (i.e. purposeless non-goal directed activity)
7. Excessive involvement in pleasurable activities that have a high potential for painful consequences (e.g. engaging in unrestrained buying sprees, sexual indiscretions, or foolish business investments)

c. The mood disturbance is sufficiently severe to cause marked impairment in social or occupational functioning or to necessitate hospitalization to prevent harm to self or others, or there are psychotic features.
d. The episode is not attributable to the physiological effects of a substance (e.g. a drug of abuse, a medication, or there are psychotic features)

Note: Criteria A to D constitute a manic episode. At least one lifetime manic episode is required for the diagnosis of bipolar 1 disorder.

Hypomanic Episode

a. A distinct period of abnormally and persistently elevated, expansive, or irritable mood and abnormally and persistently increased activity or energy lasting at least four consecutive days and present most of the day, nearly everyday.
   1. During the period of mood disturbance and increased energy and activity, three (or more) of the following symptoms have persisted (four if the mood is only irritable), represent a noticeable change from usual behavior and have been present to a significant degree
   2. Inflated self-esteem or grandiosity
   3. Decreased need for sleep (e.g. feels rested after only 3 hours of sleep)
   4. More talkative than usual or pressure to keep talking
   5. Flight of ideas or subjective experience that thoughts are racing distractibility (i.e. attention too easily drawn to unimportant or irrelevant external stimuli)
   6. Increase in goal-directed activity (either socially, at work or school, or sexually) or psychomotor agitation
   7. Excessive involvement in pleasurable activities that have a high potential for painful consequences (e.g. the person engages in unrestrained buying sprees, sexual indiscretions, or foolish business investments)
b. The episode is associated with an unequivocal change in functioning that is uncharacteristic of the person when not symptomatic.
c. The disturbance in mood and the change in functioning are observable by others.
d. The episode is not severe enough to cause marked impairment in social or occupational functioning, or to necessitate hospitalization, if there are psychotic features, the episode, by definition, manic.
e. The episode is not attributable to the physiological effects of a substance (e.g. a drug of abuse, a medication or other treatment).

Note: Criteria a to e constitute a hypomanic episode. Hypomanic episodes are common in bipolar 1 disorder but are not required for the diagnosis of bipolar 1 disorder.

Major Depressive Disorder

a. Five or more of the following symptoms have been present during the same two-week period and represent a change from previous functioning; at least one of the symptoms is either (1) depressed mood or (2) loss of interest or pleasure.

Note: Do not include symptoms that are clearly attributable to another medical condition.
   1. Depressed mood most of the day, nearly every day, as indicated by either subjective report or observation made by others.
   2. Markedly diminished interest or pleasure in all, or almost all, activities most of the day, nearly every day (as indicated by either subjective account or observation).
   3. Significant weight loss when not dieting or weight gain or decrease or increase in appetite every day
   4. Insomnia or hypersomnia nearly every day
   5. Psychomotor agitation or retardation nearly every day (observable by others)
   6. Fatigue or loss of energy nearly every day
   7. Feelings of worthlessness or excessive or inappropriate guilt nearly every day (not merely self-reproach or guilt about being sick)
   8. Diminished ability to think or concentrate or indecisiveness nearly every day (either by subjective account or as observed by others).
   9. Recurrent thoughts of death, recurrent suicidal ideation without a specific plan, or a suicide attempt or a specific plan for committing suicide
b. The symptoms cause clinically significant distress or impairment in social, occupational or other important areas of functioning
c. The episode is not attributable to the physiological effects of a substance or another medical condition

Note: Criteria a to c constitute major depressive episode. Major depressive episodes are common in bipolar 1 disorder but are not required for the diagnosis of bipolar 1 disorder.

Course and Prognosis

- Bipolar 1 usually starts with depression and is a recurring disorder.
- Most patients experience both depressive and manic episodes, although 10 to 20 percent experience only manic episodes.
- The manic episodes typically have a rapid onset (hours or days), but may evolve over a few weeks.
- An untreated manic episode lasts about 3 months; therefore, clinicians should not discontinue giving drugs before that time.
- Of persons who have a single manic episode, Ninety percent are likely to have another.
- As the disorder progresses, the time between episodes often decreases. After about five episodes, however, the interepisode interval often stabilizes at 6 to 9 months.
- Of persons with bipolar disorder, 5 to 15 percent have four or more episodes per year and can be classified as rapid cyclers.
- Patients with bipolar I disorder have a poorer prognosis than do patients with major depressive disorder.
- About 40 to 50 percent of patients with bipolar I disorder may have a second manic episode within 2 years of the first episode. Although lithium prophylaxis improves the course and prognosis of bipolar I disorder, probably only 50 to 60% of patients achieve significant control of their symptoms with lithium.

Treatment

- Lithium carbonate
- Valproate
- Carbamazepine and oxcarbazepine
- Clonazepam and lorazepam
- Atypical and typical antipsychotics

PSYCHOTHERAPY

Cognitive Therapy

- Cognitive therapy is a short term, structured therapy that uses active collaboration between patient and therapist to achieve therapeutic goals
- A central feature of the therapy is its emphasis over the psychological significance of peoples beliefs about
    - Themselves
    - Their personal world (including the people in their lives) Cognitive
    - Their future triad
- It is used with:
    - Depression
    - Panic disorder
    - Obsessive-compulsive disorder
    - Personality disorder
    - Somatoform disorder
- **Cognitive theory of depression** emphasizes the **cognitive dysfunctions** to be the core of depression, and affective and physical changes and other associated features of depression are consequences of cognitive dysfunctions.
- Depression can be explained by the cognitive triad, which explains that negative thoughts are about self, the world and the future.

Strategies

- Therapy is short and last for about 25 weeks.
- If the patient does not improve in this time, the diagnosis should be re-evaluated. Maintenance therapy can be carried out over years.
- Cognitive therapists set the agenda at the beginning of each session, assign homework to be performed between sessions and teach new skills.
  The three components of cognitive therapy are:
  1. Didactic aspects
  2. Cognitive techniques
  3. Behavioral techniques

Didactic Aspects
- In the therapy's didactic aspects, the therapist explains to the patient
  - The cognitive triad, schemas and faulty logic
  - That they would together with the patient formulate hypotheses
  - Test the hypotheses over the course of the treatment
- It requires full explanation of the relation between depression and thinking, affect and behavior as well as the rationale for all aspects of treatment.

Cognitive Techniques

It includes four processes:
- **Eliciting automatic thoughts (AKA cognitive distortions):**
  - Cognitions that intervene between external events and a person's emotional reaction to the event.
  - For example, is the thought "she doesn't like me" when someone passes in the hall without saying "hello".
- **Testing automatic thoughts:**
  - Acting as a teacher, a therapist helps a patient to test the validity of automatic thoughts. The goal is to encourage the patient to reject inaccurate or exaggerated automatic thoughts after careful examination
  - Generating alternative explanations for the events is another way of undermining inaccurate and distorted automatic thoughts
- **Identifying maladaptive assumptions:**
  - As the patient and therapist continue to identify automatic thoughts, patterns become apparent, which are maladaptive general assumptions that guide a persons life. Such rules inevitably lead to disappointments, failure and depression
  - For example "In order to be happy I must be perfect".
- **Testing the validity of maladaptive assumptions:**
  - Similar to the testing of validity of automatic thoughts, the therapists ask the the patients to defend the validity of their assumptions.
  - For example when the patient says that he always has to work up to his potential, the therapists test this assumption by asking why that is so important to them.

BEHAVIORAL TECHNIQUES

1. Behavioral and cognitive techniques go hand in hand. They help to test and change maladaptive and inaccurate cognitions. The overall purpose of such techniques is to help patients understand the inaccuracy of their cognitive assumptions and learn new strategies and ways of dealing with issues. Some of them are:
   - Scheduling activities
   - Mastery and pleasure
   - Graded task assignments
   - Cognitive rehearsal
   - Self-reliance training
   - Role playing
   - Diversion techniques

IMPORTANT INDICATIONS OF COGNITIVE THERAPY

Cognitive therapy can be used alone in the treatment of mild to moderate depressive disorders or in conjunction with antidepressants in major depressive disorder. It is one of the most useful psychotherapeutic interventions currently available for depressive disorders and it shows promise in the treatment of other disorders.

Criteria that justify the administration of cognitive therapy alone:
- Failure to respond to adequate trials of two antidepressants
- Partial response to adequate dosages of antidepressants
- Diagnosis of dysthymic disorder
- Variable mood reactive to environmental events
- Variable mood that correlates with negative cognitions
- Mild somatoform disorders (sleep, appetite, weight, libidinal)

Indications for combined therapies (medication plus cognitive therapy):
- Partial or no response to trial of cognitive therapy alone
- Partial but incomplete response to adequate pharmacotherapy alone
- Poor compliance with medication regimen

- Presence of severe somatoform disorders and marked cognitive distortions (e.g. hopelessness)
- Impaired memory and concentration and marked psychomotor difficulty
- Major depressive disorder with suicidal danger.

BEHAVIOR THERAPY

Systematic Desensitization
- It is based on the behavioral principle of counter conditioning, whereby a person overcomes maladaptive anxiety elicited by a situation or an object by approaching the feared situation gradually, in a psychophysiological state that inhibits anxiety.
- Patients attain a state of complete relaxation and are then exposed to the stimulus that elicits the anxiety response.
- The negative reaction of anxiety is inhibited by the relaxed state, a process called reciprocal inhibition.
- Works best in cases of a clearly identifiable anxiety provoking stimulus. Phobias, obsessions, compulsions, and certain sexual disorders.
- **Consists of three steps:** Relaxation training, hierarchy construction, and desensitization of the stimulus.
    1. *Relaxation training:* Relaxation produces physiological effects opposite to those of anxiety. Mental imagery is a relaxation method in which patients are instructed to imagine themselves in a place associated with pleasant relaxed memories.
    2. *Hierarchy construction:* When constructing a hierarchy, clinicians determine all the conditions that elicit anxiety, and then patients create a hierarchy list of 10 to 12 scenes in order of increasing anxiety.
    3. *Desensitization of the stimulus:* Patients proceed systematically through the list from the least, to the most, anxiety provoking scene while in a deeply relaxed state. The rate at which patients progress through the list is determined by their responses to the stimuli.

THERAPEUTIC GRADED EXPOSURE

Similar to systematic desensitization, except that relaxation training is not involved and treatment is usually carried out in a real-life context. This means that the individual must be brought in contact with the warning stimulus to learn firsthand that no dangerous consequences will ensue. Exposure is graded according to a hierarchy.

Flooding
- Similar to graded exposure in that it involves exposing the patient to the feared object in vivo; however, there is no hierarchy.
- Patients are encouraged to confront feared situations directly, without a gradual build up, as in systematic desensitization or graded exposure.
- The success of the procedure depends on having patients remain in the fear generating situation until they are calm and feel a sense of mastery.
- Imaginal flooding means the feared object or situation is confronted only in the imagination, not in real life. The technique works best with specific phobias.
- Flooding is based on the premise that escaping from an anxiety provoking experience reinforces the anxiety through conditioning.
- Prematurely withdrawing from the situation or prematurely terminating the fantasized scene is equivalent to an escape that reinforces both the conditioned anxiety and the avoidance behavior and produces the opposite of the desired effect.
- It is contraindicated when intense anxiety would be hazardous to patient.

Participant Modeling
- The participant-modeling technique has been used successfully with agoraphobia by having a therapist accompany a patient into the feared situation.
- Patients learn a new behavior by imitation, primarily by observation like with phobic children who are placed with other children of their own age and sex who approach the feared object or situation.
- In a variant of the procedure, called behavior rehearsal, real life problems are acted out under a therapist's observation or direction.

Assertiveness Training
- Assertive behavior enables a person to act in his or her own best interest, to stand up for herself or himself without undue anxiety, to express honest feelings comfortably, and to exercise personal rights without denying the rights of others.

Social Skills Training
- Patients with depression often experience a lack of social reinforcement because of a lack of social skills, and social skill-straining have been found to be efficacious for depression.
  Social skills training programs for patients with schizophrenia cover skills in the following areas: conversation, conflict management, assertiveness, community living, friendship and dating, work and vocation, and medication management.

CANNABIS

Preparations
- All parts of *Cannabis sativa* contain psychoactive cannabinoids, of which (-)-δ9-tetrahydrocannabinol (δ9-THC) is most abundant.
- The most potent forms of cannabis come from the flowering tops of the plants or from the dried, black-brown, resinous exudates from the leaves, which are referred to as hashish or hash.
- The common names for cannabis are marijuana, grass, pot, weed, tea, and Mary Jane, hemp, charas, bhang, ganja, dagga, and sinsemilla.

Neuropharmacology
- In humans, δ9-THC is rapidly converted into 11-hydroxy-δ9-THC, the metabolite that is active in the central nervous system (CNS).
- The cannabinoid receptor, a member of the G protein-linked family of receptors, is linked to the inhibitory G protein (Gi), which is linked to adenylyl cyclase in an inhibitory fashion.
- The cannabinoid receptor is found in highest concentrations in the basal ganglia, the hippocampus, and the cerebellum, with lower concentrations in the cerebral cortex.
- It is not found in the brainstem, a fact consistent with cannabis's minimal effects on respiratory and cardiac functions. Studies in animals have shown that the cannabinoids affect the monoamine and γ-aminobutyric acid (GABA) neurons.
- Moreover, some debate questions whether the cannabinoids stimulate the so-called reward
- Centers of the brain, such as the dopaminergic neurons of the ventral tegmental area
- When cannabis is smoked, the euphoric effects appear within minutes, peak in about 30 minutes, and last 2 to 4 hours. Some motor and cognitive effects last 5 to 12 hours.
- Cannabis can also be taken orally when it is prepared in food, such as brownies and cakes. About 2 to 3 times as much cannabis must be taken orally to be as potent as cannabis taken by inhaling its smoke.

Cannabis Intoxication
- Cannabis intoxication commonly heightens users' sensitivities to external stimuli, reveals new details, makes colors seem brighter and richer than in the past, and subjectively slows the appreciation of time.
- In high doses, users may experience depersonalization and derealization
- For 8 to 12 hours after using cannabis, users' impaired motor skills interfere with the operation of motor vehicles and other heavy machinery.

Cannabis-Induced Psychotic Disorder
- Cannabis-induced psychotic disorder is rare; transient paranoid ideation is more common.
- Florid psychosis is somewhat common in persons who have long-term access to cannabis of particularly high potency. The psychotic episodes are sometimes referred to as **hemp insanity**.

CANNABIS-RELATED DISORDER NOT OTHERWISE SPECIFIED

Flashbacks
- There are case reports of persons who have experienced at times significantly sensations related to cannabis intoxication after the short-term effects of the substance have disappeared.
- Continued debate concerns whether flashbacks are related to cannabis use alone or to the concomitant use of hallucinogens or of cannabis tainted with phencyclidine (PCP).

Cognitive Impairment
- Clinical and experimental evidence indicates that the long-term use of cannabis may produce subtle forms of cognitive impairment in the higher cognitive functions of memory, attention, and organization and in the integration of complex information.
- This evidence suggests that the longer the period of heavy cannabis use, the more pronounced the cognitive impairment.

Amotivational Syndrome
- A controversial cannabis-related syndrome is *amotivational syndrome*.
- Traditionally, the amotivational syndrome has been associated with long-term heavy use and has been characterized by a person's unwillingness to persist in a task be it at school, at work, Or in any setting that requires prolonged attention or tenacity.
- Persons are described as becoming apathetic and anergic, usually gaining weight, and appearing slothful.

Treatment

- Treatment of cannabis use rests on the same principles as treatment of other substances of abuse, abstinence and support.
- Support can be achieved through the use of individual, family, and group psychotherapies.
- Education should be a cornerstone for both abstinence and support programs.

HALLUCINOGENS

Preparations

- Hallucinogens are natural and synthetic substances that are variously called **psychedelics** or **psychotomimetics** because, besides inducing hallucinations, they produce a loss of contact with reality and an experience of expanded and heightened consciousness.
- The hallucinogens are classified as Schedule I drugs; the US Food and Drug Administration (FDA) has decreed that they have no medical use and a high abuse potential.
- The classic, naturally occurring hallucinogens are psilocybin (from some mushrooms) and mescaline (from peyote cactus). The classic synthetic hallucinogen is LSD was synthesized in 1938 by Albert Hoffman.

Neuropharmacology

- LSD can serve as a hallucinogenic prototype
- It is generally agreed that the drug acts on the serotonergic system, either as an antagonist or as an agonist. Data at this time suggest that LSD acts as a partial agonist at postsynaptic serotonin receptors.
- Tolerance for LSD and other hallucinogens develops rapidly and is virtually complete after 3 or 4 days of continuous use. Tolerance also reverses quickly, usually in 4 to 7 days.
- Neither physical dependence nor withdrawal symptoms occur with hallucinogens, but a user can develop a psychological dependence on the insight-inducing experiences of episodes of hallucinogen use.

Physiological Changes from Hallucinogens

1. Pupillary dilation
2. Tachycardia
3. Sweating
4. Palpitations
5. Blurring of vision
6. Tremors
7. Incoordination

Hallucinogen Persisting Perception Disorder

- Long after ingesting a hallucinogen, a person can experience a flashback of hallucinogenic symptoms.
- The differential diagnosis for **flashbacks** includes migraine, seizures, visual system abnormalities, and posttraumatic stress disorder.
- The following can trigger a flashback:
  - Emotional stress
  - Sensory deprivation, such as monotonous driving
  - Use of another psychoactive substance, such as alcohol or marijuana.
- Flashbacks are spontaneous, transitory recurrences of the substance-induced experience.
- Most flashbacks are episodes of visual distortion, geometric hallucinations, hallucinations of sounds or voices, false perceptions of movement in peripheral fields, flashes of color, trails of images from moving objects, positive after images and halos, macropsia, micropsia, time expansion, physical symptoms, or relived intense emotion.
- The episodes usually last a few seconds to a few minutes, but sometimes last longer.
- Suicidal behavior, major depressive disorder, and panic disorders are potential complications.

Hallucinogen-induced Psychotic Disorders

- If psychotic symptoms are present in the absence of retained reality testing, a diagnosis of hallucinogen induced psychotic disorder may be warranted
- The most common adverse effect of LSD and related substances is a **bad trip**, an experience resembling the acute panic reaction to cannabis but sometimes more severe; a bad trip can occasionally produce true psychotic

- Occasionally, the psychotic disorder is prolonged, a reaction thought to be most common in persons with
  - Preexisting schizoid personality disorder
  - Prepsychotic personalities
  - An unstable ego balance
  - Much anxiety.
- Such persons cannot cope with the perceptual changes, body-image distortions, and symbolic unconscious material stimulated by the hallucinogen.
- The bad trip generally ends when the immediate effects of the hallucinogen wear off.

Treatment
- Reassurance and supportive care, 'talking down the patient', Quiet environment, verbal reassurance and the passage of time
- Rapid relief of intense anxiety can be relieved by oral or iv administration of benzodiazepines
- Treatment for hallucinogen persisting perception disorder is palliative.
  - The first step in the process is correct identification of the disorder.
  - Pharmacological approaches include long-lasting benzodiazepines
  - A second dimension of treatment is behavioral. The patient must be instructed to avoid gratuitous stimulation in the form of over-the-counter drugs, caffeine, and alcohol, and avoidable physical and emotional stressors
- Three comorbid conditions are associated with hallucinogen persisting perception disorder: panic disorder, major depression, and alcohol dependence. All these conditions require primary prevention and early intervention.

STIMULANTS

Amphetamines
- The major amphetamines dextroamphetamines are dextroamphetamine, methamphetamine, a mixed dextroamphetamine-amphetamine salt, and the amphetamine-like compound-methylphenidate.
- These drugs go by such street names as ice, crystal, crystal meth, and speed; the amphetamines are referred to as analeptics, sympathomimetics, stimulants, and psychostimulants.
- The typical amphetamines are used to increase performance and to induce a euphoric feeling, for example, by students studying for examinations, by long-distance truck drivers on trips, by business people with important deadlines, by athletes in competition, and by soldiers during wartime.
- Other amphetamine-like substances are ephedrine, pseudoephedrine, and phenylpropanolamine (PPA). These drugs, PPA in particular, can dangerously exacerbate hypertension, precipitate a toxic psychosis, cause intestinal infarction, or result in death.
- The safety margin for PPA is particularly narrow, and three to four times the normal dose can result in life-threatening hypertension.

Cocaine
- Cocaine is an alkaloid derived from the shrub *Erythroxylon coca*, which is indigenous to South America
- The cocaine alkaloid was first isolated in 1860 and first used as a local anesthetic in 1880. It is still used as a local anesthetic, especially for eye, nose, and throat surgery, for which its vasoconstrictive and analgesic effects are helpful
- It was the active ingredient in the beverage Coca-Cola until 1903
- Most studies of comorbidity in patients with cocaine-related disorders have shown that major depressive disorder, bipolar II disorder, cyclothymic disorder, anxiety disorders, and antisocial personality disorder are the most commonly associated psychiatric comorbidities.

Etiology
- Genetic factors and unique (unshared) environmental factors contribute about equally to the development of stimulant dependence.
- Social, cultural, and economic factors are powerful determinants of initial use, continuing use, and relapse. Excessive use is far more likely in countries where cocaine is readily available.
- Learning and conditioning are also considered important in perpetuating cocaine use. Each inhalation or injection of cocaine yields a rush and a euphoric experience that reinforce the antecedent drug taking behavior.
- In addition, the environmental cues associated with substance use become associated with the euphoric state so that long after a period of cessation, such cues (e.g., white powder and paraphernalia) can elicit memories of the euphoric state and reawaken craving for cocaine.

NEUROPHARMACOLOGY

Amphetamines

- The **classic amphetamines** (i.e. dextroamphetamine, methamphetamine, and methylphenidate)
  - Produce their primary effects by causing the release of catecholamines, particularly dopamine, from presynaptic terminals.
  - The effects are particularly potent for the dopaminergic neurons projecting from the ventral tegmental area to the cerebral cortex and the limbic areas.
  - This pathway has been termed the *reward circuit pathway*, and its activation is probably the major addicting mechanism for the amphetamines.
- The **designer amphetamines**
  - Cause the release of catecholamines (dopamine and norepinephrine) and of serotonin, the neurotransmitter implicated as the major neurochemical pathway for hallucinogens.
  - Therefore, the clinical effects of designer amphetamines are a blend of the effects of classic amphetamines and those of hallucinogens.
- Tolerance develops with both classic and designer amphetamines and they are less addictive than cocaine.

Cocaine

- Cocaine's primary pharmacodynamic action related to its behavioral effects is competitive blockade of dopamine reuptake by the dopamine transporter. This blockade increases the concentration of dopamine in the synaptic cleft and results in increased activation of both dopamine type 1 (D1) and type 2 (D2) receptors.
- Although the behavioral effects are attributed primarily to the blockade of dopamine reuptake, cocaine also blocks the reuptake of norepinephrine and serotonin
- Cocaine is associated with decreased cerebral blood flow and possibly with the development of patchy areas of decreased glucose use. PET scans of the brains of patients being treated for cocaine addiction show high activation in the mesolimbic dopamine system activation and in areas from the amygdala and the anterior cingulate to the tip of both temporal lobes. The D2 receptors in the mesolimbic dopamine system have been held responsible for the heightened activity during periods of craving
- Cocaine has powerful addictive qualities. Because of its potency as a positive reinforcer of behavior, psychological dependence on cocaine can develop after a single use. With repeated administration, both tolerance and sensitivity can arise.
- Physiological dependence on cocaine does occur, although cocaine withdrawal is mild compared with withdrawal from opiates and opioids.

ADVERSE EFFECTS

Amphetamines

- Amphetamine abuse can produce a cerebrovascular, cardiac, and gastrointestinal effects, myocardial infarction, severe hypertension, cerebrovascular disease, and ischemic colitis.
- A continuum of neurological symptoms, from twitching to tetany to seizures to coma and death, is associated with increasingly high amphetamine doses.
- They can induce symptoms of anxiety disorders, such as generalized anxiety disorder and panic disorder, as well as ideas of reference, paranoid delusions, and hallucinations.

Cocaine

- A common adverse effect associated with cocaine use is nasal congestion; serious inflammation, swelling, bleeding, and ulceration of the nasal mucosa can also occur. Long-term use of cocaine can also lead to perforation of the nasal septa.
- The IV use of cocaine can result in infection, embolisms, and the transmission of human immunodeficiency virus (HIV).
- The major complications of cocaine use, however are cerebrovascular, epileptic, and cardiac. About two-thirds of these acute toxic effects occur within 1 hour of intoxication, about one-fifth occur in 1 to 3 hours, and the remainder occurs up to several days later.

SIGNS AND SYMPTOMS OF STIMULANT INTOXICATION

1. Mydriasis
2. Psychomotor agitation or retardation
3. Tachycardia or bradycardia

4. Perspiration or chills
5. Cardiac arrhythmia or chest pain
6. Elevated or lowered blood pressure
7. Dyskinesis or dystonias
8. Weight loss
9. Nausea or vomiting
10. Muscular weakness
11. Respiratory depression
12. Confusion, seizures and coma

"Club Drugs"

- The use of a certain group of substances popularly called *club drugs* is often associated with dance clubs, bars, and all-night dance parties (raves).
  The group includes:
  - LSD
  - γ-hydroxybutyrate (GHB)
  - Ketamine
  - Methamphetamine
  - MDMA (ecstasy)
  - Rohypnol or roofies (flunitrazepam).

Nicotine

- The World Health Organization (WHO) estimates there are 1 billion smokers worldwide, and they smoke 6 trillion cigarettes a year. The WHO also estimates that tobacco kills more than 3 million persons each year
- Approximately 50% of all psychiatric outpatients, 70% of outpatients with bipolar I disorder, almost 90% of outpatients with schizophrenia, and 70% of substance use disorder patients smoke
- The high percentage of patients with schizophrenia who smoke has been attributed to nicotine's ability to reduce their extraordinary sensitivity to outside sensory stimuli and to increase their concentration. In that sense, such patients are self-monitoring to relieve distress.
- Death is the primary adverse effect of cigarette smoking. The causes of death include chronic bronchitis and emphysema, bronchogenic cancer, 35% of fatal myocardial infarctions, cerebrovascular disease, cardiovascular disease, and almost all cases of chronic obstructive pulmonary disease and lung cancer.
- The increased use of chewing tobacco and snuff (smokeless tobacco) has been associated with the development of oropharyngeal cancer.
- These substances are not all in the same drug class, nor do they produce the same physical or subjective effects.
- GHB, ketamine, and Rohypnol have been called **date rape drugs** because they produce disorienting and sedating effects, and often users cannot recall what occurred during all or part of an episode under the influence of the drug.

Neuropharmacology

- The psychoactive component of tobacco is nicotine, which affects the central nervous system (CNS) by acting as an agonist at the nicotinic subtype of acetylcholine receptors.
- Nicotine is believed to produce its positive reinforcing and addictive properties by activating the dopaminergic pathway projecting from the ventral tegmental area to the cerebral cortex and the limbic system.
- Nicotine causes an increase in the concentrations of circulating norepinephrine and epinephrine and an increase in the release of vasopressin, β-endorphin, adrenocorticotropic hormone (ACTH), and cortisol. These hormones are thought to contribute to the basic stimulatory effects of nicotine on the CNS.

Adverse Effects

Nicotine is a highly toxic alkaloid. Doses of 60 mg in an adult are fatal secondary to respiratory paralysis; doses of 0.5 mg are delivered by smoking an average cigarette.

Signs of Nicotine Toxicity

1. Nausea
2. Vomiting
3. Salivation
4. Pallor (caused by peripheral vasoconstriction)

5. Weakness
6. Abdominal pain (caused by increased peristalsis)
7. Diarrhea
8. Dizziness
9. Headache
10. Increased blood pressure
11. Tachycardia
12. Tremors
13. Cold sweats
14. Inability to concentrate
15. Confusion
16. Sensory disturbances

Treatment

Psychosocial therapies:
- Behavior therapy.
- Skills training and relapse prevention–identify high-risk situations and plan and practice behavioral or cognitive coping skills for those situations in which smoking occurs.
- Stimulus control–eliminating cues for smoking in the environment.
- Aversive therapy—effective but requires a good therapeutic alliance and patient compliance.
- Hypnosis.

PSYCHOPHARMACOLOGICAL THERAPIES

Nicotine Replacement Therapies

- All nicotine replacement therapies double cessation rates, presumably because they reduce nicotine withdrawal. These therapies can also be used to reduce withdrawal in patients on smoke-free wards.
- Replacement therapies use a short period of maintenance of 6 to 12 weeks often followed by a gradual reduction period of another 6 to 12 weeks.
- Nicotine polacrilex gum (Nicorette) is an OTC product that releases nicotine via chewing and buccal absorption
- Nicotine lozenges, Nicotine patches, Nicotine nasal spray and the nicotine inhaler are other available nicotine replacement therapy forms.

Non-nicotine Medications

- Non-nicotine therapy may help smokers who object philosophically to the notion of replacement therapy and smokers who fail replacement therapy.
- Bupropion (Zyban) (marketed as Wellbutrin for depression) is an antidepressant medication that has both dopaminergic and adrenergic actions.
- Clonidine (Catapres) decreases sympathetic activity from the locus ceruleus and, thus, is thought to abate withdrawal symptoms
- A nicotine vaccine that produces nicotine-specific antibodies in the brain is under investigation at the National Institute on Drug Abuse (NIDA).

ALCOHOL SIGNS OF ALCOHOL INTOXICATION

1. Slurred speech
2. Dizziness
3. Incoordination
4. Unsteady gait
5. Nystagmus
6. Impairment in attention or memory
7. Stupor or coma
8. Double vision

IMPAIRMENT SEEN AT VARIOUS BLOOD ALCOHOL CONCENTRATIONS

Level	Likely impairment
20-30 mg/dL	Slowed motor performance and decreased thinking ability
30-80 mg/dL	Increases in motor and cognitive problems
80-200 mg/dL	Increases in incoordination and judgment errors Mood lability Deterioration in cognition
200-300 mg/dL	Nystagmus, marked slurring of speck, and alcoholic blackouts
>300 mg/dL	Impaired vital signs and possible death

- A single drink is usually considered to contain about 12 g of ethanol, which is the content of 12 ounces of beer (7.2 proof, 3.6% ethanol in the United States), one 4-ounce glass of nonfortified wine, or 1 to 1.5 ounces of an 80-proof (40% ethanol) liquor (e.g. whiskey or gin).
- A single drink increases the blood alcohol level of a 150-pound man by 15 to 20 mg/dL, which is about the concentration of alcohol that an average person can metabolize in 1 hour.
- About 10 percent of consumed alcohol is absorbed from the stomach, and the remainder from the small intestine. Peak blood concentration of alcohol is reached in 30 to 90 minutes, depending on whether the alcohol was ingested on an empty stomach (which enhances absorption) or with food (which delays absorption).
- The time to peak blood concentration also depends on the time during which the alcohol was consumed; rapid drinking reduces the time to peak concentration, slower drinking increases it.
- About 90 percent of absorbed alcohol is metabolized through oxidation in the liver; the remaining 10 percent is excreted unchanged by the kidneys and lungs. The rate of oxidation by the liver is constant and independent of the body's energy requirements.
- The body can metabolize about 15 mg/dL per hour.
- Alcohol is metabolized by two enzymes: alcohol dehydrogenase (ADH) and aldehyde dehydrogenase. ADH catalyzes the conversion of alcohol into acetaldehyde, which is a toxic compound; aldehyde dehydrogenase catalyzes the conversion of acetaldehyde into acetic acid. Aldehyde dehydrogenase is inhibited by disulfiram (Antabuse), often used in the treatment of alcohol-related disorders.

Delirium tremens—the most severe form of the withdrawal syndrome; medical emergency
- Untreated, DTS has a mortality rate of 20 percent,
- The essential feature of the syndrome is delirium occurring within 1 week after a person stops drinking or reduces the intake of alcohol.
- In addition to the symptoms of delirium, the features of alcohol intoxication delirium include autonomic hyperactivity such as tachycardia, diaphoresis, fever, anxiety, insomnia, and hypertension; perceptual distortions, most frequently visual or tactile hallucinations; and fluctuating levels of psychomotor activity, ranging from hyper excitability to lethargy.
- About 5 percent are hospitalized
- The syndrome usually develops on the third hospital day
- Episodes of DTS usually begin in a patient's 30s or 40s after 5 to 15 years of heavy drinking, typically of the binge type. Physical illness (e.g. hepatitis or pancreatitis) predisposes to the syndrome.

Treatment
- Prevention
- Benzodiazepines
- Avoid antipsychotics that can lower threshold for seizures
- High calorie/ carbohydrate diet with multivitamin supplementation
- Anticonvulsant medication not useful
- Supportive psychotherapy

Alcohol Withdrawal: It can include seizures and autonomic hyperactivity.
- Conditions that predispose include fatigue, malnutrition, physical illness, and depression.
- The DSM-5 criteria for alcohol withdrawal require
- The cessation or reduction of alcohol use that was heavy and prolonged as well as the presence of specific physical or neuropsychiatric symptoms.
- The classic sign is tremulousness; it can include psychotic and perceptual symptoms (e.g. delusions and hallucinations), seizures, and the symptoms of delirium tremens (DTs), called alcohol delirium in DSM-5.

- Tremulousness develops 6 to 8 hours after the cessation of drinking
- The psychotic and perceptual symptoms begin in 8 to 12 hours
- Seizures in 12 to 24 hours, and DTs anytime during the first 72 hours
- Other symptoms of withdrawal include general irritability, gastrointestinal symptoms (e.g. nausea and vomiting), and sympathetic autonomic hyperactivity, including anxiety, arousal, sweating, facial flushing, mydriasis, tachycardia, and mild hypertension.

Diagnosis and Clinical Features DSM-5

- A need for daily use of large amounts of alcohol for adequate functioning
- A regular pattern of heavy drinking limited to weekends, and long periods of sobriety interspersed with binges of heavy alcohol intake

The drinking patterns are often associated with certain behaviors:

- The inability to cut down or stop drinking;
- Repeated efforts to control or reduce excessive drinking by periods of temporary abstinence or by restricting drinking to certain times of the day;
- Binges (remaining intoxicated throughout the day for at least 2 days);
- Occasional consumption of a fifth of spirits (or its equivalent in wine or beer);
- Amnestic periods for events occurring while intoxicated (blackouts);
- The continuation of drinking despite a serious physical disorder that the person knows is exacerbated by alcohol use
- Drinking nonbeverage alcohol, such as fuel and commercial products containing alcohol.
- Impaired social or occupational functioning because of alcohol use (e.g., violence while intoxicated, absence from work, job loss)
- Legal difficulties (e.g., arrest for intoxicated behavior and traffic accidents while intoxicated)
- Arguments or difficulties with family members or friends about excessive alcohol consumption.

FETAL ALCOHOL SYNDROME

- The alcohol inhibits intrauterine growth and postnatal development.
- Microcephaly, craniofacial malformations, and limb and heart defects are common in affected infants.
- Short adult stature; development of adult maladaptive behaviors
- Women with alcohol-related disorders have a 35% risk of having a child with defects.
- Damage seems to result from exposure in utero to ethanol or to its metabolites; hormone imbalances due to alcohol consumption increase the risk of abnormalities.

TREATMENT OF ALCOHOL WITHDRAWAL

Tremulousness and mild to moderate agitation	Chlordiazepoxide	Oral	25-100 mg every 4-6 hrs
	Diazepam	Oral	5-20 mg every 4-6 hrs
Hallucinosis	Lorazepam	Oral	2-10 mg every 4-6 hrs
Extreme agitation	Chlordiazepoxide	Intravenous	0.5 mg/kg at 12.5 mg/min
Withdrawal seizures	Diazepam	Intravenous	0.15 mg/kg at 2.5 mg/min
Delirium tremens	Lorazepam	Intravenous	0.1 mg/kg at 2.0 mg/min

OPIOID

Neuropharmacology

- The primary effects of the opioid drugs are mediated via the opioid receptors
- The μ-opioid receptors are involved in the regulation and mediation of analgesia, respiratory depression, constipation, and drug dependence;
- K-opioid receptors, with analgesia, diuresis, and sedation;
- Δ-opioid receptors, with analgesia.
- In 1975, the enkephalins were identified; three classes of endogenous opioids: the endorphins, the dynorphins, and the enkephalins.
- The term "endorphin" was coined by Dr. Eric simon
- Endorphins are involved in neural transmission and pain suppression, released naturally in the body when a person is physically hurt or severely stressed accounting for the absence of pain during acute injuries.

- The addictive rewarding properties of opioids are mediated through activation of the ventral tegmental area dopaminergic neurons that project to the cerebral cortex and the limbic system
- About 90% of persons with opioid dependence have an additional psychiatric disorder.
- MC—major depressive disorder, alcohol use disorders, antisocial personality disorder, and anxiety disorders.
- 15%—attempt suicide at least once.

Morphine and Heroin

- The morphine and heroin withdrawal syndrome begins 6 to 8 hours after the last dose, usually after a 1- to 2- week period of continuous use or after the administration of a narcotic antagonist.
- The withdrawal syndrome reaches its peak intensity during the second or third day and subsides during the next 7 to 10 days, but some symptoms may persist for 6 months or longer.
- **Meperidine:** The withdrawal syndrome from meperidine begins quickly, reaches a peak in 8 to 12 hours, and ends in 4 to 5 days.
- **Methadone:** Methadone withdrawal usually begins 1 to 3 days after the last dose and ends in 10 to 14 days.

Clinical Features

The physical effects of opioids include respiratory depression, pupillary constriction, smooth muscle contraction (including the ureters and the bile ducts), constipation, and changes in blood pressure, heart rate, and body temperature. The respiratory depressant effects are mediated at the level of the brainstem reason.

Opioid Overdose

- Death—respiratory arrest from the respiratory depressant effect of the drug.
- The symptoms of overdose include marked unresponsiveness, coma, slow respiration, hypothermia, hypotension, and bradycardia. (clinical triad of coma, pinpoint pupils, and respiratory depression) penis.

MPTP-Induced Parkinsonism

- In 1976, after ingesting an opioid contaminated with methyl-phenyltetrahydropyridine (MPTP), several persons developed a syndrome of irreversible parkinsonism.
- The mechanism for the neurotoxic effect is as follows: MPTP is converted into 1-methyl-4 phenylpyridinium (MPP+) by the enzyme monoamine oxidase and is then taken up by dopaminergic neurons.
- Because MPP+ binds to melanin in substantia nigra neurons, MPP+ is concentrated in these neurons and eventually kills the cells.

Opioid Agents for Treating Opioid Withdrawal

Methadone

- Synthetic narcotic that substitutes for heroin; can be taken orally
- The drug suppresses withdrawal symptoms.
- A daily dose of 20 to 80 mg suffices to stabilize a patient,
- The duration of action for methadone exceeds 24 hours; thus, once-daily dosing is adequate.
- Methadone maintenance is continued until the patient can be withdrawn from methadone, which itself causes dependence. An abstinence syndrome occurs with methadone withdrawal, but patients are detoxified from methadone more easily than from heroin.
- Clonidine (0.1 to 0.3 mg three to four times a day) is usually given during the detoxification period.

Advantages
- Frees persons with opioid dependence from using injectable heroin
- Reduces the chance of spreading HIV through contaminated needles.
- Produces minimal euphoria and rarely causes drowsiness or depression when taken for a long time.
- Allows patients to engage in gainful employment instead of criminal activity.

Disadvantage of methadone use is that patients remain dependent on a narcotic.

Other Opioid Substitutes

Levomethadyl (LAAM)

- LAAM is an opioid agonist that suppresses opioid withdrawal.
- It is no longer used because some patients developed prolonged QT intervals associated with potentially fatal arrhythmias (*torsades de pointes*).

Buprenorphine
- Opioid agonist
- Buprenorphine in a daily dose of 8 to 10 mg appears to reduce heroin use.
- Buprenorphine also is effective in thrice-weekly dosing because of its slow dissociation from opioid receptors.
- After repeated administration, it attenuates or blocks the subjective effects of parenterally administered opioids such as heroin or morphine.
- A mild opioid withdrawal syndrome occurs if the drug is abruptly discontinued after chronic administrations.

OPIOID ANTAGONISTS

- Opioid antagonists block or antagonize the effects of opioids.
- They do not exert narcotic effects and do not cause dependence.
- Opioid antagonists include:
  - Naloxone, which is used in the treatment of opioid overdose because it reverses the effects of narcotics,
  - Naltrexone, the longest-acting (72 hours) antagonist.
  - The theory for using an antagonist for opioid-related disorders is that blocking opioid agonist effects, particularly euphoria, discourages persons with opioid dependence from substanceseeking behavior and, thus, deconditions this behavior.

INHALANTS

- Inhalant drugs (*volatile substances* or *solvents*) are volatile hydrocarbons that vaporize to gaseous fumes at room temperature and are inhaled through the nose or mouth to enter the bloodstream via the transpulmonary route.
- Commonly found in many household products
- Divided into four commercial classes:
  - Solvents for glues and adhesives
  - Propellants (e.g., for aerosol paint sprays, hair sprays, and shaving cream)
  - Thinners (e.g., for paint products and correction fluids)
  - Fuels (e.g., gasoline, propane).

NEUROPHARMACOLOGY

- 15 to 20 breaths of 1 percent gasoline vapor produce several hours of intoxication.
- Inhalants generally act as a central nervous system (CNS) depressant.
- Their effects are similar and additive to the effects of other CNS depressants it has been suggested that inhalants operate by enhancing the γ-aminobutyric acid (GABA) system. Others have suggested that inhalants work through membrane fluidization, which has also been hypothesized to be a pharmacodynamic effect of ethanol.

Clinical Features

- Small initial doses—disinhibiting, feelings of euphoria and excitement, pleasant floating sensations
- High doses—fearfulness, sensory illusions, auditory and visual hallucinations, and distortions of body size.
- Neurological symptoms—slurred speech, decreased speed of talking, and ataxia.
- Long-term use—irritability, emotional lability, and impaired memory.
- Withdrawal syndrome—sleep disturbances, irritability, jitteriness, sweating, nausea, vomiting, tachycardia, and (sometimes) delusions and hallucinations.
- The intoxicated state—apathy, diminished social and occupational functioning, impaired judgment, and impulsive or aggressive behavior, and it can be accompanied by nausea, anorexia, nystagmus, depressed reflexes, and diplopia.
- A recent user of inhalants can be identified by rashes around the patient's nose and mouth; unusual breath odors; the residue of the inhalant substances on the patient's face, hands, or clothing; and irritation of the patient's eyes, throat, lungs, and nose.

DISSOCIATIVE DISORDERS

Dissociative Amnesia

- The essential feature of dissociative amnesia is an inability to recall important personal information, usually of a traumatic or stressful nature, that is too extensive to be explained by normal forgetfulness

- It is frequently found in those who have experienced extreme acute trauma
- It also commonly develops, however, in the context of profound intrapsychic conflict or emotional stress
- Many of these patients have histories of prior adult or childhood abuse or trauma
- It has been reported in approximately 6 percent of the general population
- No known difference is seen in incidence between men and women. Cases generally begin to be reported in late adolescence and adulthood.

ETIOLOGY

Amnesia and Extreme Intrapsychic Conflict
The psychosocial environment out of which the amnesia develops is massively conflictual, with the patient experiencing intolerable emotions of shame, guilt, despair, rage, and desperation. These usually result from conflicts over unacceptable urges or impulses, such as intense sexual, suicidal, or violent compulsions.

Betrayal Trauma
Betrayal trauma attempts to explain amnesia by the intensity of trauma and by the extent that a negative event represents a betrayal by a trusted, needed other. This betrayal is thought to influence the way in which the event is processed and remembered.

Types of Dissociative Amnesia
- **Localized amnesia:** Inability to recall events related to a circumscribed period of time
- **Selective amnesia:** Ability to remember some, but not all, of the events occurring during a circumscribed period of time
- **Generalized amnesia:** Failure to recall one's entire life
- **Continuous amnesia:** Failure to recall successive events as they occur
- **Systematized amnesia:** Amnesia for certain categories of memory, such as all memories relating to one's family or to a particular person.

Differential Diagnosis
- Ordinary forgetfulness and nonpathological amnesia
- Dementia
- Delirium, and organic amnestic disorders
- Post-traumatic amnesia
- Seizure disorders
- Substance-related amnesia
- Transient global amnesia
- Acute stress disorder, post-traumatic stress disorder
- Somatoform disorders
- Malingering and factitious amnesia

Course and Prognosis
- Acute dissociative amnesia frequently spontaneously resolves once the person is removed to safety from traumatic or overwhelming circumstances.
- Some patients do develop chronic forms of generalized, continuous, or severe localized amnesia and are profoundly disabled and require high levels of social support, such as nursing home placement or intensive family caretaking.

Treatment
- Cognitive therapy
- Hypnosis
- Somatic therapies
- Group psychotherapy

Dissociative Fugue
- Sudden, unexpected travel away from home or one's customary place of daily activities, with inability to recall some or all of one's past.

- This is accompanied by confusion about personal identity or even the assumption of a new identity.
- The disturbance does not occur exclusively during the course of dissociative identity disorder
- It is not due to the direct physiological effects of a substance or a general medical condition.
- The symptoms must cause clinically significant distress or impairment in social, occupational, or other important areas of functioning.

Etiology
- Traumatic circumstances (i.e. combat, rape, recurrent childhood sexual abuse, massive social dislocations, natural disasters), leading to an altered state of consciousness dominated by a wish to flee, are the underlying cause of most fugue episodes
- The patients are usually struggling with extreme emotions or impulses (i.e., overwhelming fear, guilt, shame, or intense incestuous, sexual, suicidal, or violent urges) that are in conflict with the patient's conscience or ego ideals.

Course and Prognosis
Most fugues are relatively brief, lasting from hours to days. Most individuals appear to recover, although refractory dissociative amnesia may persist in rare cases.

Treatment
- Dissociative fugue is usually treated with an eclectic, psychodynamically oriented psychotherapy that focuses on helping the patient recover memory for identity and recent experience.
- Hypnotherapy and pharmacologically facilitated interviews are frequently necessary adjunctive techniques to assist with memory recovery.
- Family treatment and social service interventions.

Dissociative Identity Disorder
- Dissociative identity disorder, previously called **multiple personality disorder**, is characterized by the presence of two or more distinct identities or personality states that recurrently take control of the individual's behavior accompanied by an inability to recall important personal information that is too extensive to be explained by ordinary forgetfulness.
- The identities or personality states, sometimes called *alters*, *self-states*, *alter identities*, or *parts*, among other terms, differ from one another in that each presents as having its own relatively enduring pattern of perceiving, relating to, and thinking about the environment and self.

Epidemiology and Etiology
- Female to male ratios between 5 to 1 and 9 to 1 for diagnosed cases.
- Dissociative identity disorder is strongly linked to severe experiences of early childhood trauma, usually maltreatment.
- Physical and sexual abuse are the most frequently reported sources of childhood trauma.

Memory and Amnesia Symptoms
- Dissociative time loss experiences are too extensive to be explained by normal forgetting and typically have sharply demarcated onsets and offsets.
- Patients with dissociative disorder often report significant gaps in autobiographical memory, especially for childhood events.
- Dissociative gaps in autobiographical recall are usually sharply demarcated and do not fit the normal decline in autobiographical recall for younger ages.

Dissociative Alterations in Identity
- Clinically, dissociative alterations in identity may first be manifested by odd first-person plural or third person singular or plural self-references.
- In addition, patients may refer to themselves using their own first names or make depersonalized self-references, such as the body, when describing themselves and others.

Course and Prognosis
- Prognosis is poorer in patients with:
  - Comorbid organic mental disorders
  - Psychotic disorders (*not* dissociative identity disorder pseudo-psychosis severe medical illnesses.
  - Refractory substance abuse
  - Eating disorders
  - Significant antisocial personality features

- Current criminal activity
- Ongoing perpetration of abuse and current victimization, with refusal to leave abusive relationships
- Repeated adult traumas with recurrent episodes of acute stress disorder.

Treatment
- Psychoanalytical psychotherapy
- Cognitive and behavioral therapy
- Hypnosis
- Psychopharmacological interventions
- Electroconvulsive therapy
- Adjunctive treatments
- Group therapy
- Family therapy
- Self-help groups
- Expressive and occupational therapies.

Depersonalization/Derealization Disorder
- The essential feature of depersonalization as the persistent or recurrent feeling of detachment or estrangement from one's self
- Derealization refers to feelings of unreality or of being detached from ones environment.

Epidemiology
- Commonly seen in
  - Normal and clinical populations
  - Seizure patients and migraine sufferers
  - Use of psychedelic drugs; side effect of some medications, such as anticholinergic agents
  - After certain types of meditation, deep hypnosis, extended mirror or crystal gazing, and sensory deprivation experiences
- The third most commonly reported psychiatric symptoms, after depression and anxiety.

Etiology
- **Psychodynamic:** Traditional psychodynamic formulations have emphasized the disintegration of the ego or have viewed depersonalization as an affective response in defense of the ego.
- **Traumatic stress:** One-third to one-half, of patients in clinical depersonalization case series report histories of significant trauma
- **Neurobiological theories:**
  - Studies strongly implicate the *N*-Methyl-D Aspartate (NMDA) subtype of the glutamate receptor as central to the genesis of depersonalization symptoms
  - The association of depersonalization with migraines and marijuana, its generally favorable response to selective serotonin reuptake inhibitor (SSRI) drugs point to serotoninergic involvement.

Diagnosis and Clinical Features
- A number of distinct components comprise the experience of depersonalization, including a sense of:
  1. Bodily changes
  2. Duality of self as observer and actor
  3. Being cut off from others
  4. Being cut off from one's own emotions.
- Patients experiencing depersonalization often have great difficulty expressing what they are feeling.

Course and Prognosis
- Depersonalization after traumatic experiences or intoxications commonly remits spontaneously after removal from the traumatic circumstances or ending of the episode of intoxication
- Depersonalization accompanying mood, psychotic, or other anxiety disorders commonly remits with definitive treatment of these conditions.

Treatment
Patients with depersonalization disorder are often found to be a singularly clinically refractory group.

- **Pharmacotherapy:**
  - Antidepressants
  - Mood stabilizers
  - Typical and atypical neuroleptics
  - Anticonvulsants
- **Psychotherapy:**
  - Psychodynamic
  - Cognitive
  - Cognitive-behavioral
  - Hypnotherapeutic
  - Supportive stress management strategies
  - Distraction techniques
  - Reduction of sensory stimulation
  - Relaxation training
  - Physical exercise

Ganser Syndrome

- Ganser syndrome is a poorly understood condition characterized by the giving of **approximate answers** (paralogia) together with a clouding of consciousness, and frequently accompanied by hallucinations and other dissociative, somatoform, or conversion symptoms.
- Men outnumber women by approximately 2 to 1 and Three of Ganser's first four cases were **convicts**, leading some authors to consider it to be a disorder of penal populations and an indicator of potential malingering.
- The symptom of *passing over* (***vorbeigehen***) the correct answer for a related, but incorrect one, is the hallmark of Ganser syndrome. The approximate answers often just miss the mark but bear an obvious relation to the question, indicating that it has been understood.
- Neurological examination may reveal what Ganser called **hysterical stigmata**, for example, a nonneurological analgesia or shifting hyperalgesia. It must be accompanied by other dissociative symptoms, such as amnesias, conversion symptoms, or trance-like behaviors.
- Usually, a relatively rapid return to normal function occurs within days, although some cases may take a month or more to resolve. The individual is typically amnesic for the period of the syndrome.

Note

- The tenth edition of the *International Statistical Classification of Diseases and Related Health Problems* (ICD-10) classifies the dissociative disorders among the *neurotic*, *stress-related*, and *somatoform disorders*.
- The ICD-10 explicitly states that the term *hysteria* should be avoided because of its lack of precision.
- The ICD-10 dissociative [conversion] disorders include.
  - Dissociative amnesia
  - Dissociative fugue
  - Dissociative stupor
  - Trance and possession disorder
  - Dissociative disorders of movement and sensation.
- The latter includes dissociative motor disorders, dissociative convulsions, and dissociative anesthesia and sensory loss.
- Ganser syndrome and multiplex personality disorder are classified under *other* dissociative disorders. Depersonalization disorder is classified separately.

Anorexia Nervosa

- Anorexia nervosa is a syndrome characterized by three essential criteria.
- The onset of anorexia nervosa usually occurs between the ages of 10 and 30 years.
- It is present when
  - An individual voluntarily reduces and maintains an unhealthy degree of weight loss or fails to gain weight proportional to growth—a behavior
  - An individual experiences an intense fear of becoming fat, has a relentless drive for thinness despite obvious medical starvation, or both–a psychopathology
  - An individual experiences significant starvation-related medical symptomatology, often, but not exclusively, abnormal reproductive hormone functioning, but also hypothermia, bradycardia, orthostasis, and severely reduced body fat stores a physiological symptomatology
  - The behaviors and psychopathology are present for at least 3.

- The most common age of onset is between 14 and 18 years. Anorexia nervosa is estimated to occur in about 0.5 to 1% of adolescent girls.
- It occurs 10 to 20 times more often in females than in males
- It seems to be most frequent in developed countries, and it may be seen with greatest frequency among young women in professions that require thinness, such as modeling and ballet.

Comorbidity

Anorexia nervosa is associated with depression in 65% of cases, social phobia in 35% of cases, and obsessive-compulsive disorder in 25% of cases.

Etiology

Biological Factors

- Starvation produces amenorrhea, which reflects lowered hormonal levels (luteinizing, follicle-stimulating, and gonadotropin-releasing hormones). Some patients with anorexia nervosa, however, become amenorrheic before significant weight loss.
- Endogenous opioids may contribute to the denial of hunger in patients with anorexia nervosa a hypothalamic-pituitary axis (neuroendocrine) dysfunction.
- Some studies have shown evidence for dysfunction in serotonin, dopamine, and norepinephrine, three neurotransmitters involved in regulating eating behavior in the paraventricular nucleus of the hypothalamus.
- Other humoral factors that may be involved include corticotropin-releasing factor (CRF), neuropeptide Y, gonadotropin-releasing hormone, and thyroid-stimulating hormone.

Social Factors

- Patients with anorexia nervosa find support for their practices in society's emphasis on thinness and exercise.
- These patients have close, but troubled, relationships with their parents.
- Families of children who present with eating disorders, may exhibit high levels of hostility, chaos, and isolation and low levels of nurturance and empathy.

Psychological and Psychodynamic Factors

- Anorexia nervosa appears to be a reaction to the demand that adolescents behave more independently and increase their social and sexual functioning.
- These patients typically lack a sense of autonomy and selfhood.
- A projective identification process is involved in the interactions between the patient and the patient's family.
- These young patients have been unable to separate psychologically from their mothers. The body may be perceived as though it were inhabited by the introject of an intrusive and unempathic mother. Starvation may unconsciously mean arresting the growth of this intrusive internal object and thereby destroying it.

Pathology and Laboratory Examination

- In emaciated patients with anorexia nervosa.
- A complete blood count often reveals leukopenia with a relative lymphocytosis.
- If binge eating and purging are present, serum electrolyte determination reveals hypokalemic alkalosis.
- Fasting serum glucose concentrations are often low
- Serum salivary amylase concentrations are often elevated if the patient is vomiting.
- The ECG may show ST segment and T-wave changes, which are usually secondary to electrolyte disturbances; patients have hypotension and bradycardia.
- Young girls may have a high serum cholesterol level.
- All these values revert to normal with nutritional rehabilitation and cessation of purging behaviors.
- Endocrine changes that occur, such as amenorrhea, mild hypothyroidism, and hypersecretion of corticotrophin-releasing hormone are caused by the underweight condition and revert to normal with weight gain.

Subtypes

- Anorexia nervosa has been divided into two subtypes:
    - The food-restricting category
    - The binge eating or purging category.
- **In the food-restricting category:**
    - Present in approximately 50% of cases
    - Food intake is highly, and the patient may be relentlessly and compulsively overactive, with overuse athletic injuries.

- **In the binge-eating or purging subtype**:
  - Patients alternate attempts at rigorous dieting with intermittent binge or purge episodes
  - Purging represents a secondary compensation for the unwanted calories, most often accomplished by self-induced vomiting, frequently by laxative abuse, less frequently by diuretics, and occasionally with emetics.
  - Sometimes, repetitive purging occurs.

Course and Prognosis
- Restricting-type anorectic patients seemed less likely to recover than those of the binge eating-purging type.
- **Indicators of a favorable outcome**:
  - Admission of hunger
  - Lessening of denial and immaturity
  - Improved self-esteem
- **Indicators of a poor outcome:**
  - Childhood neuroticism
  - Parental conflict
  - Bulimia nervosa
  - Vomiting
  - Laxative abuse
  - Various behavioral manifestations (e.g. obsessive-compulsive, hysterical, depressive, psychosomatic, neurotic, and denial symptoms).
- About half of patients with anorexia nervosa eventually will have the symptoms of bulimia, usually within the first year after the onset of anorexia nervosa.
- In general, the prognosis is not good. Studies have shown a range of mortality rates from 5 to 18 percent.

Treatment
- Hospitalization
- Psychotherapy
- Cognitive-behavioral therapy
- Dynamic psychotherapy
- Family therapy
- Pharmacotherapy
  - Cyproheptadine
  - Amitriptyline
  - Clomipramine
  - Pimozide
  - Chlorpromazine

Bulimia Nervosa
- Bulimia nervosa is present when
  1. Episodes of binge-eating occur relatively frequently (twice a week or more) for at least 3 months
  2. Compensatory behaviors are practiced after binge eating to prevent weight gain, primarily self-induced vomiting, laxative abuse, diuretics, or abuse of emetics (80% of cases), and, less commonly, severe dieting and strenuous exercise (20% of cases);
  3. Weight is not severely lowered as in anorexia nervosa;
  4. The patient has a morbid fear of fatness, a relentless drive for thinness, or both and a disproportionate amount of self-evaluation depends on body weight and shape.
- When making a diagnosis of bulimia nervosa, clinicians should explore the possibility that the patient has experienced a brief or prolonged prior bout of anorexia nervosa, present in approximately half of those with bulimia nervosa.
- Binging usually precedes vomiting by about 1 year.
- Bulimia nervosa is more prevalent than anorexia nervosa.
- Estimates of bulimia nervosa range from 2 to 4% of young women.
- More common in women than in men, but its onset is often later in adolescence.

Etiology

Social Factors
- Patients with bulimia nervosa, as with those with anorexia nervosa, tend to be high achievers and to respond to societal pressures to be slender.
- Families of patients with bulimia nervosa are generally less close and more conflictual than the families of those with anorexia nervosa.
- Patients with bulimia nervosa describe their parents as neglectful and rejecting.

Psychological Factors
- Patients with bulimia nervosa are more outgoing, angry, and impulsive than those with anorexia nervosa. Alcohol dependence, shoplifting, and emotional lability (including suicide attempts) are associated with bulimia nervosa.
- These patients generally experience their uncontrolled eating as more ego-dystonic than do patients with anorexia nervosa and so seek help more readily.

Biological Factors
- Because antidepressants often benefit patients with bulimia nervosa and because serotonin has been linked to satiety, serotonin and norepinephrine have been implicated increased frequency of bulimia nervosa is found in first-degree relatives of persons with the disorder.
- Plasma endorphin levels are raised in some bulimia nervosa patients.

Subtypes
- The diagnosis of bulimia nervosa is subtyped into:
  - Purging type–for those who regularly engage in self-induced vomiting or the use of laxatives or diuretics
  - Nonpurging type–for those who use strict dieting, fasting, or vigorous exercise but do not regularly engage in purging
- Patients with the purging type of bulimia nervosa may be at risk for certain medical complications, such as hypokalemia from vomiting or laxative abuse and hypochloremic alkalosis.
- Those who vomit repeatedly are at risk for gastric and esophageal tears, although these complications are rare.
- Patients who purge may have a different course from that of patients who binge and then diet or exercise.

Pathology and Laboratory Investigations
- Dehydration and electrolyte disturbances are likely to occur in patients with bulimia nervosa who purge regularly. These patients commonly exhibit hypomagnesemia and hyperamylasemia.
- Although not a core diagnostic feature, many patients with bulimia nervosa have menstrual disturbances.

Course and Prognosis
- Bulimia nervosa is characterized by higher rates of partial and full recovery compared with anorexia nervosa.
- A history of substance use problems and a longer duration of the disorder at presentation predicted worse outcome.

Treatment
- Psychotherapy
- Cognitive-behavioral therapy
- Dynamic psychotherapy
- Pharmacotherapy: antidepressants, mood stabilizers.

NEUROLEPTIC MALIGNANT SYNDROME
- Neuroleptic malignant syndrome (NMS) is a rare, potentially fatal, consequence of neuroleptic administration.
- The syndrome consists of autonomic instability, hyperpyrexia, severe extrapyramidal symptoms (i.e. rigidity), and delirium.
- Sustained muscle contraction results in peripheral heat generation and muscle breakdown. Muscle breakdown contributes to elevated levels of creatine kinase (CK). Peripheral heat generation with impaired central mechanisms of thermoregulation results in hyperpyrexia.
- Myoglobinuria and leukocytosis are common.
- Hepatic and renal failure may occur. Liver enzymes become elevated with liver failure.
- Patients may die from hyperpyrexia, aspiration pneumonia, renal failure, hepatic failure, respiratory arrest, or cardiovascular collapse.

- **Treatment** includes discontinuation of the neuroleptic, hydration, administration of muscle relaxants, and general supportive nursing care.
- A typical **laboratory workup** for NMS includes a CBC, serum electrolytes, BUN, Cr, and CK. A urinalysis, including an assessment of urine myoglobin, is also usually performed.
- Pronounced elevations in the white blood cell (WBC) count may occur in NMS. White blood cell counts are typically in the range from 10,000 to 40,000 per mm^3.

TRICHOTILLOMANIA

Coined by a French dermatologist Francois Hallopeau in 1889.

Epidemiology
- The most serious, chronic form begins in early to mid-adolescence, with a lifetime prevalence 0.6 percent to as high as 3.4 percent in general populations and with female to male ratio as high as 10 to 1.
- An estimated 35 to 40 percent of patients with hair-pulling disorder chew or swallow the hair that they pull out at one time or another - one-third develop potentially hazardous bezoars—hairballs accumulating in the alimentary tract.

Comorbidity
Obsessive-compulsive disorder (OCD); anxiety disorders; Tourette's disorder; depressive disorders; eating disorders; personality disorders—particularly obsessive-compulsive, borderline, and narcissistic personality disorders.

Etiology
Disturbances in mother–child relationships, fear of being left alone, and recent object loss are often cited as critical factors contributing to the condition.

DIAGNOSIS AND CLINICAL FEATURES

The Fifth edition of the *Diagnostic and Statistical Manual of Mental Disorders* (DSM-5) includes diagnostic criteria from hair-pulling disorder.
- Before engaging in the behavior, patients with hair-pulling disorder may experience an increasing sense of tension and achieve a sense of release or gratification from pulling out their hair All areas of the body may be affected, most commonly the scalp
- Two types of hair pulling–
  - *Focused pulling* is the use of an intentional act to control unpleasant personal experiences, Such as an urge, bodily sensation (e.g., itching or burning), or thought.
  - *Automatic pulling* occurs outside the person's awareness and most often during sedentary activities. Most patients have a combination of these types of hair pulling.
- Hair loss is characterized by short, broken strands appearing together with long, normal hairs in the affected areas. No abnormalities of the skin or scalp are present.
- Trichophagy, mouthing of the hair, may follow the hair plucking. Complications of trichophagy include trichobezoars, malnutrition, and intestinal obstruction.
- Head banging, nail biting, scratching, gnawing, excoriation, and other acts of self-mutilation may be present.

Course and Prognosis
- An early onset (before age 6) tends to remit more readily and responds to suggestions, support, and behavioral strategies.
- Late onset (after age 13) is associated with an increased likelihood of chronicity and poorer prognosis than the early-onset form.

Treatment
- Psychopharmacological methods include topical steroids and hydroxyzine hydrochloride (Vistaril), an anxiolytic with antihistamine properties; antidepressants; and antipsychotics.
- Successful behavioral treatments, such as biofeedback, self-monitoring, desensitization, and habit reversal, insight-oriented psychotherapy, hypnotherapy

BODY DYSMORPHIC DISORDER

- Body dysmorphic disorder is characterized by a preoccupation with an imagined defect in appearance that causes clinically significant distress or impairment in important areas of functioning.
- If a slight physical anomaly is actually present, the person's concern with the anomaly is excessive and bothersome.

Diagnosis

The DSM-5 diagnostic criteria for body dysmorphic disorder stipulate
- Preoccupation with a perceived defect in appearance or overemphasis of a slight defect.
- The patient performs compulsive behaviors (i.e. mirror checking, excessive grooming) or mental acts (e.g. comparing their appearance to that of others).
- The preoccupation causes patients significant emotional distress or markedly impairs their ability to function in important areas.

Clinical Features
- The most common concerns involve facial flaws, particularly those involving specific parts (e.g., the nose).
- Patients had concerns about four body regions during the course of the disorder. Other body parts of concern are hair, breasts, and genitalia.
- Common associated symptoms include ideas or frank delusions of reference (usually about persons' noticing the alleged body flaw), either excessive mirror checking or avoidance of reflective surfaces, and attempts to hide the presumed deformity (with makeup or clothing).
- The effects: Almost all affected patients avoid social and occupational exposure; patients may be housebound because of worry about being ridiculed for the alleged deformities; and one-fifth of patients attempt suicide.
- Comorbid diagnoses of depressive disorders and anxiety disorders are common, and patients may also have traits of OCD, schizoid, and narcissistic personality disorders.

Course and Prognosis
- Body dysmorphic disorder usually begins during adolescence.
- The onset can be gradual or abrupt.
- The disorder usually has a long and undulating course with few symptom-free intervals.
- The part of the body on which concern is focused may remain the same or may change over time.

Treatment
- Treatment of patients with body dysmorphic disorder with surgical, dermatological, dental, and other medical procedures to address the alleged defects is almost invariably unsuccessful.
- Serotonin-specific drugs reduce symptoms in at least 50 percent of patients. In any patient with a coexisting mental disorder, the coexisting disorder should be treated with the appropriate pharmacotherapy and psychotherapy.

EXCORIATION (SKIN-PICKING) DISORDER
- Excoriation or skin-picking disorder is characterized by the compulsive and repetitive picking of the skin. It can lead to severe tissue damage and result in the need for various dermatological treatments.
- Skin-picking disorder has had many names: skin-picking syndrome, emotional excoriation, nervous scratching artifact, epidermotillomania, and para-artificial excoriation.

Epidemiology
- 1 to 5 percent in the general population.
- It is more prevalent in women than in men.

Comorbidity
OCD, trichotillomania, substance dependence, major depressive disorder, anxiety disorders, body dysmorphic disorder, borderline and obsessive-compulsive personality disorder

Diagnosis
- DSM-5 it was called trichotillomania. It was also known as skin-picking syndrome.
- Diagnostic criteria for skin-picking disorder requires recurrent skin-picking resulting in skin lesions and repeated attempts to decrease or stop picking.
- The skin-picking must cause clinically relevant distress or impairment in functioning.
- The skin-picking behavior cannot be attributed to another medical or mental condition and cannot be a result of a substance use disorder (e.g. cocaine or methamphetamine use).

Clinical Features
- The face is the most common site of skin-picking.
- Other common sites are legs, arms, torso, hands, cuticles, fingers, and scalp.

- In severe cases, skin-picking can result in physical disfigurement and medical consequences that require medical or surgical interventions (e.g., skin grafts or radiosurgery).
- Patients may experience tension prior to picking and a relief and gratification after picking.
- In spite of the relief felt from picking, patients often feel guilty or embarrassed at their behavior and avoid social situations.
- Many patients use bandages, makeup, or clothing to hide their picking.

Treatment

- Skin-picking disorder is difficult to treat.
- Most patients do not actively seek treatment due to embarrassment or because they believe their condition is untreatable. There is support for the use of selective serotonin reuptake inhibitors (SSRIs).
- The opioid antagonist naltrexone (Revia) has proven to reduce the urge to pick, particularly in patients who experience pleasure from the behavior.
- Nonpharmacological treatments include habit reversal and brief cognitive-behavioral therapy (CBT).

Factitious Disorder

- Patients with factitious disorder simulate, induce, or aggravate illness to receive medical attention, regardless of whether or not they are ill.
- Thus, they may inflict painful, deforming, or even life-threatening injury on themselves, their children, or other dependents.
- The primary motivation is not avoidance of duties, financial gain, or anything concrete.
- The motivation is simply to receive medical care and to partake in the medical system.
- Factitious disorders can lead to significant morbidity or even mortality. Therefore, even though presenting complaints are falsified, the medical and psychiatric needs of these patients must be taken seriously.
- Richard Asher coined the term "Munchausen syndrome" to refer to a syndrome in which patients embellish their personal history, chronically fabricate symptoms to gain hospital admission, and move from hospital to hospital. The syndrome was named after Baron Hieronymus Friedrich Freiherr von Münchausen a German cavalry officer.

Factitious Disorder by Proxy

- In this diagnosis, a person intentionally produces physical signs or symptoms in another person who is under the first person's care, hence the DSM-5 diagnosis of "Factitious Disorder Imposed on Another." One apparent purpose of the behavior is for the caretaker to indirectly assume the sick role;
- Another is to be relieved of the caretaking role by having the child hospitalized.
- The most common case of factitious disorder by proxy involves a mother who deceives medical personnel into believing that her child is ill.
- The deception may involve a false medical history, contamination of laboratory samples, alteration of records, or induction of injury and illness in the child.

DD: **Malingering**

- Factitious disorders must be distinguished from malingering.
- Malingerers have an obvious, recognizable environmental goal in producing signs and symptoms. They may seek hospitalization to secure financial compensation, evade the police, avoid work, or merely obtain free bed and board for the night, but they always have some apparent end for their behavior.
- Moreover, these patients can usually stop producing their signs and symptoms when they are no longer considered profitable or when the risk becomes too great.

CLUES THAT SHOULD TRIGGER SUSPICION OF FACTITIOUS DISORDER

- Unusual, dramatic presentation of symptoms that defy conventional medical or psychiatric understanding
- Symptoms do not respond appropriately to usual treatment or medications
- Emergence of new, unusual symptoms when other symptoms resolve.
- Eagerness to undergo procedures or testing or to recount symptoms.
- Reluctance to give access to collateral source of information (i.e. refusing to sign releases of information or to give contact information for family and friends).
- Extensive medical history or evidence of multiple surgeries
- Multiple drug allergies
- Medical profession
- Few visitors
- Ability to forecast unusual progression of symptoms or unusual response to treatment.

PRESENTATION IN FACTITIOUS DISORDER WITH PREDOMINANTLY PSYCHOLOGICAL SIGNS AND SYMPTOMS

- Bereavement
- Depression
- Posttraumatic stress disorder
- Pain disorder
- Psychosis
- Bipolar I disorder
- Dissociative identity disorder
- Eating disorder
- Amnesia
- Substance-related disorder
- Paraphilias
- Hypersomnia
- Transsexualism.

IMPULSE CONTROL DISORDERS

Kleptomania

- The essential feature of kleptomania is recurrent, intrusive, and irresistible urges or impulses to steal unneeded objects for personal use or for monetary value. Persons with kleptomania usually have the money to pay for the objects they impulsively steal.
- As with other impulse-control disorders, kleptomania is characterized by mounting tension before the act, followed by gratification and lessening of tension with or without guilt, remorse, or depression after the act. The stealing is not planned and does not involve others.
- Patients with kleptomania may also be distressed about the possibility or actuality of being apprehended and may manifest signs of depression and anxiety. Patients feel guilty, ashamed, and embarrassed about their behavior
- Furthermore, when the object stolen is the goal, the diagnosis is not kleptomania; in kleptomania, the act of stealing is itself the goal
- They often have serious problems with interpersonal relationships and often show signs of personality disturbance
- The onset of the disorder generally is late adolescence.
- The course of the disorder waxes and wanes, but tends to be chronic. Persons sometimes have bouts of being unable to resist the impulse to steal, followed by free periods that last for weeks or months; new bouts of the disorder may be precipitated by loss or disappointment.

Treatment

- Insight-oriented psychotherapy and psychoanalysis have been successful
- Behavior therapy, including systematic desensitization, aversive conditioning, and a combination of aversive conditioning and altered social contingencies.

INTERMITTENT EXPLOSIVE DISORDER

a. Recurrent behavioral outbursts representing a failure to control aggressive impulses as either of the following:
   1. Verbal aggression temper tantrums, tirades, verbal arguments or fights) or physical aggression towards property, animals, or other individuals, occurring twice weekly, on average, for a period of 3 months. The physical aggression does not result in damage destruction of property and does not result in physical injury to animals or other individuals.
   2. Three behavioral outbursts involving damage or destruction of property and/or physical assault involving physical injury against animals or other individuals occurring within a 12 month period.
b. The magnitude of aggressiveness expressed during the recurrent outbursts is grossly out of proportion to the provocation or to any precipitating psychosocial stressors
c. The recurrent aggressive outbursts are not premeditated (i.e. they are impulsive and/or anger-based) and are not committed to achieve some tangible objective (e.g. money, power, intimidation).
d. The recurrent outbursts cause either marked distress in the individual or in occupational or interpersonal functioning, or are associated with financial or legal consequences.
e. Chronological age is at least 6 years (or developmental level).
f. The recurrent aggressive outbursts are not better explained by another mental disorder

Note: This diagnosis can be made in addition to the diagnosis of ADHD, conduct disorder, oppositional disorder, or autism spectrum disorder when recurrent impulsive aggressive outbursts are in excess of those usually seen in these disorders and warrant independent clinical attention.

PYROMANIA

- Pyromania is the recurrent, deliberate, and purposeful setting of fires.
- Associated features include tension or affective arousal before setting the fires; fascination with, interest in, curiosity about, or attraction to fire and the activities and equipment associated with fire fighting; and pleasure, gratification, or relief when setting fires or when witnessing or participating in their aftermath. Patients may make considerable advance preparations before starting a fire.
- Pyromania differs from arson in that the latter is done for financial gain, revenge, or other reasons and is planned beforehand.
- Persons with pyromania often regularly watch fires in their neighborhoods, frequently set off false alarms, and show interest in fire fighting paraphernalia; they show no remorse and may be indifferent to the consequences for life or property.
- Fire setters may gain satisfaction from the resulting destruction; frequently, they leave obvious clues.
- Commonly associated features include alcohol intoxication, sexual dysfunctions, below-average intelligence quotient (IQ), chronic personal frustration, and resentment toward authority figures.
- Some fire setters become sexually aroused by the fire.

ELECTROPHYSIOLOGY OF SLEEP

- Sleep is made up of two physiological states: non-rapid eye movement (NREM) sleep and rapid eye movement (REM) sleep.
- NREM sleep, (stages 1–4), most physiological functions are markedly lower
- The disorganization during arousal from stage 3 or stage 4 may result in enuresis, somnambulism, and stage 4 nightmares or night terrors.
- REM sleep—high level of brain activity and physiological activity levels (similar to wakefulness)
- REM latency is usually 90 minutes - shortening of REM latency - narcolepsy and depressive disorders.
- The first REM period tends to be the shortest, usually lasting less than 10 minutes; later REM periods may last 15 to 40 minutes each.
- Most REM periods occur in the last third of the night, whereas most stage 4 sleep occurs in the first third of the night.
- REM sleep has also been termed *paradoxical sleep:* Pulse, respiration, and blood pressure in humans are all high during REM sleep— Brain oxygen use increases during REM sleep.
- Thermoregulation is altered during REM sleep— a poikilothermic condition prevails during REM sleep. Poikilothermia, results in a failure to respond to changes in ambient temperature with shivering or sweating, whichever is appropriate to maintaining body temperature.
- Almost every REM period in men is accompanied by a partial or full penile erection. This finding is clinically significant in evaluating the cause of impotence;
- Another physiological change that occurs during REM sleep is the near-total paralysis of the skeletal (postural) muscles. Because of this motor inhibition, body movement is absent during REM sleep.
- Probably the most distinctive feature of REM sleep is dreaming. Dreams during REM sleep are typically abstract and surreal; a REM period occurs about every 90 to 100 minutes during the night.

SLEEP

	Electroencephalogram	Electrooculogram	Electromyogram
Wakefulness	Low-voltage, mixed frequency activity; Alpha (8-13 cps) activity with eyes closed	Eye movements and eye blinks	High tonic activity and voluntary movements
Nonrapid eye movement sleep			
Stage I	Low-voltage, mixed frequency activity; Theta (3-7 cps) activity, vertex sharp waves	Slow eye movements	Tonic activity slightly decreased from wakefulness
Stage II	Low-voltage, mixed frequency background with sleep spindles (12-14 cps bursts) and K complexes (negative sharp wave followed by positive slow wave)	None	Low tonic activity
Stage III	High-amplitude (≥75 μV) slow waves (≤2 cps) occupying 20 to 50% of epoch	None	Low tonic activity
Stage IV	High-amplitude slow waves occupy > 50% of epoch	None	Low tonic activity
REM sleep	Low-voltage, mixed frequency activity; Saw-tooth waves, theta activity, and slow alpha activity	REMs	Tonic atonia with phasic twitches

SLEEP DISORDER CLASSIFICATION

DSM-5

The sleep-wake disorders' current classifications in accordance with the DSM-5 include the following:
1. Insomnia disorder
2. Hypersomnolence disorder
3. Narcolepsy
4. Breathing-related sleep disorders:
   a. Obstructive sleep apnea hypopnea
   b. Central sleep apnea
      i. Idiopathic central sleep apnea
      ii. Cheyne-Stokes breathing
      iii. Central sleep apnea comorbid with opioid use
   c. Sleep-related hypoventilation
5. Circadian rhythm sleep-wake disorders:
   a. Delayed sleep phase type
   b. Advanced sleep phase type
   c. Irregular sleep-wake type
   d. Non-24-hour sleep-wake type
   e. Shift work type
   f. Unspecified type
6. Parasomnias
7. Non-rapid eye movement sleep arousal disorders:
   a. Sleep walking type
   b. Sleep terror type
8. Nightmare disorder
9. Rapid eye movement sleep behavior disorder
10. Restless legs syndrome
11. Substance/medication-induced sleep disorder.

TOOLS USED IN SLEEP MEDICINE: POLYSOMNOGRAPHY

- Polysomnography is the continuous, attended, comprehensive recording of the biophysiological changes that occur during sleep. Each 30-second segment of the recording is considered an "epoch."
- A polysomnogram is typically recorded at night and lasts between 6 and 8 hours.
- Brain wave activity, eye movements, submental electromyography activity, nasal–oral airflow, respiratory effort, oxyhemoglobin saturation, heart rhythm, and leg movements during sleep are measured. Body position is usually noted, and snoring sounds may be recorded.
- Brain wave activity, eye movements, and submental electromyogram are important for identifying sleep stages.
  Indications for polysomnography include.
  1. Diagnosis of sleep-related breathing disorders
  2. Positive airway pressure titration and assessment of treatment efficacy, and
  3. Evaluation of sleep-related behaviors that are violent or may potentially harm the patient or bed partner.
- Polysomnography can also be used to diagnose atypical parasomnias, sleep-related problems secondary to neuromuscular disorders, periodic limb movement disorder, and arousals secondary to seizure disorder. In addition, patients with excessive daytime sleepiness or those who wake up gasping or choking should be referred for polysomnography.
- Referrals for polysomnography should be considered in cases in which sleeplessness has been present for 6 months or more for a minimum of four nights a week.
- It should also be considered when insomnia has not responded to pharmacological or behavioral therapy, sleep-promoting medications are contraindicated, or a medical or psychiatric cause has been excluded. Referral should also be made if the treatment of an underlying medical or psychiatric comorbidity has failed to resolve the insomnia.
- Polysomnography is also recommended to assess sleep quality and quantity on the night just prior to a multiple sleep latency test being conducted to diagnose narcolepsy.

MULTIPLE SLEEP LATENCY TEST

- The multiple sleep latency test (MSLT) is indicated for diagnosing narcolepsy.
- Beginning 2 hours after morning awakening, 20-minute nap opportunities are provided during which the patient is instructed to let himself or herself fall asleep and not resist falling asleep.
- Electroencephalographic, electro-oculographic, and submental electromyography activity is recorded to determine sleep stage.
- The latency to sleep is used to assess the level of sleepiness, and the appearance of REM sleep on two or more nap opportunities confirms narcolepsy, especially when other ancillary symptoms are present (e.g. cataplexy, sleep paralysis, hypnagogia, and excessive sleepiness).
- If the patient falls asleep on a given nap opportunity, the nap is terminated 15 minutes after initial sleep onset.
- If the patient does not fall asleep, the session is terminated after 20 minutes of recording. Five nap opportunities are provided at 2-hour intervals across the day.

Sleep-Related Bruxism

- Sleep-related bruxism is diagnosed when an individual grinds or clenches the teeth during sleep.
- Sleep bruxism can produce abnormal wear on the teeth, damage teeth, provoke tooth and jaw pain, or make loud unpleasant sounds that disturb the bed partner. Sometimes atypical facial pain and headache also result.
- It is clinically significant in only about 5 percent.
- Teeth grinding occurs most common at transition to sleep, in stage 2 sleep, and during REM sleep.
- It worsens during periods of stress.
- Sleep bruxism may occur secondary to sleeprelated breathing disorders, the use of psychostimulants (e.g. amphetamine, cocaine), alcohol ingestion, and treatment with SSRIs.
  DD: Rule out nocturnal seizures.
  Severity is judged on the basis of sleep disruption, consequent pain, and dental damage.

Treatment

- Oral appliance to protect the teeth during sleep. The soft one (mouth guard) is typical used in the short term, whereas the hard acrylic one (bite splint) is used longer term and requires regular follow-up.
- Relaxation, biofeedback, hypnosis, physical therapy, and stress management are also used to treat sleep bruxism.

SLEEP-RELATED MOVEMENT DISORDERS

Restless Legs Syndrome

- Restless legs syndrome (RLS) (also known as *Ekbom syndrome*) is an uncomfortable, subjective sensation of the limbs, usually the legs, sometimes described as a "creepy crawly" feeling, and the irresistible urge to move the legs when at rest or while trying to fall asleep.
- It tends to be worse at night and moving the legs or walking helps to alleviate the discomfort.
- Uremia, neuropathies, and iron and folic acid deficiency anemias can produce secondary RLS. RLS is also reported in association with fibromyalgia, rheumatoid arthritis, diabetes, thyroid diseases, and COPD.

Treatment

- Dopaminergic agonists Pramipexole and Ropinirole are FDA approved-TOC.
- Nonpharmacological treatments include avoiding alcohol use close to bedtime, massaging the affected parts of the legs, taking hot baths, applying hot or cold to the affected areas, and engaging in moderate exercise.

Periodic Limb Movement Disorder

- Periodic limb movement disorder (PLMD), previously called *nocturnal myoclonus*, involves brief, stereotypic, repetitive, nonepileptiform movements of the limbs, usually the legs.
- It occurs primarily in NREM sleep and involves an extension of the big toe. A partial flexion of the ankle, knee, and hip may also occur.
- These movements range from 0.5 to 5 seconds in duration and occur every 20 to 40 seconds.
- The leg movements are frequently associated with brief arousals from sleep and as a result can (but do not always) disturb sleep architecture.
- The prevalence of PLMD increases with aging and can occur in association with folate deficiency, renal disease, anemia, and the use of antidepressants.
- Pharmacotherapy for PLMD associated with RLS is the same as for RLS; Benzodiazepines, especially clonazepam, and opiates improve sleep in patients with PLMD.

Parasomnias Usually Associated with REM Sleep

REM Sleep Behavior Disorder

- REM behavior disorder (RBD) involves a failure of the patient to have atonia (sleep paralysis) during the REM stage sleep.
- Under normal circumstances, the dreamer is immobilized by REM-related hypopolarization of alpha and gamma motor neurons. Without this paralysis or with intermittent atonia, punching, kicking, leaping, and running from bed during attempted dream enactment occur.
- Patients and bed partners frequently sustain injury, which is sometimes serious (e.g., lacerations, fractures).
- There is a suggestion that RBD may result from diffuse hemispheric lesions, bilateral thalamic abnormalities, or brainstem lesions.
- Clonazepam has been used successfully to treat RBD.

Recurrent Isolated Sleep Paralysis

- Sleep paralysis is, an inability to make voluntary movements during sleep. It becomes a parasomnia when it occurs at sleep onset or on awakening
- This inability to move can be extremely distressing, especially when it is coupled with the feeling that there is an intruder in the house or when hypnagogic hallucinations are occurring.
- Sleep paralysis is one of the tetrad of symptoms associated with narcolepsy.
- Sleep paralysis is a feature of normal REM sleep briefly intruding into wakefulness. The paralysis may last from 1 to several minutes.
- Irregular sleep, sleep deprivation, psychological stress, and shift work increase the occurrence of sleep paralysis
- Occasional sleep paralysis: 7–8%; one experience of sleep paralysis during the lifetime: 25–50%
- First-line therapies: Improved sleep hygiene and assurance of sufficient sleep.

Nightmare Disorder

- Nightmares are frightening or terrifying dreams which produce sympathetic activation and ultimately awaken the dreamer.
- Nightmares occur in REM sleep
- The person having been aroused to wakefulness, he or she typically remembers the dream (in contrast to sleep terrors). Some nightmares are recurrent, and reportedly when they occur in association with posttraumatic stress disorder they may be recollections of actual events.
- Common in children ages 3 to 6 years (10–50%), nightmares are rare in adults (<1%).
- Individuals at risk for nightmares include those with schizotypal, borderline, and schizoid personality disorders, as well as those with schizophrenia; traumatic events are known to induce nightmares;
- Medications including L-DOPA and β-adrenergic blockers, withdrawal from REM suppressant medications, drug or alcohol abuse are associated with nightmares.
- Frequently occurring nightmares often produce a "fear of sleeping" type of insomnia. In turn, the insomnia may provoke sleep deprivation, which is known to exacerbate nightmares. In this manner, a vicious cycle is created.
- Universal sleep hygiene, stimulus control therapy, lucid dream therapy, and cognitive therapy reportedly improve sleep and reduce nightmares.
- In patients with nightmares related to posttraumatic stress disorder, Nefazodone reportedly provides therapeutic benefit.
- Prazosin significantly increased total sleep time and REM sleep time and significantly reduced trauma-related nightmares and distressed awakenings.

NREM Sleep Arousal Disorders

Sleepwalking (somnambulism)

- A condition in which an individual arises from bed and ambulates without fully awakening.
- Individuals can engage in a variety of complex behaviors while unconscious—range from sitting up and attempting to walk to conducting an involved sequence of semipurposeful actions.
- Sleepwalks characteristically begin toward the end of the first or second slow wave sleep episodes.
- Sleep deprivation and interruption of slow wave sleep appear to exacerbate, or even provoke, sleepwalking in susceptible individuals.
- An individual who is sleepwalking is difficult to awaken. Once awake, the sleepwalker will usually appear confused.
- Sleepwalking is very common in children and has peak prevalence between ages 4 and 8 years. After adolescence, it usually disappears spontaneously.

Sleep Terrors

- Sleep terror disorder is an arousal in the first third of the night during deep NREM (stages 3 and 4) sleep.
- It is characterized by a sudden arousal with intense fearfulness—begin with a piercing scream or cry and are accompanied by behavioral manifestations of intense anxiety bordering on panic.

- An individual experiencing a sleep terror usually sits up in bed, is unresponsive to stimuli, and, if awakened, is confused or disoriented.
- Amnesia for the episodes usually occurs.
- Fever and CNS depressant withdrawal sleep deprivation potentiate sleep terror episodes.
- Sleep terrors may contain only fragments of very brief but frighteningly vivid static images. It is sometimes called *pavor nocturnus*, incubus, or night terror,
- History of traumatic experience or frank psychiatric problems is often comorbid in adults with this disorder.

Severity ranges from less than once per month to almost nightly occurrence (with injury to the patient or others).

GENERAL PSYCHIATRY

The World Health Organization (WHO) considers normality to be a state of complete physical, mental, and social well-being. The fourth edition of Diagnostic and Statistical Manual of Mental Disorders (DSM-IV-TR) states:

- A mental disorder is a behavioral or psychological syndrome or pattern associated with distress (e.g. a painful symptom), or with a significantly increased risk of suffering, death, pain, disability, or an important loss of freedom. In addition, the syndrome or pattern must not be merely an expected and culturally sanctioned response to a particular event, such as the death of a loved one.
- Normality has been defined as patterns of behavior or personality traits that are typical or that conform to some standard of proper and acceptable ways of behaving and being.
- Psychically normal persons are those who are in harmony with themselves and with their environment. They conform to the cultural requirements or injunctions of their community. They may possess medical deviation or disease, but as long as this does not impair their reasoning, judgment, intellectual capacity, and ability to make a harmonious personal and social adaptation, they may be regarded as psychically sound or normal.

Psychoanalytic Concepts of Normality	
Theorist	Concept
Sigmund Freud	Normality is an idealized fiction
Kurt Eissler	Absolute normality cannot be obtained because the normal person must be totally aware of his or her thoughts and feelings
Melanie Klein	Normality is characterized by strength of character, the capacity to deal with conflicting emotions, the ability to experience pleasure without conflict, and the ability to love
Erik Erikson	Normality is the ability to master the periods of life: trust vs mistrust; autonomy vs shame and doubt; initiative vs guilt; industry vs inferiority; identity vs role confusion; intimacy vs isolation; generativity vs stagnation; and ego integrity vs despair
Laurence Kubie	Normality is the ability to learn by experience, to be flexible, and to adapt to a changing environment
Heinz Hartmann	Conflict-free ego functions represent the person's potential for normality; the degree the ego can adapt to reality and be autonomous is related to mental health
Karl Menninger	Normality is the ability to adjust to the external world with contentment and to master the task of acculturation
Alfred Adler	The person's capacity to develop social feeling and to be productive is related to mental health; the ability to work heightens self-esteem and makes one capable of adaptation
R. E. Money-Kryle	Normality is the ability to achieve insight into one's self, an ability that is never fully accomplished
Otto Rank	Normality is the capacity to live without fear, guilt, or anxiety and to take responsibility for one's own actions
W. Somerset Maughn	The normal is an ideal. It is a picture that one fabricates and to find them all in a single man is hardly to be expected

DEFENCE MECHANISMS

The Mature Defenses

- *Altruism:* The vicarious but constructive and instinctually gratifying service to others.
- *Anticipation:* The realistic anticipation of, or planning for, future inner discomfort; implies overly concerned planning, worrying, and anticipation of dire and dreadful possible outcomes.
- *Asceticism:* The elimination of directly pleasurable affects attributable to an experience. It is directed against all pleasures perceived consciously, and gratification is derived from the renunciation.
- *Humor:* The overt expression of feelings without personal discomfort or immobilization and without unpleasant effect on others.
- *Sublimation:* The gratification of an impulse, whose goal is retained, but whose aim or object is changed from a socially objectionable one to a socially valued one. Libidinal sublimation involves desexualization of drive impulses and placing a value judgment that substitutes what is valued by the superego or society. Sublimation of aggressive impulses takes place through pleasurable games and sports. Unlike neurotic defenses, sublimation allows instincts to be channeled rather than to be dammed up or diverted. Thus, in sublimation, feelings are acknowledged, modified, and directed toward a relatively significant person or goal so that modest instinctual satisfaction results.
- *Suppression:* The conscious or semiconscious decision to postpone attention to a conscious impulse or conflict.

DEVELOPMENT

- Development is a lifelong, dynamic process that is basically the same in childhood and adulthood. The eight conventional stages of development are as follows:
  1. The prenatal period (from conception to birth)
  2. Infancy (from birth to about 15 months)
  3. The toddler period (15 months to 2½ years)
  4. The preschool period (2½ to 6 years)
  5. The middle years (6 to 12 years)
  6. Adolescence (12 to 19 years)
  7. Adulthood (20 to 65), and
  8. Late adulthood (old age).
- Piaget described four major stages leading to the capacity for adult thought. Each stage is a prerequisite for the following one, but the rate at which different children move through different stages varies with their native endowment and environmental circumstances.
- **Piaget's four stages are:**
  1. Sensorimotor
  2. Preoperational thought
  3. Concrete operations, and
  4. Formal operations.

PSYCHIATRISTS AND THEIR WORKS

- Psychoanalytical Theory—Sigmund Freud
- Old Age Developmental Theorists—Sigmund Freud, Erik Erikson [Epigenetic Principle], Heinz Kohut, Bernice Neugarten, Daniel Levinson.
- Death theories—Kubler ross, Stages of Death and Dying - Shock and Denial, Anger, Bargaining, Depression and Acceptance.
- Attachment Theory—John Bowlby, Harry Harlow, Mary Ainsworth
- Learning Theory—Petrovich Pavlov, J.B. Watson, B.F. Skinner (concept of operant conditioning), E.L. Thorndike (the law of effect)
- Aggression—Konrad Lorenz.

Ego Psychology: Sigmund Freud advocated the three provinces id, ego, and superego which are distinguished by their different functions. Id refers to a reservoir of unorganized instinctual drives; the ego spans all three topographical dimensions of conscious, preconscious, and unconscious and superego establishes and maintains an individual's moral conscience on the basis of a complex system of ideals and values internalized from parents.

TERMS AND DEFINITIONS

Circumstantiality	Cannot seem to get to the point because of excess of trivia or details
Clang	Thoughts proceed from one to another by sound of words, such as rhyming
Echolalia	Repeating words just spoken
Flight of ideas	Thoughts seem to move quickly from idea to idea; often with pressured speech
Hallucinations	Perceptual abnormalities: auditory, tactile, gustatory, visual, olfactory, cenesthetic (visceral)
Ideas of reference	Belief that one is the topic or subject of media or other people's thoughts or Conversations
Impaired abstraction	Concrete qualities to actions and/or objects
Loose associations	Rapid shift from one unrelated topic to another
Neologisms	Use of "made-up" or new words
Perseveration	Thinking about something over and over
Tangentiality	Thoughts begin in logical fashions, then get further off track
Thought blocking	Train of thought stops, usually because of hallucinations
Word salad	Jumbled, unrelated words/phrases

PSYCHIATRIC GENETICS

Alcoholism

Several linkage studies have been completed in sizeable populations. Genes predisposing to alcohol dependence appear to be located on chromosomes 1, 2, 4, 7, and 16. Variants in GABRA2 on chromosome 4p have been shown to be associated with the power of **beta** oscillations in the EEG (which are inversely, related to inhibitory neuronal activity in the cortex) and to alcohol dependence. single nucleotide polymorphisms in some of the ADH enzymes (genes for several isoenzymes of ADH are located on chromosome 4q) have been associated.

Alzheimer Disease

Chromosomal location	Clinical correlate	Frequency	Gene name
21q	Early onset	Rare	APP
1	Early onset	Rare	Presenilin II
19	Late onset	Common	ApoE
14	Early onset	Rare	Presenilin I

Autism

What is striking about the genetics of autism is its association with multiple single-gene disorders. The most clearly documented of these disorders is the fragile X syndrome. There are also probable associations between autism and tuberous sclerosis, neurofibromatosis, and phenylketonuria. A consistent finding is seen on the long arm of chromosome 7 from 7q22. It is notable that the linked region includes the gene recently dubbed "speech 1" also known as FOXP2 and known to be a transcription factor.

Schizophrenia

- Twin studies: nearly 50% monozygotic, 17% dizygotic
- Chromosomes implicated: 3p, 5q, 6p, 6q, 8p, 10p, 13q, 15q, 18p, 22q
- Trinucleotide repeat (CAG/CTG) on chromosomes 17 and 18.

1. PSYCHOTIC DISORDERS

Schizophrenia

A prototype psychotic illness characterized by chronic course, deterioration in social and occupational functions, and positive (delusion, hallucination) and negative (flat affect, alogia, avolition) symptoms.

Diagnosis:

a. Two or more of the following each present for a significant portion of time during a one month period or less if successfully treated. At least one of these must be 1, 2 or 3
   1. Delusions
   2. Hallucinations
   3. Disorganized speech (e.g. Frequent derailment or incoherence)
   4. Grossly disorganized or catatonic behavior
   5. Negative symptoms (diminished emotional expression or avolition)
b. For a significant portion of time since the onset of disturbance, level of functioning in one or more major areas is below level achieved before the onset
c. Continuous signs of illness persist for at least 6 months. This 6 month period must include at least 1 month of symptoms that meet criterion A (active phase symptoms) and may include periods of prodromal or residual symptoms (negative symptoms/attenuated forms of symptoms in criterion A)
d. Schizoaffective disorder and depressive or bipolar disorder with psychotic features have been ruled out
e. Disturbance not attributable to effects of substance or another medical condition
f. If there is a history of autism spectrum disorder or communication disorder of childhood onset, the additional diagnosis of schizophrenia is made only if prominent delusions/hallucinations present in addition to other required symptoms of schizophrenia for at least one month.

Clinical Findings

a. Psychotic symptoms: Hallmarks of schizophrenia (patients experience a confusion of boundaries between themselves and the world surrounding them, often called "a loss of ego boundaries"). Schneider's first rank symptoms are hallucinations, delusional perception, thought alienation phenomena and passivity phenomena. Bleuler's 4 A's of schizophrenia are ambivalence, autism, affect disturbance and association disturbance.

b. Positive symptoms (hallucinations and delusions)
- **Hallucinations**
  a. Perceptual experiences that have no external stimulus (e.g. hearing voices but no one is speaking)
  b. Auditory (e.g. voices commenting, arguing, repeating patient's thoughts), visual, tactile, gustatory, or olfactory—auditory hallucinations are the most common.
- **Delusions**
  a. Disturbance of thought
  b. Firmly held false beliefs that can be bizarre or nonbizarre (beliefs unique to certain cultural or religious groups are not synonymous with delusions)
  c. Somatic, grandiose, paranoid, religious, nihilistic, sexual, persecutory, delusions of reference, delusions of thought (insertion, withdrawal, control, broadcasting)
  d. Delusions with special reference (Capgras' syndrome, koro, prison psychosis, van Gogh's syndrome)

c. Symptoms of disorganization
- Disorganized speech or thought
- Blocking of thought, clanging, distractibility, derailment, neologisms, poverty of speech and content of speech, preservation of thought, tangential speech
- Disorganized or bizarre behavior, catatonic stupor or excitement, stereotypy (repeated purposeless movements), odd mannerisms, echopraxia
- Negativism, incongruous affect, inappropriate smiling
- Deterioration of social functioning, inappropriate social behaviors, unkempt in appearance, messy or has much clutter in surroundings.
- Halstead-Reitan Battery of Neuropsychological Tests can be useful.

d. Negative symptoms
- Alogia: speech that is empty or with decreased spontaneity
- Affective blunting: sparsity of emotional reactivity
- Avolition: unable to initiate or complete goals
- Other common negative symptoms: anhedonia (unable to experience pleasure), inability to concentrate or "attend," inappropriate affect, poor hygiene.

Delusion	Definition
Capgras' syndrome	Belief that a person closely related to him or her has been replaced by a double
Erotomanic	de Clérambault's syndrome, that another person is in love with the individual
Grandiose	Conviction of having some great (but unrecognized) talent, insight, discovery, relationship, religious purpose
Jealousy	Belief that one's spouse or lover is unfaithful
Persecutory	Person believes he or she is subject of conspiracy, is being spied upon, followed, poisoned, harrassed, etc.
Somatic	Involves bodily functions and sensations (e.g., emits foul odor, insects in skin, organs not functioning)
Fregoli syndrome	Identifies a familiar person in various other people he or she encounters; even if no physical resemblance
Van Gogh's syndrome	Self-mutilation driven by delusions

Subtypes
- Five subtypes of schizophrenia have been described based predominantly on clinical presentation: paranoid, disorganized, catatonic, undifferentiated, and residual.
- DSM-5 no longer uses these subtypes but they are listed in the 10th revision of the (ICD-10).

Paranoid Type
- Preoccupation with one or more delusions (persecution or grandeur) or frequent auditory hallucinations.
- Patients are typically tense, suspicious, guarded, reserved, and sometimes hostile or aggressive
- Their intelligence in areas not invaded by their psychosis tends to remain intact.
- Patients usually
  - Have their first episode of illness at an older age than do patients with catatonic or disorganized schizophrenia
  - Have usually established a social life that may help them through their illness
  - The ego resources of paranoid patients tend to be greater
  - They show less regression of their mental faculties, emotional responses, and behavior than do patients with other types of schizophrenia.

Disorganized Type
- Characterized by a marked regression to primitive, disinhibited, and unorganized behavior and by the absence of symptoms that meet the criteria for the catatonic type.
- The onset is early, before age 25 years.
- Disorganized patients are usually active but in an aimless, nonconstructive manner. Their thought disorder is pronounced, and their contact with reality is poor.
- Their personal appearance is disheveled, and their social behavior and their emotional responses are inappropriate. They often burst into laughter without any apparent reason.
- Incongruous grinning and grimacing are common in these patients.

Catatonic Type
- The classic feature is a marked disturbance in motor function; this disturbance may involve stupor, negativism, rigidity, excitement, or posturing.
- Sometimes the patient shows a rapid alteration between extremes of excitement and stupor.
- Associated features include stereotypies, mannerisms, and waxy flexibility. Mutism is particularly common.

CATATONIA
- Catatonia is a clinical syndrome characterized by striking behavioral abnormalities that may include motoric immobility or excitement, profound negativism, or echolalia (mimicry of speech) or echopraxia (mimicry of movement).
- A diagnosis of catatonic disorder due to a general medical condition can be made if there is evidence that the condition is due to the physiological effects of a general medical condition.
- The diagnosis is not made if the catatonia is better explained by a primary mental disorder, such as schizophrenia or psychotic depression, or if catatonic symptoms occur exclusively within the course of delirium.

Epidemiology
- Catatonia is an uncommon condition mostly seen in advanced primary mood or psychotic illnesses.
- 25 to 50 percent are related to mood disorders (e.g., major depressive episode, recurrent, with catatonic features).
- 10 percent are associated with schizophrenia.

Etiology
- Medical conditions that can cause catatonia include neurological disorders (e.g., nonconvulsive status epilepticus, and head trauma), infections (e.g., encephalitis), and metabolic disturbances (e.g., hepatic encephalopathy, hyponatremia, and hypercalcemia).
- Medications that can cause catatonia include corticosteroids, immunosuppressants, and antipsychotic (i.e., neuroleptic) agents.
- Catatonic symptoms may be seen in extreme forms of neuroleptic-induced parkinsonism or neuroleptic malignant syndrome,

DSM-5 DIAGNOSIS
a. The clinical picture is dominated by three (or more) of the following symptoms:
   1. Stupor (i.e. no psychomotor activity; not actively relating to environment)
   2. Catalepsy (i.e. passive induction of a posture held against gravity)
   3. Waxy flexibility (i.e. slight, even resistance to positioning by examiner)
   4. Mutism (i.e. no, or very little, verbal response to instructions or external stimuli)
   5. Negativism (i.e. opposition or no response to instructions or external stimuli)
   6. Posturing (i.e. spontaneous and active maintenance of a posture against gravity)
   7. Mannerism (i.e. odd, circumstantial caricature of normal actions)
   8. Stereotypy (i.e. repetitive, abnormally frequent, non-goal-directed movements)
   9. Agitation, not influenced by external stimuli
   10. Grimacing
   11. Echolalia (i.e. mimicking another's speech)
   12. Echopraxia (i.e. mimicking another's movement)
b. There is evidence from the history, physical examination, or laboratory findings that the disturbance is the direct pathophysiological consequence of another medical condition.
c. The disturbance is not better explained by another mental disorder (e.g. manic episode).
d. The disturbance does not occur exclusively during the course of a delirium.
e. The disturbance causes clinically significant distress or impairment in social, occupational, or other important areas of functioning.

Coding note: Include the name of the medical condition in the name of the mental disorder (e.g. 2983,89[F06.1]) catatonic disorder due to hepatic encephalopathy). The other medical condition should be coded and listed separately immediately before the catatonic disorder due to the medical condition (e.g., 572.2 [K71.90] hepatic encephalopathy; 293.89[F06.1] catatonic disorder due to hepatic encephalopathy).

Differential Diagnosis

Hypoactive delirium, end-stage dementia, and akinetic mutism, as well as catatonia due to a primary psychiatric disorder.

Course and Treatment

- Catatonia impairs a person's ability to care for himself or herself and therefore requires hospitalization. In an excited state, the catatonic patient may represent a danger to others; hence, close supervision is needed.
- Fluid and nutrient intake must be maintained.
- The primary treatment modality is identifying and correcting the underlying medical or pharmacological cause. Offending substances must be removed or minimized.
- Benzodiazepines can provide temporary improvement in symptoms.

ECT is appropriate for catatonia due to a general medical condition, especially if the catatonia is life threatening or has developed into lethal (malignant) catatonia.

Undifferentiated Type

- Frequently, patients who clearly have schizophrenia cannot be easily fit into one type or another.
- These patients are classified as having schizophrenia of the undifferentiated type.

Residual Type

- Characterized by continuing evidence of the schizophrenic disturbance in the absence of a complete set of active symptoms or of sufficient symptoms to meet the diagnosis of another type of schizophrenia.
- Emotional blunting, social withdrawal, eccentric behavior, illogical thinking, and mild loosening of associations commonly appear in the residual type.
- When delusions or hallucinations occur, they are neither prominent nor accompanied by strong affect.

Other Subtypes

Bouffée Délirante (Acute Delusional Psychosis)

- This French diagnostic concept differs from a diagnosis of schizophrenia primarily on the basis of a symptom duration of less than 3 months.
- The diagnosis is similar to the DSM-5 diagnosis of schizophreniform disorder.

Latent

- Latent schizophrenia, was often the diagnosis used for what are now called borderline, schizoid, and schizotypal personality disorders.
- These patients may occasionally show peculiar behaviors or thought disorders but do not consistently manifest psychotic symptoms.
- In the past, the syndrome was also termed *borderline schizophrenia.*

Oneiroid

- The oneiroid state refers to a dream-like state in which patients may be deeply perplexed and not fully oriented in time and place.
- The term *oneiroid schizophrenia* has been used for patients who are engaged in their hallucinatory experiences to the exclusion of involvement in the real world.
- When an oneiroid state is present, patients should be carefully examined for medical or neurological causes of the symptoms
  Propf: Schizophrenia with mental retardation.

ETIOLOGY

Genetics

- Twin studies: Nearly 50% monozygotic, 17% dizygotic
- Chromosomes implicated: 3p, 5q, 6p, 6q, 8p, 10p, 13q, 15q, 18p, 22q
- Trinucleotide repeat (CAG/CTG) on chromosomes 17 and 18.

Findings on Imaging
- Most consistent finding is ventricular enlargement, especially third and lateral ventricles
- Selective reduction in size of frontal lobe, basal ganglia, thalamus, and limbic regions, including the hippocampus and medial temporal lobe
- Possible decrease in volume of neocortical and deep gray matter
- Sulcal widening, especially frontal and temporal areas
- Some studies indicate small but significant difference in brain and intracranial volume
- Increased incidence of Cavum septum pellucidum and Partial callosal agenesis.
- **Functional neuroimaging:**
  - Hypofrontality (frontal and prefrontal cortex): negative symptoms and neurocognitive deficits
  - Positron emission tomographic (PET) studies implicate frontal cortex (orbital, dorsolateral, medial), anterior cingulated gyrus, thalamus, several temporal lobe subregions, and cerebellum.

Neuropathology
- Decreased cell density in the dorsomedial nucleus of thalamus
- Displacement of interneurons in frontal lobe cortex.

Neurochemical Considerations
- **Dopamine hypothesis: excess of dopamine linked to psychotic symptoms**
  1. Dopamine-blocking drugs seemed to lessen psychotic symptoms (antipsychotics)
  2. Drugs stimulating dopamine release caused psychotic symptoms (amphetamine, cocaine)
  3. Five types of dopamine receptors: D1, D2, D3, D4, D5
     a. D1: located in cerebral cortex and basal ganglia
     b. D2: located in striatum
     c. D3 and D4: high concentration in the limbic system
     d. D5: located in thalamus, hippocampus, and hypothalamus
  4. Hyperactivity of dopamine system (especially D2 receptor): thought important to positive symptoms of schizophrenia
- **Others implicated**
  1. Serotonin: Hyperactivity
  2. Norepinephrine: Hyperactivity
  3. Gabba: Aminobutyric acid (GABA): Loss of GABAergic neurons in hippocampus (decreased GABA, increased dopamine).

Clinical Management
(See Psychopharmacology under Neuropharmacology Section)

OTHER PSYCHOTIC DISORDERS

Schizoaffective Disorder
- Prominent mood symptoms with psychosis
- At least 2 weeks of psychosis without mood symptoms
- Prognosis: better than schizophrenia, worse than mood disorder
- Prevalence: <1% ; Suicide risk: 10%

Delusional Disorder
- Delusions are nonbizarrre, persistent
- Difficult to treat: denial of illness, difficulty with trust
- Prevalence: 0.03%, F>M, onset in middle age
- Functioning usually not impaired

Brief Psychotic Disorder
- Psychotic symptoms last <1 month
- Usually due to precipitating event
- Brief, sudden onset of psychosis
- Usually 20 to 30-year-old age group

SCHIZOPHRENIFORM DISORDER

Duration of clinical signs and symptoms is less than 6 months.

Overview of Criteria

a. At least two of the following: delusions, hallucinations, disorganized speech, disorganized behavior or catatonia, or negative symptoms
b. Symptoms not caused by schizoaffective disorder, mood disorder with psychotic features, substance-induced disorders, or general medical condition
c. Symptoms last at least 1 month, but less than 6 months.

Clinical Findings

Similar to schizophrenia except for duration, 33% fully recover within 6 months, 66% usually progress to schizophrenia or schizoaffective disorder.

Premenstrual Dysphoric Disorder

- 80 percent of all women experience some alteration in mood, sleep, or somatic symptoms during the premenstrual period.
- 40 percent of these women have at least mild to moderate premenstrual symptoms.
- Only 3 to 7 percent of women have symptoms that meet the full diagnostic criteria for PMDD.

Criteria

a. In a majority of menstrual cycles at least 5 symptoms must be present in the final week before the onset of menses, start to improve within a few days after the onset of menses and become minimal or absent in the week post menses.
b. One or more of the following symptoms must be present:
   - Marked affective lability (e.g. Mood swings, feeling suddenly sad or tearful, increased sensitivity to rejection)
   - Marked irritability or anger or increased interpersonal conflicts
   - Marked depressed mood, feelings of hopelessness or self deprecating thoughts
   - Marked anxiety, tension, feelings of being keyed up or on the edge
c. One or more of the following symptoms must additionally be present to reach a total of five symptoms when combined with symptoms from criterion B above
   1. Decreased interest in usual activities (e.g. Work, school, friends, hobbies)
   2. Subjective difficulty in concentration
   3. Lethargy, easy fatiguability or marked lack of energy
   4. Marked change in appetite; over eating; specific food cravings
   5. Hypersomnia or insomnia
   6. Absence of being overwhelmed or out of control
   7. Physical symptoms such as breast tenderness or swelling, joint or muscle pain, a sensation of bloating or weight gain
   The symptoms in criteria A-C must have been met for most menstrual cycles that occurred in the preceding year
d. The symptoms are associated with clinically significant distress or interference with work, school, usual social activities, or relationships with others
e. The disturbance is not merely an exacerbation of the symptoms of another disorder (e.g. Panic disorder, MDD, dysthymia, personality disorder).
f. Criterion A should be confirmed by prospective daily ratings during at least two symptomatic cycles.
g. The symptoms are not attributable to the physiological effects of substance or another medical condition.

Postpartum Psychosis (*puerperal psychosis*)

- Characterized by the mother's depression, delusions, and thoughts of harming either herself or her infant.
- Data suggest a close relation between postpartum psychosis and mood disorders, particularly bipolar disorder and major depressive disorder. It is coded as a subtype of bipolar disorder in DSM-5.
   - Incidence—1 to 2 per 1,000 childbirths.
   - 50 to 60% of affected women have just had their first child
   - 50% of cases involve deliveries associated with nonpsychiatric perinatal complications.
   - 50 percent of the affected women have a family history of mood disorders.
   - Two thirds of the patients have a second episode of an underlying affective disorder during the year after a baby's birth.
- The delivery process may best be seen as a nonspecific stress that causes the development of an episode of a major mood disorder, perhaps through a major hormonal mechanism.
- Mean time to onset is within 2 to 3 weeks and almost always within 8 weeks of delivery.

- The onset of florid psychotic symptoms is usually preceded by prodromal signs such as insomnia, restlessness, agitation, lability of mood, and mild cognitive deficits. Later, suspiciousness, confusion, incoherence, irrational statements, and obsessive concerns about the baby's health and welfare may be present.
- Delusional material may involve the idea that the baby is dead or defective. Hallucinations with similar content may involve voices telling the patient to kill the baby or herself.
- Subsequent pregnancies are associated with an increased risk of another episode (50%)
- Postpartum psychosis is a psychiatric emergency. Antipsychotic medications and lithium (eskalith), often in combination with an antidepressant, are the treatments of choice.
- No pharmacological agents should be prescribed to a woman who is breastfeeding.
- Psychotherapy is indicated after the period of acute psychosis, and therapy is usually directed at helping the patient accept and be at ease with the mothering role.

BABY BLUES AND POSTPARTUM DEPRESSION

Characteristic	Baby blues	Postpartum depression
Incidence	30%–75% of women who given birth	10%–15% of women who give birth
Time of onset	3 to 5 days after delivery	Within 3 to 6 months after delivery
Duration	Days to weeks	Months to years, if untreated
Associated stressors	No	Yeas, especially lack of support
Sociocultural influence	No; present in all cultures and socioeconomic classes	Strong association
History of mood disorder	No association	Strong association
Family history of mood disorder	No association	Some association
Tearfulness	Yes	Yes
Mood lability	Yes	Often present, but sometimes mood is uniformly depressed
Anhedonia	No	Often
Sleep disturbance	Sometimes	Nearly always
Suicidal thoughts	No	Sometimes
Thoughts of harming the baby	Rarely	Often
Feelings of guilt, inadequacy	Absent or mild	Often present and excessive

Multiple Choice Questions

1. Children with autism exhibit all of the following *except*:
   a. They have difficulty with change
   b. They may be very sensitive to specific sounds
   c. They often prefer imaginative play with dolls
   d. They often perform repetitive stereotyped behaviors

2. Autism may be associated with other neurologic disorders *except*:
   a. Tuberous sclerosis
   c. Wilson's disease
   b. Seizure disorders
   d. Fragile X syndrome

3. Which of the following is true about the biology of panic disorder?
   a. Clonidine (alpha-2 agonist) provokes panic
   b. Lactate infusions prevent panic by stimulating the substantia nigra
   c. CO, inhalation prevents panic
   d. Yohimbine (alpha-2 antagonist) provokes panic by stimulating the locus ceruleus

4. All of the following statements about treatment of depression are false *except*:
   a. Cognitive behavioral therapy has been shown to be an effective treatment
   b. Antidepressant monotherapy is effective 95% of the time
   c. Antidepressants usually works within 1 to 2 weeks
   d. Antidepressants medication is not lethal in overdose

5. Which of the following is incorrect symptoms of PMDD?
   a. They may include impaired concentration, Insomnia or hypersomnia
   b. They have been reported to be absent during non-ovulatory cycles
   c. They may be related to how an individual's brain reacts to normal variations in the serum levels of gonadotropins
   d. They may be caused by late luteal phase falls in the levels of progesterone and estradiol

6. Which of the following lab tests may indicate a pattern of heavy drinking?
   a. Decreased triglycerides
   b. Decreased carbohydrate–deficient transferrin
   c. Elevated γ glutamyltransferase
   d. Decreased uric acid

7. Which of the following groups is not at increased risk of postpartum psychiatric disorder?
   a. Primiparous women
   b. Those with a history of psychiatric illness postpartum
   c. Those with a family history of mood disorders
   d. Those who experience obstetrical complications during delivery

8. Which of the following false concerning delirium?
   a. There is a disturbance of consciousness, impaired attention or ability to focus
   b. It develops over a short period tending to fluctuate
   c. It may be hyperactive hypoactive or mixed in type
   d. Patients are usually oriented to place

9. In delirium which of the following is true:
   a. The EEG usually shows increased alpha activity
   b. There is evidence that it is caused by hyperfunctioning of the cholinergic neurons
   c. Impairment usually resolves neurons
   d. There may be increased mortality

10. Which of the following is false concerning steroid induced psychosis:
    a. Hallucination is usually visual in nature
    b. It has been reported that postmenopausal women may be at greater risk
    c. Resolution usually occurs rapidly with discontinuation or reduction of the steroids
    d. A history of mood disorder appears to be a risk factor

Answers

| 1. c | 2. c | 3. d | 4. a | 5. d | 6. c | 7. d |
| 8. d | 9. d | 10. d | | | | |

11. Which of the following is false concerning withdrawal from heroin?
    a. Symptoms usually develop within 6 hours after the last dose of the drug
    b. If severe may include dilated pupils irritability, and muscle bone aches
    c. Generally any severe symptoms will peak at 48 hours after the last dose of drug
    d. It may be followed by symptoms for many weeks

12. Abnormalities in which of the following systems have not been reported in catatonia:
    a. Dopamine
    b. GABA
    c. Acetylcholine
    d. Glutamate

13. Which is not a criterion for borderline personality disorder BPD?
    a. Chronic feelings of emptiness
    b. Anhedonia
    c. Recurrent self-mutilatory behavior
    d. Marked impulsivity

14. Which of the following is true of postpartum psychosis:
    a. Early treatment can decrease episode length and it may last than a week
    b. In general those who have the disorder a poor prognosis
    c. Women with this illness may be at decreased risk of psychiatric admission
    d. Antipsychotics are contraindicated

15. Which of the following is false about the biology of PTSD:
    a. There are increased circulating catecholamines
    b. There is hippocampal shrinkage
    c. Hippocampal size is negative correlated with trauma severity
    d. The corpus callosum is hypertrophied

16. Which of the following is false about late onset schizophrenia?
    a. It occurs more frequently in older women
    b. Those with this disorder tend to have fewer negative symptoms
    c. Neuropsychological testing may reveal deficits
    d. It does not respond to the usual treatments

17. All of the following may directly cause or mimic depression except:
    a. Iron deficiency anemia
    b. Pancreatic cancer
    c. Laryngeal cancer
    d. CVAs

18. Which of the following may not have depression as a presenting symptoms?
    a. Carcinoma of the pancreas
    b. Diabetes mellitus
    c. Hypothyroidism
    d. Hypoparathyroidism

19. Risk factor for suicide in depression are all except:
    a. Female
    b. Male > 40 years
    c. With conduct disorder
    d. Family history of suicide

20. A 61-year-old male had undergone cardiac surgery 2 days back. Now he started forgetting things not able to recall names and phone numbers of his relatives. What is the probable diagnosis?
    a. Post-traumatic psychosis
    b. Cognitive dysfunction
    c. Depression
    d. Alzheimer's disease

21. A smoker is worried about side effect of smoking but he does not stop smoking thinking that he smokes less as compared to others and takes a good diet. This thinking is called as:
    a. Self exemption
    b. Cognitive behavior
    c. Self-protection
    d. Distortion

22. All are seen in Nicotine withdrawal, except:
    a. Hyperhidrosis
    b. Anxiety
    c. Tachycardia
    d. Insomnia

23. Which metabolite of nicotine is observed in urine of passive smokers?
    a. Cotinine
    b. Anabasine
    c. Nornicotine
    d. Polycyclic aromatic hydrocarbons

24. The effects of Marijuana cigarette are seen within minutes. How long does the effect last?
    a. 2-4 hours
    b. 6-8 hours
    c. 4-6 hours
    d. 10-12 hours

25. Reciprocal inhibition is done by:
    a. Flooding
    b. Systematic desensitization
    c. Exposure and response prevention
    d. Psychoanalysis

26. Which is not seen in a hyperkinetic child?
    a. Decreased attention span
    b. Soft neurological signs
    c. Left-to-right disorientation
    d. Aggressive behavior

27. Not an associated comorbid condition in children with hyperkinetic attention deficit disorder is:
    a. Sleep disorder
    b. Language disorder
    c. Anxiety disorder
    d. Elimination disorder

Answers

11. a	12. c	13. b	14. a	15. d	16. d	17. c
18. d	19. a	20. b	21. a	22. c	23. a	24. a
25. b	26. d	27. c				

28. A middle aged male complained of lack of sleep during the night time. The duration of time he is truly asleep or awake can be ascertained by which of the following?
    a. Plethysmography
    b. Actigraphy
    c. Kymography
    d. Barography

29. The Halstead-Reitan battery involves all except:
    a. Finger oscillation
    b. Constructional praxis
    c. Rhythm
    d. Tactual performance

30. Sleep deprivation leads to:
    a. Psychotic behavior
    b. Decreased mental alertness
    c. Emotional disturbances
    d. Anxiety neurosis

31. A 42-year-old woman comes to the psychiatrist with complaints of short-term memory loss. She has lost her way home several times in past weeks. Mini mental status exam scores 18 of 30 points. An MRI shows the loss of brain volume. The patient's mother died of the same disease at age Which of the following genes in this patient (and her mother) are likely to show a mutation on chromosome14?
    a. Presenilin 1
    b. Presenilin 2
    c. B-Amyloid precursor protein(APP)
    d. Apolipoprotein E (Apo E)

32. 'Marchiafava-Bignami' syndrome is:
    a. Also called hospital addiction
    b. Related to alcoholism
    c. Congenital
    d. Related to opium withdrawal

33. All are true regarding LSD abuse except:
    a. Perceptual changes in clear consciousness
    b. Produce pupillary constriction
    c. May produce acute panic reaction
    d. Flash back phenomenon is a feature

34. 'Hemp insanity' is due to intake of:
    a. Cocaine
    b. Cannabis
    c. Opioid
    d. Heroin

35. A factory worker is required to submit to random drug tests as part of the drug-free policy his employers have adopted. If he used cocaine 3 days before the test was administered, which assay is most likely to detect cocaine metabolites?
    a. Blood
    b. Hair
    c. Saliva
    d. Urine

36. Doppelganger is:
    a. Shadow following person
    b. Feeling of double of oneself
    c. Identification of stranger as familiar
    d. None of the above

37. All are required to diagnose major depression except:
    a. Depressed mood
    b. Insomnia
    c. Nihilistic ideas
    d. Decreased concentration

38. Endocrine disorders associated with depression are all except:
    a. Hypothyroidism
    b. Hyperthyroidism
    c. Pheochromocytoma
    d. Acromegaly

39. Kleine-Levin syndrome:
    a. Insomnia
    b. Anxiety
    c. Depression
    d. Hypersomnia

40. Which of the following is not an environmental risk factor for schizophrenia?
    a. Cannabis use
    b. Migration
    c. Higher socioeconomic status
    d. Obstetric complications

41. Schizophrenia is a common presentation in which genetic disease?
    a. Down's syndrome
    b. DiGeorge syndrome
    c. Klinefelter's syndrome
    d. Neurofibromatosis

42. Higher cortisol levels are seen in which of the following conditions?
    a. Depression
    b. Phobia
    c. Schizophrenia
    d. Parkinsonism

43. All of the following are true about bipolar disorder except:
    a. Prevalence is more amongst females than males
    b. Lifetime prevalence is around 1%
    c. Mean age of onset is 21 years
    d. Prevalence varies according to socioeconomic status

44. Which of the following is not a feature of mania?
    a. Disorientation
    b. Delusion of grandeur
    c. Elation
    d. Pressure of speech

45. False statement regarding myocardial infarction and depression is:
    a. Depression is a risk factor for MI
    b. MI is a risk factor for depression
    c. SSRIs can be used post MI for treatment of depression
    d. Only cognitive behavioral therapy is used after MI

Answers

28. b	29. b	30. b	31. a	32. b	33. b	34. b
35. d	36. b	37. c	38. c	39. d	40. c	41. b
42. a	43. a	44. a	45. d			

46. Brain areas involved with obsessive compulsive disorder include all *except*:
    a. Claustrum
    b. Orbitofrontal cortex
    c. Basal ganglia
    d. Head of caudate nucleus

47. All are true statements about PTSD, *except*:
    a. Women are more likely to develop PTSD than men
    b. Children are less likely to experience PTSD after trauma than adults
    c. War veterans are commonly at risk for PTSD
    d. Most people having experienced a traumatizing event will develop PTSD

48. Which of the following is NOT a somatic symptom:
    a. Anhedonia
    b. Constipation
    c. Impotence
    d. Numbness

49. A 30-year-old lady presented to physician with complaints of hematuria, On evaluation RBCs were found in urine but no cause was found. On further enquiry it was found that she has gone to many doctors with the same complaints and would demand inpatient care. She would prick her finger and mix blood in urine sample. Her diagnosis is:
    a. Malingering
    b. Factitious illness
    c. Dissociative disorder
    d. Hypochondriasis

50. An 18-year-old boy presented with a belief that his penis is retracting in the abdomen and he will die when it complete retracts. What is this disorder called as?
    a. Dhat syndrome
    b. Koro
    c. Latah
    d. Munchausen syndrome

51. Diagnosis of alcohol dependence includes all of the following *except*:
    a. Impaired occupational and social functioning
    b. Need for daily drinking to function adequately
    c. Lack of tolerance for alcohol
    d. Inability to cut down on alcohol intake

52. Which is not a feature of caffeine withdrawal?
    a. Headache
    b. Hallucination
    c. Depression
    d. Weight gain

53. Area of brain resistant to neurofibrillary tangles Alzheimer's disease:
    a. Visual association area
    b. Entorhinal cortex
    c. Lateral geniculate body
    d. Cuneal gyrus area VI/temporal lobe

54. Frontotemporal dementias include all *except*:
    a. Pick's disease
    b. Nonfluent aphasia
    c. Semantic dementia
    d. Alzheimer's disease

55. True regarding FTD are all *except*:
    a. Semantic dementia
    b. Nonfluent aphasia
    c. Apathetic, disinhibited personality
    d. Rapid onset static course

56. All are true regarding frontotemporal dementia *except*:
    a. Stereotypic behavior
    b. Disorientation
    c. Age less than 65 years
    d. Apathy

57. Not true about anorexia nervosa:
    a. Loss of 15% of body weight
    b. Amenorrhea
    c. Over consciousness about body structure
    d. Loss of weight according to patient

58. Which of the following is not true about bulimia nervosa?
    a. Invariable weight loss with endocrine disorder
    b. Occurrence of both binge eating and inappropriate compensatory behaviors at least twice weekly on an average for 3-months
    c. Recurrent episodes of binge eating
    d. Recurrent self-induced vomiting

59. False regarding anorexia nervosa:
    a. Psychiatric symptoms such as depression may be as
    b. Excessive exercising can be a feature
    c. Weight loss is a feature
    d. Decreased appetite is a feature

60. Not true about nocturnal penile tumescence is:
    a. Totals about 100 min/night
    b. Normal phenomenon
    c. Occurs in NREM sleep
    d. Can be used to distinguish between psychological or impotence

61. Somnambulism is mostly seen in which age group?
    a. Children
    b. Adolescents
    c. Adults
    d. All age group

62. Regarding, Kleine-Levin syndrome which of the following is not true?
    a. Hypersomnia
    b. Hyposexually
    c. Spontaneous resolutiorn
    d. Also called sleeping beauty syndrome

63. Tourette's syndrome is associated with all of the following *except*:
    a. Depression
    b. Obsessive compulsive disorder
    c. ADHD
    d. Parkinson's disease

Answers

46. a	47. d	48. a	49. b	50. b	51. c	52. b
53. c	54. d	55. d	56. b	57. d	58. a	59. d
60. c	61. a	62. b	63. d			

64. A 14-year-old boy has difficulty in expressing himself in writing and makes frequent spelling mistakes. He passes his examination with poor marks. However his mathematical ability and social adjustment are appropriate for his age. Which of the following is the most likely diagnosis?
    a. Mental retardation
    b. Specific learning disability
    c. Lack of interest in studies
    d. Examination anxiety

65. According to Sigmund Freud, primary process thinking is:
    a. Illogical and bizarre
    b. Rational
    c. Absent during sleep
    d. Logical and unconscious

66. Wrong statement about psychoanalysis is:
    a. Parapraxis is useful
    b. Transference is patient's feeling for therapist
    c. Counter transference is clinician's feelings for patient
    d. Unguided communication has no meaning

67. Anaesthetic agent used in ECT is:
    a. Ketamine
    b. Thiopentone
    c. Propofol
    d. Methohexital

68. A 70-year-old man is brought to the physician by his wife. She notes that over the past year he has experienced a slow, stepwise decline in his cognitive functioning. One year ago she felt his thinking was normal but now he gets lost around the house and can't remember simple directions. The patient insists that he feels fine, though he is depressed about his loss of memory. He is eating and sleeping well. Which of the following is the most likely diagnosis?
    a. Major or mild vascular neurocognitive disorder
    b. Mood disorder due to another medical condition
    c. Degenerative neurocognitive disorder
    d. Major depressive disorder

69. A 26-year-old woman with panic disorder notes that during the middle of one of her attacks she feels as if she is disconnected from her body, and feels as if she is floating above it. Which of the following terms best describes this symptom?
    a. Illusion
    b. Hallucination
    c. Depersonalization
    d. Derealization

70. A 45-year-old man with chronic psychotic disorder is interviewed after being admitted to a psychiatric unit. He mimics the examiner's body posture and movements during the interview. Which of the following terms best characterizes this patient's symptom?
    a. Perseveration
    b. Palilalia
    c. Echolalia
    d. Echopraxia

71. Organic causes for mental disorder are more the following *except* those with:
    a. Visual hallucinations
    b. A family history of psychiatric illness
    c. Onset in the last 2 days
    d. Age >30 years

72. A 48 Years old woman has ingested an unknown amount of Lithium carbonate 2 hours ago. This had been started 3 weeks ago by her psychiatrist. Which of the following is TRUE?
    a. A lithium level should be taken at 4 hours post ingestion
    b. The first signs of toxicty are sually gastrointestinal symptoms
    c. The most common ECG abnormality is QRS prolongation
    d. Ataxia is a late sign of significant toxicity

73. With personality disorders, the following are true *except*:
    a. Cluster 'C' represents the 'anxious & fearful' group of personality disorders
    b. Personality disorder is a 'Axis III' diagnosis
    c. Both anti-social and Histrionic personality disorders are found in Cluster 'B
    d. A person with avoidant personality disorder is socially withdrawn but actually would like to have friends

74. An 18-year-old boy is admitted to the hospital with a diagnosis of pain of unknown origin. His parents tell the physician that the child has complained about pain in his legs for about 1 month. Neurologic and orthopedic examination fail to identify any pathology. The history reveals that the child was hospitalized on two previous occasions for other pain symptoms for which no cause was found. After 4 days in the hospital, the nurse reports that the child shows little evidence of pain and seems remarkably content. She reports that she found a medical textbook in the boy's bedside table with a bookmark in the section entitled skeletal pain of unknown origin. Which of the following best describes symptom production and motivation in this case?
    a. Symptom production conscious, motivation primarily conscious
    b. Symptom production unconscious, motivation primarily conscious
    c. Symptom production conscious, motivation primarily unconscious
    d. Symptom production unconscious, motivation primarily unconscious

Answers

| 64. b | 65. a | 66. d | 67. d | 68. a | 69. c | 70. d |
| 71. b | 72. b | 73. b | 74. c | | | |

75. Post stroke depression is more commonly seen with:
    a. Lesion of right hemisphere
    b. Lesion of left hemisphere
    c. Equal in both right & left
    d. Does not depend on what hemisphere is involved

76. A 4-year-old girl who has been in foster care since is very friendly and affectionate with strangers. She puts arms out to them to be picked up and then cuddles up to them. the foster mother states that the child has behavior problems and then notes that she has never felt close to the child. The most likely explanation for this child behavior towards strangers is:
    a. Autism
    b. Rett's disorder
    c. Reactive attachment disorder, inhibited type
    d. Reactive attachment disorder, disinhibited type

77. A terminally ill-patient who uses a statement such as,"it is the doctor's fault that I became ill, she didn't do an electrocardiogram when I came for my last office visit," is most likely in which stage of dying, according to Kübler-Ross?
    a. Denial   b. Anger
    c. Bargaining   d. Depression

78. When an 80-year-old man who has had a stroke attempts to reproduce a clock face, he does the tasks like this effectively neglecting the left of the drawings. The area(s) of the brain most likely to be affected in this patient is (are) the:
    a. Right parietal lobe   b. Basal ganglia
    c. Left parietal lobe   d. Left frontal lobe

79. A 3-year-old girl who had been developing typically since birth begins to withdraw socially and then stops speaking altogether. Also, instead of purposeful hand movements, the child has begun to show repetitive hand wringing behavior. The chromosome most likely to be involved in this disorder is chromosome:
    a. 21   b. 16
    c. 18   d. X

80. A very anxious 25-year-old patient is examined in the emergency room. There is no evidence of physical Ilness. If it could be measured, the γ-aminobutyric acid (GABA) activity in the brain of this patient would most likely be:
    a. Increased
    b. Decreased
    c. Unchanged
    d. Higher than the activity of serotonin

81. After 20 years of smoking, a 45-year-old female patient has decided to quit. Of the following, what physical effect is most likely to be seen as a result of this patient's withdrawal from nicotine?
    a. Weight gain   b. Euphoria
    c. Excitability   d. Delirium tremens

82. A 72-year-old man with Alzheimer disease is be treated with memantine. What is believed to be the basis of the therapeutic action of memantine on neurons in the brain:
    a. To inhibit the action of acetylcholinesterase
    b. To block the influx of calcium
    c. To increase the influx of glutamate
    d. To facilitate the influx of calcium

83. A 36-year-old female patient comes to the physician complaining of extreme fatigue and depression. Physical evaluation reveals a darkening of her skin, particularly in the creases of her hands as well as darkening of the buccal mucosa. The most likely cause of this picture is:
    a. Hypocortisolism
    b. Hypercortisolism
    c. Hypothyroidism
    d. Hyperthyroidism

84. A 40-year-old woman reports that over the past 6 months she has had little appetite, sleeps poorly, and has lost interest in her normal activities. Physical exam is unremarkable. Which of the following is the most likely laboratory finding in this woman?
    a. Positive dexamethasone suppression test (DST)
    b. Normal growth hormone regulation
    c. Increased 5-hydroxyindoleacetic acid (5-HIAA) levels
    d. Normal melatonin levels

85. A 55-year-old male patient with no history of psychiatric illness is admitted to the hospital complaining of intense abdominal pain. He states that over the past few days his wife has been giving him food that is poisoned so that she can kill him and be with another man. The wife states that she loves her husband and would never harm him or leave him. When the patient's urine is collected, it appears purplish red in color. Urine testing is most likely to reveal an elevated level of:
    a. Vanillylmandelic acid (VMA)
    b. 5-hydroxyindoleacetic acid (5-HIAA)
    c. Porphobilinogen
    d. Cortisol

Answers

| 75. b | 76. d | 77. b | 78. a | 79. d | 80. b | 81. a |
| 82. b | 83. a | 84. a | 85. c | | | |

86. A 55-year-old woman was diagnosed with schizophrenia at the age of 22. If this diagnosis was appropriate, the volume of the hippocampus, the size of the cerebral ventricles, and glucose utilization in the frontal cortex of this patient are now most likely to be, respectively:
    a. Increased, increased, increased
    b. Decreased, decreased, decreased
    c. Decreased, decreased, increased
    d. Decreased, increased, decreased

87. A 57-year-old male patient who has had a stroke cannot copy a design drawn by the examiner. The test that the examiner is most likely to be using to evaluate this patient is the:
    a. Bender Visual Motor Gestalt Test
    b. Luria-Nebraska neuropsychological battery
    c. Halstead-Reitan battery
    d. Dexamethasone suppression test (DST)

88. A 27-year-old female patient shows a sudden loss of motor function below the waist that cannot be medically explained. To determine whether psychological factors are responsible for this symptom, the most appropriate diagnostic technique is:
    a. PET
    b. CT
    c. Amobarbital sodium (Amytal) interview
    d. EEG

89. A 45-year-old female patient reports that over the last 3 months she has lost her appetite and interest in her usual activities, and often feels that life is not worth living. Compared with typical sleep, in this patient the percentage of REM sleep, percentage of delta sleep, and sleep latency, respectively, are most likely to:
    a. Increase, decrease, decrease
    b. Increase, decrease, increase
    c. Decrease, stay the same, increase
    d. Decrease, decrease, increase

90. A 28-year-old man comes in complaining of headaches and a variety of other aches and pains that have been present for the past 6 months. He denies that he is sad or hopeless. After a 4-week trial of antidepressant medication, the patient's physical complaints have disappeared. The most appropriate diagnosis for this patient is:
    a. Dysthymic disorder
    b. Major depressive disorder
    c. Masked depression
    d. Hypochondriasis

91. Although he is scolded by his father for television when he should be doing his homework, a 9-year-old boy increases his television watching. The father then decides to ignore the boy's television-watching behavior. Within a week, the boy has stopped watching television when he should be doing homework. The father's intervention, improvement in the boy's "doing his homework" behavior best be described as:
    a. Positive reinforcement
    b. Punishment
    c. Negative reinforcement
    d. Extinction

92. A grade school principal has 1 week to try out a new fire-alarm system or the school. He decides to test the system three times during the week. The first time the alarm is sounded, all of the students leave the school within 5 minutes. The second time, it takes the students 15 minutes to leave the school. The third time the alarm is sounded, the students ignore it. The students' response to the fire alarm the third time it is sounded is most likely to have been learned by:
    a. Sensitization   b. Habituation
    c. Classical conditioning   d. Punishment

93. A 4-year-old child who has received beatings in the past, from which he could not escape, appears unresponsive and no longer tries to escape new beatings. This behavior by the child is an example of:
    a. Stimulus generalization
    b. Extinction
    c. Positive reinforcement
    d. Learned helplessness

94. Although a father spanks his child when she hits the dog, the child continues to hit the dog. This child's hitting is most likely to be a result of behavior:
    a. Punishment
    b. Negative reinforcement
    c. Positive reinforcement
    d. Classical conditioning

95. A patient with diabetes increases her time spent exercising in order to reduce the number of insulin injections she must receive. The increased exercising behavior is most likely to be a result of:
    a. Punishment
    b. Negative reinforcement
    c. Positive reinforcement
    d. Classical conditioning

Answers

86. d	87. a	88. c	89. b	90. c	91. d	92. b
93. d	94. c	95. b				

Question Bank

1. GTLA GQIB antiganglioside antibodies are characteristically associated with:
   a. Acute motor and sensory axonal neuropathy
   b. Acute motor axonal neuropathy (AMAN)
   c. Acute inflammatory demyelinating polyneuropathy
   d. Miller Fisher syndrome

2. Most common posterior fossa brain tumor in children:
   a. Medulloblastoma
   b. Pilocytic astrocytoma
   c. Hemangioblastoma
   d. Occipital fossa tumor

3. Aquaporin-4 has been proposed as the primary autoimmune target in:
   a. Neuromyelitis optica
   b. Diabetes insipidus
   c. Congenital cataract
   d. Multiple sclerosis

4. A 25-year-old female with 16 weeks of gestation presents with excess vomiting, apathy, ataxia, nystagmus and ophthalmoplegia. The diagnosis is:
   a. Wernicke's encephalopathy
   b. Hyperemesis gravidarum
   c. Chorea gravidarum
   d. Korsakoff gravidarum

5. Brighton's criteria is used for:
   a. Guillain-Barrè syndrome
   b. Myasthenia gravis
   c. Polymyositis
   d. Muscular dystrophy

6. Which of the following medication in the treatment of Parkinson's disease is an NMDA antagonist?
   a. Entacapone
   b. Amantadine
   c. Ropinirole
   d. Selegiline

7. Subacute combined degeneration of spinal cord is associated with all except:
   a. Ataxia with spasticity
   b. Sensory impairment from thoracic level
   c. Optic atrophy
   d. Cognitive impairment is frequently associated

8. Right frontal lobe lesion leads to:
   a. Impaired left conjugate gaze
   b. Impaired right conjugate gaze
   c. Impaired upward conjugate gaze
   d. Impaired downward conjugate gaze

9. Deficiency of arylsulphatase is seen in:
   a. Gaucher's disease
   b. Metachromatic leukodystrophy (MLD)
   c. Tay-Sachs's disease
   d. Niemann-Pick disease

10. The following neuropathy is associated with temperature dependence and predominantly sensory loss:
    a. Leprosy
    b. Guillain-Barre' syndrome
    c. Charcot-Marie-Tooth disease
    d. Hereditary sensorimotor neuropathy Type II

11. When to do retinopathy screening in a patient with diabetic neuropathy?
    a. Immediately
    b. After 4 weeks
    c. After 4 months
    d. After 1 year

12. All are features of LMN lesion except:
    a. Plantar flexion
    b. Absent DTR
    c. Hypertonia
    d. Hypotonia

13. The antiepileptic drug, Phenytoin therapeutic blood level is:
    a. 0–9 mcg/mL
    b. 10–19 mcg/mL
    c. 20–29 mcgmL
    d. 30–39 mcgmL

14. Intracranial tension is decreased by all of the following methods except:
    a. ICT monitoring
    b. Craniotomy
    c. Tumor removal
    d. CSF removal

15. NOT a feature of Horner's syndrome:
    a. Loss of taste sensation
    b. Ptosis
    c. Anhydrosis
    d. Miosis

16. Most common cause of intracerebral haemorrhage in adults is:
    a. Hypertension
    b. Ruptured berry aneurysm
    c. Arteriovenous malformation
    d. Trauma

Answers

1. d	2. b	3. a	4. a	5. a	6. b	7. b
8. a	9. b	10. a	11. a	12. c	13. b	14. a
15. a	16. a					

17. Which of following measures cannot reduce incidence of head injuries?
    a. Setting up of neurological centers
    b. Education about safety
    c. Strict safety rules
    d. Wearing helmets

18. FALSE about vomiting due to increased ICT:
    a. Occur due to vomiting centre in medulla
    b. Frequently occurs before sleeping
    c. Vomiting precedes headache
    d. It is projectile

19. Most common disorder in females when compared to:
    a. Conduct disorder
    b. Eating disorder
    c. Oppositional defiant
    d. Antisocial personality disorder

20. The percent of suicidal deaths in Schizophrenia is:
    a. 10%   b. 30%
    c. 50%   d. 70%

21. In MMSE maximum score is given for:
    a. Recall   b. Place orientation
    c. Language   d. Excessive appetite

22. NOT a paranoid symptom:
    a. Delusion of persecution
    b. Delusion of infidelity
    c. Delusion of grandeur
    d. Thought alienation

23. Visual hallucinations are associated with:
    a. Frontotemporal dementia (FTD)
    b. Alzheimer's disease
    c. Progressive supranuclear palsy (PSP)
    d. Lewy body dementia

24. Which of this is FALSE about Varenicline?
    a. Drug is started at 0.5 mg
    b. Suicidal ideation is a side effect
    c. Treatment is given for 6 weeks only
    d. Acts as partial agonist on nicotinic receptors

25. A person hears voices before falling asleep, history of falls in day time sleep attacks. The probable diagnosis:
    a. Narcolepsy   b. Schizophrenia
    c. Delusion   d. Insomnia

26. How would diagnosis of agoraphobia be made?
    a. Patient has panic attack when left alone
    b. Patient will have fear if she is in open space
    c. She would be able to get into lift alone
    d. She complains of insomnia

27. A 35-year-old patient having history of taking marijuana constantly since 20 years. Now he comes to you with withdrawal symptoms, which is the most frequently encountered symptom?
    a. Yawning   b. Seizures
    c. Irritability d. None

28. Not a side effect of lithium:
    a. Leukopenia   b. Hypothyroidism
    c. Polyuria   d. Hypercalcemia

29. de Clerambault's syndrome is associated with the behavior:
    a. Erotic   b. Jealous
    c. Aggressive   d. Hallucinative

30. Marijuana withdrawal syndrome is associated with:
    a. Irritability b. Seizures
    c. Increased sleep d. Excessive appetite

31. Which of this is correctly matched?
    a. Clozapine—Dryness of mouth
    b. Mirtazapine—Akathisia
    c. Bupropion—Premature ejaculation
    d. Sertraline—Delayed ejaculation

32. Part of the brain most commonly affected in Alzheimer:
    a. Locus coeruleus b. Entorhinnal cortex
    c. Prefrontal cortex d. Temporal cortex

33. All of the following are associated with better prognosis in schizophrenia, except:
    a. Late onset   b. Married
    c. Negative symptoms d. Acute onset

34. True about Trichotillomania is:
    a. Irresistible desire to set fire
    b. Irresistible desire to steal things
    c. Associated with patchy hair loss
    d. Pathological gambling

35. Transitional objects is seen between the ages of:
    a. 6 months to 1 year b. 2 to 5 years
    c. 6 to 9 years   d. 9 to 12 years

36. Antipsychotic associated with LEAST extrapyramidal side effects is:
    a. Haloperidol b. Thioridazine
    c. Thiothixine d. Pherphenazine

37. A 25-year-old female living as a paying guest presents to casualty with H/O consumption of 30 tablets of Diazepam. Which of the following is NOT included in suicide risk factor assessment?
    a. Hopelessness b. Insomnia
    c. Social isolation d. Substance abuse

Answers

17. a	18. b	19. b	20. a	21. b	22. b	23. d
24. c	25. a	26. b	27. d	28. a	29. a	30. a
31. a; b; d	32. b	33. c	34. c	35. a	36. a	37. d

38. Which is NOT true about Internal capsule?
    a. Continues above as corona radiata
    b. Continues below as tectum
    c. Corticobulbar and corticonuclear fibres occupy genu and anterior part of posterior limb
    d. Corticospinal tract is carried by posterior limb of internal capsule

39. Lateral geniculate body is a part of:
    a. Pons
    b. Midbrain
    c. Thalamus
    d. Hypothalamus

40. The Broca's area is situated in the:
    a. Temporal lobe
    b. Posterior part of inferior frontal gyrus
    c. Occipital calcarine fissure
    d. Mammillary body region

41. UNTRUE about corticospinal tract:
    a. Uncrossed fibres are responsible for mirror action
    b. Represents phylogenetically oldest tract
    c. Descends from the origin through the corona radiata
    d. Anterior corticospinal tract is responsible for the control of the proximal musculature

42. Which one of the following pituitary hormones is an opioid peptide?
    a. ACTH
    b. Beta endorphin
    c. Alpha melanocyte stimulating hormone
    d. Beta melanocyte stimulating hormone

43. Most common type of benign orbital tumour in adults is:
    a. Lipoma
    b. Dermoid
    c. Haemangioma
    d. Schwannoma

44. Sunflower cataract is seen in:
    a. Galactosemia
    b. Diabetes mellitus
    c. Laurence-Moon-Biedl syndrome
    d. Wilson's disease

45. FALSE about open angle glaucoma is:
    a. Mild to moderate increase in IOP
    b. Shallow anterior chamber
    c. Progressive peripheral visual field loss
    d. Cupping of optic disc

46. Cataract is NOT seen with:
    a. Steroids
    b. Vitamin B12 deficiency
    c. Diabetes mellitus
    d. Homocystinuria

47. FALSE statement about Pterygium:
    a. Causes astigmatism and diplopia
    b. Bare sclera method is most preferred
    c. Conjunctival autograft is associated with lower recurrences
    d. For recurrent cases best treatment is lamellar keratectomy/keratoplasty

48. Action of superior oblique muscle is:
    a. Depression, Extorsion, Adduction
    b. Intorsion, Depression, Adduction
    c. Intorsion, Depression, Abduction
    d. Depression, Extorsion, Abduction

49. Which of the following is earliest and shortest acting skeletal muscle relaxant?
    a. Rocuronium
    b. Vecuronium
    c. Atracurium
    d. Suxamethonium

50. Brain dead individuals have all of the following features *except:*
    a. Dolls eye movement is absent
    b. Oculovestibular reflex is absent
    c. Only pain is preserved
    d. Corneal reflex is absent

51. A patient appears awake and is not talking. No voluntary movements. He can signal with vertical eye movements. The CT scan shows infarction of ventral pons. The diagnosis is:
    a. Coma
    b. Abulia
    c. Locked in state
    d. Catatonia

52. All of the following are true about Neurocysticercosis *except:*
    a. Albendazole is the drug of choice
    b. More common in vegetarians
    c. Produces intracerebral calcification
    d. Man is the definitive host

53. Bilateral facial nerve palsy is seen:
    a. Herpes zoster
    b. Ramsay Hunt syndrome
    c. Guillain-Barre syndrome
    d. Melkersson-Rosenthal syndrome

54. EEG with eyes closed, in normal alert adult predominantly shows:
    a. Alpha waves
    b. Beta waves
    c. Theta waves
    d. Delta waves

55. FALSE statement regarding aneurysms is:
    a. True aneurysm contains all the 3 layers
    b. In dissecting aneurysms media is defective
    c. Charcot-Bouchard aneurysms are seen in brain
    d. Saccular aneurysm involves the entire circumference

Answers

38. c	39. c	40. b	41. a	42. b	43. c	44. d
45. b	46. b	47. a	48. c	49. d	50. c	51. c
52. b	53. c	54. a	55. d			

56. Fluent aphasia with preserved comprehension and impaired repetition is:
    a. Broca's aphasia
    b. Wernicke's aphasia
    c. Anomic aphasia
    d. Conduction aphasia

57. Frontal lobe lesion can cause all except:
    a. Grasping reflex
    b. Personality changes
    c. Acalculia
    d. Emotional alteration

58. Intention tremor is seen in:
    a. Head injury
    b. Cerebellar disease
    c. Parkinsonism
    d. Wilson's disease

59. Lesion in Gerstmann syndrome is:
    a. Left parietal lobe
    b. Left occipital lobe
    c. Left frontal lobe
    d. Right temporal lobe

60. A patient presented with chronic neck pain and minor hyperextension trauma. Now complaints of disproportionate weakness of bilateral upper limbs and sensory loss is minimal. Lower limbs are normal. The probable diagnosis is:
    a. Anterior cord syndrome
    b. Posterior cord syndrome
    c. Central cord syndrome
    d. Brown-Sequard syndrome

61. Metabolic syndrome includes all of the following features, except:
    a. Hypertension
    b. Coronary heart disease
    c. Hyperinsulinism
    d. Increased hip/waist ratio

62. Most common site for hypertensive intracerebral hemorrhage is:
    a. Frontal lobe
    b. Temporal lobe
    c. Occipital lobe
    d. Putamen

63. Most common intracranial tumor of over 60-year-old:
    a. Meningioma
    b. Schwannoma
    c. Ependymoma
    d. Glioblastoma multiforme

64. Pall anesthesia is:
    a. Loss of vibration sense
    b. Loss of pain sensation
    c. Loss of position sense
    d. Loss of temperature

65. Pathogenesis of frontal lobe disorders entails with all except:
    a. Foster Kennedy syndrome
    b. Rett syndrome
    c. Anton syndrome
    d. Disinhibition syndrome

66. Person having cerebellar signs on the same side with hearing loss. Site of damage is:
    a. Left cerebellopontine angle
    b. Left pons
    c. Left medulla
    d. Middle ear

67. Poisoning causing pure motor/sensory neuropathy is:
    a. Lead
    b. Thallium
    c. Cisplatin
    d. Arsenic

68. Prophylaxis of tension type of headache is:
    a. NSAID
    b. Tricyclic antidepressants
    c. Triptans
    d. Propranolol

69. Tension headache is:
    a. The rarest form of headache
    b. Commonly occipitonuchal in distribution
    c. Diagnosed by an abnormal electromyographic study
    d. Best treated with Alprazolam

70. Thiamine dose in alcoholic with Korsakoff's psychosis:
    a. 50 mg IV daily for 5 days
    b. 300–500 mg IV for 3 days
    c. 100 mg IV twice a day for the first 3–5 days
    d. 200 mg IV twice a day for the first 3–5 days

71. Waddling gait is seen in:
    a. Cerebral palsy
    b. Lower motor neuron disease
    c. Muscular dystrophy
    d. Sensory ataxia

72. What is the most common loss of sense above 70 years:
    a. Proprioception
    b. Vibration
    c. Touch
    d. Pressure

73. EDH least common possibility is in:
    a. Middle cerebral artery
    b. Middle meningeal artery
    c. Venous sinuses
    d. Saccular aneurysm

74. Most common cause of SAH is due to:
    a. Traumatic aneurysm
    b. Saccular aneurysm
    c. Mycotic aneurysm
    d. Aortic aneurysm

75. Subdural Hematoma (SDH) is caused by:
    a. Bridging veins
    b. Carticocavernous fistula rupture
    c. Middle meningeal artery
    d. None

Answers

56. d	57. c	58. b	59. a	60. c	61. c	62. d
63. d	64. a	65. c	66. a	67. d	68. b	69. b
70. c	71. c	72. b	73. d	74. b	75. a	

76. A patient on treatment for psychiatric disorder takes overdosage of a drug, develops bradycardia, hypotension, decreased sweating and salivation. The likely drug is:
    a. Amitriptyline
    b. Lithium
    c. Selegiline
    d. Amphetamine

77. Adjustment disorder. False is:
    a. Pharmacotherapy is invariably needed
    b. Psychotherapy much useful
    c. Group therapy is useful
    d. Adjustment disorder is a permanent condition not caused by stress

78. All are true regarding non-dependent chronic alcohol consumption except:
    a. Increase in dopamine levels from ventral tegmental area
    b. Increased GABA receptor density
    c. Excitation of NMDA receptors involved
    d. Release of Beta endorphins

79. Most common type of Delusion associated with Schizophrenia is:
    a. Delusion of persecution
    b. Delusion of grandiosity
    c. Delusion of nihilism
    d. Delusion of Reference

80. Most common psychiatric disorder in community is:
    a. Depression
    b. Schizophrenia
    c. Paranoid disorders
    d. Obsessive compulsive neurosis

81. Neuroleptic malignant syndrome is characterized by all except:
    a. Autonomic deregulation
    b. Increased BP and heart rate
    c. Hypothermia
    d. Muscle rigidity

82. Brain areas involved with obsessive-compulsive disorder include all except:
    a. Claustrum
    b. Orbito-frontal cortex
    c. Basal ganglia
    d. Head of caudate nucleus

83. The following symptoms are common in Anorexia nervosa except:
    a. Weight loss
    b. Mood changes
    c. Dehydration
    d. Menorrhagia

84. True about schizophrenia is all except:
    a. Ambivalence
    b. Hypodopaminergic
    c. Hyperdopaminergic
    d. Autism

85. True statement regarding delirium includes:
    a. Insidious onset
    b. Clear consciousness
    c. Irreversible
    d. Decreased attention

86. Visual hallucinations are most common in:
    a. Lewy body dementia
    b. Alzheimer's disease
    c. Early parkinsonism
    d. Delirium

87. Wernicke-Korsakoff syndrome is seen in chronic alcohol abuse and is characterized by all the following symptoms, except:
    a. Confabulation
    b. Loss of remote memory
    c. Ataxia
    d. Nystagmus and paralysis of certain ocular muscles

88. Child was seen taking off clothes while watching TV he suddenly closes eyes for sometime and was lethargic after sometime. He had probably:
    a. GTCS
    b. Absence seizures
    c. Temporal lobe epilepsy
    d. Febrile seizures

89. Gyrus not on the lateral aspect is:
    a. Superior temporal gyrus
    b. Middle frontal gyrus
    c. Cingulate gyrus
    d. Inferior frontal gyrus

90. Lateral ventricle is connected to third ventricle by:
    a. Aqueduct of Sylvius
    b. Foramen of Luschka
    c. Interventricular foramen of Monro
    d. Foramen of Magendie

91. Pain insensitive structure in brain is:
    a. Falx cerebri
    b. Dural venous sinuses
    c. Choroid plexus
    d. Middle meningeal artery

92. The classic anatomy of the circle in Circle of Willis is only seen in % of cases:
    a. 40%
    b. 60%
    c. 20%
    d. 10%

93. All of the following are branches of internal carotid artery except:
    a. Anterior cerebral artery
    b. Posterior cerebral artery
    c. Ophthalmic artery
    d. Middle cerebral artery

Answers

76. a	77. d	78. c	79. a	80. a	81. c	82. a
83. d	84. b	85. d	86. d	87. b	88. c	89. c
90. c	91. c	92. a	93. b			

94. All of the following are true about CSF protein except:
    a. More protein in basal cisterns than lumbar spine
    b. Normal proteins: 20-40 mg/dL
    c. Normal CSF proteins concentration in children to 4 years of age: 24 mg/dL
    d. Albumin is main component

95. All of the following hormones are produced by anterior pituitary, except:
    a. TSH
    b. Gonadotropic hormone
    c. Growth hormone
    d. MSH

96. IPSP is due to:
    a. Cl influx
    b. Na influx
    c. K⁺ influx
    d. Ca influx

97. Lobe of civilization:
    a. Frontal lobe
    b. Parietal
    c. Temporal
    d. Occipital

98. True regarding sleep pattern in people with age > 50 years all except:
    a. Increased REM sleep
    b. Increased sleep latency
    c. Decreased total sleep duration
    d. Decreased REM sleep

99. Drug of choice for the treatment of negative symptoms of schizophrenia is:
    a. Chlorpromazine
    b. Haloperidol
    c. Clozapine
    d. Doxepine

100. Which phenothiazine does not have a piperazine side chain:
    a. Trifluoperazine
    b. Prochlorperazine
    c. Chlorpromazine
    d. Fluphenazine

101. Gamma knife surgery for all conditions for except:
    a. Acoustic neuroma
    b. Pituitary adenoma
    c. Brain tumors or lesions 4 cm or larger in diameter
    d. Trigeminal Neuralgia

102. According to WHO, the most common cause of preventable blindness in India?
    a. Keratomalacia
    b. Cataract
    c. Refractive error
    d. Glaucoma

103. Area of Retina where only cones are concentrated:
    a. Fovea
    b. Macula
    c. Optic nerve
    d. Foveola

104. Distance of patient while reading Snellen chart is:
    a. 6 feet
    b. 25 cm
    c. 6 meters
    d. 25 feet

105. Increased Left Internuclear Ophthalmoplegia is seen:
    a. Impaired adduction and nystagmus of left
    b. Impaired adduction and nystagmus in right eye
    c. Impaired adduction of right eye and nystagmus in left eye
    d. Impaired adduction of left eye and horizontal nystagmus of right eye

106. Posterior subcapsular stellate cataract seen:
    a. Wilson's disease
    b. DM
    c. Myotonic dystrophy
    d. SLE

107. Retinoblastoma is associated with which chromosome?
    a. 13
    b. 11
    c. 17
    d. 15

108. Sudden painless loss of vision is seen in:
    a. Vitreous hemorrhage
    b. Optic atrophy
    c. Developmental cataract
    d. Acute angle closure glaucoma

109. 100% oxygen therapy is used in:
    a. Cluster headache
    b. Migraine
    c. Congenital spherocytosis
    d. COPD

110. Heubner arteritis is associated with:
    a. Endarteritis obliterans
    b. Cerebral syphilitic arteritis
    c. Hypersensitivity arteritis
    d. Giant cell arteritis

111. Embolism of posterior cerebral artery leads to memory impairment because of damage to:
    a. Hippocampal gyrus
    b. Angular gyrus
    c. Premarginal area
    d. Superior temporal gyrus

112. Axonal neuropathy differentiating from demyelinating neuropathy in nerve conduction study:
    a. H reflex
    b. Conduction block
    c. F wave
    d. None

113. Prosapagnosia is associated with lesion of:
    a. Cingulate cortex gyrus
    b. Posterior parietal cortex
    c. Hippocampus, amygdale and entorhinal cortex
    d. Fusiform gyrus and lingual gyrus

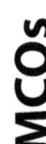

Answers

94. a	95. b	96. a	97. a	98. a	99. c	100. c
101. c	102. c	103. d	104. c	105. d	106. c	107. a
108. a	109. a	110. b	111. a	112. b	113. d	

114. **ATM mutation is seen in:**
    a. Ataxia telangiectasia
    b. Fragile X syndrome
    c. Joubert syndrome
    d. Spinocerebellar ataxia

115. **Parietal lobe lesion presented with Sensory seizures, motor deficits, visual disorders, no touch perception on opposite side and on simultaneous bilateral touch. This is associated with:**
    a. Unilateral parietal lobe dysfunction
    b. Dominant parietal lobe dysfunction
    c. Non-dominant parietal lobe dysfunction
    d. Bilateral parietal lobe dysfunction

116. **Causes of Bell's palsy include all *except*:**
    a. HIV
    b. Diabetes mellitus
    c. Multiple sclerosis
    d. Frontal sinusitis

117. **NOT a feature of Horner's syndrome:**
    a. Exophthalmos
    b. Ptosis of upper eyelid
    c. Miosis
    d. Anhydrosis

118. **Multiple brain abscesses are characteristic of:**
    a. Cyanotic heart disease
    b. Otitis media
    c. Hematogenous
    d. Hemorrhage

119. **Consider the statement about trigeminal neuralgia:**
    a. Maxillary division is most frequently affected
    b. Mandibular division is most frequently affected
    c. Ophthalmic V is most frequently affected
    d. All of the above divisions are equally affected

120. **Progressive multifocal leukoencephalopathy is due to:**
    a. JC virus
    b. Papova virus
    c. Measles
    d. Japanese encephalitis

121. **Itch sensation from skin is carried by:**
    a. A alpha
    b. A gamma
    c. Nerve fibre
    d. Central itch centre

122. **MPTP (2-methyl-1,2, 3,4'-tetrahydro-p-earbolines) is a causative factor for:**
    a. Parkinson's
    b. Schizophrenia
    c. Alzheimer's
    d. Huntington's chorea

123. **"Ocular bobbing" is seen in:**
    a. Lesion in midbrain
    b. Lesion in pons
    c. Lesion in posterior frontal lobe
    d. Lesion in medulla

124. **Loss of memory, urinary incontinence and abnormal gait are seen in:**
    a. Temporal lobe lesion
    b. Paraneoplastic encephalomyelitis
    c. Normal pressure hydrocephalus
    d. None of the above

125. **Crossed aphasia is associated with:**
    a. Lt. Hemisphere damage in Rt. handed person
    b. Lt. Hemisphere damage in Lt. handed person
    c. Rt. Hemisphere damage in Rt. handed person
    d. Lt. Hemisphere damage in Rt. handed person

126. **Which of the following HIV complications is the least affected by antiretroviral therapy?**
    a. Progressive multifocal leukoencephalopathy
    b. AIDS dementia
    c. CNS toxoplasmosis
    d. Cryptococcal meningitis

127. **Which of the following is NOT seen in morbidly obese sleep apnea patient?**
    a. Polycythemia
    b. Hypoxemia
    c. Rt. Ventricular failure
    d. Lt. Ventricular failure

128. **Most common presentation of neurocysticercosis is:**
    a. Seizures
    b. Focal neurological deficits
    c. Dementia
    d. Radiculopathy

129. **A patient came with diplopia when he sees up and out, the defective extraocular muscle:**
    a. Right superior rectus
    b. Right superior oblique
    c. Left superior oblique
    d. Right inferior rectus

130. **Selected trinucleotide repeat disorders are all *except*:**
    a. Machado Joseph disease
    b. Friedreich's ataxia
    c. Spinocerebellar ataxia type 2
    d. Huntington's disease

131. **Intermittent muscular weakness is a feature of:**
    a. Myasthenia gravis
    b. Mitochondrial myopathies
    c. Duchenne muscular dystrophy
    d. Lambert-Eaton syndrome

132. **Muscle fatigue, which increases progressively from start of the day to evening includes:**
    a. Myasthenia gravis
    b. Hypothyroidism
    c. Duchenne muscular dystrophy
    d. Limb girdle dystrophy

Answers

114. a	115. a	116. d	117. a	118. c	119. a	120. a
121. c	122. a	123. b	124. c	125. c	126. b	127. c
128. a	129. a	130. d	131. a	132. a		

133. Both upper and lower limbs are in extended position, when the lesion is at:
    a. Lower midbrain
    b. Above red nucleus
    c. Upper medulla
    d. Caudal diencephalon

134. Cause of dysphonia and hoarseness of voice includes:
    a. Thiamine
    b. Pyridoxine
    c. Vitamin B12
    d. Folic acid

135. In raised CSF pressure which is NOT seen?
    a. Tachycardia
    b. Respiratory depression
    c. Hypertension
    d. Altered consciousness

136. Drugs which can NOT reduce the CSF pressure:
    a. Acetazolamide
    b. 20% mannitol
    c. Ketamine
    d. Thiopentone

137. Loss of pain and motor activity with preserved proprioception is a clinical feature of:
    a. Anterior cord syndrome
    b. Posterior cord syndrome
    c. Brown-Sequard syndrome
    d. All of the above

138. A child presented with weakness of limbs cannot sit properly and swaying both sides while walking. The lesion is in:
    a. Cerebellar vermis
    b. Cerebellar hemisphere
    c. Cerebellopontine area
    d. Neocerebellum

139. Cabergoline is the drug of choice for:
    a. Parkinsonism
    b. Alzheimer's
    c. Prolactinoma
    d. Galactorrhea

140. Brain dead patient has:
    a. Pupillary light reflex
    b. Vestibular ocular reflex
    c. Cough reflex
    d. None of the above

141. In the lower motor neuron lesion diseases, there is:
    a. Spastic paralysis
    b. There may be wasting of muscles in long standing cases
    c. Exaggerated tendon reflexes
    d. Absence of fasciculations

142. Absence seizures are characterized on EEG by:
    a. 3 Hz spike and wave
    b. 1-2 Hz spike and wave
    c. Generalized polyspikes
    d. Hypsarrhythmia

143. Condition associated with prolonged muscle contraction followed by slow muscle relaxation includes:
    a. Myotonia
    b. Dystonia
    c. Mitochondrial myopathies
    d. Hypotonia

144. Autism is:
    a. Neurodevelopmental disorder
    b. Social and language communication problem
    c. Metabolic disease
    d. Mainly due to hypothalamus damage

145. Parinaud's syndrome is associated with all *except*:
    a. Collier's sign may be present
    b. Can be caused by hydrocephalus with aqueductal stenosis
    c. Light near dissociation of pupil
    d. Nuclear gaze palsy

146. All of the following statements about Creutzfeldt Jakob disease are true, *except*:
    a. It is a neurodegenerative disease
    b. It is caused by infectious proteins
    c. Myoclonus is rarely seen
    d. Brain biopsy is specific for diagnosis

147. Unilateral motor weakness is due to lesion in:
    a. Basal ganglia
    b. Pons
    c. Cerebral cortex
    d. Superior cervical cord

148. Ideomotor apraxia is due to damage of all of the following *except*:
    a. Left prefrontal area
    b. Left parietal lobe
    c. Premotor cortex
    d. Subcortical vascular injury

149. A 29-year-old man, with IDDM for the last 14 years develops sudden vision loss and has non-proliferative diabetic retinopathy, cause is:
    a. Macular edema
    b. Vitreous hemorrhage
    c. Subretinal hemorrhage
    d. Retinal traction

150. Area of damage in temporal cortex leads to difficulty in face recognition. The lesion is at:
    a. Amygdala
    b. Fusiform gyrus
    c. Brainstem
    d. Hippocampus

Answers

133. a	134. a	135. a	136. c	137. a	138. a	139. c
140. d	141. b	142. a	143. a	144. b	145. d	146. c
147. c	148. a	149. a	150. b			

151. A 45-year-old woman with Intracranial extradural hemorrhage is presented with all *except:*
    a. Lucid interval present
    b. Not commonly seen in old age
    c. Middle meningeal artery involvement
    d. Temporoparietal region fracture

152. NOT a neuroglial tumor:
    a. Shwannoma
    b. Astrocytoma
    c. Medulloblastoma
    d. Ependymoma

153. The most malignant brain tumor is:
    a. Ependymoma
    b. Medulloblastoma
    c. Oligodendroglioma
    d. Glioblastoma multiforme

154. Bilateral raccoon eye is seen in:
    a. Fracture of anterior cranial fossa
    b. Fracture of posterior cranial fossa
    c. Fracture of mastoid process
    d. Diastatic skull fracture

155. Dopaminergic imbalance in which connections causes positive symptoms of Schizophrenia?
    a. Frontolimbic
    b. Hippocampal
    c. Mesolimbic
    d. Nigrostriatal

156. Which one of the following usually differentiates Hysterical symptoms from Hypochondriacal symptoms?
    a. Symptoms do not normally reflect understandable physiological or pathological mechanism
    b. Physical symptoms are prominent which are not explained by organic factors
    c. Personality traits are significant
    d. Symptoms run a chronic course

157. Hypoceruloplasminimia is associated with which abnormality?
    a. Menke's disease
    b. Alzheimer's disease
    c. Schizophrenia
    d. Obsessive compulsive disorder

158. Environmental risk factor for Schizophrenia is:
    a. Cannabis
    b. Obstetrical complication
    c. Sexual abuse
    d. Migration

159. All are true statements about post-traumatic stress disorder (PTSD), *except:*
    a. Women are more likely to develop PTSD than men
    b. Children are less likely to experience PTSD after trauma than adults
    c. War veterans are commonly at risk for PTSD
    d. Most people having experienced a traumatizing event will develop PTSD

160. Antipsychotic drugs act through:
    a. Dopamine Dl receptor blockade
    b. Dopamine D2 receptor blockade
    c. Dopamine D3 receptor blockade
    d. Dopamine D4 receptor blockade

161. Rorschach test measures:
    a. Intelligence
    b. Creativity
    c. Personality
    d. Neuroticism

162. Diagnosis of alcohol dependence include all of the following, *except:*
    a. Impaired occupational and social functioning
    b. The need for daily drinking to function adequately
    c. Lack of tolerance for alcohol
    d. Inability to cut down or stop drinking

163. Agoraphobia commonly occurs with:
    a. Bipolar affective disorder
    b. Schizophrenia
    c. Panic attacks
    d. Depression

164. All of the following are true about obsessive disorder *except:*
    a. Washers
    b. Checkers
    c. Thought insertion causes distress
    d. Insight is absent

165. Episodic disorder is seen in:
    a. Schizoeffective disorder
    b. Depression
    c. Autism
    d. Attention deficit hyperactivity disorder

166. Epidemiology of generalized anxiety disorders include:
    a. Failure to thrive
    b. OCDs
    c. Only peripheral actions of anxiety acted upon propranolol
    d. None of the above

167. Therapy with empathy listening offering solution to:
    a. Builds trust and respect
    b. Enables the disputants to release their emotions
    c. Reduces tensions
    d. All of the above

Answers

151. a	152. a	153. d	154. a	155. c	156. a	157. a
158. d	159. d	160. b	161. c	162. c	163. c	164. d
165. a	166. b	167. d				

168. Which of the following will be LEAST useful in treating obsessive compulsive disorder?
    a. Clomipramine
    b. SSRIs
    c. Cognitive behavioral therapy
    d. Systematic desensitization

169. Drug that is mostly used to decrease the suicidal tendencies in Maniac Bipolar Disorder:
    a. Fluoxetine
    b. Lithium
    c. Carbamazepine
    d. Risperidone

170. "Angel dust" is the common name given for:
    a. LSD
    b. PCP
    c. Heroin
    d. Cocaine

171. Scientist who won Nobel prize for research in split brain personality?
    a. Penfield
    b. Roger Sperry
    c. Michael Morris
    d. George D Snell

172. Most common psychiatric condition is:
    a. Anxiety related
    b. Depressive related
    c. Phobias
    d. Schizophrenia

173. Ego centric and magical thinking, excessive emotionality and attention seeking pattern is associated with which type of personality?
    a. Schizoid
    b. Schizotypal
    c. Avoidant
    d. Narcissistic

174. FALSE statement about REM sleep:
    a. Comprises about 20% in total sleep
    b. Comprises more than 50% of sleep in infants
    c. First cycle starts within 1-2 hrs of sleep onset
    d. Slow wave sleep increases with age

175. FALSE statement about Hallucinations:
    a. Perceived as not real
    b. Appears to be coming from external world
    c. Sensory organs are not involved
    d. It occurs in the absence of perceptual stimulus

176. Ebstein's anomaly is caused by:
    a. Lithium
    b. Carbamazapine
    c. Imipramine
    d. Amphetamine

177. De la Tourette syndrome is associated with all except:
    a. Depression
    b. Obsessive compulsive disorder
    c. ADHD
    d. Parkinson's disease

178. A girl feels very depressed, as her father died one month back. She feels moody and won't join with others, and she thinks about joining her father. This is a case of:
    a. Post-traumatic stress reaction
    b. Grief reaction
    c. Depressive psychosis
    d. Bipolar disorder

179. All are correct. Match pairs except:
    a. Continuous irrelevant intrusive thoughts about having HIV and hand washing—Hypochondriac
    b. Loss of limb movement—Conversion disorder
    c. Abnormal social behavior and failure to recognize what is real—Schizophrenia
    d. Unmanageable emotional excesses—Phobia

180. A person restricts himself to house and fears about trains, elevators, and shopping malls. It is a feature of:
    a. Generalized Anxiety disorder
    b. Agoraphobia
    c. Claustrophobia
    d. Acrophobia

181. All of the following are indications for electroconvulsive therapy except:
    a. Depression with suicidal tendencies
    b. Residual schizophrenia
    c. Catatonia
    d. Psychotic depression

182. All of the following are true about Cocaine addiction, except:
    a. Myocardial infarction
    b. Seizures
    c. Addicted to alcohol also
    d. Amantadine is the drug of choice

183. The individuals using following antipsychotic drug are at greatest risk for developing neuroleptic malignant syndrome (NMS):
    a. Clozapine
    b. Olanzapine
    c. Ziprasidone
    d. Haloperidol

184. Agoraphobia is:
    a. Fear of open spaces
    b. Fear of closed spaces
    c. Fear of heights
    d. Fear of crowded places

185. The specific laboratory finding often reflect the clinical manifestations of neuroleptic malignant syndrome (NMS) is:
    a. Elevated creatine kinase
    b. Hypocalcemia
    c. Increased alkaline phosphatase
    d. Leukocytosis

Answers

168. d	169. b	170. b	171. b	172. a	173. d	174. d
175. c	176. a	177. d	178. b	179. d	180. b	181. b
182. d	183. d	184. a	185. a			

186. All of the following are essential features of attention deficit hyperactivity disease (ADHD) except:
    a. Lack of concentration
    b. Impulsivity
    c. Mental retardation
    d. Hyperactivity

187. Classic tetrad of Narcolepsy are all except:
    a. Hypnogogic hallucination
    b. Sleep attacks
    c. Sleep paralysis
    d. Cataplexy

188. False about cocaine:
    a. Tactile hallucinations
    b. Its a local anaesthetic
    c. Causes vasoconstriction
    d. Bradycardia

189. Antidepressant increase which transmitters in brain:
    a. Imipramine
    b. Sertraline
    c. Mirtazapine
    d. Fluoxetine

190. Social etiological factors of schizophrenia are all except:
    a. Higher socioeconomic status
    b. Early developmental insults
    c. Winter birth
    d. Increasing parental age

191. All of the following are associated with better prognosis in schizophrenia except:
    a. Late onset
    b. Married
    c. Negative symptoms
    d. Acute onset

192. Mitral cells are seen in:
    a. Olfactory bulb
    b. Basal ganglia
    c. Hippocampus
    d. Hypothalamus

193. Structures in the lateral wall of the cavernous sinus include all except:
    a. Oculomotor nerve
    b. Trochlear nerve
    c. Optic nerve
    d. Abducens nerve

194. Node of Ranvier means:
    a. Gap between two Schwann cells
    b. Indentation Schwann cell due to synapsing of adjacent unipolar neuron
    c. Gaps between dendrites and Schwann cells
    d. Gaps between Schwann cell and axon

195. Notochord develops by:
    a. 8 weeks of pregnancy
    b. 24 weeks of pregnancy
    c. 14-21 days post conception
    d. 2 weeks post conception

196. Position of corticobulbar fibres in internal capsule:
    a. Anterior limb
    b. Genu
    c. Posterior limb
    d. All of the above

197. Dorsal motor nucleus location of 10th cranial nerve are all except:
    a. Medulla
    b. Floor of the fourth ventricle
    c. Nucleus ambiguous
    d. Pons

198. Cerebellum:
    a. Axons of the Purkinje cells are the efferents from the cerebellar cortex
    b. All its arteries are derived from vertebral artery
    c. Inferior cerebellar peduncle is the most medial of the peduncles entering through the anterior cerebellar
    d. Dentate nucleus is the largest and phylogenetically oldest of its nuclei

199. All veins are valveless except:
    a. Inferior vena cava
    b. Superior vena cava
    c. Portal vein
    d. External iliac vein

200. Which of the following does NOT present in auditory Pathway?
    a. Superior olivary nucleus
    b. Lateral lemniscus
    c. Medial genicualte body
    d. Trapezoid body

201. Long-term potentiation means:
    a. Enhancement of signal transmission
    b. Increased number of receptors
    c. Increased number of neurons
    d. Increased muscle tone

202. A patient is on both Clomipramine and Escitalopram. We should monitor him for:
    a. Parkinson's disease
    b. Serotonin syndrome
    c. Neuroleptic malignant syndrome
    d. Hyperpyrexia

203. The mechanism of action of haloperidol is the blockage of:
    a. Serotonin receptor
    b. GABA receptor
    c. Dopamine receptor
    d. Adrenergic receptor

204. Which drug does NOT cause chorea as a side effect:
    a. Phenytoin
    b. OCP
    c. Carbamazepine
    d. Clozapine

Answers

186. c	187. d	188. b	189. c	190. a	191. c	192. a
193. d	194. a	195. c	196. b	197. d	198. a	199. d
200. b	201. a	202. b	203. c	204. d		

205. Patient treated with Ropinirol 8 mg, came with fever and muscle rigidity: Tests to be done are:
    a. Hemogram, CPK, Renal function tests
    b. Hemogram, X-ray, Creatinine
    c. Hemogram, Creatinine
    d. Hemogram, Liver function tests

206. Aripiprazole is a:
    a. 5-HT2 antagonist
    b. 5-HTIA antagonist
    c. 5-HT2 agonist
    d. None of the above

207. Homonymous Hemianopia may be seen in lesion of all of the following *except:*
    a. Optic nerve
    b. Optic chiasma
    c. Optic tract
    d. Optic radiation

208. Cause of progressive painless loss of vision:
    a. Anterior optic neuropathy
    b. CRAC
    c. CRVO
    d. Retinal detachment

209. A 35-year-old insulin Dependent Diabetes Mellitus (IDDM) patient on Insulin for the past 10 years complains of gradually progressive painless loss of vision. Superior sagittal sinus thrombosis causes. Most likely he has:
    a. Cataract
    b. Vitreous hemorrhage
    c. Total rhegmatogenous retinal detachment
    d. Tractional retinal detachment not involving the macula

210. Most common cause for vitreous hemorrhage in elderly:
    a. Diabetic retinopathy
    b. Retinal detachment
    c. Eale's disease
    d. Hypertension

211. Wilson's KF ring is associated with following:
    a. Oil drop cataract
    b. Rosette cataract
    c. Snow Flake cataract
    d. Sunflower cataract

212. The core protein of plaques in Alzheimer's disease:
    a. Synuclein
    b. Tau
    c. Apo-E
    d. A beta

213. Hyponatremia is caused by which antiepileptic drug?
    a. Magnesium valproate
    b. Phenytoin
    c. Carbamazepine
    d. Ethosuximide

214. Pure motor neuropathy includes:
    a. Dapsone intoxication
    b. Amyloidosis
    c. Tangier disease
    d. Fabry's disease

215. On an average Clonus beat frequency to range from:
    a. 1 to 3 HZ
    b. 3 to 8 Hz
    c. 9 to 11 Hz
    d. 10 to 15 Hz

216. Spinocerebellar ataxia with CTG repeats are seen in:
    a. Type 3
    b. Type 4
    c. Type 8
    d. Type 10

217. Total score in Glasgow Coma Scale of a conscious:
    a. 8
    b. 3
    c. 15
    d. 10

218. A 25-year-old female presents with the acute onset of cessation of lactation. She delivered her first child several months ago and has been breastfeeding since then. She reports that she has not menstruated since the delivery: She also says that lately she has been tired and has been feeling cold all of the time. Laboratory workup reveals a deficiency of ACTH and other anterior pituitary hormones. What is the most likely cause of this patient's signs and symptoms?
    a. Craniopharyngioma
    b. Cushing's disease
    c. Empty sella syndrome
    d. Sheehan's syndrome

219. Perinaud syndrome is associated with lesion in:
    a. Brainstem
    b. Pons
    c. Cerebellum
    d. Thalamus

220. Dopamine and Cholinergic blockade are NOT associated with following side effect:
    a. Parkinsonism
    b. Galactorrhea
    c. Akathesia
    d. Mydriasis

221. Grossly incongruous, incomplete (contralateral) Homonymous Hemianopia causing lesion is:
    a. Optic nerve
    b. Lateral optic chiasm
    c. Central optic chiasm
    d. Optic tract

222. Most common cause of neuropathy is:
    a. Leprosy
    b. Guillain-Barre syndrome
    c. Amyloidosis
    d. Diabetes mellitus

223. Lesion in Meyer's loop of optic radiation causes:
    a. Homonymous hemianopia
    b. Superior quadrantanopia
    c. Inferior quadrantanopia
    d. Central scotoma

Answers

205. a	206. a	207. a	208. a	209. a	210. a	211. d
212. d	213. c	214. a	215. b	216. c	217. c	218. d
219. a	220. a	221. b	222. d	223. b		

224. Brain death is said to occur if there is:
    a. Absent spinal reflexes
    b. Cortical death following widespread brain injury
    c. Absence of brainstem reflexes
    d. Core temperature of the body is below 35°C

225. Most common Primary Brain tumor is:
    a. Glioma
    b. Glioblastoma
    c. Meningioma
    d. Medulloblastoma

226. Differentiating feature between Tay-Sachs disease and Sandhoff's disease includes:
    a. Mild hepatosplenomegaly
    b. Startle response to noise
    c. Macular cherry red spot
    d. Gelastic (laughing) seizures

227. Incongrous contralateral hemianopia is seen in:
    a. Optic tract lesion
    b. Optic chiasm lesion
    c. Medial geniculate lesion
    d. Lateral geniculate lesion

228. Devic's disease is associated with:
    a. Aquaporin 0
    b. Aquaporin I
    c. Aquaporin 2
    d. Aquaporin 4

229. Characteristic of Gerstmann syndrome include all *except*:
    a. Aphonia/ dysphonia
    b. Left-right disorientation
    c. Dysgraphia/Agraphia
    d. Dyscalculia/Acalculia

230. Typically the Tuberculous Meningitis evolves over:
    a. 1–2 weeks
    b. 6–12 weeks
    c. 1–6 months
    d. 6–12 months

231. "Waxy flexibility" is a feature of:
    a. Catatonic schizophrenia
    b. Dystonia
    c. Myotonia
    d. Hebephrenic schizophrenia

232. Most common manifestation of multiple sclerosis is:
    a. Weakness
    b. Ataxia
    c. Optic neuritis
    d. Internuclear ophthalmoplegia

233. Chorea is NOT seen in:
    a. Huntington's disease
    b. Creutzfeldt-Jakob disease
    c. Rheumatic fever
    d. Tourette syndrome

234. rtPA is NOT a contraindication in stroke with:
    a. BP 185/110 mm Hg
    b. Heparin in the past 24 hrs
    c. Coma
    d. Lesion occupying 1/3 of middle cerebral artery territory

235. Child with infratentorial tumour with spinal seeding is:
    a. Medulloblastoma
    b. Meningioma
    c. Astrocytoma
    d. Glioblastoma

236. Reversible cause of Dementia includes:
    a. Alzheimer's disease
    b. Dementia pugilistica
    c. Normal pressure hydrocephalus
    d. Multi-infarct dementia

237. Most common cause of seizures in an elderly with Cerebrovascular Stroke is:
    a. Alcohol withdrawal
    b. Cerebrovascular stroke
    c. Uremia
    d. Meningitis

238. "Reward pathway" is associated with:
    a. Nucleus accumbens
    b. Nucleus ambiguus
    c. Dentate nucleus
    d. Substantia nigra

239. Autism is characterized by all *except*:
    a. Motor abnormalities
    b. Less eye contact
    c. High intelligence
    d. Unusual gestures

240. Not a feature seen in Wernicke's encephalopathy:
    a. III CN palsy
    b. Anterograde amnesia
    c. Nystagmus
    d. Ataxia

241. Which one of the following is a correct matching:
    a. Neurofibromatosis—Osteogenesis imperfecta
    b. Sturge-Weber syndrome—Faber's disease
    c. Tuberous selerosis (TS)—von Hippel-Lindau disease
    d. Ataxia-telangiectasia (A-T)—Dermatomyositis

Answers

224. c	225. a	226. a	227. d	228. d	229. a	230. a
231. a	232. c	233. d	234. c	235. a	236. c	237. b
238. a	239. c	240. c	241. c			

242. **NOT causing Peripheral Neuropathy:**
    a. Herpes
    b. Leprosy
    c. Syphilis
    d. Candida

243. **Following sign is seen, when brain herniates from Foramen Magnum:**
    a. Respiratory depression
    b. Papilledema
    c. Miotic pupil
    d. Altered consciousness

244. **A peripheral nerve lesion is NOT associated with:**
    a. Glove and Stocking anesthesia
    b. Muscle atrophy
    c. Tinel's sign
    d. Sensory loss

245. **Purtscher's retinopathy results from:**
    a. Trichiasis
    b. Head injuries
    c. Chest injuries
    d. All of the above

246. **"Hunt and Hess scale" is the grading system used to classify the severity of:**
    a. Hydrocephalus
    b. Extracranial hemorrhage
    c. Subarachnoid hemorrhage
    d. Increased intracranial tension

247. **A man falling from a height directy hitting his pelvis to ground and presented with urinary incontinence. The probable injury he sustained is:**
    a. Cervical spine injury
    b. Pelvic hematoma
    c. Blunt injury abdomen
    d. Injury to loin region

248. **The most prognostic sign in Glasgow Coma Scale is:**
    a. Eye movement
    b. Motor response
    c. Verbal response
    d. All of the above

249. **Battle's sign is seen in:**
    a. Linear fracture
    b. Basilar fracture
    c. Depressed fracture
    d. Diastatic fracture

250. **Agoraphobia is associated with:**
    a. OCD
    b. Bipolar disorders
    c. Stress disorders
    d. Panic disorders

251. **Waxy movement is seen in:**
    a. Dystonia
    b. Myotonia
    c. Catatonia
    d. Cataplexy

252. **Drug mimicking psychiatric and cognitive symptoms:**
    a. Fentanyl
    b. Methylphenidate
    c. Clobazam
    d. Pimozide

253. **Which one of the following is NOT a Somatic Symptom:**
    a. Anhedonia
    b. Constipation
    c. Impotence
    d. Numbness

254. **Somatic symptoms of Depression include all except:**
    a. Feelings of guilt
    b. Reduced libido
    c. Insomnia
    d. Weight change

255. **Waxy flexibility is characteristic of:**
    a. OCD
    b. Excitatory catatonia
    c. Stupurous catatonia
    d. All of the above

256. **Drug effect mimicking 'Schizophrenia' includes:**
    a. Barbiturates
    b. Cocaine
    c. Phencyclidine
    d. Levodopa

257. **Alcohol specific enzyme is:**
    a. AST
    b. ALT
    c. GGT
    d. ALP

258. **"Systematic desensitization" behavioral therapy is used to treat:**
    a. Depression
    b. Anxiety disorders
    c. Attention deficit hyperactivity disorder
    d. Anterograde amnesia

259. **Most common psychiatric disorder in the:**
    a. Stress disorder
    b. Depression
    c. Schizophrenia
    d. Mixed anxiety and depression

260. **Therapeutic dose of Lithium is:**
    a. 1–2 mEq/L
    b. 0.8–1.2 mEq/L
    c. 0.3–0.6 mEq/lit
    d. 2–3 mEq/L

261. **Drugs used in bipolar disorder:**
    a. Benzodiazepines
    b. Lithium
    c. Sodium valproate
    d. All of the above

262. **Schizophrenia is a common presentation in which genetic disease?**
    a. Down's syndrome
    b. Di George syndrome
    c. Klinefelter's syndrome
    d. Neurofibromatosis

Answers

242. d	243. a	244. a	245. (b, c)	246. c	247. b	248. a
249. b	250. d	251. c	252. b	253. b	254. a	255. c
256. c	257. a	258. b	259. d	260. b	261. d	262. b

263. FALSE statement regarding MI and Depression is:
    a. Depression is a risk factor for MI
    b. MI increases chances of depression
    c. SSRIs can be used in post MI patients
    d. Cognitive behavior therapy is only given after MI

264. Definition of Bipolar Disorder includes:
    a. Alternating periods of mania and depression
    b. Depression is more common than mania
    c. Mania is the prominent feature
    d. Depression or mania are present in bipolar

265. Drug of choice for Psychosis in Parkinson's disease is:
    a. Clozapine
    b. Lithium
    c. Haloperidol
    d. Chlorpromazine

266. "Magical thinking" is characteristically seen in:
    a. Schizophrenia
    b. Obsessive compulsive disorder
    c. Schizotypal personality
    d. Anxiety disorder

267. A 50-year-old guy presented with 25 years of married life, having 5 years of established doubt on his wife's fidelity, despite proof to the contrary, and his other aspects of life are normal. The probable diagnosis is:
    a. Panic disorder
    b. Depressive disorder
    c. Delusional disorder
    d. Phobias

268. NOT an atypical antipsychotic is:
    a. Risperidone
    b. Pimozide
    c. Asenapine
    d. Quetiapine

269. All are risk factors for Schizophrenia except:
    a. Family history
    b. Viral infection
    c. Social isolation
    d. Age related

270. NOT seen in Narcolepsy:
    a. Sleep paralysis
    b. Ataxia
    c. Catalepsy
    d. Abnormal REM sleep

271. Obsessive Compulsive Disorder is NOT associated:
    a. Repetitive behavior
    b. Thought insertion
    c. Anxiety
    d. Paranoid behavior

272. Which one of the following is usually NOT called as Atypical Antipsychotic'?
    a. Clozapine
    b. Asenapine
    c. Sulpiride
    d. Ziprasidone

273. Schizophrenia is associated with the following Genet:
    a. Apert syndrome
    b. Turner's syndrome
    c. Di George syndrome
    d. Down's syndrome

274. Cranial nerves II, IIV, V, VI lesions are associated a covalenly inked to:
    a. Sphenoparietal sinus
    b. Occipital sinus
    c. Occipital sinus
    d. Cavernous sinus

275. Not a content of jugular foramen:
    a. Hypoglossal nerve
    b. Glossopharyngeal nerve
    c. Occipital arteries
    d. Sigmoidal sinus

276. Purtscher's retinopathy due to acute pancreatitis is:
    a. Laser therapy to the retina
    b. Vitamin a supplementation
    c. Ciprofloxacin and metranidazole
    d. All of the above

277. An Antiepileptic drug, but NOT a mood stabilizer includes:
    a. Topiramate
    b. Lamotrigine
    c. Sodium valproate
    d. Levetiracetam

278. Clonidine acts on:
    a. Sympathetic nerve via presynaptic end
    b. Vasomotor centre
    c. Sympathetic ganglion
    d. Postsynaptic beta receptors

279. Felbamate acts by:
    a. GABa antagonist
    b. NMDa blockade
    c. Glutamate receptor antagonist
    d. Glycine receptor agonist

Answers

263. d	264. a	265. a	266. c	267. c	268. b	269. d
270. c	271. b	272. c	273. c	274. d	275. a	276. c
277. d	278. b	279. b				

280. **An Antiepileptic drug NOT used in BPAD includes:**
    a. Carbamazepine
    b. Sodium valproate
    c. Topiramate
    d. Lamotrigine

281. **Mechanism of action of Memantine includes:**
    a. GABa nergic action
    b. Glutaminergic action
    c. Adrenergic action
    d. Dopaminergic action

282. **Drug side effect and its right pair:**
    a. Vigabatrin—Renal stones
    b. Lamotrigine—Stevens Johnson syndrome
    c. Gabapentin—hepatitis
    d. Valproic acid—visual field defects

283. **Prolactin is inhibited by:**
    a. Dopamine
    b. Neurophysin
    c. Serotonin
    d. Glutamate

284. **Alcoholic liver disease is associated with:**
    a. AST>ALT
    b. ALT>AST
    c. GGT is specific to alcohol fatty liver
    d. AST/ALT usually < 1

285. **MRI finding of Schizophrenia false is:**
    a. Increased ventricular volume
    b. Cortical thickening
    c. Reduced volume of temporal lobe
    d. Reduced volume of hippocampal lobe

286. **Lumbar puncture preceded by CT include all except:**
    a. Positive Kernig sign
    b. Age > 65
    c. Focal neurological signs
    d. Recent history of seizures

Answers

| 280. d | 281. b | 282. b | 283. a | 284. a | 285. b | 286. a |

Milton Keynes UK
Ingram Content Group UK Ltd.
UKHW030629020824
446397UK00001B/2

9 789390 020034